Gilles de la Tourette Syndrome
Second Edition

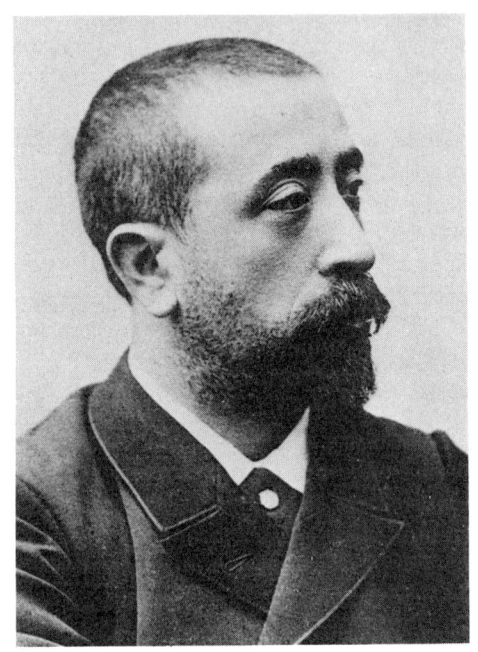

Gilles de la Tourette (1857–1904)
(*Courtesy of Dr. Alexander Lucas*)

Gilles de la Tourette Syndrome
Second Edition

Arthur K. Shapiro, M.D.
*Clinical Professor
Department of Psychiatry; and
Director
Tourette and Tic Laboratory
and Clinic
Mount Sinai School of Medicine
New York, New York*

Elaine S. Shapiro, PH.D.
*Clinical Associate Professor
of Psychology
Department of Psychiatry; and
Co-Director
Tourette and Tic Laboratory
and Clinic
Mount Sinai School of Medicine
New York, New York*

J. Gerald Young, M.D.
*Director
Department of Child Psychiatry; and
Professor, Pediatrics and Psychiatry
Mount Sinai School of Medicine
New York, New York*

Todd E. Feinberg, M.D.
*Physician-in-Charge
Neurobehavior Center
Beth Israel Medical Center; and
Assistant Professor of Psychiatry
and Neurology
Mount Sinai School of Medicine
New York, New York*

Raven Press ◆ New York

Raven Press, 1185 Avenue of the Americas, New York, New York 10036

© 1988 by Raven Press, Ltd. All rights reserved. This book is protected by copyright. No part of it may be reproduced, stored in a retrieval system, or transmitted, in any form or by any means, electronical, mechanical, photocopying, or recording, or otherwise, without the prior written permission of the publisher.

Made in the United States of America

Library of Congress Cataloging-in-Publication Data

Gilles de la Tourette syndrome.

  Bibliography: p.
  Includes indexes.
  1. Gilles de la Tourette's syndrome. I. Shapiro, Arthur K., 1923–. [DNLM: 1. Gilles de la Tourette's Disease. WM 197 G4771]
RC375.G54   1988   616.8′3   87-45465
ISBN 0-88167-340-4

  The material contained in this volume was submitted as previously unpublished material, except in the instances in which credit has been given to the source from which some of the illustrative material was derived.
  Great care has been taken to maintain the accuracy of the information contained in the volume. However, neither Raven Press nor the editors can be held responsible for errors or for any consequences arising from the use of the information contained herein.

9 8 7 6 5 4 3 2 1

Preface

The First Edition of our book provided clinicians and researchers in neurology, psychiatry, genetics, and neurosciences, as well as patients and their families, with a greater understanding of a rare and complex illness. The clinical insights grew out of 10 years of clinical experience and detailed study of only 145 patients. The first volume stimulated interest in Tourette's syndrome, facilitated more frequent and earlier diagnosis of this disorder, and contributed to a phenomenal increase in research and studies. Since its publication, references in the literature have more than doubled, and our current data base is more than 1,600 patients.

The published history of Tourette's syndrome spans five centuries and is distributed in many journals and languages throughout the world. Despite the enormous growth of the literature, in this Second Edition, we attempt to review, summarize, and discuss all relevant studies and papers. We are fortunate in having the collaboration of Drs. J. Gerald Young and Todd E. Feinberg in this undertaking.

The illness is referred to as Gilles de la Tourette syndrome in the title of this book, which is the classic appellation by which it is known throughout the world. In the United States, however, it is called Tourette's disorder because of the decision by the framers of the influential Diagnostic and Statistical Manual (DSM) of the American Psychiatric Association to use the term "disorder" instead of "syndrome" for illnesses of unknown etiology. In this book we use the latest version of the DSM nomenclature, which classifies the general category as "tic disorders" and includes four subtypes: Tourette's disorder, chronic motor or vocal tic disorder, transient tic disorder, and tic disorder not otherwise specified.

As in the previous Edition, we continue to use a data-oriented approach to the study of clinical disorders of unknown etiology. This approach attempts to verify clinical observations and impressions by subjecting them to testing of hypotheses. We refer to this approach as data-oriented, an orientation that slowly matured and became established in the early 1970s following the accumulation of data derived from controlled scientific studies and the remarkable development of research methodology during the past 30 years.

A data-oriented approach may help mitigate the potentially horrendous consequences of this illness by correcting the myths and fallacies that have haunted patients for centuries. It is hoped that providing reliable and valid data about this condition, suggestions about how to study clinical conditions of unknown etiology, and illustrative clinical examples will contribute to more meaningful research that will help liberate patients from the affliction of Tourette's syndrome and other tic disorders.

In the present volume the sample for our studies is 666 consecutive Tourette patients evaluated between 1965 and 1981; this is the largest carefully studied group of patients in the literature with a verified diagnosis of Tourette's disorder.

We begin this volume with a review of the seminal papers from the past because of their historical importance. The extensive literature review of the first volume is not duplicated nor do we review the current literature in Chapter 1. Instead, published literature that is germane to the topic is reviewed in each chapter. We have decided on this approach because the number of papers published on Tourette's disorder is so extensive and subject-specific that it is no longer possible to meaningfully abstract the literature as a whole. The bibliography lists all the published material referred to and its size is convincing proof of the profusion of investigators who are now studying Tourette's disorder.

This is followed in Chapter 2 by a description of the sample used in our studies, the procedures used in the collection of data, the type of data collected, description of measures, variables, statistical analyses, and the hypotheses and purposes of the study. Subsequent Chapters 3, 4, and 5 summarize the data about the epidemiology, demography, family, birth, development, signs, symptoms, and clinical course of TS.

Chapter 6 summarizes the psychological and central nervous system findings, Chapter 7 (written by T.E.F.) summarizes the neurological and electroencephalographic findings, and Chapter 8 (written by J.G.Y.) discusses the genetics. Chapter 9 (written by J.G.Y.) reviews the literature and discusses current concepts about neurophysiology, neurochemistry, and neuropathology of Tourette's disorder. The differential diagnosis of tic syndromes and proposed changes in nosology and criteria for diagnosis are discussed in Chapter 10. Chapter 11 reviews studies of treatment, and Chapter 12 describes the use of specific medications for the treatment of the disorder and the identification and remediation of adverse effects. Chapter 13 discusses problems and presents two studies about the measurement of severity and change in Tourette's disorder and the cognitive adverse effects of treatment with neuroleptic drugs. Finally, our conclusions are summarized in Chapter 14.

This volume is a totally revised edition of our previous book on Tourette syndrome; most analyses and studies have not been published previously.

Arthur K. Shapiro, M.D.
Elaine Shapiro, Ph.D.
J. Gerald Young, M.D.
Todd E. Feinberg, M.D.

Preface to the First Edition

This book was developed to provide clinicians and researchers, as well as patients and their families, with a greater understanding of a rare and complex illness. The clinical insights have grown out of ten years of experience in diagnosing, treating, and studying over 500 patients with Tourette syndrome. Our extensive collection of data was used to establish criteria for early identification and treatment of patients. Our data and clinical observations are presented in great detail so that they can be useful to all.

The published history of Tourette syndrome spans 165 years, and the literature is distributed in many journals and languages. To make this work more useful we have attempted to review, summarize, and describe the history and accumulated knowledge about the illness.

The book also provided us with an opportunity to demonstrate the usefulness of a data-oriented approach in psychiatry. This approach attempts to verify clinical observations and impressions by subjecting them to testing of hypotheses, the use of large samples, replication of retrospective observations, and the use of other appropriate research methodology. We attempt to differentiate conclusions drawn from tentative clinical impressions and reliable and valid analysis of data. We refer to this approach as data-oriented psychiatry, an orientation now made possible because of the slow accumulation of data derived from controlled scientific studies and the extraordinary development of methodology.

We have attempted to use this approach in analysis of the data and understanding of Tourette syndrome. It may help to mitigate the potentially horrendous consequences of this illness by correcting some of the myths and fallacies that have haunted patients for centuries. Providing reliable and valid data about this condition, suggestions about how to study chemical conditions of unknown etiology, and many illustrative clinical examples hopefully will contribute to meaningful research that will liberate patients from the affliction of Tourette syndrome.

Arthur K. Shapiro
Elaine S. Shapiro
Ruth D. Bruun
Richard D. Sweet
1978

Acknowledgments

In our first book on Tourette syndrome, now called Tourette's disorder, we expressed our gratitude to many collaborators who participated in the studies at the Tourette Studies Laboratory from 1965 to 1977 at the Payne Whitney Psychiatric Clinic, Cornell University Medical College, and New York Hospital: Drs. Richard D. Sweet, Ruth D. Bruun, Henrietta Wayne, Gail Solomon, John Clarkin, and many others cited in the first volume. We are indebted to Dr. William T. Lhamon, Chairman of the Department of Psychiatry at the time, for providing facilities as well as his consistent support and encouragement of our early studies.

In 1977, shortly before the publication of the book, we joined the Department of Psychiatry, Mount Sinai School of Medicine, Mount Sinai Hospital. Here we established the Tourette and Tic Laboratory and Clinic, with Dr. Arthur K. Shapiro, Clinical Professor of Psychiatry, as Director, and Dr. Elaine Shapiro, Associate Clinical Professor, as Co-Director. Although the authors primarily responsible for this volume are Drs. Arthur K. and Elaine Shapiro, Dr. J. Gerald Young and Dr. Todd E. Feinberg contributed important chapters. Dr. Young is Director of the Division of Child and Adolescent Psychiatry, Professor of Psychiatry and Pediatrics, Mount Sinai School of Medicine, and Dr. Feinberg is Assistant Professor of Psychiatry and Neurology, Mount Sinai School of Medicine, and Physician-In-Charge of the Neurobehavior Center, Beth Israel Medical Center. Other collaborators at Mount Sinai include George Fulop, M.D., Gail Eisenkraft, M.A., Johanna Nordlie, M.A., Rebecca Levine, M.A., John Thornton, Ph.D., Michael Hubbard, Ph.D., Andrew Shenker, M.D., Ph.D., Ronald Dworken, M.D., Hadassah Gurfein, Ph.D., Melvin Van Woert, M.D., and Ivan Bodis-Wollner, M.D. Several of the genetic studies described in this volume required the meaningful collaboration of Miron Baron, M.D. and Morton Levitt, Ph.D., Department of Medical Genetics, Columbia University. Statistical support for initial analysis of our computerized data was provided by programmers G. Abernathy, M.S., K. Lempit, J. Raab, Ph.D., J. Pittman, M.S., and Dr. Elmer (Moose) Struening, Head, Epidemiology of Mental Disease Unit, Department of Epidemiology, New York State Psychiatric Institute, Columbia University. We are particularly indebted to our very good friend Moose, who was always available for informal consultations and served on the Medical Advisory Committee and the Board of Directors of the Tourette Research Foundation.

The publication of the first volume on Tourette's disorder catalyzed a deepened commitment to research on this disorder. The book stimulated physician awareness about Tourette syndrome and resulted in a rapid increase in referrals of patients for study and treatment. In addition, recognizing that we were totally dependent on outside sources for funding, a group of families made a commitment to support our research year after year. We particularly cite Marvin Wolf, Estelle Wolf, Elaine and Mandell Shimberg, Mr. and Mrs. Herman Stein, Mr. and Mrs. Herman Sarkowsky, Marvyn Gould, Esq., and Edna Kamin Gould, Ph.D., who made a continuing commitment to support our studies. Even more important has been their loyal friendship and belief in our work, especially during many discouraging periods of lean finances. We are especially grateful to Mr. Harold Stein, who not only provided financial support, friendship, and sustained encouragement, but also encouraged others to support our work. He illustrates the aphorism by Maimonides that "He who pursues others to give alms and moves them to act thus, his reward is greater than the reward of him who gives alms himself . . . "

In 1980, some of these and other families joined together to establish the Tourette Research Foundation, 17 Colvin Road, Scarsdale, New York 10583, to serve as a conduit for research funds. It is a nonprofit, public foundation governed by a 15-member Board of Directors comprising individuals from many parts of the country with diverse backgrounds in medicine, psychology, law, and business. Through contributions from them and others we have been able to pursue our research on Tourette's disorder. Financial support to the Tourette Research Foundation was provided by Faye and Herman Sarkowsky for genetic studies, treatment strategies, measurement and nosology; by Kyle Bahre, who provided general support; and by the Gateposts Foundation, who provided partial support for initial keypunching of the Tourette's disorder data and a study of the effect of medication on cognitive functioning. We would like to acknowledge as well the contribution of the Braun Foundation to assist us in the preparation of this book. Mr. and Mrs. Braun expressed to us their continuing interest in the dissemination of information concerning Tourette's disorder to professionals, parents of afflicted children, and the children themselves. We are also grateful to members of the Research Advisory Board of the Foundation, who provided advice on medical matters and research strategies. They include Drs. Richard D. Sweet, Elmer Struening, Alvin Mesnikoff, James Eisenkraft, Joseph Kochin, and Mr. Robert Belitto, Esq.

McNeil Pharmaceuticals provided a small grant to conduct a study of the efficacy of pimozide (ORAP) compared to placebo in the treatment of patients with Tourette's disorder, which led to its approval by the Food and Drug Administration, and generously supplied medication for the continuing study of treatment with pimozide and penfluridol in open clinical trials. The results of these studies are presented in this volume. In 1984 we were awarded a 3-year grant from the National Institute for Neurological Diseases and Stroke (NIH-NICDS 5RO1 NS20529) to compare the efficacy and cognitive adverse effects of haloperidol, pimozide, and placebo in the treatment of

Tourette's disorder. Preliminary results of this study, currently in progress, are presented in this volume. The Medical Fellows Program of the Office of Mental Retardation and Developmental Disabilities of the State of New York provided support to Dr. J. G. Young for the work described in Chapters 8 and 9. A small grant to study psychopathology in patients with Tourette's disorder was awarded by the Tourette Syndrome Association. Preliminary results are described in this volume.

Many other individuals and foundations have supported our research. We are deeply grateful to them. Unfortunately, the number is too great and the space too limited to mention all of them by name. Some of the contributors include: Goldring Foundation, Harold L. Perlman Foundation, Joseph and Gertrude Baumgarten Foundation, Charles W. Lubin, Zolie and Elaine Frank Fund, C. and R. Levy Foundation, Kristina Barr and George Barr Foundation, Chai Foundation, Theodore Horwich, Sanford Lassers, Wanda Cygan, Milton Fish, Louis S. Kanne, and Robert Novak. One of our very faithful contributors has been Larry Miller of Littleton, Colorado, who consistently sent a monthly contribution for research. Donations such as these have been instrumental in fortifying our continuing resolve to learn as much as we can about this illness, to help patients overcome the potential handicap of having the illness, and to use our research skills for its eventual eradication.

We also thank the many patients who have participated in our studies. Without their collaboration none of this would have been possible. Finally we owe our gratitude to Cynthia Carpenter, Julie Miller, and Anita Cooper, the secretaries responsible for typing our many research grants, papers, and, finally, the contents of this book.

With publication of this book, the clinical services and research of the Tourette and Tic Laboratory and Clinic, previously located at Mount Sinai School of Medicine, will be located at 35 East 85th Street, New York, NY 10028, and at 17 Colvin Road, Scarsdale, NY 10583.

Contents

Introduction *xvii*

1 History of Tourette and Tic Disorders *1*
Hereditary Antecedents • Psychological Etiology • Psychoanalysis • Epidemiology • Reviews of Hospital Records • Review of the Literature • Psychochemotherapy • Important Achievements Over the Past Twenty-five Years • Consensual Areas of Agreement and Controversies

2 Samples, Procedures, and Variables *29*
Sample • Clinical Procedure • Diagnostic Criteria • Data Management • Variables • Missing Data • Contrast Samples • Statistical Analysis • Data-Oriented Approach to the Study of Tic Disorders

3 Epidemiology *45*
Tics • Tourette's Disorder • Chronic Motor Tic Disorder • Tourette and Chronic Motor Tic Disorders • Conclusion

4 Patient Characteristics *61*
Sample Changes Over Time • Age • Sex • Race and Place of Birth • Ethnic and Religious Background • Genetics • Birth History • Medical History • Social Class • Marital Status • Organic Stigmata • Situational Events Preceding the Onset of Tourette's Disorder

5 Signs, Symptoms, and Clinical Course *127*
Patient Characteristics • Symptomatology • Sampling Problems in Studies of Tourette's Disorder • Clinical Course • Severity of Symptoms • Stimuli-Induced Changes in Severity of Symptoms • Natural Course and Prognosis • Differences Between Questionnaire Surveys and Clinical Samples

6 Psychology, Psychopathology, and Neuropsychology *195*
Psychopathology • Obsessions, Compulsions, and Impulsions • Psychometric and Neuropsychological Testing • Speech and Language • Conclusion

7 Neurology *253*
Postmortem Studies • Tic-like Symptoms Associated with Other Disorders • Treatment Interventions • Electroencephalograms • Neurological Examination • Evoked Potentials • Bereitschafts (Premovement) Potential • Computerized Axial Tomography, Positive

Emission Tomography, and Magnetic Resonance Imaging Studies •
Sleep and Arousal Disturbance • Conclusion

8 **Genetics** *289*
Familial Aggregation, Classic Pedigree Method, and Segregation
Analysis • Clinical Research on Family Aggregation in Tourette's
Disorder • Twin Research • Associated Psychiatric Disorders • Genes
and Environment • Conclusion

9 **Neural Mechanisms** *313*
General Organization of the Motor System • Regulatory Control and
Coordination of the Motor System • Neuronal Localization of
Neurotransmitters: Perspectives on Pathophysiology and
Neuropharmacology • Clinical Neurochemical Research • Neural
Function and Dysfunction in Tourette's Disorder: Hypotheses for
Research

10 **Proposed Nosology, Criteria, and Differential Diagnosis** *343*
History • Change of Diagnostic Classification from Stereotyped
Movement Disorders to Tic Disorders • Criteria for Tics • Motor Tics •
Vocal Tics • Echophilia • Coprophilia • Sensory Tics • Obsessive
Compulsive Disorder, Obsessive Compulsive Symptoms, and
Impulsions • Organic Factors • Behavioral Symptoms and
Psychopathology • Diagnostic Criteria for Tic Disorders • Tic Disorder
Not Otherwise Specified • Tic Disorders as a Continuum or Spectrum

11 **Studies of Treatment** *381*
Early History of Treatment • Pharmacotherapy • Controversy About
Stimulants and Tic Disorders • Psychotherapy • Treatment History of
Patients in Current Study • Spontaneous, Nonspecific, and Placebo
Effects • Conclusion

12 **Treatment of Tic Disorders** *423*
Indications for Treatment • General Principles of Treatment •
Haloperidol • Pimozide • Other Drugs • Psychotherapy or Counseling
for Associated Behavioral Problems • Conclusion

13 **Measurement in Tic Disorders** *451*
Reliability and Validity of Measurement in Tourette's Disorder •
Effect of Neuroleptics on Cognition

14 **Conclusions** *481*
Inadequate Support of Research • Homage to Researchers • Critique
of Research in Tourette's Disorder • Summary of Results

Appendix	*503*
Bibliography	*513*
Subject Index	*547*

Introduction

I did not know at the time, and it may be hard to believe, that my interest in Gilles de la Tourette syndrome began on January 17, 1949, at 7:20 p.m., in the 8th Street Bookstore in New York City's Greenwich Village. While browsing through Horney's *The Neurotic Personality of Our Time,* I heard peculiar noises, which initially sounded like "shi, pi, fu," and then sounded like obscenities. At first I thought I was projecting some of my evil thoughts, and I listened more carefully. Out of the corner of of my eye, I saw a woman in her early twenties, shaking and jerking spasmodically, and erupting with "shit, piss, fuck." I dismissed the thought that it was a Greenwich Village prank as I continued to observe the young woman. She was well dressed, wore a conventional seal fur coat, and was not otherwise bizarre. She was also browsing through a book; I strained my eyes: It was the collected poetry of Keats.

I do not remember thinking about this young woman again during 10 years of training and 6 years of subsequent clinical experience, nor do I recall hearing lectures or reading about tics or Tourette syndrome—not until April 21, 1965.

A colleague in neurology referred a 24-year-old unmarried female for treatment. The diagnosis was "habit tic with hysterical personality associated with 'la belle indifference'," and the treatment recommended was "psychotherapy."

Her symptoms were striking and bizarre: spasmodic jerking of the head, neck, shoulders, arms and torso; various facial grimaces; odd barking and grunting sounds; frequent throat clearing; periodic forceful protrusion of the tongue; and occasional shrill screams and coprolalia, such as "cocksucker." I instantly recalled the young woman, and I thought, "So that's what I saw in Greenwich Village 16 years ago."

Over the next several months a thorough and careful clinical evaluation was conducted. It included interviews with the family, obtaining previous records, and arranging for psychological testing. The family and developmental history, psychodynamics, ego strengths and weaknesses, and defenses were carefully assessed. The most striking aspect of the illness was that the bizarre symptoms could not be explained by the patient's developmental history or psychological assessment. The symptoms suggested a malignant psychological illness. I remember seeing such bizarre symptoms in only two groups of patients. Chronic schizophrenics, usually diagnosed as hebephrenic, with bizarre, incongruous, and incomprehensible behavior, and patients with general paresis, the tertiary stage of syphilis, who tended to be older, have delusions of grandeur, and occasionally without provocation erupt with obscenities.

This patient did not have general paresis and simply was not psychotic, schizophrenic, or even disturbed.

Another possibility was that the manifest symptomatology reflected a massive unconscious conflict. Psychodynamic reasoning would infer the underlying etiology from the manifest symptomatology. If the symptoms included vigorous muscular jerking, primitive sounds, and socially unacceptable coprolalia, the inference could be made that the patient suffered from a massive conflict about the expression of aggressive impulses. Reaction formation leading to a passive personality and obsessive-compulsive defenses would be likely to develop, but would be inadequate to control the conflict. The symptoms would break through, but be experienced as ego alien and beyond voluntary control. Thus, underlying impulses could be expressed but defensively disowned.

Such a major conflict, inadequately warded off by more socially acceptable defenses, could only mean that the unconscious conflict represented a psychotic process and that the patient should be characterized as having an underlying psychosis.

This formulation was readily available to psychodynamically oriented psychiatrists as an explanation for many symptoms, including those of Gilles de la Tourette syndrome. The only problem was that clinical observation of the patient did not fit the theoretical postulates. The patient, by history, present functioning, psychological testing, and observation for several months, could not be characterized as psychotic or as having an underlying psychosis. Although she did have some reaction formation, inhibition of aggression, and depression, possibly caused by reaction to her increasing symptomatology, these traits were not severe enough to explain the symptomatology. In addition, other expected defenses or character development, namely, obsessive-compulsive symptoms, defenses, or character, were absent. The patient did not manifest isolation, undoing, rationalization, intellectualization, thriftiness, difficulty with decisions, or the expression of affect.

Only the repetitive muscular movements, noises, and words could possibly be interpreted as obsessive-compulsive symptoms. Clinically, however, even these symptoms were not clearly obsessions or compulsions. Usually, obsessive-compulsive symptoms are cognitive, deliberate, and voluntary, although unwanted. Obsessive-compulsive patients usually say: "I know it's silly, but I have to do it." With more severe obsessive-compulsive symptoms, they say: "It may be silly, but I don't want to take a chance on being wrong." With severe symptomatology, the obsessions and compulsions become delusionary, and patients may say: "If I don't count things three times I'll get a brain tumor." In my patient, the movements, noises, and words were rapid, spasmodic, unwanted, uncontrollable, and involuntary. The definition of these terms in psychiatric dictionaries supports the clinical observation, namely, that an obsession or compulsion is a voluntary, unwanted, and repetitive thought or act.

It is difficult to know to what extent these observations or thoughts came from clinical observations or from reading the literature, which I began to do soon after the initial evaluation of the patient. In fact, I did not know before reading the literature that the condition was called Gilles de la Tourette syndrome. I looked up "tics" in textbooks on neurology and psychiatry and soon came upon the diagnosis. This led me to read everything I could find about this strange disorder.

Most of the literature generally recounted the same history of Tourette's disorder, which is discussed more fully in Chapter 1 and is referred to only briefly in this chapter.

Although other neurologists had previously described several patients, the most comprehensive and brilliant characterization of the disorder was by George Gilles de la Tourette (1884, 1885). Tourette characterized the condition as the onset of multiple tics in childhood, with a fluctuating chronic course, associated with verbal tics and echolalia. Coprolalia occurred in five (56%) of his patients. He noted that patients did not deteriorate intellectually or become psychotic, and was impressed that they were able to maintain their sanity despite their horrible affliction.

However, in the ensuing years an unfortunate error crept into the literature. Both Meige and Feindel, in their 1902 book on tics, and Brissaud, in his introduction to the book, were responsible for the error that Tourette's disorder was associated with severe mental disorder and dementia. Tourette's disorder was defined subsequently in medical literature and texts as a chronic illness involving muscular and verbal tics, coprolalia, and echolalia that may result in dementia. Ferenczi (1921) noted that in texts on psychiatry tics were labeled as a symptom of degeneration.

During the next 80 years (1885 to 1965), only approximately 50 cases, primarily single case reports, were described in English literature. Several factors contributed to the small number of reported cases. Physicians generally were unfamiliar with the syndrome and never had seen a patient with Tourette's disorder. Inadequate familiarity with the syndrome led to infrequent diagnoses. Another factor was that the erroneous diagnostic criteria in medical literature and texts were absorbed by clinicians and contributed to the infrequency with which Tourette's disorder was diagnosed and reported. The recognition of the disorder would decrease if coprolalia, echolalia, intellectual deterioration, and eventual psychosis were required for the diagnosis. Coprolalia occurs in only 30% to 60% of patients and may appear an average of 6.3 (range 0–23) years after the onset of the illness; and it spontaneously disappears in approximately one-third of patients, an average of 10.3 (range 1.5–17.0) years after its onset. Echolalia occurs in only 35% of patients. Intellectual deterioration is not associated at all with the syndrome, and psychotic deterioration is unrelated to Tourette's disorder and infrequent. If these criteria were rigidly applied, it would exclude practically all patients from the diagnosis of Tourette's disorder. The development of specific criteria for the diagnosis (American Psychiatric Association, DSM-III, 1980), has facilitated diagnosis and the number of identified Tourette's disorder patients has increased manyfold in recent years. The diagnosis has now reached almost epidemic proportions.

Another factor contributing to underdiagnosis is a condition frequently observed in children by pediatricians and general practitioners, diagnosed formerly as habit tic and currently as transient tic disorder. The frequency is estimated at 4% to 25% and the distribution for the age of onset is approximately the same as for Tourette's disorder. Physicians generally advise parents that the tic is temporary and will disappear within a year. In several surveys, 25% to 50% of tics disappeared by or during adolescence, 46% were markedly improved, and 6% were unchanged (Zausmer, 1954; Torup, 1962; Corbett et al., 1969; Pasamanick and Kawi, 1956). It is difficult to differentiate between Tourette's disorder and transient tics because the initial histories are indistinguishable in all respects.

Also contributing to the massive underdiagnosis of Tourette's disorder in the past is the recurrent theme in the history of medicine of theory outpacing empiricism. Theory becomes overelaborated and is imposed on clinical practice and treatment but is eventually replaced by clinical observation, empiricism, and research. This theme was detected by Hippocrates, who advised that the overelaborate theoretical formulations of his day be replaced by observation of patients. Despite this universally accepted injunction, Galen's pharmacopeia of 820 animal, vegetable, and mineral matter, all of which were placebos, was imposed on medicine for 1,000 years. Sydenham, sometimes referred to as the second Hippocrates, advocated that the overelaborate theory of his day be replaced with empirical observation of patients.

In the nineteenth century the etiology of mental phenomena included vague references to inheritance or abnormal brain function, and followed the dictum: Where there is a crooked thought there is a crooked molecule. Throughout the succeeding years, in part associated with the popularity of psychoanalysis, the dictum became: Where there is a crooked molecule there is a crooked thought. Psychiatry and medicine became psychologically oriented, and diseases of unknown etiology were attributed to unconscious psychological conflicts. However, the postulate of the unconscious is, by definition, unavailable to the patient and can only be interpreted by a psychoanalyst, himself psychoanalyzed, through psychoanalytic interpretation of the patient's free association, slips, dreams, and transference. In time these formulations became more accepted and assumed the status of verifiable facts. This led to the interpretation that symptomatology for many conditions was caused by unconscious conflicts, and to the hazardous tendency to infer etiology from symptomatology.

During the 20th century it became increasingly fashionable to attribute diseases of unknown origin to a psychological etiology, characterized by the dictum: When in doubt it is psychological. Thus many illnesses, such as duodenal ulcer, bronchial asthma, irritable bowel, ulcerative colitis, neurodermatitis, dysmenorrhea, stiff-man syndrome, dystonia musculorum deformans, and many other so-called psychosomatic illnesses, were labeled as psychogenic in origin. The evidence from an increasing number of carefully controlled studies provides little support for a psychological etiology for these and many other conditions.

The history of Tourette's disorder during the twentieth century was influenced by the prevailing psychological beliefs, and is another example of the harmful consequences of substituting psychological theory for careful clinical observation. The deductions based on erroneous psychological assumptions then influence and obscure the clinical data. These assumptions then influence concepts about diagnosis, etiology, clinical course, prognosis, and treatment. The tendency to burden medicine with overdeveloped theories has always impaired medical progress, interfered with the treatment of patients, and led to fruitless years of treatment and hardship for many afflicted patients.

The literature on the treatment of Tourette's disorder can be characterized by the statement: Name a treatment and a Tourette patient has had it. Patients may have consulted 100 physicians, spent $100,000, and received every known sedative, stimulant, antidepressant, anticonvulsant, or psychotomimetic, antianxiety, antipsychotic, and/or other drug. Surgical procedures included phrenic nerve ligation, chryothalomotomy, and various types of lobotomies. Patients were treated with megavitamins, allergic desensitization, insulin coma treatment, electroconvulsive treatment, narcosis treatment, acupuncture, and substances to correct hypoglycemic states and nutritional deficiencies. Patients have tried every type of psychotherapy, including classic Freudian psychoanalysis, intensive psychotherapy, supportive psychotherapy, group therapy, family therapy, hypnosis, gestalt therapy, primal scream therapy, and behavior therapies. Although there are many case reports in the literature about the success of these therapies, they always describe single patients for whom the *post hoc ergo propter hoc* fallacy applies. One of the criteria for the diagnosis of Tourette's disorder is a waxing, waning, and fluctuating clinical course. These spontaneous changes are frequently misinterpreted as therapeutic effects. For some treatments, especially hypnosis and behavior therapy, symptoms decrease during the session when the patient is comfortable and absorbed in the process of therapy.

Psychotherapists unfamiliar with the natural waxing, waning, and fluctuating clinical course of the illness frequently misinterpret a decrease in symptoms as a therapeutic effect. Frequently in psychotherapy a new symptom suddenly appears following the disappearance of an older symptom. The new symptom is either ignored or erroneously interpreted as symptom substitution.

The reviewed literature was totally unconvincing about the effectiveness of any psychological, physiological, or drug therapy in Tourette's disorder, except for phenothiazine and butyrophenone drugs.

These conclusions about medicine and psychiatry in general and Tourette's disorder in particular were slowly arrived at while reviewing the literature and observing the patient for many months. I then told the patient that her condition was called Gilles de la Tourette syndrome. She touchingly responded, "What a beautiful name for such a horrible disease." I fully informed the patient about what I had learned about the disorder. I told her that the cause of the illness was unknown but my impression was that it was related to an abnormality in the central nervous system and not to psychological conflicts. I explained that although there was no known cure, some patients had been helped by treatment. We both agreed that the best approach was to try a number of drugs that had been reported as helpful. A description of the treatment and the results has been published elsewhere (Shapiro and Shapiro, 1968), and only the outline of the treatment is presented here. During the next several months, 36 drugs, in different dosages or various combinations, were tried. Each drug was tried two or three times and alternated periodically with placebos. Several of the phenothiazines decreased some of the symptoms, but caused adverse effects that interfered with functioning and prevented further increase in drug dosage.

From the review of the literature, I came across several reports that described a promising chemotherapeutic treatment for Tourette's disorder (Seignot, 1961; Caprini and Melotti, 1961; Challas and Brauer, 1963; Chapel et al., 1964). Haloperidol, a butyrophenone drug introduced in Europe in 1959, similar to the piperazine group of phenothiazine antipsychotic drugs, had been established as effective in the treatment of psychotic and schizophrenic patients. The initial results were consistently promising to warrant a trial on haloperidol.

Haloperidol was not approved by the Food and Drug Administration (FDA) at the time. An application was made for the use of this drug; it was approved by the FDA and the drug was provided by McNeil Pharmaceuticals. The drug was started at a very low dosage (0.5 mg b.i.d) and resulted in dramatic improvement on the first day. However, the improvement was associated with akinesia, a profound body lethargy, which sometimes occurs with initial ingestion of this and similar drugs. An antiparkinsonian drug was used to control the akinesia; as the akinesia wore off during the next several days, the symptoms returned. The dosage was slowly titrated upward for maximal relief of symptoms with minimal adverse effects. During the next 11 months the dosage was varied between 1 and 10 mg/day. It became apparent that the best overall dosage was 3 mg/day. At that dosage 90% of symptoms were controlled and adverse effects were minimal.

Ten months after beginning treatment, a double-blind trial was conducted. Haloperidol was slowly withdrawn. Many symptoms returned but not as intensely as before treatment. The patient was given one bottle containing 0.5-mg tablets of haloperidol and another of matching placebos. Instructions were to use either bottle at a beginning dosage of one tablet t.i.d.; the dosage was to be increased and the medication changed at the discretion of the patient for the next 2 months.

The initial medication blindly chosen by the patient was 1.5 mg/day placebo for 8 days, 2 mg/day haloperidol for 7 days, 3 mg/day placebo for 4 days, and, finally, 3 mg/day haloperidol. Symptoms markedly decreased at the last dosage.

There was a remarkable change in the personality and functioning of the patient after approximately 1 year of treatment. She was no longer depressed, was happy, outgoing, and socially responsive. She subsequently married and had two children. On periodic follow-ups during the past 22 years, the patient reported that she has very few tics, perhaps one in a week or two, and only with tension. Her symptoms are so infrequent that she no longer thinks of herself as having Tourette's disorder, except when she forgets to take her medication, which varies in dosage between 1 and 2 mg/day haloperidol. Occasionally during the past 22 years she became curious about what effect stopping the medication would have on her symptoms. Each time the medication was stopped, symptoms reappeared at their original intensity in approximately 4 days.

Subsequent publicity in the lay press, especially a report in the *New York Post* (1967) entitled *Weird Psychosis Cured by New Drug,* led patients to contact McNeil Pharmaceuticals or Dr. George Challas in Iowa. Since I was one of the few physicians using haloperidol as an investigatory drug in the northeastern United States at the time, these patients were referred to me for treatment. This contributed to a slow but steady increase in the number of patients evaluated during the subsequent 6 years. By 1971, 34 patients had been evaluated, studied, and treated. Many detailed papers describing our findings were published in medical, psychiatric, and psychological journals. These studies included more patients than any study heretofore. Previous reports described 15 patients by Lucas (1967), seven by Feild et al. (1966), seven by Eisenberg et al. (1959), and approximately 50 clinical studies of one or two patients.

At the same time, in January 1970, a letter appeared in the *New York Post* from Mr. Martin A. Levey, a father who had spent $50,000 fruitlessly to obtain a diagnosis of Tourette's disorder, pleading for other families to contact him to exchange information and support.

Plea for Help
We write to you in quiet desperation. We have a son who has a very rare neurological disorder called "Gilles de la Tourette." There are probably 75–100 cases known at present. Doctors know very little, no previous usable case history of consequence. Believe me if I say we have made the rounds over the years. As the saying goes "He helps those who help themselves." We would like to contact others in this situation so as to exchange mutual information and to possibly form an organization for this rare disorder. We have exhausted our resources in this lonely battle. Would parents of children who have this syndrome please contact us through the *New York Post?*
Martin A. Levey

Five parents responded to his letter. Mr. Levey asked if I would contact the patients I had been seeing to join in the formation of a Tourette organization. Twenty-two of my patients agreed, and 27 individuals met in June of 1971 at the Payne Whitney Clinic and Cornell Medical Center to form the Tourette Syndrome Association (TSA) with Martin Levey as the first president. We provided advice and counsel for many years to the fledgling organization. Since then, the TSA has grown and now comprises 32 official chapters with an additional 200 representatives throughout the United States, Canada, Denmark, England, Australia, Spain, and France.

In addition, several reports in the media of our work stimulated considerable publicity and referral of more patients. The first major report appeared in the *Wall Street Journal* (1972), followed by the *New York Daily News* (1972), *Newsweek* (1972), *Reader's Digest* (1973), and many other newspapers and journals throughout the United States. Our work was also shown and described on television stations, such as ABC, NBC, CBS, and WNET (PBS).

All of these factors contributed to a steady increase in patients referred to us for treatment over the years. Since the publication of our first book, the increase in the number of patients evaluated by us, as well as the number of patients diagnosed by other physicians, has been dramatic, almost epidemic. This is graphically illustrated by the number of centers in major medical schools that have established clinics for treatment and research and the proliferation of publications on this disorder in the last 8 years.

Although Tourette's disorder was thought to be a rare illness, recent evidence indicates that it is considerably more common than previously estimated. Current estimates of its prevalence is at least five per thousand, or over one million individuals in the United States.

Our contribution to the phenomenal increase in identified patients was the development of specific criteria for the diagnosis of Tourette's disorder, the specification that despite Tourette's original papers and those of other early investigators, coprolalia and echolalia were not necessary for the diagnosis. We demonstrated that patients with the disorder do not deteriorate psychologically and intellectually and that Tourette's disorder has an organic rather than a psychological etiology. Further, we have developed methods of treatment with haloperidol, pimozide, and other medications and have provided evidence of their effectiveness.

Arthur K. Shapiro, M.D.

Gilles de la Tourette Syndrome
Second Edition

1

History of Tourette and Tic Disorders

Important historical papers on Tourette's disorder published before 1974 are reviewed in this chapter. In the first edition, the literature was summarized in the form of an annotated chronological bibliographical review to provide readers with a summary of the Tourette literature. Unfortunately, or fortunately, the published literature on Tourette's disorder has increased astronomically since our initial volume so that a complete summary of all the published literature is no longer possible. We estimate that approximately 500 articles have been published on all aspects of Tourette's disorder since publication of our 1978 book. In this volume, each chapter includes a review of the literature germane to the content of the chapter. We believe that this approach is more meaningful, since it provides the reader with a handy reference to all published material on genetics, biochemistry, epidemiology, and so on.

HEREDITARY ANTECEDENTS

Roughly from 1825 to the end of the nineteenth century, including the papers by Gilles de la Tourette, the literature focused on the separation of this illness from other neurological conditions, and the identification and range of its symptomatology. The etiology of Tourette's disorder was attributed to neuropathic heredity by early investigators, and later to mental instability. As we shall see, Tourette's original evaluation of patients, possibly in response to the work of Charcot and Guinon, changed from characterizing the mental status of Tourette's disorder patients as good to a concern with their mental instability, and to differentiating the disorder from hysteria.

All mental illness during this period was believed to be hereditary, although it is not clear from the literature what was inherited. Certainly, the authors looked closely at the family background and described what they called "neuropathic" antecedents in the patient's background; how these "neuropathic" tendencies resulted in motor and verbal tics, however, was not defined. Concepts of heredity were primitive and the mechanisms poorly understood.

Prior to the first major work on movement disorders by Bouteille in 1810, we have not found any reference to Tourette's disorder. There are several isolated references in the literature to individuals with symptoms that might have been part of the syndrome. Sprenger (1489), in the *Malleus Maleficarum* (*Witch's Hammer*), describes

> A sober priest without any eccentricity . . . no sign of madness or any immoderate action [who was said to be possessed of the devil] . . . when he passed any church, and genuflected in honour of the Glorious Virgin, the devil made him thrust his tongue far out of his mouth; and when he was asked whether he could not restrain himself from doing this, he answered: "I cannot help myself at all, for so he used all my limbs and organs, my neck, my tongue, and my lungs, whenever he pleases, causing me to speak or to cry out; and I hear the words as if they were spoken by myself, but I am altogether unable to restrain them; and when I try to engage in prayer he attacks me more violently, thrusting out my tongue" [pp.128,129].

Whether the good priest had Tourette's disorder or not is problematic, but fortunately he was cured by exorcism. A rejuvenated interest in exorcism was stimulated by the movie *The Exorcist*, which is reputedly based on an exaggerated and distorted interpretation of a patient with Tourette's disorder who was hospitalized at Georgetown University (1974).

Another possible early case was cited by Stevens (1971) who, in an historical paper describing some of the notable achievements of Georges Gilles de la Tourette, mentions an

> affected Prince de Conde who was compelled to stuff his mouth with any nearby object, including a curtain, to suppress an involuntary bark in the presence of Louis XIV.

Lees (1985) cites several other early references to individuals who may have suffered from this condition; Mary Hall of Gadsden in Hertford described by William Drage in 1663 and a family of barking girls by Friend in 1701:

> The awful sight of the yelping girls confronted me directly, each of them replying to the other in absolutely strict alternation with a violent shaking of her head, as if encouraging the others by her nod—like a common country piper—to sing their unpleasant tune together. They were not affected by any spasms in the face except for movements which frequently made their mouths go to and fro; and their pulse was like that of the healthy except that it was slightly weak just before the end. The sound, as it seemed to me, resembled not so much the barking of dogs as their howling, except that it was more rapidly repeated. Often, between these howlings, they enjoyed the power of speech and full possession of their senses.

More compelling evidence for a diagnosis of Tourette's disorder was presented by McHenry (1967) and Murray (1978, 1982) for the symptoms exhibited by Samuel Johnson which included tics of the mouth, head, hands, feet, and torso; sounds; echolalia; counting and touching.

Until the end of the nineteenth century, movement disorders, referred to as motor incoordinations, were diagnosed as chorea, a Greek word meaning dance. Movements were a prominent symptom in many illnesses; Bouteille (1810), in his book *Traite de Chorée,* described and characterized them. Of interest to us historically was the specification of a separate movement disorder, which he labeled as pseudo- or false chorea. Although false chorea resembled a true chorea in its motor component, other components were different. Pseudochorea might have included Tourette's disorder.

The first description of a patient with Tourette's disorder appeared 15 years later in a paper by Itard (1825), who described a French noblewoman who displayed not only movements but also obscene vocalizations. This noblewoman, the Marquise de Dampierre, subsequently seen by Charcot and discussed by his pupil Gilles de la Tourette, has become a famous historical case. She had involuntary convulsive spasms in the arms and hands since the age of 7. These movements were followed by movements in the muscles of the shoulder and neck and contortions and grimaces of the face. Her symptoms also involved the organs of speech and voice. She was reported to make bizarre noises and utter words that made no sense and were also of an obscene nature. During her teens, her symptoms remitted and only slight twitching of the face and neck were observed, but they reappeared again, becoming progressively worse.

Itard provided an excellent description of how difficult Tourette symptoms can be for patients:

> Thus in the middle of a conversation that interests her suddenly without being able to avoid it, she interrupts that which she says or hears by bizarre cries and extraordinary words which make deplorable contrast to her distinguished manner. These words are mostly rude oaths, obscene adjectives which are no less embarrassing for herself as for the other . . .

Obscenities were referred to as coprolalia for the first time 70 years later by Gilles de la Tourette. Itard explained this illness as an idiopathic irritation of the brain.

Reference to Itard's patient was made by Roth (1850) and Sandras (1851). However, no detailed report on this illness appeared again until Trousseau (1873) became interested in refining the distinctions between various movement disorders, then referred to as the tic illness (*maladie des tics*), which was later renamed Gilles de la Tourette syndrome. Trousseau described the muscular and motor tics, the bizarre nature of the vocalizations, and he was the first to describe palilalia.

> Non-dolorous tic consists of brief and momentary muscular contractions, more or less limited as a general rule, involving preferably the face, but affecting also the neck, trunk and limbs. Their exhibition is a matter of everyday experience. In one case it may be a blinking of the eyelids, a spasmodic twitch of the cheek, nose and lip; in another it is a toss of the head; in the third, it is a shrug of the shoulder, a convulsive movement of the diaphragm or abdominal muscles. In time, the term

embodies an infinite variety of bizarre actions that defy analysis. These tics are not infrequently associated with a highly characteristic scream, cry, or bark, a sort of laryngeal or diaphragmatic chorea, which may itself constitute the condition, or there may be a more complicated symptom of a curious impulse to repeat the same word or the same exclamation. Sometimes the patient is driven to utter aloud what he would conceal.

Trousseau did not conclude that these symptoms constituted a disorder distinct from chorea and never actually differentiated it as a separate entity. He did, however, emphasize the hereditary nature of tics, recounting the case of a mother with three daughters, all of whom had tics, and a boy with loud cries, a brother with tics, and diverse antecedents with neuropathic qualities.

It is of interest historically that the current use of massed practice in behavior modification therapy for the tics of Tourette's disorder was anticipated by Trousseau. His therapy consisted of using a metronome to exercise the movements in the affected part of the body. Interestingly enough, he noted that if the tic subsided in the exercised muscle, it would reappear in another part of the body.

Another contribution was made by Friedrich (1881), who referred to the illness as a subgroup of the choreas. His was the first systematic attempt to develop a theoretical explanation. Of crucial importance he believed was the influence of sudden and violent psychic anxiety on the origin of tics. Cortical and psychological causation were involved. He characterized the movements as "remembrance spasms," postulating that at the moment of an actual intense fright experienced by the person, usually in childhood, the person had reacted with a series of combined movements. When other events in some way replicate this experience and its state of excitability, the initial movement is reproduced spontaneously. Ultimately, if the excitability is maintained, the movements occur without an external stimulus, then become involuntary, and eventually become coordinated spasms. In retrospect, the cases described by Friedrich were more consistent with a panic state with some choreiform movements than with Tourette's disorder.

During the latter part of the 1800s a new phenomenon, not a tic but rather a variety of the tic illness, was described in the medical literature. Beard (1880) reported experiments with what he called a most incredible nervous phenomenon: "the jumping Frenchman of Maine." When startled by an abrupt command, these "jumpers" would perform the command as well as repeat the words of the command. These symptoms were expressed suddenly, ended quickly, and did not begin or persist independent of stimulation. The most prominent characteristic was repeating language, or echolalia. A similar condition, called latah, was described by O'Brien (1883) in Malaysia, which also included coprolalia. The Russian equivalent, called myriachit, was incompletely described by Hammond (1884). The movements occurred in response to startle. Echo phenomena or imitative movements were also involved, such as imitating the actions of others and echoing sounds or words. Hammond did not mention coprolalia as a symptom.

All three conditions, jumpers of Maine, latah, and myriachit, are startle reactions; namely, the symptoms are not spontaneous but must be precipitated, and they are imitative, resulting in echolalia, automatic obedience, and sometimes echopraxia. They are clearly different from Gilles de la Tourette syndrome, in which the motor tic is spontaneous. Only in latah is coprolalia reported, but it always accompanies a startle reaction.

These illnesses are important historically because in 1884 Gilles de la Tourette thought they were similar to the convulsive tic illness and grouped them together diagnostically. Gilles de la Tourette proposed that the symptoms observed in nine patients, six of whom were his, constituted a new disease category which should be separated from the choreas. He called the illness a nervous affliction characterized by generalized motor incoordination and noises, accompanied by echolalia and coprolalia. In his opinion, the jumping Frenchman, latah, and myriachit were similar manifestations of the convulsive tic illness in other countries.

Because Tourette did not differentiate his syndrome from the jumping Frenchman, latah, and myriachit, in which echolalia was a prominent symptom, the frequency and importance of echolalia were exaggerated. Echolalia was not observed in all of Tourette's patients. Gilles de la Tourette's major contribution, aside from his brilliant clinical characterization of the illness, was to classify Tourette's disorder as separate from other movement disorders. He was rewarded for his contribution by Charcot who named the new disease entity after him (Shapiro and Shapiro, 1984d).

A brief description of the nine patients described by Tourette in his 1885 paper, six of whom were observed personally, will help to clarify the symptomatology.

The first, the Marquise de Dampierre, seen by both Itard and Charcot, was a female characterized by convulsions of the hands and arms, shoulders, neck, and face which began at the age of 7. These were followed by bizarre cries. The symptoms persisted through puberty, but at 17 she experienced a remission which lasted for approximately 18 to 20 months. The symptoms returned, including the onset of coprolalia, and persisted throughout her life. Coprolalia caused her to become a social recluse. This case provided an excellent example of the lifelong nature of this disorder, since the Marquise lived to be 86 years old.

The symptoms in a second male patient (Tourette's patient) began at the age of 16 with rapid movements of the right leg and left side. At 17 he began to utter a light cry, "hm" and "ouah." He also developed echolalia and coprolalia, but the coprolalia disappeared at age 20, as did the large disorganized movements. Only limited movements of the upper limb and tongue protrusion persisted.

The third patient (Tourette's patient) was a male whose symptoms began at age 9 with rapid flexion and extension of the head and neck. Soon afterward, facial grimaces and movements of the arms and shoulders developed. Complex movements appeared in the form of running and getting down on his knees, raising himself, and performing various contortions. Coprolalia developed at age 14. Echopraxia and echolalia were also noted.

Patient four (Tourette's patient) was a male in whom symptoms developed at 8 or 9 years of age, which consisted of movements of the muscles of the face, trunk, and limbs. Echolalia, complex jumping movements, clicking of the teeth, and biting of the tongue, but not coprolalia, were described.

The fifth patient (Tourette's patient), a male, developed twitches of the face, followed by arm and leg movements at age 8. Complex knee bends, jumps, and lip biting, but not sounds or coprolalia, were also described. The absence of vocalizations (based on our criteria, which are described later) suggests the diagnosis of chronic motor tic (CMT) rather than Tourette's disorder.

The sixth patient (Tourette's patient), also a male, began to grimace at age 7, followed by twitches of all the muscles. Also noted was a strident cry of "ouh! ouh!," but not coprolalia.

A seventh patient (Tourette's patient) was again a male whose symptoms began at 8 or 9 years of age with eye blinking followed by contortions of the body which led to a changed style of walking. The patient's aunt was reported to have had the same symptoms, and an aunt of the mother was reported to have had chorea. This patient also jumped if brushed accidentally. The absence of vocalizations suggests a diagnosis of CMT rather than Tourette's disorder.

A female whose symptoms began at age 9, the eighth patient, was a patient of Professor Pitres. Movement of the limbs and face, a guttural sound, coprolalia, echolalia in the form of imitating the barking of dogs, and echopraxia were described.

The ninth patient (Dr. Fere's patient) was a male with onset at age 14 of movements of the arms and legs. The movements were described as fits or convulsions, with the patient turning around and around, falling, and biting his tongue, but without loss of consciousness. To this was added the symptom of repeating his own words or the same syllables of the same word. At night or with tiredness he uttered an obscenity. Because the symptoms included convulsions, there is a diagnostic question as to whether this patient had Tourette's disorder, or whether Tourette's disorder and epilepsy coexisted.

In his 1885 paper, Tourette identified the unique development of the symptoms. Motor symptoms were the first to appear, most frequently of the face, specifically eye blinking, and then the upper limbs. These movements appeared suddenly and were executed rapidly and at close intervals. Facial tics appeared with greatest frequency and intensity, whereas the more complicated movements occurred less frequently. The next symptoms were verbal, cries such as "hm," "ouh," "ouah," and "ah." Tourette erroneously described vocalizations as always occurring simultaneously with a motor symptom. Echolalia followed and was considered by Tourette to be one of the most persistent symptoms. The third symptom category identified by Tourette was coprolalia, which he considered to be pathognomonic. Despite the fact the coprolalia existed in only five (55%) of the patients reported by Tourette, he stated " . . .we would be tempted that in a majority of cases, and in a variable period of the disease, it will almost certainly appear."

Tourette noted that some patients had only motor symptoms, in contrast to the later opinion that verbal tics are necessary for the diagnosis of Tourette's disorder. He observed that other symptoms such as echolalia and coprolalia may appear many years later in some cases, making diagnosis difficult. The exact time of their appearance was variable, but Tourette felt they would appear eventually as last symptoms.

Intellectual or psychological deterioration did not occur according to Tourette, although many subsequent writers described a poor outcome as the ultimate course for Tourette patients, possibly because of the absence of effective treatment. Tourette was less pessimistic about the psychological state of patients which he related to the severity of Tourette's disorder.

> As for the mental state it is perfectly regular and normal: The subjects are reasonable, in no way do their acts resemble those of madmen; they are totally aware of their state; most are very intelligent . . . In all our patients, the general sensitivity was absolutely normal. As for the physical, moral, and mental state of the patient . . . it is excellent in all respects, except of course, for the disadvantages which such an abnormal state can create . . . when it occurs in children, it induces habits of laziness and prevents their intellectual development by suppressing work, or by bringing serious obstacles. It is easy besides, to understand that as these sick people advance in age, their situation becomes more and more disagreeable. But even here there are questions of degree . . ."

Other factors identified by Tourette were its childhood onset, usually before puberty, the male predominance, and that the symptoms are progressive, new ones added to or replacing old ones. He believed social class as well as geography to be of no importance because all social classes and people from many different areas were affected.

As to the cause, Tourette believed, as did Trousseau and Beard, that it was hereditary. The case histories included only one patient with a history of tics in the family, one with a grandfather with chorea, and one with a father with a nonpainful facial tic.

In his 1899 paper, Tourette revised some of his original ideas about the illness, stating that the disease was likely to occur equally in both sexes, whereas previously he thought it was more frequent in boys. Another revision concerned his original classification of the movements as motor incoordinations. He now agreed with the observation of Guinon (1886) that the movements were systematized and coordinated. In fact, he believed the distinction between coordination and uncoordination was crucial when making a differential diagnosis between *maladie des tics convulsif* and Sydenham's chorea.

Perhaps the most significant revision in Tourette's thinking about this syndrome concerned his focusing on the mental instability of the patient and the nervous or mental disorders in the family background, in contrast to his earlier belief that the illness was not a psychiatric disorder. He had previously been impressed with the excellence of the patient's mental state. In the 1899 paper, Tourette observed that there was always some nervous disorder in the family and that the patient had numerous anxieties, fantasies, and fears. These emotional stigmata signified to him that the patients were mentally unstable or "degenerate." In arriving at this conclusion, Tourette acknowledged the influence on his thinking of Guinon's observation that tiqueurs almost always exhibited a state of mental instability characterized by countless phobias, arithromania, and agoraphobia.

Another change, also an outgrowth of Guinon's influence, was the specification of coprolalia as a psychic stigmata. Although Guinon believed that there was an emotional significance to the motor component of the illness as well, Tourette disagreed. As to coprolalia, however, Tourette was convinced that there was an irresistible psychic impulsion that forced the patient to utter filthy words. Echolalia was also labeled a psychic stigmata, and Tourette acknowledged that it was less frequent among tiqueurs than he had previously thought.

He concluded that the symptoms of coprolalia, echolalia, impulsions, and phobias that plagued these patients indicated that they could be classified as "degenerates." Nevertheless, his own observations that they were frequently above average in intelligence and had high social positions caused him to reconsider this classification. His compromise was to label them "higher degenerates."

It was unfortunate historically that Tourette revised his evaluation of the mental stability of these patients and failed to heed his own astute observations about how well many of these patients functioned apart from the tic symptomatology.

The balance of the paper discussed the differential diagnosis between Tourette's disorder, Sydenham's chorea, hysteria, and variable chorea. Features differentiating Sydenham's chorea from the tic illnesses include the age at onset, length of time the symptoms persisted, and their presence after puberty. Tics were brief, jerky, convulsive, sometimes systematized, and could be inhibited for a variable period in the tic illness, whereas they were rounded off and lacked coordination in Sydenham's chorea.

He believed that the prognosis for patients with the tic illness was dependent on the severity of the symptomatology and the recurrence of the symptoms after periods of remission. These variables would determine how much the symptoms interfered with the physical and social life of the patient. However, he categorically stated that despite the variability in symptomatology and severity, tics persisted throughout a person's life: "Once a tiqueur, always a tiqueur." He believed, however, that the psychic stigmata implied a fairly severe prognosis. As for treatment, he impotently recommended rest, isolation, and avoiding fatigue.

Three lectures by Charcot were published by G. Melloti (1885) in an Italian medical journal. These lectures were of some importance since Charcot disagreed with Tourette that jumping Frenchman, latah, and myriachit were identical with the illness described by Tourette in 1885. He observed that coprolalia was not found in jumping Frenchman or in myriachit, although it was reported in latah. Similarly, he noted with some surprise that Beard and Hammond had not described the choreal movements in these disorders, which were the cornerstone of the tic illness. He stated: ". . .it is a mistake to consider it all one thing with jumpers or latah in which the tic is not mentioned while in the illness of Gilles de la Tourette it is the foundation."

The differentiation of the three conditions from Tourette's disorder was important because it lessened the prominence of echo phenomena as a symptom of Tourette's disorder. Unfortunately, this change was not reflected in the literature and the importance of echo phenomena was exaggerated. Charcot differentiated between a simple tic and a more severe, morbid type. The common variety was characterized by a facial grimace accompanied by a slight movement of the arm or fingers, and a monosyllabic exclamation, "heu, heu." This disorder did not prevent the person's normal development socially or vocationally and was considered to be an infirmity, not an illness. Gilles de la Tourette illness, according to Charcot, was more serious because of its intensity and its complicated movements, which did limit a person's development.

The characteristics of the illness described by Charcot included age at onset at 7, 8, or 9, the appearance of a single tic following a violent emotion or fright, and the gradual addition of other movements. In the morbid state, as opposed to the common tic, he noted that patients were not able to function, and in some way their lives were endangered. The common or simple tic imitates reflex acts, such as pulling one's beard.

The development of the illness was insidious. It might appear benign at certain stages; but underneath this benign appearance, the illness continued and could not be cured. The importance of heredity was emphasized by Charcot; he believed that a hereditary factor could be found in all cases of tics, especially if coprolalia was present. The hereditary element may be a history of tics in the family or psychopathic antecedents, especially family members with hysteria or insanity.

Charcot was the first neurologist to identify involuntary impulsive ideas as part of the illness. These involuntary ideas have also been called *folie du doute,* or doubting mania, and compel a person to doublecheck each action; other involuntary ideas include the craze of touching, or arithromania, repeating an action a certain number of times. According to Charcot these impulsive ideas in the mental sphere are physical, coming from the brain. He saw a union between the impulsive ideas and the impulsive movements, the mental and the physical; thus he resolved the two aspects of the illness.

Guinon (1886, 1887) and Chabbert (1893) stressed the hereditary nature of the illness. Guinon believed that the illness was always an expression of a hereditary defect and that its cause was a "hereditary degeneration."

Catrou (1890) in a thesis on *maladie des tics convulsif* described some of the changes suggested by Charcot, namely the substitution of the term convulsive tic for motor incoordination, and the introduction of the term *idee fixes* to describe certain types of impulsions. Grasset (1890) was concerned with differentiating habits or mannerisms from tics.

Hammond's (1892) paper is historically important because it implicates for the first time a specific lesion of the motor cerebral cortex in the thalamus, striatum, and cell area of the pons and medulla. He believed that the initial cause was an irritant rather than a destructive lesion, but that structural cell changes might occur with persistent irritation.

Summaries of one or more cases were also reported by Dana and Wilken (1886), Railton (1886), Osler (1891), Bresler (1896), Brissaud (1899), and Koester (1899). These reports are summarized in the 1978 volume.

PSYCHOLOGICAL ETIOLOGY

Shortly before 1900, physicians, neurologists, and psychiatrists, as part of the *zeitgeist*, became interested in the psychology of patients, illnesses, and people in general. Influenced by Bernheim, Charcot, Janet, Dejeraine, Dubois, Freud, Breuer, and others, it resulted in creative speculation about presumed underlying psychological mechanisms that determined or influenced sickness and personality. These speculations, based on clinical observation and without empirical support, in retrospect quite naive, were applied to the etiology of tics, dystonia, Tourette's disorder, and many other conditions, replacing the emphasis on neuropathic hereditary factors.

The earliest paper discussing the relationship between the psychic and motor components of the illness was by Guinon (1886, 1887); we have already noted his influence on Tourette's thinking. He observed that many of the distinguishing characteristics of the convulsive tic were almost identical to those seen in hysteria, thus making it difficult to separate the hysteric from the convulsive tic. Criteria were established to differentiate the two conditions. If the symptoms had an early age of onset, were multiple, complex, and resistant to treatment, the diagnosis should be convulsive tics. Prognosis was thought to be poor in the convulsive tic disorder, which was absolutely tenacious and incurable. The tics could be hysterical in nature or superimposed on a hysterical nature.

Interest in the contribution of hysteria to the development of tics continued to be a dominant theme in a paper by Chabbert (1893). He described tics in a mother and son in whom emotional factors were thought to be more etiologically important for the son than for the mother. The first patient had an unchanging facial tic following an injury, with no further development except occasional coprolalia later in life. The second patient had a delayed age of onset and failed to show the usual progression of symptomatology characteristic of Tourette's disorder. Chabbert believed that the illness was hereditary, whether it was a local, minor or generalized convulsive tic, but did not specify whether the tic condition or the "neurosis" was inherited.

Freud briefly commented on *maladie des tics* in 1893 (1966). Freud attended Charcot's Tuesday lectures and agreed with Charcot that the only difference between *tic convulsif* and hysteria was that the hysterical tic disappears, whereas the genuine tic persists. Freud characterized *tic convulsif* as a neurosis with so much symptomatic similarity to hysteria that it may be a partial manifestation of hysteria. He was intrigued by coprolalia, which he felt could be explained in the following way. The patient perceived that he was unable to repress a particular sound, and this led him to fear that he would lose control not only of sounds but of words as well, and ultimately result in what he feared coming true. Freud was convinced of this following his experience with a patient who did not have Tourette's disorder but whose need to keep from saying a name was reversed into a counter-will, that is, saying the name aloud. Freud suggested that the same mechanism may underlie coprolalia since obscene words are secrets everyone knows and which they feel compelled to acknowledge to each other. This concept was previously described by Trousseau (1873) who said of the obscenities: "Sometimes a patient is driven to utter aloud what he would conceal." Freud characterized coprolalia as a mental phenomenon and thus speculated that the cause of the behavior could be found in the patient's psyche. However, Ferenczi (1921) quoted Freud as believing there was an organic factor in tics: "When I incidentally discussed the meaning and significance of tics with Professor Freud he mentioned that apparently there was an organic factor in the question."

Interest in psychological causation culminated in the treatise on tics by Meige and Feindel in 1902, translated into English by Wilson in 1907, which subsequently had a powerful influence on solidifying the belief that tics were a mental illness. In their treatise, a tic was defined as:

> a coordinated purposive act, provoked in the first instance by some external cause or by an idea; repetition leads to its becoming habitual, and finally to its involuntary reproduction without cause and for no purpose, at the same time as its form, intensity, and frequency are exaggerated; it thus assumes the character of a convulsive movement, inopportune and excessive; its execution is often proceded by an irresistible impulse, its suppression associated with malaise. The effect of distraction or of volitional effort is to diminish its activity; in sleep it disappears. It occurs in predisposed individuals, who usually show other indications of mental instability.

This definition was used by most authors for tics and Tourette's disorder in succeeding years. The book by Meige and Feindel was classic on the subject, but unfortunately was responsible for propagating many erroneous ideas about tics and Tourette's disorder.

Meige and Feindel defined tics as originating in a purposive act which had been provoked by a cause or idea. It is now clear that tics, in fact, serve no purpose, and that they are not an intended or voluntary response to an external stimulus. In most patients the tic begins without a specific stimulus, although there is a subgroup of patients who report a sensory stimulus which precipitates a dystonic voluntary movement. That tics become habitual is also incorrect, because the natural course is fluctuating, waxing and waning of tics, with new ones added to or replacing old ones. The idea that tics are preceded by an irresistible impulse is also incorrect. Tics can best be described as sudden, involuntary, frequent, and unrelated to need. If inhibited for too long, patients must release the resulting build-up of tension; but despite this limited or partial ability to control tics, they are involuntary. Possibly of greatest harm to patients with tics was the erroneous belief of the authors that tics occur in predisposed individuals who usually show other indications of mental instability. Tiqueurs were characterized as mentally infantile, as evidenced by the fickleness of their minds and the inconsequence of their ideas. Meige and Feindel characterized the ticqueur as having a pronounced hereditary psychiatric or neuropathic tendency, multifarious psychic or physical anomalies, and numerous phobias and obsessions. In fact, the authors state: "A tic cannot be a tic unless it is associated with a certain degree of mental instability and imperfection."

Etiologically, they rely on heredity to explain the illness, but their concept of heredity is, at best, hazy. The evidence of a family member with mental instability is certainly inadequate to etiologically explain tic behavior; nor is the presented evidence specific as to what was inherited.

In addition, we know that most individuals with tics and Tourette's disorder have average intellectual abilities and that many have superior intelligence or have achieved considerable professional, academic, and vocational success. They cannot be characterized as more maladjusted than a neurotic outpatient psychiatric group; psychological factors are not etiologic to Tourette's disorder. We also have not replicated Meige and Feindel's finding of physical anomalies, such as a lack of sexual growth, in our sample. As for the obsessions, some of the touching phenomena described by the authors are tics and not true obsessions.

It is of interest that Meige and Feindel credit Charcot with demonstrating the pathogenic significance of the psychic factor in tiqueurs. They quote him as saying that tics are physical only in appearance; in all other respects it should be considered a mental disease, a sort of hereditary aberration.

Although the authors were concerned primarily with tics and not Tourette's disorder, many of the patients they described clearly should have been diagnosed as having Tourette's disorder. In other cases, the symptoms are difficult to categorize and many patients appeared to have psychiatric disabilities.

They believed that Gilles de la Tourette syndrome constitutes a separate entity which they designated as a disease of convulsive tics. This term should include only

> those cases whose progressive evolution ends in the generalization of the convulsive movements, to the accompaniment of coprolalia, and sometimes echolalia . . . From the psychical aspect, moreover, the development it undergoes may culminate in actual insanity.

Other authors who published papers on tics during the period include Johnson (1905), Patrick (1905), Prince (1906), Ross (1909), Fleischner (1911), Williams (1912), Barbour (1913), Wilson (1927), Brain (1928), and Selling (1929).

PSYCHOANALYSIS

The interest in psychological causation was continued and further refined in the flurry of papers on tics and Tourette's disorder by psychoanalysts from the 1920s through the 1960s. Psychoanalytic writers were impatient with the superficial psychological writings by Meige and Feindel, and sought to explain tics as a symbolic expression of underlying or intrapsychic conflicts.

There were occasional references to possible "constitutional" or "organic" substrata, but these authors were interested in identifying the specific personality types or dynamic conflicts in patients with tics and Tourette's disorder. Support for the resulting concepts was based on the study of individual patients. The organic or constitutional component was usually characterized as an increased eroticism of the musculature or a constitutional hyperkinesis, which created an organ neurosis of the neuromuscular system. The tic symbolically expressed an underlying conflict. There was little unanimity among psychoanalysts, however, about the "specific" underlying conflict, some of whom characterized the illness as a narcissistic disorder, and others as an anal-sadistic disorder. These theories were based almost exclusively on the study of a single case during psychiatric treatment or interviews.

An early paper by Sadger (1914) characterized tics in a female patient as a source of erotic pleasure and an expression of unconscious sexual striving. In contrast, Oberndorf (1916) felt that the tic represented a defense against a primarily autopleasurable act.

The first extensive psychoanalytic discussion of tics and Tourette's disorder was by Ferenczi (1921), who considered many tics to be stereotyped equivalents of onanism. In a tic, libido connected with genital sensation was displaced onto other parts of the body, resulting in increased pleasure in muscular movements. Coprolalia represented the spoken expression of the same erotic emotion which previously had been abreacted in a symbolic movement.

Ferenczi hypothesized a relationship between tics, narcissism, and catatonia. He considered tics to be a narcissistic disorder. The narcissism was the pleasure derived by the tiqueur from his muscular movements. He believed, too, that psychosis and tic had the same root, since many paranoiacs and schizophrenics had tics. In addition, the tendency to echolalia, echopraxia, stereotype, grimacing, and mannerisms was common to tics and catatonia. The tic is a momentary and paroxysmal defense against all external stimuli analogous to the principal symptoms of negativism and rigidity in catatonia, the summation of numberless clonic defensive convulsions (tics), and would lead to tonic rigidity and climax in catatonia. They noted a tendency for tiqueurs to retain positions that their limbs adopt or in which they are placed without the smallest muscular resistance. Ferenczi suggested that the similarity between tics and catatonia was supported by Meige and Feindel's observations.

Abraham (1927), Klein (1925), and Fenichel (1945) discussed tics from a psychoanalytic prospective but disagreed about their psychogenesis.

Historically, the papers by Mahler and her co-workers offer the most thorough delineation of the psychoanalytic theory of tics and Tourette's disorder (Mahler and Rangell, 1943; Mahler, 1944, 1949; Mahler et al., 1945; Mahler and Gross, 1945; Mahler and Luke, 1946). These papers differed from previous psychoanalytic papers by presenting many case studies which were not purely theoretical. Their influence was profound since they presented a psychoanalytic theory of etiology and treatment of tics at a time when psychoanalytic theory was fashionable and influential.

The first problem is to untangle the number of patients observed and the criteria for inclusion of patients in the sample. The authors described two samples (Mahler et al., 1945; Mahler and Luke, 1946) that included 18 patients in the first sample and 16 patients in the second sample. The number of patients observed included 18 patients who are referred to as the follow-up group. They were selected by a retrospective review of 541 admissions to the children's ward of the New York State Psychiatric Institute and Hospital of Columbia University between 1930 and 1943, and 16 patients, described as patients with "actual tic syndromes," who were referred from various hospitals and diagnosed by "consultation between neurologists and psychiatrists as suffering from a psychogenic or functional tic syndrome." One of the patients was included in both the follow-up and clinical study so that the total number of patients was 33. Selection criteria included explicit agreed-upon diagnosis of psychogenic or functional tic syndrome, and some patients with a similar personality make-up as the first group but without tics. Patients with mild tics were excluded, as were patients with organic psychosis or other psychosis and those with a psychoneurotic or symptomatic tic.

From the previously described inclusion and exclusion criteria, the sample comprised a heterogeneous group of patients with and without tics, some of whom had Tourette's disorder. Throughout the papers, these patients were described as having a tic syndrome, Tourette's disorder, incipient, not yet crystallized tics and the personality of the ticqueur. It is probable, therefore, that many subjects do not fulfill the criteria for the diagnosis of Tourette's disorder. Support for this likelihood is suggested by a subsequent paper on the tic syndrome (Mahler and Luke, 1946), in which only 11 of the 18 retrospective follow-up group were described as "suffering from a typical and severe tic syndrome at the time of their hospitalization." The remaining seven did not suffer from a tic syndrome ". . .but had . . . symptomatic tics in association with other neurotic traits of the primary behavior disorder type . . ." These 11 patients were discussed in the paper on outcome by Mahler and Luke (1946). Another indication of poor sampling or criteria is suggested by details about three female patients. The diagnosis for one patient was torsion spasm or psychogenic tic; a second patient had a single eye tic and logorrhea; a third patient was "in an early stage of development." These sparse details suggest that these patients do not fulfill the criteria for the diagnosis of Tourette's disorder. How many of the four other female and 26 male patients fulfill the criteria is unknown since the authors merely state that the diagnosis was Tourette's disorder.

Also contributing to, or perhaps determining, the reported psychopathology and psychodynamics is the selection of the first 18 patients from a hospitalized psychiatric sample. These patients may have been psychiatrically ill in addition to having Tourette's disorder and would not be representative of most Tourette patients, who are infrequently hospitalized for general psychopathology.

Bearing these methodological problems in mind, and perhaps making the heuristic assumption that the sample was more similar to patients with Tourette's disorder than reflected in the descriptive criteria, we can now consider the major psychoanalytic conclusions of Mahler and her colleagues.

Mahler (1944) differentiated three types of tics. The first results from a conflict between a vicariously used and overtaxed affective motility, hyperactivity, and the need for control. These tics are characterized by interchangeability, can be controlled voluntarily, and disappear before latency.

The second type occurs at about school age in children with a history of hyperactivity. Usually in response to trauma or threat (guilt), a volitional habit, such as blinking, develops and is associated with anxiety states. The real tic appears following relinquishing of autoerotic activities. These children do not have the abundance of expressive motility characteristic of the first type of ticqueur.

The third type of tic appears in adolescents and adults. The affected muscle group is used as symbolization and the tic has an organ neurotic character. These tics are difficult to treat because they are isolated from the ego function.

Thus the dynamic formulation about tics is that, in the first phase, a conflict exists between the motor-mindedness or constitution of the ticqueur and the environmental interference with motor activity, which then results in the hyperkinesis and generalized motor restlessness. Parents who are rigid and overprotective indirectly and subtly restrict motor activity. In the second phase, aggression is suppressed because of the restrictive environment, and an internalized conflict begins between the active and passive elements. In the third phase, referred to as the final crystallized tic, the tic represents "both provocative erotic aggression toward mother or father in the gestural idiomotor vocal sphere, and a defense against the mother or father as aggressor."

The psychodynamic explanation is that the tic is the expression of a conflict between the gratification of and defense against instinctual impulses. It is difficult to extrapolate any consistent dynamic formulation since the basic conflict is different for each patient.

In their 1943 paper, Mahler and Rangell clearly state: "While we believe we are dealing with an underlying organic pathology of the central nervous system, this somatic nucleus is acted upon and activated by psychodynamic forces similar to those found operating in cases of defensively functional tics." There is a constitutional inferiority of the subcortical structures. However, the organic substrata is insufficient to cause the syndrome. The organic factors make the individual susceptible and defenseless to emotional and psychodynamic factors. Because Mahler and her co-workers were concerned mainly with psychodynamic factors, the postulated organic factors were obscured by the psychoanalytic superstructure, and the belief that this disorder was predominantly psychological in origin unfortunately became predominant for the next 30 years.

The authors postulate an environmental need for increased motor outlets and an inherent constitutional factor of the somatic type for the habits of the ticqueur. Nine of the males were asthenic or hypoplastic, 11 were described as having a dysplastic hypogenital habitus, five were classified as having Froelich type of dystropia adiposogenitalis, five had bilateral cryptorchidism, microphallus, tall dysplastic stature, and feminine distribution of the subcutaneous fat, and seven were well built, sturdy, and athletic. The authors found no relationship between body type and severity or character of the tic syndrome. They quote Woodward's description of the personality of the ticqueur as a "peculiar mixture of affability, diffidence, shyness, and timidity, with self-indulgence, suppressed aggressivity, and tempers, and often crudely sadistic and erotic fantasies in the girls as well as the boys."

Some of the findings and observations were similar to those obtained by us, and others were quite different. Over 50% of our initial sample had a history of hyperactivity and perceptual problems and other indices of central nervous system (CNS) abnormality. We found no evidence for environmental restriction of movement through either physical illness or excessive infantilization, or evidence of a strong somatic type. Some, but not most, of our patients had delayed sexual maturation. We found no evidence for the authors' explanation of the underlying meaning of the symptom, e.g., the progression of symptoms represents "an additional gratification and an additional attempt to ward off and dissemble the previous tics", and that the specific symptoms were related to a specific emotional situation which represented a specific affective expression. As we describe in detail later, the type of tic, the part of the body affected, and the sequence of the tics are remarkably similar among patients, although some variability occurs as the tics emerge.

We find no support, fully described in Chapter 6, for the concept that psychodynamic forces are associated with the cause or development of the illness. Our findings suggest that the development of this illness follows a natural course and that it will occur without precipitants, such as psychodynamic factors, stress, trauma, illness, or family dynamics.

Treatment with psychotherapy was advocated, although in their 1946 paper (Mahler and Luke), deep psychotherapy with undue emphasis on release of erotic and aggressive material was considered harmful to patients.

A series of single case reports using psychoanalytic or other psychodynamic approaches appeared during this period (Latimer, 1945; Menaker, 1945; Ascher, 1948, 1966; Gerard, 1946; Rosenheim, 1948; Heuscher, 1953; Kanner, 1957; Michael, 1957; Aarons, 1958; Milman, 1960; Tobin and Reinhardt, 1961; Mazur, 1953a,b; MacDonald, 1963; Downing et al., 1964; Kurland, 1965; Polites et al., 1965; Faux, 1966; Robinson, 1966; Bai, 1966; Elkisch, 1968; and Lindner and Stevens, 1967). Family dynamics were stressed by Bruch and Thum (1968), Latimer (1945), Dunlap (1960), Downing et al. (1964), Kurland (1965), Robinson (1966), and Bradnan (1972).

Other papers discussed various etiological theories, diagnostic problems and surgical procedures (Brown, 1957; Bockner, 1959; Savin, 1961; Baker, 1962; Eriksson and Persson, 1969; Mersky, 1974; Araneta et al., 1975).

EPIDEMIOLOGY

Following the psychoanalytic period, psychoanalytically oriented papers about tics and Tourette's disorder diminished, but interest in the condition resumed with the publication of several epidemiological studies. The data are derived from sources such as population surveys, hospital records, and literature reviews. Although these studies are methodologically flawed from today's prospective, the data are of historical importance. This review focuses on epidemiological studies that describe demography, family psychological test data, and outcome information. This phase was anticipated by the studies of Boncour (1910) and Bonheim (1930). More recent epidemiological studies with data about the prevalence of tics and Tourette's disorder are described in Chapter 3.

Population Surveys

The earliest of these studies is that by Boncour (1910) who surveyed 1,759 students between the ages of 2 and 13. Boncour was interested in the assumed correlation between certain personality traits and the presence of tics in children. Details about the prevalence are provided in Chapter 3 but it is interesting that Boncour did not confirm the belief that children with tics were vicious, degenerate, and weak-minded. The majority of the children were characterized as average in their application to work, their conduct, and their intelligence. Only three children were classified as degenerate although 35 were classified as backward intellectually.

Bonheim (1930) compared his findings on 49 children with tics to those of Boncour. He found a family history of nervousness expressed as motor excitement and restlessness in the parents of 22 children. Eighteen families had other signs of nervousness, two had a history of psychosis, and a family history of tics was present in two children. Thirty-nine children were described as hyperactive, fidgety, with most having excitable conduct, restlessness in school, faulty concentration, and distractability. It is difficult to ascertain how many of these children would be classified as having Tourette's disorder or attention deficit disorder (ADD) because the symptomatology was not well delineated.

REVIEWS OF HOSPITAL RECORDS

Zausmer (1954) studied two samples: a retrospectively collected group of 53 patients referred to the psychiatric department of the Royal Liverpool Children's Hospital from May 1947 and 1952, and 43 patients seen by the author after May, 1952. The total sample consisted of 96 consecutive tiqueurs (not further defined) who were referred to the psychiatric department between 1947 and 1954. The mean annual referral rate was approximately 5% of the total number of all referred cases. Methodological shortcomings of the study included retrospective study of half of the sample (probably the first group primarily), lack of information about the source of referral or whether other problems led to the referral and failure to specify the criteria for the type of tic. Diagnoses could range from a transient tic to Tourette's disorder.

The sex ratio was approximately 2:1, consisting of 63 boys and 33 girls, a lower ratio of boys to girls than the expected 3:1 found in most Tourette's disorder samples. The age of onset varied between 3.5 and 12.5 years with a well-defined peak at 7 years of age, similar to our mean age of onset. At the time of examination, 34% had symptoms for 6 months and 56% for 1 year. The longest interval between onset and referral was 8 years.

Intelligence quotient (IQ) was approximately normal in distribution. The personality of the patients was described as restless, sensitive, irritable, stubborn, excitable, phobic, apprehensive, and quick-tempered, but the frequencies of these behaviors were not provided. Family history of tics was reported in 38 families (40.4% of the sample). Diagnosis of Tourette's disorder was not established at follow-up for 41 of the first 53 patients who were followed for 3 to 8 years after the onset of tics. Ten (24%) had a spontaneous remission, 21 (52%) had considerable improvement, and 10 (24%) were unchanged; the total improvement was approximately 76%. Patients were both untreated and treated with a variety of techniques, including lengthy psychotherapy or a few hours of educational guidance. The results were not related to the type of treatment. Thus, approximately 25% were cured, the criteria being freedom from symptoms for at least 1 year. Although not supported by the data, the author concluded that psychotherapy might be helpful. The results probably reflect naturally occurring spontaneous changes that take place during the course of this illness, as suggested by the data summarized in Chapters 5 and 11.

Pasamanick and Kawi (1956) studied the association between paranatal factors and tics. Impressed with the evidence that cerebral injury was implicated in the etiology of tics, they noted the increased frequency of hyperactivity among children with tics, the relationship of tics to epidemic encephalitis, and that more males than females had tics. They postulated a continuum of reproductive causality in which the effect of damage to the brain varies from minimal cerebral damage resulting in minor behavioral dysfunction to death.

For their study, they examined the records of all children diagnosed as ticqueurs at the Children's Psychiatric Clinic of the Harriet Lane Home, Johns Hopkins Hospital, who were born since 1926. The birth certificates of these children were then examined. The control group comprised the next recorded birth from the same place as the child with tics matched by race, sex, and age.

Of the 83 patients with tics, 65 (78%) were male, similar to the ratio found in our study, and 8% were black. Twenty-one complications of pregnancy and parturition were recorded for the mothers of tiqueurs, compared with only ten such complications for the control mothers ($p < 0.05$). Prematurity was infrequent in both groups and even less frequent for patients with tics. The number with neonatal abnormalities was too small for discerning trends. When all the birth hazards were grouped, 37.3% of the ticqueurs were exposed to one or more of these abnormalities, contrasted with 25.5% of the controls.

Although the authors were impressed with the evidence suggesting an association between brain damage and tics, they expressed reservations about interpreting retrospective data because both prematurity and neonatal abnormalities were absent.

Eisenberg et al. (1959) described seven patients seen at the Henry Phipps Psychiatric Clinic between 1951 and 1958. All the patients were males, exhibiting numerous muscular tics and vocalizations, and five had coprolalia. Three of four tested patients had IQs above 120. Outcome for five of the patients with follow-up evaluations included state hospitalization for one, increasing difficulties with some deterioration in academic performance for two, improvement with psychotherapy but deterioration in school performance in one, and improvement with psychotherapy for one. The father of one patient had tics, such as facial grimacing and eye-blinking, as well as nail biting and compulsions to touch and avoid. With the exception of eye-blinking, they disappeared at age 14. Another patient had a brother with chorea. The authors concluded that pharmacological therapy, such as sedatives, muscle relaxants, and tranquilizers, are ineffective. They suggested the continued use of psychotherapy, although not believing that intrapsychic tensions caused the symptoms and that the etiology of the illness was obscure.

Torup (1962) studied 237 children who were treated for tics between 1946 and 1947 in the inpatient and outpatient services of the Pediatrics and Child Psychiatry Departments at Rigshospitalet Hospital, Copenhagen, Denmark. The sample included children in whom tics were diagnosed incidentally as well as those who were referred because of them. Information about the patients was obtained from a retrospective inspection of hospital records, occasionally supplemented by records from other hospitals, personal interviews with 217 families, and by letters to the three remaining families. The interviews, 26 at the hospital and the remainder at home, were with mothers, family, and usually the afflicted child.

There were 163 boys and 57 girls, a ratio of 3:1, which is similar to the sex ratio in our study. The children were of average intelligence. Family history of tics was found in 30 to 40% of the closest family members. Eleven to 30% of the parents had tics.

Two hundred twenty patients with a history of tics were followed for 1 to 15 years (average approximately 9 years) after treatment in the Rigshospitalet Hospital. The age at follow-up ranged from 6 to 26 years. Tics had disappeared in approximately 50% and were unchanged in approximately 6%; they had decreased and were often insignificant in the remainder. Tics often ceased at puberty. Among those cured, the cure lasted for 1 month to 14 years. These results are more applicable to a sample of children with tics who were referred for this symptom together with an unknown number who may have had psychological difficulties. The results are not generalizable to a sample of children with tics who may or may not have other psychological or physical difficulties.

Feild et al. (1966) described seven cases diagnosed as Tourette's disorder at the Mayo Clinic between 1935 and 1966, from a total of approximately 1.5 million patients newly admitted during that period. Detailed case reports were presented for the seven patients. The age of onset ranged from 4 to 13 years. Progression of symptoms, not confirmed by us, was reported as going from the muscles of the neck and shoulders to the arms and finally to the lower extremities. All of the patients had vocalization, six had articulated words, and five had coprolalia. The authors reported that uniform psychological characteristics were not found for the seven patients, but that the paucity of neurological abnormalities argued against an organic etiology. Six patients had electroencephalographic (EEG) abnormalities that were not specific for Tourette's disorder. Tic symptoms persisted in six of the followed-up patients, although the severity and period of remission varied. Although the authors state that 40% of patients develop schizophrenia, mental deterioration, and serious personality disorders, none of their seven patients developed such psychopathology.

Challas et al. (1967) briefly described the clinical histories of six new and six previously described children with Tourette's disorder treated at the Psychiatric Clinic of Iowa from 1962 to 1967. EEGs were normal in most of the patients whose symptoms began between 5 and 11 years of age. The literature was briefly and selectively reviewed and the author concluded that the illness was not inherited and did not provide conclusive evidence for an organic etiology. Challas advanced the notion that symptoms developed under conditions encouraging regression, and observed among his patients that at least one parent was controlling and punitive while the other parent was overindulgent or overprotective.

Lucas et al. (1967) described four patients evaluated since 1949 at the Children's Service at the Neuropsychiatric Institute in Ann Arbor and 11 patients of a total of 10,000 children and adolescents seen since 1956 in the outpatient department at the Hawthorn Center in Michigan.

Of the 15 patients, 73% were boys and 27% were girls. Similar to our results, the sex ratio of boys to girls was approximately 3:1, and the age of onset ranged from 4 to 10 years (mean, 6.6 years). The length of follow-up for 13 patients varied from 2 to 15 years (mean, 11 years). The greatest number of patients were middle children, unlike our findings and other reports in the literature.

Three case histories were presented to illustrate three types of family dynamics or patterns—a severe and diffuse expression of aggression, excessive emphasis on the inhibition of aggression and negativism, and absence of disturbance.

The IQ scores ranged from 85 to 146, similar to our results. No common individual or family psychodynamics were found. The authors considered the possibility that psychological factors might influence the development of tics or that psychogenic factors may be associated with milder tics. They concluded that psychological factors did not adequately explain the pathophysiology. The evidence for an organic etiology is also considered by the authors to be unconvincing and inconclusive. They postulate an interaction of organic and psychological factors, both factors modifying or exacerbating the symptomatology.

The authors recommend that children with learning disabilities be treated as inpatients in a residential school. Individual psychotherapy for the patient and case work with the parents were recommended. Haloperidol was effective for two patients. A variety of other drugs was used in eight patients; tics were rated as improved in four, almost absent in three, and absent in one. Information about the drug therapy for three patients was not provided; symptoms improved for one, were almost absent for a second, and persisted in the third. Two patients had recently begun chemotherapy. For two patients not treated with drugs, one was reported to be improved.

Corbett et al. (1969) studied the relationship between tics and psychiatric disturbance and the prognosis for tics. The authors retrospectively examined case records of 170 patients who attended the children and adolescent department of Maudsley Hospital and Brixton Child Guildance Unit between 1948 and 1965, and an additional nine cases from the adult department of psychiatry at Maudsley Hospital. Of the 179 patients, a minority (but an unknown number) had Tourette's disorder. This study, as most previously described, was therefore largely concerned with tics.

The ratio of boys to girls was 3.6:1, similar to the 3:1 ratio found in our sample. The age of onset was 7.3 years, similar to our study; the age at which the patients were examined was 10.2 years, whereas the present age for our sample was 25.5 years.

The authors were able to rule out the relationship of tics to chronic sinusitus. The movements had a descending order of frequency from the upper part of the face to the feet. Isolated or single tics occurred in the face alone in 51.8% of patients, in the whole head, neck, or shoulder in 10.4%, and in the limb, thorax, and abdomen in 4.8%. Isolated vocal tics were reported in 11.6%, and in combination with other tics in 23%. The significantly lower percentage of vocal tics, compared with our finding of 100%, is probably because the sample was composed of patients with tics, whereas our sample consisted only of patients with Tourette's disorder.

Symptoms of emotional disturbance were based on retrospective examination of case records. The data for these children were compared with a sample of disturbed but nonpsychotic children attending the Maudsley Hospital for Children, which included 7% who were identified as ticqueurs. A higher proportion of boys were found in the disturbed group but other symptoms were found in both groups. Thirty percent in both groups had sleep disorders, tension habits, temper, aggression, disturbed relationships with parents and peers, and disobedience and anxiety in school. Habit disorders, such as gratification habits, speech disorders, defecation disorders, and obsessional and hypochondriacal symptoms, occurred more frequently in the tic group, whereas aggression and depression occurred more frequently in the disturbed group. Some of the symptoms cited as disturbed behavior, such as speech disturbances and obsessional symptoms, may have been tic symptomatology. Since the research was dependent on the data reported in the patients' charts, the percentages reported must be considered as approximations only. The IQ scores were within the normal range.

A family history of tics was found in 10% of the cases; the percentage in our sample was considerably higher. Thirty-one percent of the parents of the children with tics had a history of psychiatric illness, as compared to 19.3% of the General Maudsley Hospital population, and 6.2% of the dental clinic sample.

Follow-up data were presented for 73 primary tiqueurs who were children with tics as their primary symptom when they applied to the center. The ratio of boys to girls increased to 4:1, and the age of onset decreased to 6.9 years. The follow-up varied from 1 to 18 years after the initial visit. The mean duration of illness was 5.4 years, and the mean age was 15 years.

Total recovery was unrelated to whether patients were treated or not treated. Treatment with haloperidol was reported to be effective; the authors report 6% unimproved, 53% improved to a varying extent, and 40% completely recovered. A significant association was found between outcome and duration of follow-up. The group followed the longest showed the greatest improvement. A significant association was also found between outcome and age at onset. More patients whose tics began between 6 and 8 years of age recovered completely.

There were trends suggesting a poor prognosis for obsessional patients and those with tics in the limbs or lower body, vocal tics, and coprolalia, and a more favorable prognosis for those with sleep disturbances. The authors indicate that chance alone could account for these trends.

Psychiatric symptoms at follow-up included 11 patients with anxiety, five with phobias, three with obsessive-compulsive symptoms, and 10 with depressive symptoms. The worst outcome occurred for the two most severely disturbed patients. For 18 patients with improvement of tic symptoms, psychiatric symptoms were present in 14 and absent in four. For nine patients without psychiatric symptoms, tics were present in three and absent in six.

A series of important papers by Abuzzahab and Ehlen (1971) and Abuzzahab and Anderson (1973, 1974) described an exhaustive search of the world's literature and the development of an international registry for cases of Gilles de la Tourette syndrome. The first paper (Abuzzahab and Ehlen, 1971) described the clinical data and management of seven patients. The two papers by Abuzzahab and Anderson (1973, 1974) consolidated the data derived from 430 published cases and 55 case reports from the international registry for a total of 485 cases. The national origin of patients was related to variations in onset, symptomatology, and treatment. The age at onset for 90% of the sample was between 3 and 16 years of age with 75% between the ages of 5 and 12. Patients from the United States had a younger age at onset than those from other countries. The sex distribution was approximately 3 males to 1 female. Ninety-two percent of the patients had facial tics, 78% arm tics, 54% leg tics, 53% neck tics, and 31% eye tics. Vocal symptoms were reported in 90% of the patients, with 58% reporting coprolalia. Patients in the United States had more coprolalia and neck tics than those in France, Germany, the United Kingdom, and Italy. French patients had fewer neck tics and less eye tics but more echokinesis, whereas the Italians had more eye tics, and patients from the United Kingdom had less echo phenomena. No significant differences were reported for the German group. Abnormal EEG findings were reported in 45 (44.1%) of 102 patients and intelligence was normal for most of the 44 patients tested. Although psychopathology was reported in 33% of patients, criteria for psychopathology were not described except for the inclusion of phenomena such as arithromania, abnormal desire to touch, and abnormal doubts, which are more likely symptoms of Tourette's disorder than primary psychological psychopathology.

The major shortcoming of these studies is that data analysis was retrospective and heavily dependent on the thoroughness with which the data was originally recorded and the sensitivity of the reviewer. Another shortcoming is that adequate diagnostic criteria were not available at the time for meaningful differential criteria of transient tic disorder (TTD), CMT, or Tourette's disorder.

REVIEW OF THE LITERATURE

Kelman (1965) summarized 44 cases of Tourette's disorder published during the past 60 years. Her review did not include the patients described by Mahler et al. (1945) since, as she points out, and we concur, it is not possible to distinguish which patients had generalized tics and which had Tourette's disorder. A major shortcoming of this review was its retrospective reliance on published reports, which vary considerably in their completeness and accuracy in describing the symptomatology, clinical course, and history of Tourette's disorder. Nevertheless, it was a historically important paper because many more patients with Tourette's disorder were described than previously in the literature.

For 34 patients, 82.4% had eye-blinking, neck movements, and facial twitching; 50% had coprolalia; and only two had echolalia. The percentages for our sample were somewhat higher for eye-blinking and coprolalia, but roughly similar for sex ratio and age at onset below 10 years of age. We could not confirm her sequence for the development of symptoms from facial tics to head, neck, upper limb, body movements, and vocalizations. A family history of tics was present in 11.8%, infrequent enough to be of little significance in comparison with 43% of patients in our sample who had a family history of tics or Tourette's disorder. There were no apparent relationships between precipitating factors and onset of symptoms. Abnormal neurological and EEG findings were reported in 42% of the 19 patients with such data. Although treatment included psychotherapy, electroconvulsive treatment, drugs, and many other modalities, only phenothiazines were found to be effective. Most of the patients treated with haloperidol improved. Kelman's review did not substantiate a poor prognosis for these patients. She felt that although the evidence was inadequate to support an organic etiology, she was convinced that future research would do so.

Fernando (1967), in an extensive survey confined to the English language literature, found 85 cases published between 1894 and 1965. Correctly, in our opinion, using the criteria of age at onset before 16 and multiple motor and verbal tics, he excluded 20% of the cases. In addition to the remaining 65 cases, Fernando added four of his own patients. The main shortcoming of this comprehensive review was the methodological problems associated with all retrospective studies. Similar to our data, the ratio of males to females was almost 3:1, and 85% had an age at onset before the age of 11. The distribution of symptoms was most frequent in the head, followed by the neck and limbs. Complex movements were rarely reported. Vocalizations appeared within 5 years after the onset of motor movements. In many patients, vocalization was either the first symptom to appear or appeared shortly after the onset of movements. Coprolalia, present in 26.1%, was reported as early as 10 years of age. Nevertheless, the IQ for patients was normally distributed. Nonspecific EEG abnormalities were found in about 25% of the patients. Neurotic symptoms in childhood were reported in 59%, and 20 patients had obsessional symptoms. He concluded, based on a history of tics in the family and the number of abnormal EEGs, that the etiology was organic.

In the review of the literature by Morphew and Sim (1969), 90 cases were found, but only 37 were considered sufficiently well documented to be included in the paper. Six cases seen by the authors were added to the sample, which totaled 43. The sex ratio was almost 2:1, less males than reported in other reviews. Facial tics were the most frequent initial symptom, followed by limb jerking. For 30 patients about whom birth order information was available, 46.4% were first-born. A variety of neurotic symptoms were reported, with enuresis being most frequent. The parents were characterized as neurotic, the fathers being obsessional and the mothers being overprotective and anxious. The intelligence of the patients appeared normally distributed. Most of the patients (71.5%) were characterized as obsessional. Precipitating factors were noted in 18 patients.

The authors concluded that the absence of EEG or physical abnormalities, normal intelligence, and the sex ratio of patients supported a functional etiology. Although the specific psychopathological factor could not be identified, they suggested that the symptom of stammering was a displacement upward of the anal sphincter. The symptom was associated with hostility, aggression, and a marked obsessional preoccupation, since the hostility uttered in disguise or secret was not available for analysis. However, most patients (39.3%) improved on phenothiazines. Psychotherapy was reported to be effective in four patients, and all nonorganic types of treatment together resulted in improvement in 14 patients. The authors favored treatment with both drug and nondrug treatments, considering them effective since they worked on the ego disintegration rather than the organic state.

PSYCHOCHEMOTHERAPY

With the introduction of psychochemotherapy in 1954, it was inevitable that these drugs would be used to treat patients with Tourette's disorder. It led to the first successful use of haloperidol in Europe in a single patient by Seignot (1961), in another patient wiht Tourette's disorder by Caprini and Melotti (1961), and in two patients with Tourette's disorder in the United States by Challas and Brauer (1963).

However, most available drugs including sedatives, antianxiety agents, anticonvulsants, antipsychotics, and antidepressants have been tried (Abuzzahab and Anderson, 1973). In the 1978 volume we reviewed published reports of treatment with various classes of drugs from 1964 to 1975 (Chapel et al., 1964; Healy and Fisher, 1965; Stevens and Blachly, 1966; Challas et al., 1967; Connell et al., 1967; Lucas, 1964, 1967; Boris, 1968; Levy and Asher, 1968; Shapiro and Shapiro, 1968; Fernando, 1967; Craven, 1969; Morphew and Sim, 1969; Bieren, 1969; Ford and Gottlieb, 1969; Healey, 1970; Shapiro, 1970 a,b,c; Shapiro and Shapiro, 1971; Messiha et al. 1971; Moldofsky, 1971, Stam, 1971; DiGiacomo et al., 1971; Abuzzahab and Ehlen, 1971; Fisarova, 1972; Sand, 1972; Barr et al., 1972; Clements, 1972; Sand and Carlson, 1973; Jeste et al., 1973; Friel, 1973; Sanders, 1973; Shapiro et al., 1973a; Logue et al., 1973; Carroll, 1974; Clement, 1974; Teoh, 1974; Moldofsky et al., 1974; Goforth, 1974; Golden, 1974; Lerman and Nussbaum, 1974; Milman, 1975; Abuzzahab and Anderson, 1976). Early studies using a combination of drugs and psychotherapy included those of Mesnikoff (1959), Schneck (1960), and Milman (1960). Our experience treating the first 34 patients with haloperidol was described in our 1968, 1970, and 1976 papers and in the 1978 volume. The literature on psychopharmacologic treatment of Tourette's disorder since the 1978 volume is reviewed in Chapter 11.

IMPORTANT ACHIEVEMENTS OVER THE PAST TWENTY-FIVE YEARS

In our opinion, five achievements stand out in the history of Tourette's disorder in the last 25 years: (a) Development of effective pharmacotherapy for patients with Tourette's disorder; (b) recognition that drugs that bind to D_2 receptors are effective for the treatment of the syndrome and implicate a dopamine (DA) etiology for Tourette's disorder; (c) development of specific criteria facilitating diagnosis and leading to an epidemic increase in diagnosed patients and to the establishment of Tourette laboratories and clinics throughout the world; (d) refocusing from a psychological to an organic central nervous system etiology; and (e) establishing a familial genetic basis for some forms of Tourette's disorder. Finally, all of these factors decreased the time from onset to diagnosis, increased the number of physicians treating Tourette's disorder and the number of available facilities for treatment.

CONSENSUAL AREAS OF AGREEMENT AND CONTROVERSIES

There are now many consensual areas of agreement about Tourette's disorder: criteria for tic disorders; organic etiology for tic disorders; similar etiology for Tourette's disorder, CMT, and TTD; the effectiveness of neuroleptics with DA blocking properties; the ineffectiveness of psychologic treatment as a primary treatment for tics; the clinical course and natural history of Tourette's disorder; and the inadequacy of the DA hypothesis as an adequate explanation for Tourette's disorder.

However, there are still areas of disagreement: Is the etiology of the disorder solely organic or are psychologic factors or triggers necessary for its expression? Are attention deficit disorder, psychopathology, and obsessive-compulsive disorder intrinsically associated with Tourette's disorder? Do stimulants cause, provoke, or permanently exacerbate tics or Tourette's disorder? Is there a sensory tic subtype of the disorder and does it have the same etiology as Tourette's disorder?

We hypothesize, based on currently available evidence, that Tourette's disorder does not require psychologic factors for its expression, that attention deficit disorder, obsessive-compulsive disorder, and other psychopathologies are not intrinsic to Tourette's disorder, and that stimulants do not cause or permanently exacerbate tics or Tourette's disorder. These hypotheses are evaluated in subsequent chapters of this book. Resolution of these controversies is necessary to minimize the problem of heterogeneity in studies, to insure progress in research, and to facilitate appropriate treatment and management of patients with Tourette's disorder.

2

Samples, Procedures, and Variables

SAMPLE

The findings described in this book are derived from a unique sample of 1,610 patients who were evaluated for a movement disorder between May 1965 and December 1984. Because increased knowledge about the diagnosis and treatment has resulted in more physicians treating tic disorders, it is unlikely that a comprehensive data set of this size will ever be duplicated by a single research group. The separation of clinical care from research has made it increasingly difficult for one group of researchers to acquire sufficient subjects for research.

Prior to 1965 only 50 Tourette's disorder patients were described in the English language literature (Fernando, 1976). From 1965 to 1974 we evaluated 145 Tourette's disorder patients who served as the sample for our first book on Tourette's disorder, (Shapiro et al, 1978). Between 1974 and 1986 we evaluated 1,117 Tourette's disorder patients, or 89% of our total sample of 1,262 Tourette's disorder patients. Over 50% of these patients were evaluated in the last 6 years, illustrating the dramatic increase in identification of patients with this syndrome.

Of the total sample of 1,610 patients, 1,262 (78.4%) were diagnosed as having Tourette's disorder, 205 (12.7%) were diagnosed as having a tic disorder, and 141 (8.8%) were diagnosed as having another disorder (Table 2.1). The results described in this book are for 828 consecutive patients evaluated by us between 1965 and 1981, and for 237 patients who completed our Movement Disorder Questionnaire (MDQ), but were not personally evaluated by us. The sample of 545 patients evaluated from 1981 to 1986 are not systematically described, except for selected subsamples, because funds were not available to computerize these data.

Our studies of Tourette's disorder were conducted between 1966 and 1976 at the Special Studies Laboratory and the Tourette Studies Laboratory at the

TABLE 2.1. Tic categories for patients evaluated from 1965 to 1984

	Clinical data[a]						Questionnaire data[b] 1972–1979	Total	
	1965–1981[c]	1981–1984		Total					
	N	N		N	%		N	N	%
Tic disorders									
Tourette's disorder	666	390		1,056	76.9		206	1,262	78.4
Chronic motor tic disorder[e]	5	4		9	0.7		8	17	1.1
Chronic multiple motor tic disorder[f]	27	25		52	3.8		5	57	3.5
Transient tic of childhood	11	22		44	2.4		9	42	2.6
Sensory dystonia Tourette's disorder subtype[g]	15	36		51	3.7		1	52	3.2
Atypical tic (or movement) disorder[h]	18	18		36	2.6		1	37	2.3
Total	742	495		1,237	90.1		230	1,467	91.1
Other movement disorders									
Atypical stereotyped movement disorder	29	7		36	2.6		2	37	2.3
Paroxysmal myophonoclonus[i]	2	3		5	0.4		—	5	0.3
Cough of adolescence[j]	4	1		5	0.4		—	5	0.3
Laryngeal dystonia	0	3		3	0.2		—	3	0.2
Focal dystonia	6	3		9	0.7		1	9	0.6
Huntington's chorea	2	0		2	0.1		—	2	0.1

Tardive dyskinesia	12		13	0.9	1	14	0.9
Hemifacial spasm	0	1	1	0.1	—	1	0.1
Essential tremor	8	3	11	0.8	—	11	0.7
Myoclonus	0	1	1	0.1	—	1	0.1
Myoclonus epilepsy	1	0	1	0.1	—	1	0.1
Total	64	23	87	6.3	4	89	5.5
No movement disorder[k]	22	27	49	3.9	3	52	3.2
Total	828	545	1,373	100.0	237	1,610	100.0

[a] Clinical data: Patients completing Movement Disorder Questionnaire and clinical evaluation interview.
[b] Questionnaire data: Patients completing Movement Disorder Questionnaire but not clinically evaluated, 1972–1979.
[c] June 1965 to May 1981.
[d] June 1981 to December 1984.
[e] Diagnosis in DSM-III.
[f] Diagnosis not included in DSM-III.
[g] Diagnostic criteria in DSM-III not fulfilled, classified as subtype of Tourette's disorder.
[h] Signs and symptoms resemble tic disorder, but movements do not fulfill criteria for tic disorder.
[i] Postulated new diagnostic entity.
[j] Diagnosis described clinically in the literature; referred to as psychological cough in WHO.
[k] Patients referred for evaluation but who did not have a movement disorder; diagnoses included obsessive compulsive disorder, attention deficit disorder with and without hyperactivity, mental retardation, pervasive developmental disorder, drug addiction, and schizophrenic disorder.

Payne Whitney Psychiatric Clinic, Cornell University Medical College, New York, and from 1977 to 1986, as the Tourette and Tic Laboratory and Clinic, Mount Sinai School of Medicine, New York. We strove for completeness, accuracy, and comprehensiveness in the data collection. Patients were evaluated, studied, or treated in either the private offices of the PIs (A.K.S., E.S.) or in the clinical and research laboratories at Cornell University Medical College or Mount Sinai School of Medicine.

CLINICAL PROCEDURE

Appointments are made within 1 month after initial inquiry. Patients complete a comprehensive MDQ and provide relevant information, such as birth certificates, hospital birth records, previous medical and psychiatric records, results of X-rays, computerized axial tomography (CAT) scans, EEGs and other laboratory measures, psychometric, projective, and neuropsychological test results, and the results of previous treatment. The Minnesota Multiphasic Personality Inventory (MMPI) for adults and the Child Behavior Checklist (Achenbach, 1978) for children and adolescents are administered. Initial evaluation includes a semistructured 2-hr session during which the movement disorder history and records are reviewed, clarified, and verified. The history of possible precursors, the onset, development, and course of each symptom, and response to treatment are carefully elicited; the psychological history and other associated factors are reviewed and evaluated; a screening physical and neurological examination is performed; the severity of the tic condition is rated; and a diagnosis, differential diagnosis, and possible associated diagnoses based on DSM-III criteria are made. The results of the evaluation, diagnosis, recommendation about management and treatment, and disposition are discussed with the patient and summarized in a narrative report which becomes a part of the record and is provided to the patient and relevant professionals.

In our early work with Tourette's disorder, patients were evaluated and treated by one investigator (A.K.S.). Psychiatric evaluations were thorough, careful, detailed, and included many sessions, occasionally up to 100, with the patient and often with the family. Patients were encouraged to undergo neurological, electroencephalographic, psychological, and other examinations. With increased experience and development of the MDQ and other routine procedures, there was less need for extensive psychiatric evaluation, and most patients were evaluated in a 2-hr session.

DIAGNOSTIC CRITERIA

The diagnosis of Tourette's disorder and other tic disorders is based on criteria in Shapiro et al. (1978) and DSM-III (American Psychiatric Association, 1980). Revised criteria proposed for DSM-III-R (1987), are essentially similar to those in DSM-III. Our proposed revision of the nosology and criteria for the symptoms, diagnosis, and differential diagnosis for tic disorders is discussed in Chapter 10.

Tourette's Disorder

1. Age at onset between 1 and 17 years of age. Although DSM-III specifies onset between 2 and 15 years, the age at onset for our sample ranges from 1 to 17 years of age. Onset is specified as before 21 years in DSM-III-R.
2. Presence of recurrent, involuntary, repetitive, rapid, purposeless motor movements affecting multiple muscle groups.
3. Multiple vocal tics. Although the criteria in DSM-III-R will require only one or more vocal tics some time during the course of the illness, all patients in our sample had at least two vocal tics.
4. Ability to suppress movements intentionally or voluntarily for minutes to hours.
5. Spontaneous variations of the type, complexity, number, frequency, location, or intensity of tics over weeks or months. DSM-III specifies only variations in the intensity of the symptoms.
6. Duration of more than 1 year.

Transient Tic Disorder

1. Onset during childhood or early adolescence.
2. Presence of recurrent, involuntary, repetitive, purposeless motor movements (tics).
3. Ability to suppress the movements voluntarily for minutes to hours.
4. Spontaneous variation of the type, complexity, number, frequency, location, or intensity of tics over weeks or months. DSM-III specifies only variation in the intensity of the symptoms.
5. Duration of at least 1 month but not more than 1 year.

Chronic Motor Tic Disorder

1. Onset during childhood or adolescence. DSM-III does not specify age of onset.
2. Presence of recurrent, involuntary, repetitive, purposeless movements (tics). DSM-III specifies no more than three muscle groups at any one time.
3. Ability to suppress the movements voluntarily for minutes to hours. DSM-III specifies inability to suppress the movements for more than a few seconds.

4. Spontaneous variation of the type, number, frequency, location, or intensity of tics during the course of the illness. DSM-III specifies unvarying symptoms.
5. Duration of at least 1 year.

Atypical Tic or Movement Disorder

The category atypical tic disorder in DSM-III is reserved for the diagnosis of tics that cannot be adequately classified in any of the previous categories. We have added the category atypical movement disorder; the rationale for this diagnosis is discussed in Chapter 10.

Sensory Tic Subtype of Tourette's Disorder

Forty patients in our sample have only intentional or voluntary, usually tonic, movements in response to sensory stimuli that are experienced as dysphoric. The intentional or voluntary movement relieves the disturbing internal sensation. We refer to this category of symptoms as sensory tic subtype of Tourette's disorder. In addition, 45 patients in our sample have typical motor and vocal tics characteristic of Tourette's disorder and also have similar sensory tics. These subtypes are discussed more fully in Chapter 10.

Attention Deficit Disorder with Hyperactivity

The diagnosis of attention deficit disorder with hyperactivity (ADD+H) in patients with Tourette's disorder (TS+ADD+H) requires fulfillment of criteria for Tourette's disorder, and DSM-III criteria for the diagnosis of ADD+H. A semistructured interview, covering the following clinical features, listed in DSM-III, is used for diagnosis.

Inattention

At least three of the following:

1. Often fails to finish things he or she starts;
2. often doesn't seem to listen;
3. easily distracted;
4. has difficulty concentrating on schoolwork or other tasks requiring sustained attention; and
5. has difficulty sticking to a play activity.

Impulsivity

At least three of the following:

1. Often acts before thinking;
2. shifts excessively from one activity to another;
3. has difficulty organizing work (not due to cognitive impairment);
4. needs a lot of supervison;
5. frequently calls out in class; and
6. has difficulty awaiting turn in games or group situations.

Hyperactivity

At least two of the following:

1. Runs about or climbs on things excessively;
2. has difficulty sitting still or fidgets excessively;
3. has difficulty staying seated;
4. moves about excessively during sleep;
5. duration of at least 6 months; and
6. not due to schizophrenia, affective disorder, or severe or profound mental retardation.

An additional criteria for diagnosis, not part of DSM-III, is a score of 15 points or more on the Abbreviated Parent-Teacher Questionnaire (Conners Hyperactivity Score) completed by the parent or teacher (Conners, 1969, 1970).

In addition, the 17 items making up the criteria for ADD+H in DSM-III were rated on a four-point scale (see description of ratings in the section on Behavioral Symptoms): (0) not at all; (1) just a little; (2) pretty much; and (3) very much. The scores are summed and referred to as the Total ADD score.

Attention Deficit Disorder Without Hyperactivity

The criteria for the diagnosis of attention deficit disorder without hyperactivity (TS+ADD−H) are the same as those for TS+ADD+H except for the absence of hyperactivity and a Hyperactivity Score less than 12.

Attention Deficit Disorder, Residual Type

1. The individual once met the criteria for ADD+H. This information was obtained from individual family members and previous records when available.
2. Signs of hyperactivity are no longer present, but other signs of the illness

have persisted to the present without periods of remission, as evidenced by signs of both attentional deficits and impulsivity (e.g., difficulty organizing work and completing tasks, difficulty concentrating, being easily distracted, making sudden decisions without thought of the consequences).
3. The symptoms of inattention and impulsivity result in some impairment in social or occupational functioning.
4. Not due to schizophrenia, affective disorder, severe or profound mental retardation, or schizotypal or borderline personality disorders.

Reliability of Diagnoses

The PIs (A.K.S., E.S.) conducted 97% of the evaluations; the remainder were conducted by experienced clinical collaborators. Both PIs reviewed the records to confirm diagnoses. The diagnosis required agreement by both clinicians, independently or after discussion. Although a more reliable procedure would include an independent and blind interview by a second clinician, this was not feasible, and since both clinicians have had extensive experience with tic disorders, the likelihood of diagnostic error is minimal. The reliability and validity for the diagnosis of ADD+H is a problem that has been extensively discussed in the literature (Ullman et al., 1981; Shaffer et al., 1985). Our ability to diagnose this disorder, however, was improved by careful and thorough collection of previous evaluations by teachers, psychologists, psychiatrists, neurologists, and pediatricians.

DATA MANAGEMENT

The data for 1,065 patients, studied between June 1965 and May 1981, were coded, key punched, verified, and stored in the Mount Sinai computer facilities. All patients were identified only by number and not by name. From these data, which included twenty-two 80-column cards per patient, 878 variables were derived, although not all variables were used in analyses. Because the number of items and ratings in the MDQ have changed over the years, the sample size varies for selected variables. The sample size is specified in the variable list (Table A.1) and in specific analyses. Data for additional patients ($N = 545$) studied between June 1981 and December 1986 have not been keypunched because of financial limitations. Selected analyses for this group of patients are described in later sections.

VARIABLES

The initial or basic questionnaire was used for the total sample of patients. Therefore, the following variable categories were completed for the total sample: study information; demography; family history; birth history; sibling status; maturational milestones; patient medical history; axis I, II, or III diagnoses; illness-related variables; situational factors at onset of Tourette syndrome; age at onset, persistence or disappearance of symptoms; clinical course; severity of Tourettee's disorder; and treatment history. The theoretical sample size for these variables is equal to the total sample. However, the actual sample size for some variables is reduced because of missing data due to adoption, death of informants, and so on.

The following variables were added to the MDQ in 1977: nine intellectual and psychosocial assets items; five behavioral items; and 21 stimuli-induced symptom change items. Variables added in 1978 include a ten-item hyperactivity scale (Conners, 1969, 1970) and a 12-item obsessive-compulsive scale with ratings of resistance and interference. Twenty-one additional behavioral items were added in 1981. In 1984, we added a 17-item (DSM-III) total attention deficit disorder scale; 39 items describing characteristics of symptoms; 24 additional items for rating of stimuli-induced change of symptoms; and an 18-item rating scale for Tourette's disorder severity.

Complete data were available for most consecutive patients evaluated between 1965 and 1974. Most were given psychometric and projective psychological tests, MMPIs, EEGs, and neurological evaluations. Although these evaluations were not routine after 1974, the results were added to our data base if they were done elsewhere or by us subsequently. All patients have had a neurologic evaluation since 1981. The Achenbach Child Behavior Checklist (CBCL) (1981), completed by parents or teachers for children 16 years or younger, and the MMPI for patients over 16 years of age, are part of the intake procedure since 1984.

Neurological Examination

A standard neurological examination was done between 1969 and 1974 on 82 consecutive patients by Dr. R. D. Sweet, who also reviewed reports by other neurologists for seven patients (Shapiro et al., 1978). Since 1974 ratings are based on reports by other neurologists and a screening neurological evaluation by A.K.S. The PIs rated the record by consensus as 1: normal; 2: borderline; and 3: definitely abnormal using the following criteria: Borderline abnormalities are subtle neurological deficits, minor motor findings, or soft or nonlocalizing neurological abnormalities such as impaired tandem walking, finger-to-finger test, finger-to-nose test, one-foot standing with eyes closed, pronation or drift of an outstretched extremity, snout reflex, dysdiadochokinesis, etc. Definite abnormalities are focal weakness, spasticity, nystagmus, rigidity, or pathological reflexes.

Electroencephalograms

A standard EEG was done on 64 patients in our original sample of 114 patients studied between 1966 and 1974 (Shapiro et al., 1978). They were rated on a three-point scale by two senior electroencephalographers, Drs. H. Wayne and G. Solomon. The correlation coefficient between raters was 0.87 and 0.83 for two samples. Ratings of abnormality were based on features described by Stevens et al. (1968), 0:normal; 1:nonspecific or borderline abnormality (mild background disorganization, slight increase in theta slowing, excessive rapid beta activity, rare asynchronous delta, very rare sharp-wave activity, or more than expected asynchronous response to hyperventilation for the age of the patient); 2 or 3: significant abnormality (increasing degrees of disorganization, theta and delta slowing, significant paroxysmal activity such as sharp waves, spikes, spike and waves, or focal abnormalities). EEGs were not done routinely by us subsequently and if done elsewhere were added to our data base. The reports were reviewed and rated by consensus by A.K.S., E.S., and T.E.F.

Psychopathology

No attempt was made to carefully evaluate the presence of clinical psychopathology after we had concluded that psychopathology was not intrinsically associated with Tourette's disorder (Shapiro et al., 1978). Only global psychopathology was noted, such as schizophrenia, affective illness, autism, Down's syndrome, etc. Studies of psychopathology, to be described in Chapter 6, are based on behavioral factor scores and psychometric scales such as the MMPI, Achenbach Child Behavior Checklist (CBCL), and projective tests.

Behavioral Symptoms

Over the years various investigators have described diverse behavioral symptoms and problems in patients with Tourette's disorder. Behavioral symptoms cited in the literature are based primarily on retrospective, clinical reports, small samples, or on ratings of single items. The behavioral items in the MDQ have similar limitations, except for the Conners Abbreviated Parent Questionnaire, a scale for obsessive-compulsive-like symptoms or impulsions and the clinical features in DSM-III criteria for ADD. Behavioral symptoms comprised 31 items (Table A.1) which are rated (0) none or not at all; (1) just a little, mild, or somewhat of a problem at times, but do not interfere with functioning; (2) pretty much, moderate difficulty, definitely a problem at times or on many occasions, with some interference with functioning; (3) very much, severe difficulty, often definitely a problem, others have commented on behavior, interferes with social, academic or occupational functioning, requires professional help. Factor analysis yielded four factor scores (FS) with adequate reliabilities (R_{xx}): hyperactivity FS ($R_{xx} = 0.88$), learning disorder FS ($R_{xx} = 0.81$), anger-moodiness FS ($R_{xx} = 0.94$) and inhibition FS ($R_{xx} = 0.94$) (see Table A.1). The Hyperactivity Scale or the Conners Abbreviated Parent Questionnaire includes ten items which are scored 0 to 3, with a potential range of 0 to 30 (Conners, 1969, 1970).

Obviously, better controlled studies are required to evaluate whether behavioral symptoms and psychopathology are intrinsically associated with Tourette's disorder. The samples for such studies, as we discuss later, should include Tourette's disorder patients with and without the associated diagnosis of ADD.

Assets and Abilities

Nine items measuring assets and abilities were rated as −1: below average; 0: average; 1: above average; and 2: excellent. Factor analysis yielded two factor scores: coordination abilities FS ($R_{xx} = 0.75$) and intellectual-psychosocial FS ($R_{xx} = 0.84$) (Table A.1).

Obsessive-Compulsive-Like Symptoms

Twelve items reflecting obsessive-compulsive-like symptoms and traits were rated as 0: not at all; 1: just a little; 2: pretty much; and 3: very much. Each item was rated for interference on a four-point scale and for resistance on a five-point scale. These items were carefully differentiated from simple and complex motor and vocal tics during the initial diagnostic evaluation based on the DSM-III and DSM-III-R criteria for tics and compulsions (e.g., a tic is involuntary, not done for a purpose, an end-in-itself; compulsions are intentional or voluntary, done for a purpose such as to avoid a dreaded consequence) (see Chapters 6 and 10 for detailed discussion of problems of differentiating a tic from a compulsion). Two FSs were derived from factor analysis of the 12 items: obsessive-compulsive-like symptoms FS ($R_{xx} = 0.73$) and compulsive personality FS ($R_{xx} = 0.80$) (Table A.1).

Medical History

Factor analysis extracted 4 FSs from 21 medical history variables: parents' age at birth FS ($R_{xx} = 0.87$), sit-walk-talk FS ($R_{xx} = 0.47$), bladder-bowel trained FS ($R_{xx} = 0.94$) and history of head trauma FS ($R_{xx} = 0.58$). Eleven other items are included in this group of variables (Table A.1).

Illness Variables

Factor analysis of illness variables resulted in two factors: Duration of illness FS ($R_{xx} = 0.99$) and previous diagnosis or consultation FS ($R_{xx} = 0.44$). Age at onset of Tourette's disorder was included as a separate item (Table A.1).

Symptoms

Only one factor, remission of Tourette's disorder FS ($R_{xx} = 0.91$), was extracted from factor analysis of 18 symptom variables (Table A.1)

Other Variables

Only 54 variables (Table A.1) are used routinely in analysis of the data. Items listed alphabetically are included in the list of variables to describe the factor structure and loadings for the factor scores and are used only occasionally in analysis of the data. Other variables (numbers 55–70), used occasionally in analyses, are described in the text.

Shapiro Tourette's Disorder Severity Scale

The Shapiro Tourette's disorder severity (TS-Sev) Scale is a simple six-item scale, with clinically derived weighted ratings that has high reliability and validity as a measure of severity of Tourette's disorder and response to treatment. It yields ratings of 1: very mild; 2: mild; 3: moderate; 4: marked; 5: severe; or 6: extreme Tourette's disorder. This scale has been used to rate the severity of all tic and Tourette's disorder patients. The TS-Sev Scale was rated by the PIs independently; rating differences, rarely more than one unit, were resolved by consensus. Details about the TS-Sev Scale are discussed in Chapter 13.

MISSING DATA

The basic data are remarkably complete, missing data averaging less than 1%. Some subsequently added variables have a smaller sample size, but the number of available subjects is adequate to fulfill most statistical power criteria. Means for the total sample were used for a small number of variables with missing data.

CONTRAST SAMPLES

The data from this study are contrasted with data from published studies whenever appropriate in an attempt to replicate findings and develop generalization about tic disorders. The specific samples or subgroups used in analyses are described in subsequent sections. These samples may include all patients with specific primary and associated diagnoses, or matching experimental, contrast, or control samples on variables such as age, sex, race, social class, year of evaluation, and duration of illness.

We previously described the major findings of published Tourette's disorder studies prior to 1974 (Shapiro et al., 1978). There were only eight studies of 76 patients with Tourette's disorder. The number of studies has increased dramatically since that time (Tables 3.1, 3.2, 3.4). They now include nine epidemiologic studies comprising 1,286 children with tics, and six clinical studies of 1,702 children with tics. Tourette's disorder studies are limited to those describing at least five patients. There are three questionnaire surveys of 707 patients with Tourette's disorder and 35 studies totaling 2,099 patients with Tourette's disorder. These studies were done for different purposes, and consequently the degree of comprehensiveness, number and types of variables, measures and scales, reliability and validity data, method of classifying Tourette's disorder symptoms, areas addressed, and types of statistical analyses varied considerably. In addition, variables once thought to be relevant have become less important, and as new questions and issues are identified new variables are developed.

Despite these limitations, available data from these studies are compared with the data from our study. An attempt is made to identify areas of consensual agreement among studies, generalizations about the data, and unresolved problems suggesting future research.

STATISTICAL ANALYSIS

More weight is given to data derived from carefully controlled, predictive or hypothesis-oriented studies. Although many retrospective analyses are done for heuristic purposes, these analyses are clearly specified in the text. Whenever possible, an attempt is made to obtain evidence supporting or rejecting the results of retrospective analyses by comparison with published data or by conducting a prospective study. Similarly, clinical experience, impressions, and conclusions are clearly differentiated from data derived from both predictive and retrospective studies.

All analyses utilized statistical procedures described in SAS/STAT Guide for Personal Computers (1985) for use on the IBM AT computer.

Hypothesized and expected relationships are stated positively and utilize two-tailed tests of significance. Alpha levels for testing contrasts are 0.05 unless specified otherwise. Specific statistical analyses and other alpha, based on the number of contrasts, are specified in subsequent sections. The large sample size in this data set will permit analyses without concern for calculating the probability of error for most statistical analyses. Such analyses are done for smaller samples.

Factor analyses were used to reduce the number of variables and to improve the reliability of measurement. Principle factors were extracted and rotated to normal varimax criteria, with commonality estimates in the diagonals. Factor loadings and generalized Spearman Brown internal consistency reliabilities for factor scales are included in Table A.1.

Stepwise regression analyses (SRA) are used to select independent variables most highly associated with various dependent variables, to eliminate those contributing redundant variance, to identify those accounting for significant and unique variance in dependent variables, to test predictive hypotheses, and to retrospectively develop hypotheses for future study. It is understood that, because of the large number of examined variables, the results must stand the test of replication (Cohen and Cohen, 1983; Kerlinger and Pedhazur, 1973). Fifty-four variables are categorized into seven groups in the list of variables (Table A.1). Independent variables within each group are introduced in a stepwise multiple regression analysis until the last variable selected does not account for a sufficient amount of dependent variance to be significant at the 5% level (5% inclusion and exclusion criteria). In a summary stepwise regression analyses, the variables selected from each of the seven variable categories are submitted to stepwise analysis to make a final selection of variables accounting for significant and unique variance in dependent variables. Tables describing the results include the simple r, R^2, parameter estimate, and significance levels for the final summary SRA, and occasionally for variables selected by SRA for each of the seven groups of independent variables.

The Duncan multiple range test and Scheffe multiple comparision procedure, with an alpha level of 0.05, are used for testing contrasts in analyses of variance (ANOVA). Contrasts for chi-square analyses utilize partitioning procedures described by Castellan (1965) and Bresnahan and Shapiro (1966). Categories are mutually exclusive and exhaustive of the population and appear only once, the same combination of categories do not appear more than once, the dividing line for partitions is invariant, and the number of partitions are limited by the df, or, more rarely, the df for all partial contrasts is equal to the total df for the chi-square.

Other statistical procedures include correlational procedures (product moment, bivariate and phi and intraclass correlation), correlated and uncorrelated t-tests, chi-square, Fisher's Exact Test, contingency coefficient, ANCOVA. Notation in the tables for analyses not done are indicated by. . . . and by ___ for nonsignificant comparisons.

DATA-ORIENTED APPROACH TO THE STUDY OF TIC DISORDERS

Our approach to the study of tics and Tourette's disorder is reflected by the aphorism, *If you cannot put it in a chart it's poetry*. The aphorism requires modification however because *Not everything that counts can be counted and not everything that can be counted counts*. The former reflects a scientific approach and the latter reflects classical clinical methods. Both approaches are required for study of syndromes of unknown etiology.

The classical clinical approach, used successfully for centuries, has resulted in important advances in medicine. This approach relies on existing scientific knowledge, clinical experience, observation, intuition, and intensive study of patients.

Our experience with Tourette's disorder illustrates both the importance and limitations of the clinical approach. Up until 1965, we had never treated a patient nor heard a discussion of this syndrome. The scarcity of information in the literature (50 recorded cases in the English language) and the emphasis on the psychogenesis and psychodynamic treatment of the disorder initially led us to evaluate the first patient in the traditional way. However, we became aware that our clinical observations did not fit the psychogenic model. We became convinced that it was necessary to discard *a priori* clinical concepts and to rely on our own clinical observations and impressions. We began to follow clinical leads about the illness provided by our initial and subsequent patients. We listened more carefully to their description of the symptoms, factors associated with change of symptoms, and to their concepts about the cause and experience with treatment of the illness. Had we continued to rely on established conceptions of the illness, inferring etiology from the bizarre symptomatology, we would have concluded as others had that this was indeed a disease caused by deep-seated psychological conflicts (Shapiro, 1970 a,b,c; Shapiro et al., 1978). The clinical approach frequently results in serious omissions, commissions, and excesses. Treatment is particularly prone to these distortions and results in placebo effects, an effect so powerful that the history of medical treatment until recently has been characterized as the history of the placebo effect (Shapiro, 1960; 1978).

Systematic and scientific methods for studying clinical conditions has developed rapidly in the last 30 years. It was initiated perhaps by Harry Gold with the introduction of the double-blind procedure in 1937 (Shapiro, 1978), and subsequently, he and others, highlighted the importance of the placebo effect in medicine (Shapiro, 1960; 1978; Shapiro and Morris, 1978). The double-blind procedure, essentially a controlled or scientific method for studying the effects of treatment, strongly resisted initially, has become the standard and definitive method for evaluating new treatments. Advances in the control of placebo effects, observer bias, bandwagon effects, and the influence of many psychosocial and situational variables, has led to the development of sophisticated methods for controlling these variables (Shapiro and Morris, 1978).

Sensitivity about the importance of controls in clinical research became evident in the studies of tuberculosis in the 1940s and poliomyelitis shortly thereafter. The introduction of psychopharmaceuticals into psychiatry in the 1950s led to the importance of reliably and validly defining psychological and subjective variables, and contributed to the development of sensitive methodology required for evaluating the effectiveness of psychochemotherapy. Other important methodological contributions came from psychology which had long been concerned with controlled experimental studies, advances in statistical methodology and the availability of computer technology.

These developments led to increased efficiency of clinical studies and to the availability of reliable and valid data in all of the medical specialties, especially in psychiatry. Sophisticated psychiatric studies of etiology, diagnosis, and treatment have slowly begun to build a firm data base. We refer to a primary reliance on data derived from carefully controlled studies as a data-oriented approach to the study of clinical conditions (Shapiro et al., 1978; Shapiro and Shapiro, 1981b).

Our studies of Tourette's disorder provided us with an opportunity to demonstrate the usefulness of a data orientation. While giving full reign to our clinical impressions and intensively studying patients for meaningful hypotheses, the data-oriented approach requires *a priori* hypothesis, differentiation between *a priori* hypotheses and retrospective analysis of data, verification of retrospective observations and clncal impressions by subjecting them to prospective testing of hypotheses, development of reliable and valid independent and dependent variables, replication of results on other samples, the use of control groups, relevant statistical procedures, and other appropriate research methodology. This approach requires that clinical impressions be differentiated from conclusions drawn from reliable and valid data analysis.

These two approaches converged in our attempt to understand and delineate the clinical course, diagnostic criteria, etiology, and treatment of tics and Tourette's disorder.

3

Epidemiology

This chapter discusses the epidemiology of tics and Tourette's disorder. Its focus is to estimate the prevalence of tic and Tourette's disorders from a thorough review of the literature, to identify factors contributing to differences between the two disorders, and to examine the question of whether they should be considered similar or separate categories.

TICS

Nine epidemiological studies with data about the prevalence of tics are summarized in Table 3.1. The table includes the authors, site of the study, age range, sample characteristics, size of sample, and percent of infrequent, frequent, and total tics by sex. Two types of prevalence rates are presented: point prevalence which is the "number of cases present at a specified moment of time," and period prevalence which is "the number of cases that occur during a specified period of time—for example, a year" (Liebenfeld, 1976). Lifetime prevalence is the number of cases that occur at any time during the lifetime of a group or sample.

There were seven epidemiological studies of development in children (studies 1–4,6,7,9) that included a single question about tics, variously described as twitches, jerks, habit spasms, unusual movements, mannerisms, body movements, or sounds. The lack of a clear symptom description tends to increase the number of responses from individuals with a variety of different disorders including transient tic of childhood, chronic motor tic, Tourette's disorder, as well as others with stereotypic movements, organic movement disorders, habits, mannerisms, and possibly obsessive-compulsive disorder. The instruments included parent questionnaires (studies 1,2,7,9), parent interviews (studies 1,3,4,6), school district survey (study 5), and medical history and examination (studies 1,8) (Table 3.1). The severity of the symptoms was rated as frequent,

TABLE 3.1. Epidemiological studies of tics, twitches, habit spasms, or mannerisms[a]

Study	Site of study	Age (years)	Sample characteristics	Total sample	Point prevalence (%): Tics, twitches, mannerisms											Period (%) prevalence Total
					Infrequent			Frequent			Total				
					Boys	Girls	Total	Boys	Girls	Total	Boys	Girls	Total	
1. Pringle et al. (1967)	England	7	Parent questionnaire[b] Medical history[b] Medical examination[b]	7,949 7,958 7,965	6.5 — —	4.8 — —	5.7 — —	2.6 — —	1.5 — —	2.0 — —	9.0 5.9 4.2	6.3 4.4 3.9	7.7 5.2 4.1	— — —
2. Abe and Oda (1980)	Japan	8	Parent questionnaire[a,c] Parents with tics Parents without tics Total	76 177 253	— — —	— — —	— — —	— — —	— — —	— — —	— — —	— — —	19.7 9.6 12.6	— — —
3. Lapouse and Monk (1958, 1964)	United States	6–12	Parent interview	482	—	—	—	13.0	11.0	12.0	—	—	—	—
4. Rutter et al. 1970	England	9–12	Parent interview, samples: Nonpsychiatric Psychiatric Nonpsychiatric epileptic Psychiatric epileptic	1,919 95 26 17	— — — —	— — — —	— — — —	— — — —	— — — —	— — — —	— — — —	— — — —	4.0 18.0 8.0 24.0	— — — —
5. Boncour (1910)	France	2–13	Survey	1,759	—	—	—	—	—	—	—	—	23.7	—
6. MacFarlane et al. (1954)	United States	1.75–14	Parent interview[b,c]	41–116	—	—	—	—	—	—	2.7	3.1	—	25.0
7. Shepherd et al. (1971)	England	5–15	Parent questionnaire[c]	6,290	8–20	8–10	—	1.2	0.5	0.9	13–28	11–20	—	20.0

8. Torup (1962)	Denmark	?	Random pediatric medical sample	50	—	—	—	—	—	—	—	—	—	16.0
9. Current study[d]	United States	6–16	Parent questionnaire											
			Normal sample	1,100	8.6	4.9	6.7	1.5	0.6	1.0	10.0	5.5	—	—
			Referred sample[b]	1,100	17.6	17.1	17.4	12.2	10.7	11.5	29.8	27.8	7.7	28.8

Comparisons (Kellmer-Pringle study)	χ_2	df	p
Parent questionnaire			
Twitches sometimes, often or not present by sex	21.9	2	0.016
Twitches sometimes or often by sex	1.5	1	NS
Twitches present or not present by sex	20.5	1	0.000
Medical history			
Twitches present or not present by sex	8.4	1	0.004
Medical examination			
Twitches present or not present by sex	0.9	1	NS

[a] See text for description of studies.
[b] Mannerisms included in the questionnaire item.
[c] Vocal tics included in the questionnaire item.
[d] Normative data for the normal sample and referred sample used to develop the Child Behavior Checklist kindly supplied by Dr. T. M. Achenbach. The referred sample were children referred for mental health services in the past 6 months. For χ_2 analysis see Table 3.2.

extreme, often, very noticeable, or as certainly applies, or as applies somewhat, moderately, and occasionally, in four of the studies (studies 1,3,7,9). Study 8 sampled a control group of 50 pediatric patients who were hospitalized for medical reasons. The salient characteristics and results for each of the studies are summarized in Table 3.1.

Review of Studies

Pringle et al. (1967). A child development epidemiological study of 7-year-old single-birth English children asked parents to indicate if their child had twitches, mannerisms, tics, or habit spasms of the face, eyes, or body movements, and to rate them present sometimes or frequent. This study included data derived from the mother's questionnaire, medical history obtained by a nurse, and medical examination.

Infrequent and frequent symptoms are recorded on the parent questionnaire. The ratio of infrequent to frequent symptoms is not significantly different between boys and girls (Table 3.1). Infrequent symptoms are reported at a higher percentage than frequent symptoms for both boys and girls ($p = 0.016$). The total percent reported for both infrequent and frequent or total symptoms is highest on the parent questionnaire (7.7%), in between on the medical history obtained by a nurse (5.2%), and lowest on the medical examination (4.1%). These data indicate that mothers probably report more symptoms than are actually present. We reported a similar trend in our current study (see Chapter 5), and this tendency has been noted in other epidemiologic studies (MacFarlane et al, 1954; Lapouse and Monk, 1964). Another indication that the data vary with the source of information is the sex ratio. The ratio of males to females is significantly higher on the mothers' questionnaire (1.4:1) ($p = 0.000$), and medical interview (1.3:1) ($p = 0.004$), and lowest and not significantly different on the medical examination (1.1:1) (NS) (Table 3.1). The relationship of the sex ratio to tics and Tourette's disorder is discussed in Chapter 4.

Abe and Oda (1980). In a sample of 1,272 3-year-old Japanese children, 76 had at least one parent who had tics. A matched sample of 177 children whose parents did not have tics served as a control. Five years later, at age 8, parents completed a questionnaire about the presence of tics in the child (repeated blinking; twitches of the face, neck and shoulder; shaking of the head; and vocal utterances). Parents with tics had significantly more children with tics (19.7%) ($\chi^2 = 4.9$, df=1, $p = 0.0262$).

Lapouse and Monk (1964). A random sample of 482 parents in Buffalo, New York, were interviewed using a structured schedule for 200 behavioral items which included one question about the presence of tics (blinking eyes, twitching mouth, movements of the head, jerking shoulders or any other part of body). Though not specifically described the study appears to be a point prevalence study of children from 6 to 12 years of age (average 8.5 years). Only percentages with extreme scores are presented. Extreme tics were present in 13% for boys, 11% for girls, and 12% for both sexes. There were no significant differences for sex, age, race, social class or number of children in the family.

Rutter et al. (1970). The epidemiologic study on the Isle of Wight, which included 2,057 9- to 12-year-old children recorded point prevalence rates for "twitches, mannerisms or tics of the face or body" that were rated "applies somewhat or certainly applies" by parents and teachers. The sample was classified into four groups: nonpsychiatric, nonpsychiatric epileptic, psychiatric epileptic, and psychiatric. Chi-square for the total distribution was significant ($\chi^2 = 40.8$, df=3, $p = 0.0000$). Partitioning the chi-square resulted in a significantly higher percentage of tics for the total psychiatric group (psychiatric epileptic and psychiatric group) compared with the total nonpsychiatric group (nonpsychiatric epileptic and nonpsychiatric group) ($\chi^2 = 38.9$, df=1, $p = 0.000$). The percentages are higher, but not significantly so, for the total epileptic group compared to the total nonepileptic group. Teacher responses were essentially identical to parent responses for the nonepileptic samples.

Boncour (1910). In a point prevalence survey of the entire student body in a township in France, which included 1,759 students between 2 and 13 years of age, 417 (23.7%) had tics that were not defined. In the 7- to 13-year age group, 47.8% were boys and 52.5% were girls. More girls were afflicted at age 7 than boys (male to female ratio, 0.9:1) ($\chi^2 = 29.6$, df=6, $p < 0.0005$). Boncour reported that tics varied considerably after 7 years, increased sharply in boys at age 12, and decreased in both sexes at age 13. Females had an earlier onset, although 50% of both sexes had an onset before 8.5 years of age. Children with tics did not have more psychological problems than children without tics.

MacFarlane et al. (1954). This longitudinal developmental study of 45 behavior problems at successive ages from 1.75 to 14 years of age included a random sample of 116 normal children who were initially interviewed at 1.75 years of age. Mothers were reinterviewed at yearly intervals until the children were 14 years old. Unfortunately, the sample size decreased from 116 at 1.75 years to 41 by the age of 14. Most mothers completed a questionnaire and all were interviewed. One question included tics or mannerisms, other than nail-biting, thumb-sucking, masturbation, and stammering that were rated on a three-point scale: "(1) compulsive, pronounced, tic-like behavior occurring daily whether obviously ritualistic or not, and whether involving only small muscle groups. Either severe or frequent or less severe, but going off many times a day. (By severe is meant involvement that compels attention of anyone); (2) persistent mannerisms, less often or severe than (1). Obvious enough to be noticed by anyone. Clearing throat, sniffing, hunching up shoulders, squinting, twitching of any facial muscles, tapping with feet, etc.; and (3) when child is fatigued or under emotional pressure, or when discussing some emotional topic, or when preoccupied, consistently resorts to mild motor tic-like behavior."

This study is noteworthy because the definition of tics is more fully described and includes vocal tics. The examples for tics are appropriate except for the use of the word "compulsive" and tapping of feet. The authors note that higher percentages are obtained from questionnaires than from interviews. Point prevalence data are presented for the number of children with tics at each successive year from 1.75 to 14 years of age. Similar to the finding of Boncour, more girls than boys had tics. The yearly average was 2.7 for boys and 3.1 for girls (male to female ratio, 0.87:1). Tics reached their peak at 6 years (10%) for girls and at 7 years (11%) for boys. The period prevalence rate between 1.75 and 14 years of age (tics present at some time during the course of the study) was 25% for both boys and girls.

Shepherd et al. (1971). A questionnaire about the mental health of children was completed by parents of a random sample of 5- to 15-year-old English children. One of the questions included twitches that were present at the time when the questionnaire was completed. Twitches were rated as "a very noticeable twitch of the face or body or mannerism which takes place most of the time; occasional twitches or mannerisms which occur when tired, bored, etc; and no twitches or mannerisms." The study is therefore a point prevalence study at each yearly age from 5 to 15 years for 3,251 boys and 3,039 girls, and included "mannerisms" as a feature of the "twitch." Specific data was provided only for "very noticeable and persistent twitches," which were more frequent in boys ($N = 40$, 1.23%) than girls ($N = 15$, 0.49%), total 55 (0.87%) (male to female ratio, 2.5:1) ($\chi^2 = 9.9$, df=1, $p = 0.0017$). The percentages for both occasional and frequent twitches varied from 13 to 28% for boys and 11 to 20% for girls during each year from 5 to 15 years of age. The yearly percentage of noticeable and persistent tics was fairly constant between 1 and 2% for 6- to 15-year-old boys and for girls up to age 9, with only two cases reported after age 9. Occasional twitches were more common than frequent twitches, and varied from 8 to 20% for boys, peaking at 20% for 12-year-old boys, and were fairly constant at 8 to 10% for girls. These symptoms reached a peak of approximately 30% for boys between the ages of 10 and 12, and 20% for girls at age 12. The male to female ratio is approximately 1.7:1 for occasional twitches (estimated from figure in study text), and 2.5:1 for very noticeable twitches.

Torup (1962). As part of a follow-up study of tics, in a control group of 50 random children who were hospitalized for medical reasons, eight (16%) had tics in the past or currently (lifetime prevalence). Tics were pronounced in only one child (12.5%). Age of patients, medical reasons for hospitalization and other information were not provided.

Current Study. The data for this analysis, kindly provided by Dr. Thomas M. Achenbach, comprised a normative sample of 6- to 16-year-old children used for development of the Child Behavior Checklist (Achenbach, 1978;

1979). The normal sample included a random group of 550 boys and 550 girls. The referred sample included 550 boys and 550 girls who had been referred to a mental health facility in the past 6 months. The Child Behavior Check List asks parents whether "nervous movements or twitches" are "present now or within the past 6 months," and to rate them as "very true or often true, somewhat or sometimes true, and not true." The results are summarized in Table 3.2.

For the normal sample, these symptoms were present in more boys (10%) than girls (5.5%) ($\chi^2 = 8$, df=1, $p = 0.005$) and totalled 7.7% for both boys and girls. Similar to the Pringle et al. study (1967), the ratings for the "very true or often true" category were very much lower (1.5% for boys, 0.6% for girls, 1.0% for both boys and girls) than for the "somewhat or sometimes true" category (8.6% for boys, 4.9% for girls, 6.7% for both groups) ($\chi^2 = 8.3$, df=2, $p = 0.016$).

Tics were significantly more frequent for all categories in the referred sample (28.8%) than in the normal sample (7.7%) ($\chi^2 = 178$, df=2, $p = 0.000$). Mild tics were more frequent (17.4%) than severe tics (11.5%), but equally frequent in males and females ($\chi^2 = 0.7$, df=2, NS).

Difficulty of Establishing the Prevalence of Tics

All authors in the cited studies discuss the difficulties of obtaining valid estimates for the prevalence of tics. Epidemiological studies usually survey many types of behavior which may include only one item about tics. The brief and varied descriptions of tics, such as tics, twitches, squints, mannerisms, habit spasms, and vocal sounds, preclude a definite diagnosis and differential diagnosis for many diverse tic conditions such as transient tic disorder, chronic motor tic disorder, Tourette's disorder, and nontic disorders such as stereotypic movement disorder, cough of adolescence, various dystonic syndromes, habits, mannerisms, and so on. For example, parents completing our Movement Disorder Questionnaire classify many symptoms as tics which are not confirmed by clinical interview. In our sample of 1,610 patients who were evaluated for a tic disorder, 141 (8.8%) were diagnosed as having another movement disorder, or no movement disorder at all (Table 2.1).

Moreover, each epidemiological study used a different rating scale for severity (frequent, often, very noticeable, very true or often true; occasional, sometimes, hardly ever, somewhat or sometimes true). Some of these problems may lead to an overestimation, others may contribute to an underestimation of the actual prevalence.

Another variable is the method of obtaining information. They include parent questionnaires (studies 1,2,7,9), parent interviews (studies 1,3,4,6), school survey (study 5) and medical examination (study 1). MacFarlane et al. (1954) noted that children have difficulty differentiating tics from other symp-

TABLE 3.2. Six months point prevalence for "twitches" during the past 6 months in normal and referred children[a]

Samples	Percent of children with twitches in age groups											Total (all ages)
	6	7	8	9	10	11	12	13	14	15	16	
Normal sample[b]												
Boys (N = 50 in each age group)												
Somewhat or sometimes true	2	10	10	12	12	16	6	10	4	6	6	8.6
Very true or often true	2	2	2	4	4	0	2	0	0	0	0	1.5
Total	4	12	12	16	16	16	8	10	4	6	6	10.0
Girls (N = 50 in each age group)												
Somewhat or sometimes true	2	10	2	8	6	8	2	2	6	4	4	4.9
Very true or often true	2	2	0	0	0	0	0	0	0	2	0	0.6
Total	4	12	2	8	6	8	2	2	6	6	4	5.5
Total (N = 100 in each age group)												
Somewhat or sometimes true	2	10	6	10	9	12	4	6	5	5	5	6.7
Very true or often true	2	2	1	2	2	0	1	0	0	1	0	1.0
Total	4	12	7	12	11	12	5	6	5	6	5	7.7
Referred sample[c]												
Boys (N = 50 in each age group)												
Somewhat or sometimes true	24	14	16	28	20	10	10	14	16	8	34	17.6
Very true or often true	12	22	2	12	6	18	12	10	12	20	8	12.2
Total	36	36	18	40	26	28	22	24	28	28	42	29.8
Girls (N = 50 in each age group)												
Somewhat or sometimes true	22	10	22	28	16	10	10	14	12	26	18	17.1
Very true or often true	8	14	14	8	12	22	10	12	8	4	6	10.7
Total	30	24	36	36	28	32	20	26	20	30	24	27.8
Total (N = 100 in each age group)												
Somewhat or sometimes true	23	12	19	28	18	10	10	14	14	17	26	17.4
Very true or often true	10	18	8	10	9	20	11	11	10	12	7	11.5
Total	33	30	27	38	27	30	21	25	24	29	33	28.8

Comparisons	χ^2	df	p
Normal sample			
Twitches sometimes, often or not present by sex	8.3	2	0.016
Twitches sometimes or often vs. sex	0.4	1	NS
Twitches present or not present by sex	8.0	1	0.005
Referred sample			
Twitches sometimes, often or not present by sex	0.7	2	NS
Twitches sometimes or often vs. sex	0.2	1	NS
Twitches present or not present by sex	0.5	1	NS
Normal vs. referred sample			
Twitches sometimes, often or not present by sex	178.0	2	0.000
Twitches sometimes or often vs. sex	21.4	1	0.000
Twitches present or not present by sex	163.0	1	0.000

[a]In 1,100 normal and 1,100 referred children between 6 and 16 years of age. The data for this analysis is from the normative samples used to develop the Child Behavior Checklist kindly provided by Dr. Thomas M. Achenbach (Achenbach and Edelbrock, 1978; 1979).
[b]Random sample of 550 boys and 550 girls.
[c]Sample of 550 boys and 550 girls referred to a mental health facility in the past 6 months.

toms and give many more positive responses to questions about tics than mothers. Both MacFarlane et al. (1954) and Pringle et al. (1967) report that mothers report more tics on questionnaires than when interviewed.

Another difficulty is the different purposes of the studies. They include studies of incidence, point, period and lifetime prevalence, and development over time. Tics may be recorded at the time of evaluation, from 2 to 6 months previously or sometime in the past, at different ages or age ranges, or at any time in the past. Seven of the studies were point prevalence studies (studies 1–7), one was a 6-month period prevalence study (study 9), and three reported essentially lifetime prevalence (studies 6,7,8). Point and period prevalence rates by definition would be lower than lifetime prevalence rates, as indicated by the range of 4 to 24% for the former and 16 to 25% for the latter. However, although the rates are higher for lifetime prevalence, very little data are presented in the three studies (studies 6–8) in support of the estimates.

Finally, none of the studies differentiate transient tics, chronic motor tics, Tourette's disorder, and many other adventitious movements (see Chapter 10). It is probable that transient tic disorder (TTD) is much more frequent than chronic motor tic disorder (CMT), which is much more frequent than Tourette's disorder. The reviewed studies, therefore, would include all of these disorders.

Conclusions

Despite the limitations and difficulties inherent in conducting epidemiological studies, several generalizations about the prevalence of tics are possible from review of epidemiological studies.

Children report more tics than mothers, who report more tics on questionnaires than when interviewed; the smallest percentage is reported by clinicians. It is probable that more reliable and valid estimates of tics in the population require a clinical interview of the parents, in the presence of the child, and conducted by a clinician who is knowledgeable about movement disorders. The estimates of frequent tics, which significantly exceed infrequent tics, are probably more reliable than estimates of infrequent tics which may include many nontic symptoms.

One of the symptoms classified as an infrequent tic in most of the questionnaires is "tics when tired," although none of the studies report the frequency of this symptom. We have never encountered tics only when tired in children or adults, or even when anxious for that matter, and it may be that other types of movements may be misinterpreted as tics. If tics occur only when tired or anxious, it may be potentially important and interesting and should be documented and studied.

Because of the variability of the type of studies and their results, the re-

TABLE 3.3 *Summary percent ranges for point, period, or lifetime prevalence for tics, twitches, mannerisms, or habit spasms reported in nine epidemiology studies[a]*

Tics, twitches, mannerisms, or habit spasms	Boys (%)	Girls (%)	Total (%)
Random Samples			
Point prevalence (age 5–16 years)			
Infrequent	7–20	5–10	6–7
Frequent	1–13	1–11	1–12
Total	4–28	4–20	4–24
Period or lifetime prevalence	—	—	16–25
Psychiatric Samples			
Point prevalence (age 6–16 years)			
Infrequent	18	17	17
Frequent	12	11	12
Total	30	28	18–29

[a]See Table 3.1.

ported ranges for all the studies are probably a better indication of the possible range for the prevalence in the population (Table 3.3).

Also, because the nine studies sampled symptoms other than tics, such as twitches, habit spasms, mannerisms, and other movements, they are collectively referred to as symptoms.

Boys appear to have more frequent, infrequent, and total tics than girls, although the range for all point prevalence studies overlaps: 4 to 28% for boys and 4 to 20% for girls (Table 3.3). The total for all tics for both sexes ranges from 4 to 24%. However, not all studies report significant sex differences (studies 1,3,5,6). Moreover, evaluation of the same children using different methods results in a significant male to female difference on the mothers' questionnaire but not by clinical interview (Pringle et al., 1967). As discussed more fully in Chapter 4, the male to female ratio is significantly lower in epidemiological studies of nonclinical samples than in studies of clinical patients with Tourette's disorder.

Lifetime prevalence appears to be higher, from 16 to 25%, although the data are not based on carefully conducted studies. Symptoms are markedly higher for psychiatric patients, ranging from 18 to 29% in two point prevalence studies (studies 4,9). However, the possible inclusion of stereotypic, hyperactive, and other awkward or manneristic symptoms in psychiatric groups may inflate the percentages.

It is clear, however, that the prevalence of tic disorders is much higher than previous estimates. Since there is increasing evidence that the etiology for all tic disorders is similar, the problem may be much more extensive than previously considered and warrants carefully designed studies.

TOURETTE'S DISORDER

A survey of the literature yielded eight citations about the prevalence of Tourette's disorder (Table 3.4). The range for the first four studies (1899–1966) varied from 0.0005 to 0.019%. Only 14 patients were cited as having Tourette's disorder from a surveyed sample of over 2 million, or 0.0007%. Surveys of the English-language literature (published between 1965 and 1969) yielded 39 to 69 patients with Tourette's disorder (Kelman, 1965; Fernando, 1967; Morphew and Sim, 1969). Abuzzahab and Anderson (1973, 1974) cited 430 cases of Tourette's disorder from the world literature published between 1825 and 1973, although many were inadequately described and may not fulfill current criteria for the diagnosis of the disorder. Subsequent estimates strongly suggest that the prevalence of Tourette's disorder has been underestimated, because, as discussed previously, the diagnosis of the disorder in the past erroneously required coprolalia, echolalia, and intellectual and psychological deterioration.

The impression that Tourette's disorder has been grossly underdiagnosed is supported by our data for 666 Tourette's disorder patients who were evaluated between 1965 and 1981: 61.7% had never been diagnosed although all had previous consultations with physicians, many at major diagnostic centers.

The last two studies in Table 3.4 tend to support the impressions of increased prevalence, although all of the cited studies have serious limitations. The Tourette Syndrome Association, based on their membership and response to publicity, loosely estimate that there are 100,000 patients with Tourette's disorder in the United States, or approximately 0.043%. Baron et al. (1981), based on data from a genetic study of 127 consecutive patients with Tourette's disorder, using a single major locus model, indirectly estimates the predicted population prevalence for Tourette's disorder and CMT, excluding TTD, as 2.3% for males and 0.8% for females, or 1.6% for both sexes combined.

Caine et al. (1985) presented the preliminary results of a survey of 5- to 18-year-old school children. All relevant professionals and the Tourette Syndrome Association in Monroe County, in the Rochester-New York area, were asked to refer 5- to 18-year-old children with Tourette's disorder for further evaluation by the authors. Diagnosis of Tourette's disorder was confirmed in 41 of an estimated sample of 142,857 children, yielding a percentage of 0.0287, with a 95% confidence level of 0.020 to 0.037. An indication that even this percent was an underestimate is that 17 patients had not been previously diagnosed, four patients with Tourette's disorder were excluded because they declined evaluation, and nine other patients with Tourette's disorder who were diagnosed within 2 years after the study period were not included in the results. Another indication of possible underestimate for Tourette's disorder is that the male to female ratio was 9.3:1, which is approximately three times higher than is usually reported, indicating that fewer females were identified.

TABLE 3.4. Prevalence of Tourette's disorder reported in studies

Studies	Site of study	Sample characteristics	Sample size	N	%	Per thousand
Koester (1899)	Leipzig	Admissions, Universitats Poliklnik	2,500	2	0.0800	0.8
Ascher (1948)	Baltimore[a]	Hospitalized and outpatients, Johns Hopkins	590,000	4	0.0007	0.007
Salmi (1961)	Finland	Educational Guidance Clinic	5,300	1	0.0190	0.19
Feild et al. (1966)	Minnesota[a]	Mayo Clinic Admissions, 1935–1965	1,500,000	7	0.0005	0.005
Baron et al. (1981)	New York[a]	Predicted prevalence of TS and CMT from genetic model	127	—	1.5500	15.5
Caine (1985)	New York[a]	Survey of referred 5- to 18-year-old children	142,000	41	0.0290	0.29
Burd et al. (1986c)	North Dakota[a]	Survey of 6 to 18-year-old children				
		Males	71,640	67	0.0935	0.935
		Females	60,910	6	0.0099	0.099
		Total	140,580	73	0.0519	0.519
Burd et al. (1986b)	North Dakota[a]	Survey of adults over 18 years of age				
		Males	223,537	17	0.0076	0.076
		Females	224,999	5	0.0022	0.022
		Total	448,556	22	0.0049	0.049

[a]United States.

This may be due to females having milder forms of the disorder resulting in fewer referrals and less frequent diagnosis of Tourette's disorder. Subjects with a diagnosis of CMT or TTD were not included.

A prevalence of 0.0519%, 1.8 times higher than the previous study, was reported by Burd et al. (1986c). Children aged 6 to 18 years, diagnosed as having Tourette's disorder and referred by professionals, were entered on a state-wide list maintained by the authors in North Dakota. Similar to the previous study, the male to female ratio was 9.3:1, much higher than the expected ratio of 3:1, again indicating underrepresentation of females and possible overrepresentation of males with attention deficit disorder plus hyperactivity (ADD+H) and other CNS disorders which are common in clinical samples. As indicated previously, since the study included only diagnosed cases and did not include children fully at risk for Tourette's disorder, the reported percentage of 0.0519% can only be considered a minimum estimate. An indication of the difficulty of assessing the prevalence of Tourette's disorder from diagnosed cases is the significantly lower percentage of 0.0049% reported for adults, which is 11 times lower than for children (Burd et al., 1986b). Symptoms tend to decrease in severity in adulthood (see Chapter 5). Adults with mild symptoms tend not to seek treatment and therefore are not identified in clinical samples.

Since all published studies are based on incomplete registers of diagnosed patients, variable referral patterns, and do not survey the occurrence within a community (Schoenberg, 1982; Cohen and Cohen 1984), all current prevalence rates for Tourette's disorder should be considered minimal estimates. These methodological limitations, and the increase in reported Tourette's disorder patients in the literature has prompted a cautious statement in DSM-III-R that "The estimated lifetime prevalence rate is at least 0.5 per thousand." Our guess is that it is much higher, somewhere between 1 to 10 per thousand, or 0.1 to 1.0% of the population.

CHRONIC MOTOR TIC DISORDER

A compelling indication that the estimates for Tourette's disorder are minimal is the marked discrepancy between the number of patients with the disorder reported in studies compared to those with CMT. The main reason for the discrepancy is that the symptoms are generally more severe in Tourette's disorder than CMT. Patients with Tourette's disorder seek help, are identified as patients, and therefore are reported in studies. Those with mild symptoms for both Tourette's disorder and CMT tend not to seek help and are infrequently recorded as patients. For example, although only 4.6% of our sample were diagnosed as having CMT, patients report 6.3 times more relatives with CMT and TTD than Tourette's disorder (Table 2.1). Other published data confirm the observation that CMT is more common than Tourette's disorder. The percent of CMT in family studies reported is 2.7 (Comings and Comings,

1984) to 7.5 (Pauls et al., 1981) times more frequent than Tourette's disorder. Mildly afflicted patients often are unaware that they have tics. During intake it is common for a parent to deny a family history of tics while at the same time displaying mild and occasionally moderately severe tics which are often obvious to other family members. A more direct assessment of the discrepancy is reported by Pauls et al. (1984) who noted that 1.6 more individuals are identified as having tics when personally interviewed compared to when a history is obtained from parents. These results were confirmed by Kurlan et al. (1986) who interviewed 159 Mennonite relatives of patients with Tourette's disorder. Although 54 relatives were diagnosed as having Tourette's disorder or CMT, 16 (29.6%) were unaware that they had tics, 28 (52.9%) were aware that they had tics but had never sought help, and only 10 (18.5%) had sought treatment. The ratio of untreated to treated tics is 4.4:1.

TOURETTE AND CHRONIC MOTOR TIC DISORDERS

It is likely that the prevalence for both Tourette's disorder and CMT is much higher in the population than the frequency estimated from clinical samples. The basis for this conclusion rests on the discrepancy between the percentage of patients with diagnoses of CMT and TTD reported in studies and the much higher percentage of relatives with a history of CMT reported in family studies. A speculative estimate of the prevalence could be derived from existing data. Burd et al. (1986c) report Tourette's disorder in 0.0935% of males. If the assumption is made that one-third are females, an estimate of Tourette's disorder for both sexes would be 0.07%. If this is then multiplied by the estimate that CMT is 7.5 times more common than Tourette's disorder (Pauls et al., 1981), the percent would be 0.5% for CMT. Since one-third of patients are unaware that they have tics (Kurlan et al., 1986), the percent of individuals with CMT would be 0.7%. Thus, the total estimate (0.07% for Tourette's disorder and 0.7% for CMT) would be 0.77% or a total of approximately 1,800,000 individuals in the United States with Tourette's disorder or CMT.

The total may be even higher. In a genetic study of a subsample of 127 consecutive patients evaluated by us during 1 year, an indirect estimate, using a single major locus model, of the predicted population prevalence for Tourette's disorder and CMT, excluding TTD, is 2.3% for males and 0.8% for females, or 1.6% for both sexes combined, or an estimated total of approximately 3,680,000 individuals in the United States (Baron et al., 1981).

CONCLUSION

Carefully controlled epidemiological studies of community or nonclinical samples are required to document the postulated extensiveness of the tic disorders in the population.

4

Patient Characteristics

We describe and compare the patient characteristics of our samples with data in the literature in this chapter. Our purpose is to examine the many domains and variables within these domains to see which have any relevance to the etiology of the disorder. The domains include demographic, perinatal, maturational, developmental, intellectual, behavioral and asset variables, genetic family and patient medical histories, and organic CNS factors. The increase in the size of our sample has given us the opportunity to study these domains in greater detail than heretofore. The analysis of the data identifies relevant and meaningful variables, variables requiring further study and those no longer germane.

SAMPLE CHANGES OVER TIME

Our clinical impression that patient characteristics have changed since the publication of our early papers and previous book on Tourette's disorder was confirmed by the following analyses: Patients evaluated since 1975 were being diagnosed at an earlier age, had a shorter duration of illness, fewer years between onset and diagnosis, were younger at time of evaluation, severity of Tourette's disorder was decreased, and fewer patients had a diagnosis of attention deficit disorder (ADD) and other CNS deficits (Tables 4.1, 4.2)).

Sample characteristics changed again since 1981, probably due to the development of reliable diagnostic criteria (Shapiro et al., 1978), and the widespread dissemination of information about Tourette's disorder. Both factors have facilitated diagnosis, resulting in an increase in the number of diverse professionals identifying, diagnosing, and treating tics and Tourette's disorder. Paradoxically, we are now referred more severely afflicted patients with complicated histories and differential diagnoses. At the same time, we

TABLE 4.1. *Tourette sample changes over time*

Patient status	Sample 1[a] (1965–1974)	Sample 2[b] (1975–1978)	Sample 3[c] (1979–1981)	ANOVA ($p =$)	Duncan Multiple Range Test		
					Sample 1 vs. 2 ($p <$)	Sample 1 vs. 3 ($p <$)	Sample 2 vs. 3 ($p <$)
Age	22.6	18.5	17.4	0.0005	0.05	0.05	—
Age at diagnosis of TS[d]	21.3	17.7	16.5	0.0020	0.05	0.05	—
Years from onset to diagnosis	14.4	10.9	10.0	0.0025	0.05	0.05	—
Duration of present illness	15.8	11.8	10.9	0.0006	0.05	0.05	—
Age first diagnosed TS	17.0	12.8	14.3	0.0281	0.05	0.05	—
Attention deficit disorder[e]	51.2%	21.4%	16.4%	0.0001	0.00	0.00	—
Conners Hyperactivity Index	20.3	12.7	11.6	0.0612	0.05	0.05	—
Severity of TS	3.4	2.6	2.3	0.0001	0.05	0.05	0.05

[a] $N = 121$.
[b] $N = 313$.
[c] $N = 232$.
[d] TS = Tourette's disorder.
[e] Chi-square.

have the impression that Tourette's disorder is being overdiagnosed. Many recently evaluated patients referred as having a tic disorder have various non-tic movements disorders (Table 2.1).

In addition, the number of Tourette's disorder patients with associated diagnoses has increased. The percent of patients with both Tourette's disorder and ADD increased from 24.9% for patients evaluated between 1965 and 1981 to 42.4% for patients evaluated between 1981 through 1985 ($\chi^2 = 28.8$, df=1, $p = 0.0000$). This increase may be due to a recent ongoing study which offered free consultation, diagnosis, and treatment at our laboratory. The number of patients referred for consultation with other diagnoses in addition to Tourette's disorder, such as severe conduct disorder, personality disorder, stereotypic movement disorder, and other CNS disorders also increased. The shift over the years in the character of samples is also reflected in published studies. Some centers, especially research units or those highly specialized to treat and hospitalize severely ill psychiatric and neurological patients, often located away from major cities, are more likely to see more disturbed and atypical Tourette's disorder patients. Moreover, patients who have severe forms of Tourette's disorder are more likely to be diagnosed and to be identified in a clinical sample. These sampling problems which may overestimate the severity of Tourette's disorder may be the source of some of the controver-

TABLE 4.2. *Variables significantly correlated with year of evaluation, age, and sex of patients with Tourette's disorder*[a]

Variables	Year of evaluation	Age	Male vs. female
Demography			
Age	−0.13[b]	−0.12[c]	—
Genetics			
Family history of TS	0.15[d]	—	—
Past History			
Parents' age at birth	−0.08[e]	—	—
Pregnancy complications	0.10[c]	−0.16[d]	—
Length of labor	—	0.09[e]	—
Age bladder-bowel trained FS	—	−0.20[d]	−0.11[c]
Past history of scarlet fever	−14[b]	—	—
Past history of chorea	—	0.12[c]	0.09[c]
Past history of allergies	—	−0.08[e]	—
Neurological			
Attention deficit disorder	−0.17[b]	−0.17[d]	−0.12[c]
EEG abnormality	−0.16[c]	−0.16[c]	—
Neurological abnormality	−0.17[b]	—	—
Behavior			
Hyperactivity FS	—	−0.21[d]	−0.20[b]
Learning disorder FS	—	−0.16[c]	−0.15[c]
Anger-moodiness FS	—	−0.19[b]	—
Inhibition FS	—	0.15[c]	—
Obsessive-compulsive-like symptoms FS	—	0.21[b]	—
Obsessive-compulsive personality FS	—	0.20[b]	—
Illness variables			
Duration of present illness FS	−0.12[e]	0.98[d]	—
Previous diagnosis-consultation FS	—	−0.11[c]	—
Age at onset of TS	—	0.31[d]	—
Symptoms			
Face	—	—	−0.10[c]
Head	—	0.08[d]	−0.09[c]
Arm	−0.10[c]	0.14[b]	—
Leg	−0.14[b]	0.19[d]	−0.08[e]
Torso	—	0.09[e]	—
Inarticulate sounds	—	0.08[e]	—
Coprolalia	−0.21[d]	—	—
Copropraxia	0.11[c]	—	—
Total current tics	−0.12[b]	0.16[d]	—
Total cumulative tics	—	0.11[c]	−0.09[e]
Remission of symptoms FS	0.19[d]	−0.09[e]	—
Severity of TS	−0.37[d]	—	—

[a] See Table A.1 for list of 54 variables. Only significant variables are included in the table. Two-tailed tests; variables at $p < .01$ considered significant.
[b] $p < 0.001$.
[c] $p < 0.01$.
[d] $p < 0.0001$.
[e] $p < 0.05$.

sial data reported in the literature and may contribute substantially to the problems of heterogeneity.

AGE

The mean age at initial evaluation for the sample of 666 Tourette's disorder patients is 18.9 (SD = 12.0), with a mode of 11 and median of 14 (range 4–69) years. The mean age for our initial sample of 114 patients was 23.2 (SD = 13.6) years (Shapiro et al., 1978). The age of patients decreased significantly over the years ($r = -0.12$, $p < 0.01$), from 22.6 years for 121 patients evaluated between 1965 and 1974, to 17.4 years for 232 patients evaluated between 1979 and 1981 ($p < 0.0005$) (Table 4.1). The earlier age at diagnosis, and decreased time from onset to diagnosis, etc., reflect increased knowledge about Tourette's disorder.

The samples described in published studies have different mean ages because some include predominantly children, others adolescents or adults. Older patients are more likely to have been previously diagnosed as having Tourette's disorder ($r = 0.20$, $p < 0.0001$), more likely to have more symptoms ($r = 0.08–0.16$, $p = 0.05–0.0001$), less likely to be diagnosed as having ADD ($r = -0.17$, $p < 0.0001$), hyperactivity ($r = -0.21$, $p < 0.0001$), learning disorders ($r = -0.16$, $p < 0.01$) and EEG abnormalities ($r = -0.16$, $p < 0.01$) (Table 4.2). However, there may be a subtle effect of age on symptom reporting. Older patients have greater difficulty dating the exact age at onset of their symptoms compared to younger patients who have a shorter duration of illness. Periods of remission, especially short periods, are more likely to be remembered by younger patients or their parents. The diagnosis of ADD, especially ADD-residual-type, is more difficult to make in adulthood as earlier symptoms abate in severity, are compensated for, or are forgotten (Wender et al., 1981, 1985). For example, in our sample the diagnosis of ADD was made in 33% of Tourette's disorder patients 16 years or younger, compared with only 15% in those over 16 years of age ($p < 0.002$) (Table 4.5). Many behavioral symptoms, which are significantly more frequent in younger patients ($r = 0.16–0.21$, $p < 0.01–0.0001$) (Table 4.27), are related to the frequency and ease of diagnosing ADD in children (Tables 4.4, 4.5). Abnormal EEGs, especially borderline EEGs, tend to normalize in adulthood and may explain the inverse correlation with age ($r = -0.16$, $p < 0.02$). Whereas 28.2% of EEGs were abnormal in the younger group, only 9.2%, within normal expectation of 5 to 15%, were definitely abnormal in older patients (Table 7.8). The effects of age also have implications for studies of obsessive-compulsive-like symptoms. These symptoms were significantly associated with age ($r = 0.20–0.21$; $p < 0.001$) (Table 4.2), confirming reports in the literature that these symptoms are less frequent in childhood. This finding suggests that studies of the relationship of obsessive-compulsive symptoms and Tourette's disorder might be more fruitful if limited to adult samples.

Despite the limitations of this retrospective analysis, it is clear that age has a significant effect on many variables. In fact, some characteristics may be a function of age and duration of illness rather than intrinsic to Tourette's disorder. The effect of age and other variables associated with age should be evaluated to minimize the problem of potential heterogeneity in studies of tic disorders and Tourette's disorder.

SEX

There is a curious variability in the percent of male to females (sex ratio) reported among and within epidemiologic and clinical studies of tics and Tourette's disorder. This section examines the data to determine the source of the variability, whether the sex ratio differs for tics and Tourette's disorder and to establish base-line estimates for the sex ratio in Tourette's disorder. We then describe differential characteristics for male and female patients with Tourette's disorder.

Male to Female Ratio

The sex ratio varies considerably in studies of both tics and Tourette's disorder. The percent of males reported in general descriptive, psychopathology and treatment studies varies from 40 to 100%. We have tested several alternative hypotheses to explain these differences. Retrospective analyses were conducted to further evaluate the effect of the male to female ratio on the results of studies. We expected that the sex ratio would vary with the source of data, and would be higher for clinical samples than for nonclinical or epidemiologic samples that include a high percentage of patients with Tourette's disorder and ADD, patients with more severe forms of tic disorders, and patients evaluated in clinics or hospitals, especially those specializing in treating seriously impaired patients. Tests of hypotheses and retrospective analyses are described in the next section.

Epidemiologic Compared with Clinical Studies of Tic Disorders

Studies of tics and Tourette's disorder in the literature which included data about the male to female ratio are summarized in Table 4.3, and are classified as studies of tics or Tourette's disorder. The tic studies are subclassified into epidemiologic and clinical studies. The six epidemiologic studies randomly sampled a past history of tics. As described previously, no distinction was made between tics associated with Tourette's disorder, transient tic disorder

TABLE 4.3. *Studies citing sex ratio for Tourette and tic disorders*

Studies	Total N	Males %	Male to female ratio	ADD[a] %
Tics				
Epidemiological studies				
Boncour (1910)	417	47.8	0.91[b]	
Lapouse and Monk (1964)	58	55.2	1.18[b]	
Pringle et al. (1967)	611	58.8	1.42	
MacFarlane et al. (1954)	@75	46.7	0.87[b]	
Current study				
Normal sample	85	68.8	1.82	
Referred sample	316	51.9	1.07[b]	
Total	1,562	54.0	1.17	
Clinical Studies				
Bonheim (1930)	49	67.3	2.07	
Zausmer (1954)	96	65.6	1.91	
Pasamanick and Kawi (1956)	83	78.3	3.55	
Torup (1962)	220	74.1	2.86	
Corbett et al. (1969)	179	78.2	3.59	
Lerman and Nussbaum (1974)	50	72.0	2.57	
Total	677	73.9	2.82	
Total tic studies	2,239	60.0	1.50	
Tourette's Disorder				
Literature reviews				
Kelman (1965)	39	76.9	3.33	
Fernando (1967)	69	73.9	2.83	
Challas et al. (1967)	57	84.2	5.33	
Morphew and Sim (1969)	43	65.1	1.87	
Abuzzahab and Anderson (1974)	430	70.9	2.44	
Total	638	72.4	2.63	
Questionnaire Surveys				
Jagger et al. (1982)	75	76.0	3.17	32.7
Stefl (1983, 1984)	425	77.6	3.47	23.2
Current study (1972–1979)	221	69.6	2.29	
Total	707	75.1	3.02	
Clinical Studies				
Tourette (1885)	9	77.8	3.50	
Eisenberg et al. (1959)	7	100.0	—	
Feild et al. (1966)	7	71.4	2.50	
Challas et al. (1967)	11	63.6	1.75	
Lucas et al. (1967)	15	73.3	2.75	
Morphew and Sim (1969)	5	40.0	0.67	
Abuzzahab and Anderson (1974)	7	57.0	1.30	
Moldofsky et al. (1974)	15	93.0	14.00	
Jenkins and Fine (1976)	18	66.7	2.00	
Fisarova (1976)	18	77.8	3.50	
Cohen et al. (1978)	6	83.3	5.00	
Singer et al. (1978)	11	90.9	10.00	
Cohen et al. (1980)	25	76.0	3.17	
Singer et al. (1981)	8	87.5	7.00	
Nee et al. (1982)	30	73.3	2.75	
Lucas et al. 1982	25	76.0	3.17	
Nomura and Segawa (1982)	97	84.5	5.67	
Asam (1982)	16	87.5	7.00	

TABLE 4.3. (Continued)

Studies	Total N	Males %	Male to female ratio	ADD[a] %
Wilson et al. (1982)	21	76.2	3.20	
Montgomery et al. (1982)	15	86.7	6.50	
Bogomolny et al. (1982)	16	87.5	7.00	
Golden (1982)	80	82.5	4.71	
Borison et al. (1983)	22	63.6	1.75	
Han-bai and Han-quin (1983)	19	78.9	3.75	
Min (1983)	24	79.2	3.80	29.2
Lees et al. (1984)	53	75.5	3.08	29.2
Leckman et al. (1983)	5	100.0	—	
Leckman et al. (1984a,b)	18	94.4	17.00	66.7
Jankovic et al. (1984)	9	88.9	8.00	
Goetz et al. (1984)	21	76.2	3.20	
Comings and Comings (1984)	250	80.4	4.10	54.0
Leckman et al. (1985)	13	92.3	12.00	69.2
Erenberg et al. (1986)	200	82.5	4.71	35.0
Caine (1985)	41	90.2	9.25	29.3
Burd et al. (1986c) (6–18 years)	73	91.8	9.42	
Burd et al. (1986b) (over 18 years)	22	77.3	3.46	
Current study (1965–1981)	666	76.3	3.22	24.9
Current study (1982–1985)	288	79.7	3.92	42.4
Total	2,187	79.6	3.90	

Comparison	χ_2	df	p
Total: TS clinical studies, TS questionnaire studies, clinical tic studies, epidemiology tic studies by sex	303.4	3	0.000
TS clinical studies vs. questionnaire studies by sex	6.5	1	0.011
TS clinical and questionnaire studies vs. clinical tic studies by sex	6.9	1	0.009
All clinical TS and tic studies vs. tic epidemiology studies by sex	292.4	1	0.000

[a]Studies reporting percent of patients with attention deficit disorder. PMR between percent males and percent ADD reported in studies: $r = 0.72$, df-9, $p = 0.0117$.
[b]Male to female ratio not significant; $p(\chi^2)$ for all other comparisons 0.05–0.0001.

(TTD), or chronic motor tic (CMT) disorder and the samples may have included patients with habits, mannerisms, stereotypic and other movement disorders. The same limitation applies to the six clinical studies of tics. For example, in the study by Corbett et al. (1969), 11.6% had only motor tics and 11.4% had both vocal and motor tics, the latter probably fulfilling the current criteria for Tourette's disorder. The Tourette's disorder samples include only clinical patients evaluated or treated for the disorder.

The Tourette's disorder studies are further classified as literature reviews, questionnaire survey studies, and clinical studies. The data from the current study of patients evaluated between 1965 and 1981 and those evaluated between 1982 and 1985 are also included. Literature reviews are included for comparative purposes but will not be used in analyses because the samples in the three English studies are not independent (Kelman, 1965; Fernando, 1967; Morphew and Sim, 1969) and probably overlap somewhat with the review by Abuzzahab and Anderson (1974).

Three studies are Tourette's disorder questionnaire surveys. The first study (Jagger et al., 1982) sampled 200 members of the national Tourette Syndrome Association (TSA), of which 37.5% responded. The second study (Stefl, 1983, 1984) includes 81.3% of 530 members of the Ohio TSA. The third study consisted of 221 patients who completed our MDQ questionnaire between 1972 and 1979 but were not clinically evaluated by us. The sample consisted of patients who voluntarily responded to requests in the TSA Newsletter and those who called our clinic for information and were asked to complete the questionnaire. Our sample probably overlaps with the Jagger et al. (1982) and Stefl (1983, 1984) samples.

The Tourette's disorder clinical studies included studies published between 1885 and 1986 that described five or more patients. The data from our current study includes 666 patients who were evaluated between 1965 and 1981, and 299 patients evaluated subsequently by us between 1982 and 1985. Table 4.3 summarizes the results and chi-square partitioning.

Several differences among the samples are striking. For Tourette's disorder studies, the male to female ratio is 3.9 for the clinical studies, 3.02 for the questionnaire studies, 2.63 for the literature reviews. The ratio is 2.82 for clinical tic studies, and 1.17 for epidemiology studies ($p = 0.0000$). The male to female ratio is significantly lower for epidemiologic tic studies compared to clinical tic studies ($p = 0.0000$), for Tourette's disorder questionnaire compared to Tourette's disorder clinical studies ($p = 0.011$), for clinical tic studies compared to Tourette's disorder studies ($p = 0.009$), and for epidemiology studies compared to clinical Tourette's disorder and tic studies ($p = 0.000$). Although interpretation of these differences cannot be definitive because of different sampling methods and characteristics, several speculations deserve consideration.

The male to female ratio in the epidemiologic tic studies, averaging 1.17:1 is significantly elevated ($p = 0.0001$) for the Pringle et al. (1967) study only. It is possible that the male to female ratio is not elevated in nonclinical random samples of patients with mild tics. The Pringle et al. study (1967) rated tic frequency as frequently or sometimes. If severity of tics is related to the male to female ratio, subjects with infrequent tics should have a lower male to female ratio than subjects with frequent tics (Table 4.3). Although the percent of males with "frequent" tics is higher (63.6%) than for males with tics "sometimes" (58.1%), the difference is not significant ($\chi^2 = 1.5$, df=1, NS).

Relationship of Source of Information to Sex Ratio

The Pringle et al. study (1967) indicates that the method of eliciting a history of tics can result in a significant difference in the sex ratio. The mother's questionnaire, which may include symptoms other than tics, yielded the highest percentage of males (59.6%), a nurse obtaining a medical history yielded a lower percent (57.8%), and the physician during a medical examination elicited the lowest percentage (53.5%). The male to female ratio is significantly different for the mother's questionnaire ($p = 0.0000$) and medical history questionnaire ($p = 0.0038$), but not for the medical examination (Table 3.1). The medical examination, which included an interview and observation, may be the most reliable and valid measure. Thus, if the male to female ratio is limited to the data derived from the medical examination, there is little difference in sex ratio.

Relationship of Clinical and Nonclinical Samples to Sex Ratio

The data for epidemiologic tic studies of random nonclinical samples suggest that males may exceed females slightly (Table 4.3).

It may be that the male to female ratio is elevated only in clinical samples which include patients with more severe forms of tic disorders. This possibility is supported by the higher male to female ratio in the clinical Tourette's disorder and tic studies than in the epidemiologic tic studies ($p = 0.0000$). It is reasonable to assume that tics would be more severe in the Tourette's disorder samples and that the male to female ratio would be higher than in the clinical tic samples. This is confirmed by higher male to female sex ratios in the Tourette's disorder samples compared to the clinical tic samples ($p = 0.009$).

These results raise a number of questions. If tics and Tourette's disorder share a common etiology, differing only on a continuum of severity, it would be expected that the sex ratio would be similar for both conditions. Since the male to female ratio is approximately equal or only slightly elevated for tics in the population compared with the significantly higher male to female ratio for Tourette's disorder, it suggests different etiologies for the two tic conditions. This explanation has to be modified, however, because the true sex ratio may be distorted by the possible inclusion of habits, mannerisms, and other non-tic movements in the epidemiologic tic samples which may distort the sex ratio. If non-tic symptoms were excluded by clinicians in the clinical studies, it would result in a more reliable diagnosis of a tic condition, and a more valid difference in the male to female ratio. These questions cannot be resolved by available data and require better designed epidemiologic studies.

However, there are other variables that influence reports of the difference in the male to female ratio for tic disorders.

Relationship of Severity of Symptoms to Sex Ratio

The data suggest that the severity of symptoms is related to the sex ratio. Patients with severe Tourette's disorder symptoms are more likely to seek help and be identified than those with less severe symptoms. CMT, although probably more frequent than Tourette's disorder, is reported much less frequently in the literature. One reason for this may be that the symptoms of CMT are less severe than those of Tourette's disorder. For example, the severity of CMT is 1.7, significantly lower than the rating of 2.2 for Tourette's disorder ($p = 0.0001$) (Table 10.10). However, although there may be a relationship of severity and sex ratio in patients with tics, it does not hold for Tourette's disorder alone in our sample since the male to female ratio is unrelated to the severity of symptoms.

Relationship of Attention Deficit Disorder to Sex Ratio

The associated diagnosis of ADD is significantly associated with both the male to female ratio and severity. Estimates in the literature of the male to female ratio for ADD varies from 4:1 to 10:1. Since more males than females have ADD, we reasoned that the number of males would be positively related to the percent of Tourette's disorder patients with ADD. Nine studies in the literature provided data about the sex ratio and percent of ADD (Table 4.3). Moreover, separating Tourette's disorder patients with ADD from those without ADD might clarify whether the male to female ratio is intrinsically elevated in Tourette's disorder patients. Our hypothesis that the sex ratio is associated with ADD was supported by a significant correlation between the male to female ratio and the percent of patients with TS+ADD ($r = 0.72$, df $= 9$, $p = 0.0117$). Although the sample size is small, the results suggest that 52% of the variability for the sex ratio is accounted for by ADD.

Other data supporting the relationship of TS+ADD to the percent of males is available in two of our studies and one by Comings and Comings (1984) (Table 4.4). The sex ratio is not significantly different in the three samples. The number of males is significantly higher, however, in the TS+ADD group for all three samples (5.68, 7.13, and 5.75) than in the TS-alone group for all three samples (2.75, 2.77, and 2.97) ($p < 0.04$–0.002), averaging 6.07 for the TS+ADD group and 2.79 for the TS-alone group ($p = 0.0000$).

Moreover, the more severely afflicted ADD group in the Comings' sample had a much higher male to female ratio (19.3:1) than the mildly afflicted ADD group (3.4:1) ($p < 0.004$). Of further interest, the sex ratio in the TS+ADD groups was not significantly different in the three samples, nor was it significantly different in the TS-alone groups.

TABLE 4.4. *Relationship of sex ratio to Tourette's disorder with and without attention deficit disorder in three studies*

Studies	Males N	Males %	Females N	Females %	Total N	Total %	Male:female ratio
1. Current study (1965–1981)							
a. TS-alone	366	73.4	133	26.6	499	74.9	2.75
b. TS + ADD	142	85.0	25	15.0	167	25.1	5.68
c. Total	508	76.3	158	23.7	666	100.0	3.22
2. Current study (1981–1984)							
a. TS-alone	122	73.5	44	26.5	166	57.6	2.77
b. TS + ADD	107	87.7	15	12.3	122	42.4	7.13
c. Total	229	79.5	59	20.5	288	100.0	3.88
3. Comings and Comings (1984)							
a. TS-alone	86	74.8	29	25.2	115	46.0	2.97
b. TS + ADD	115	85.2	20	14.8	135	54.0	5.75
c. Total	201	80.4	49	19.6	250	100.0	4.10
d. TS + ADD (mild)	57	77.0	17	23.0	74	30.0	3.35
e. TS + ADD (severe)	58	95.1	3	4.9	61	24.0	19.33
f. Total	115	85.2	20	14.8	135	54.0	5.75
4. Total							
a. TS-alone	574	73.6	206	26.4	780	64.8	2.79
b. TS + ADD	364	86.0	60	14.0	424	35.2	6.07
c. Total	938	77.9	266	22.1	1204	100.0	3.53

Comparisons	χ^2	df	$p =$
1a by 1b by 2a by 2b by 3a by 3c by sex	25.1	5	0.0033
Diagnosis (1a × 1b) by sex	10.1	1	0.0016
Diagnosis (2a × 2b) by sex	8.7	1	0.0032
Diagnosis (3a × 3b) by sex	4.3	1	0.0309
Diagnosis (4a × 4b) by sex	24.7	1	0.0001
Severity of ADD by sex	8.6	1	0.033

Interaction of Age and Attention Deficit Disorder with the Sex Ratio

Our data indicated that the diagnosis of ADD was more frequent in children than adults. TS + ADD was diagnosed significantly more frequently in children and adolescents (32.6%) than in adults (14.6%) in our sample (Table 4.5).

It is common clinical experience that the diagnosis of ADD is easier to make in children and adolescents than in adults (Wender, 1981). The symptoms of ADD, especially hyperactivity, are more prominent and disruptive in childhood and more readily detected by parents, teachers, and pediatricians. Moreover, some of the symptoms, especially manifest hyperactivity, decrease

TABLE 4.5. *Relationship of sex ratio to age and diagnosis of Tourette's disorder with and without attention deficit disorder in current sample*

| | Males | | Females | | Total | | Male: female |
Age groups	N	%	N	%	N	%	ratio
16 Years or younger							
TS-alone	193	63.3	67	82.7	260	67.4	2.88
TS + ADD	112	36.7	14	17.3	126	32.6	8.00
Total	305	100.0	81	100.0	386	100.0	3.77
Over 17 years							
TS-alone	173	85.2	66	85.7	239	85.4	2.62
TS + ADD	30	14.8	11	14.3	41	14.6	2.73
Total	203	100.0	77	100.0	280	100.0	2.64
Total all ages							
TS-alone	366	73.4	133	26.6	499	74.9	2.75
TS + ADD	142	85.0	25	15.0	167	25.1	5.68
Total	508	76.3	158	23.7	666	100.0	3.22

Comparisons	χ^2	df	$p =$
Age by diagnosis by sex	3.9	3	0.003
Diagnosis by sex for 16 years or younger	11.0	1	0.001
Diagnosis by sex for over 17 years	0.1	1	NS
Age by sex	28.1	1	0.000

in adulthood or are diverted into socially acceptable outlets. We therefore reasoned that the male to female ratio should be even higher for children and adolescents than adults. Our expectations were confirmed: the sex ratio is 3.77:1 for younger patients, compared to 2.64 for older patients (Table 4.5). Moreover, for the younger group with more reliable diagnoses of ADD, the sex ratio is 8:1 for the TS+ADD group compared to 2.88:1 for the TS-alone group ($p < 0.001$) (Table 4.5).

Male to Female Ratio for the TS-Alone Group

The data also provide a possible answer to the question of whether the male to female ratio is elevated in the TS-alone group and provide a more meaningful estimate of the magnitude of the male to female ratio. The most reliable data (Tables 4.4, 4.5) indicate that the male to female ratio is elevated in Tourette's disorder ranging from 2.6 to 3.0:1. It is likely, however, that it would be even lower in nonclinical random samples of individuals with Tourette's disorder, CMT, and TTD.

Other Variables and the Male to Female Ratio

The relationship of other variables to the sex ratio in the TS-alone group warrants further analysis. These variables include severity of Tourette's disorder, specialized clinic versus private practice settings, nonclinical epidemiological versus clinical samples, presence or absence of a family history of Tourette's disorder or CMT or both, age at onset of Tourette's disorder, presence or absence of type, location and frequency of symptoms (simple versus complex, head versus limbs versus torso, coprophilia, echophilia, etc.), presence or absence of associated psychopathology (obsessive-compulsive-like symptoms or impulsions, obsessive-compulsive disorder, learning disorders, affective disorder, and other psychopathology), and comparison among tic categories (Tourette's disorder, CMT, TTD, sensory tic subtype of Tourette's disorder, and atypical tic or movement disorder).

The relationship between the percent of ADD patients in Tourette's disorder samples, the percent in nonclinical samples, and the relationship with other variables has important consequences for studies of Tourette's disorder and the problem of heterogeneity. These issues are discussed more fully later in this chapter.

Summary and Conclusion About Sex Ratio

This review of the sex ratio suggests the following conclusions: The male to female ratio is lowest in epidemiological tic studies of nonclinical random samples, averaging 1.17:1 (range 0.91–1.82), increases significantly to 1.50:1 (range 1.91–3.59) for clinical patients with tics, increases to 2.63:1 (1.87–5.33) in literature reviews of Tourette's disorder, increases to 3.02:1 (range 2.29–3.47) in Tourette's disorder questionnaire surveys, and is highest 3.90:1 (range 0.67:1–100%) in clinical studies of Tourette's disorder. The male to female ratio increases in patients with more severe forms of tic disorder such as Tourette's disorder compared with CMT, and with severity of ADD. However, the higher male to female ratio in Tourette's disorder appears to be real because when TS+ADD patients, who have an average male to female ratio of 6.07:1 (range 5.68–7.13:1), are separated from patients with TS-alone, the male to female ratio averages 2.79:1 (range 2.75–2.97). Future study of etiology, heterogeneity, neurological mechanisms, psychopathology, and treatment should include analyses of TS-alone and TS+ADD, and both groups combined. The effect of other variables and their interaction with the male to female ratio requires further study.

Differences Between Male and Female Patients

Based on our general hypothesis that tic and Tourette's disorders are not associated with psychopathology and other variables, we hypothesized that the major differences between the sexes would be an increased percent of ADD and other neurological factors in male subjects; our expectations were confirmed when we compared the groups using correlations (Table 4.2), t-tests and the summary SRA (Table 4.6). The higher percent of facial tics in male subjects (95%) than in female (89%) and head tics in male subjects (93%) than in female (87%) may be chance results but warrant further study.

The conclusion is that male and female samples are similar and can be studied as one group if the groups are matched on variables such as ADD and other CNS disorders known to be more frequent in males.

RACE AND PLACE OF BIRTH

Most patients and their parents are white and born in the United States (Table 4.7). Although black and Hispanic patients are infrequent in tic samples, their numbers have increased considerably since 1981. We have evaluated over 50 black and Hispanic patients. A possible reason for the increase is the greater dispersal of information about tic disorders. Our impression, however, is that the proportion of black and Hispanic patients is still less than population estimates and that increased information about Tourette's disorder should be provided to these groups.

Our sample and the proliferation of reports from all parts of the world (Table 4.3) indicate that Tourette's disorder is universal and is unrelated to race or national background.

ETHNIC AND RELIGIOUS BACKGROUND

Reports in the literature prior to 1978 (Table 4.8) described samples with a higher than expected proportion of patients with East European and Jewish (Ashkenazi) background. In our previous sample of 114 patients, one or both parents were East European in 48.2% of patients and one or both parents were Jewish in 56.1% of patients, decreasing to 25% in a subsample of consecutive patients evaluated in 1980 (Shapiro and Shapiro, 1982).

When we combined this with the observation that torsion dystonia is more frequent in East Europeans, a possible vulnerability of Ashkenazim to Tourette's disorder was suggested. Although the percentage has decreased to 40.1% in our more recent sample, it is still higher than expected (Table 4.7). However, other investigators do not report a higher prevalence of East Europeans, or Ashkenazim. Nee et al. (1980) reported that the percentage of Jews with Tourette's disorder was similar to the percentage of Jews with other

TABLE 4.6. *Variables significantly differentiating male and female patients with Tourette's disorder and summary stepwise regression analysis[a]*

Variables	Mean or percent		Parameter estimate $p =$
	Males	Females	
Demography	—	—	—
Genetics	—	—	—
Past history			
Bladder-bowel trained FS	4.5	1.8	0.0008
Neurological			
Attention deficit disorder	28.0%	15.8%	0.002
Neurological abnormality	1.4	1.2	0.027
Behavior			
Hyperactivity FS	1.4	1.0	0.0003
Learning disorder FS	0.7	0.4	0.0019
Illness Variables	—	—	—
Symptoms			
History of facial tics	94.5%	88.6%	0.011
History of head tics	92.5%	86.7%	0.025
History of leg tics	42.9%	33.5%	0.036
Total current tics	7.2	6.2	0.0319
Total cumulative tics	16.2	14.2	0.0194
Other variables[b]			
Bender-Gestalt Test	0.9	0.5	0.005
Conners Hyperactivity Index	12.7	9.9	0.0065

	Summary stepwise regression analysis		
Variables	r	R^2	Parameter estimate
Facial tics	0.10	0.06	0.41[d]
Hyperactivity FS	0.20	0.11	0.08[e]
Head tics	0.09	0.13	0.22[e]
Neurological abnormality	0.10	0.15	0.12[e]
Adjusted R^2		0.13[d]	

[a]See Table A.1 for list of 54 variables. Two-tailed t-test; variables at $p < 0.01$ are considered significant.
[b]Other variables added to the list.
[c]$p < 0.01$.
[d]$p < 0.0001$.
[e]$p < 0.05$.

TABLE 4.7. Demographic features of sample[a]

Sample description	N	%
Age		
10 years or less	172	25.8
11–14 years	164	24.6
15–25 years	168	25.2
25 or more years	162	24.3
Race		
White	640	96.1
Black	11	1.7
Biracial	4	0.6
Oriental	4	0.6
Other[b]	7	1.1
Parents' place of birth		
Both parents, USA	489	73.4
One parent foreign born	72	10.8
Both parents foreign born	89	13.4
Unknown	16	2.4
Patients' place of birth		
United States	621	93.2
Other English speaking	9	1.4
Germany	3	0.5
Poland	2	0.3
Italian	2	0.3
Spain	3	0.5
Other Mediterranean	2	0.3
South America	2	0.3
Puerto Rico	6	0.9
Scandinavia	2	0.3
Other	14	2.1
Ethnic background[b]		
East European (Jewish)[c]	239	35.9
East European (Non-Jewish)	458	8.7
Other (Jewish)	28	4.2
Italian	150	22.5
Other[d]	191	28.7

	Mother		Father	
Religion	N	%	N	%
Roman Catholic	243	36.5	245	36.8
Greek Orthodox	13	2.0	16	2.4
Jewish	267	40.1	260	39.0
Protestant	123	18.5	125	18.8
Other[d]	9	1.4	8	1.2
None	7	1.1	7	1.1
Unknown	4	0.6	5	0.8

[a]$N = 666$.
[b]One or more parents.
[c]Ashkenazi.
[d]Other: American Indian, Hispanic, Arab, Mexican, Greek, Indonesian.

TABLE 4.8. Studies citing percent Tourette patients with Jewish and East European (Ashkenazi) background[a]

Study	Place of study	Total sample N	Jewish East European		Jewish Non-East European		Total Jewish	
			N	%	N	%	N	%
Mahler et al. (1945)	Columbia University Medical School, New York	33	—	—	—	—	22	66.7
Shapiro et al. (1978)[b]	Cornell University Medical School, New York	114	—	—	—	—	64	56.1
Eldridge et al. (1976)	Tourette Syndrome Association, New York	21	31	61.9	—	—	13	61.7
Wassman et al. (1978)	Minnesota	15	—	—	—	—	4	26.7
Nee et al. (1980)	National Institutes of Health, Bethesda	50	—	—	10	20.0	70	20.0
Golden (1982)	Albert Einstein College of Medicine, New York	43	12	28.0	—	—	12	28.0
Lucas et al. (1982)	University of Texas, Galveston	32	—	—	1	2.7	1	2.7
	Rochester, Minnesota	24	—	—	2	8.3	2	8.3
Coming and Comings (1984)	City of Hope Hospital, Duarte, California	250	—	—	25	10.0	25	10.0
Lees et al. (1984)	Tourette Syndrome Association, England	53	7	13.2	—	—	7	13.2
Burd et al. (1986b)	North Dakota	73	0	0.0	0	0.0	0	0.0
Current study[b]	Cornell and Mount Sinai Medical Schools, New York	666	239	35.9	28	4.2	267	40.1

[a] One or both parents.
[b] Shapiro et al. (1978) data included in current study.

medical conditions treated at the National Institutes of Health in Bethesda. Golden's (1982) percentage decreased from 28% in New York to 2.7% in Galveston, Texas. Decreased percentages also are reported in Minnesota (8.3%) (Lucas et al., 1982), California (10.0%) (Comings and Comings, 1984), England (13.2%) (Lees et al., 1984), and none in North Dakota (Burd et al., 1986 a,b). It is not known, however, whether these percentages exceed population estimates because all of the studies, with the exception of the Nee et al. (1980) study, did not use an appropriate control group. It is fairly certain, however, that the high percentages of Askhenazim in our sample is due to ascertainment bias, and it is likely that the percentage does not exceed the frequency in the population.

GENETICS

Tourette's disorder is referred to as a syndrome because the etiology is unknown and the diagnosis is based on signs, symptoms, and clinical course.

The term *syndrome* refers to a set of symptoms that occur together associated with an illness whose etiology is unknown and for which there is no specific diagnostic test (*Dorland's Illustrated Medical Dictionary*, 1981). Thus, syndromes are heuristically separated from diseases to keep open the question of whether the observed signs, symptoms, and causes are due to one or several illnesses. Historically, many syndromal illnesses were thought to be one illness, but with the accumulation of additional data it was determined that they were related to more than one disease entity. A classic example of this is the diagnosis of dropsy (edema). We now know that dropsy is a symptom of many illnesses, such as congestive heart failure, liver disease, carcinomatosis, and so on. On the other hand, some symptoms formerly believed to be associated with many different illnesses were later determined to be due to one illness. Examples of this are the diagnoses of syphilis and pellagra. Although Tourette's disorder and tics are referred to in DSM-III as disorders, the question of whether they represent one or many illnesses has not been resolved (Shapiro et al., 1978; Caine et al., 1982, 1984). Until such time, we refer to the symptoms as a syndrome. Deriving a test that is specific for the disease, or, even better, identifying the pathophysiology would resolve the issue. Without specific data, genetic studies become important. Genetic data are also potentially useful when studying etiology, management, treatment, prognosis, and for genetic counseling.

The observation that Tourette's disorder, CMT, and other tic disorders tend to cluster in families has been noted for over 100 years (Trousseau, 1873; Gilles de la Tourette, 1885; Chabbert, 1893; Koester, 1899; Zausmer, 1954; Pasamanick and Kawi, 1956; Torup, 1962; Connell et al., 1967; Shapiro et al., 1972b, 1973b, 1978; Lucas, 1973; Friel, 1973; Arena et al., 1974; Eldridge et al., 1977; Wassman et al., 1978, Guggenheim, 1979;, Hajal and Leach, 1981;

Matthews, 1981). Guggenheim (1979) described a family in which 17 of 43 members over five generations had Tourette's disorder or CMT. As the number of patients available for study increased so has the interest of geneticists and an increase in genetics studies of tic disorders (see references in Tables 4.12, 4.14; also Baron et al. 1981; Kidd et al., 1980, 1982; Pauls et al., 1981, 1984; Comings and Comings, 1984). These studies are discussed in further detail in Chapter 9.

This section focuses primarily on the data for our sample. It provides information that may be helpful to patients, families, genetic counselors, and for future genetic research. Our data are compared with published studies in an attempt to confirm or reject various hypotheses and to identify areas that require further study. Chapter 9 focuses on the development of genetic research, models, theories, and orientations for future genetic studies.

It is difficult to compare studies, especially random samples in epidemiologic studies, consecutive private or clinical samples and questionnaire surveys of TSA volunteers (Eldridge et al., 1977; Nee et al., 1980; Schoenberg, 1982; Golden, 1982; Kondo and Nomura, 1982; Stefl, 1983, 1984). Although similar diagnostic criteria for Tourette's disorder are used by most researchers, the diagnostic criteria for CMT have not been standardized. This diagnosis is a loose one and may include patients with a history in childhood of transient tics, acute or chronic single or multiple motor or vocal tics, chronic motor tic as defined in DSM III, sensory tics and atypical movement disorders, stereotypic movements, dystonic disorders, and so on. A history of CMT in the family of Tourette's disorder patients may be under- or overestimated. It is common experience for parents to deny having tics, even when they are obvious to the clinician and to their families. Historical information about tics in relatives is limited and is usually underestimated. Pauls et al. (1984) has provided some preliminary data suggesting that interviews of relatives elicit a diagnosis of Tourette's disorder 5.5 times more frequently and a diagnosis of CMT 1.5 times more frequently (1.9 times more frequently for both diagnoses) than does an interview of the patient or family about their relatives. On the other hand, some informants, motivated by their desire to be complete and inclusive, or due to lack of knowledge about what constitutes a tic, cite many transient habits, mannerisms, stereotypic movements, compulsions, and other symptoms as tics. Researchers too may be overinclusive in their zeal to study the problem. For example, a researcher cited a parent as having a vocal tic in childhood when she reported voluntarily imitating a cat sound for a short period as a child.

Another problem that may bias results is the potential differences between patients seeking a clinical evaluation compared with individuals who have never sought evaluation and treatment (Cohen and Cohen, 1984; Robins et al., 1984).

There are probably many more patients with a tic disorder than are reported in studies. This conclusion is suggested by epidemiological surveys

(Tables 3.1, 3.2, 4.3) and the finding that 70% of interviewed relatives never sought help for their symptoms (Pauls et al., 1984). It is not known how non-help-seekers, possibly with less severe symptoms, differ from those who seek help.

The diagnosis of Tourette's disorder or CMT in the patient and primary family (parents, siblings, children) in our sample is more reliable than in secondary relatives. The diagnosis of Tourette's disorder in secondary relatives is easier to make than the diagnosis of CMT. The symptoms for CMT are usually less severe, are more apt to remit, are less obvious, perhaps more intermittent, and the range of symptoms is poorly remembered or less clearly described by primary relatives. Considerable time, however, was given during the evaluation and subsequent inquiry, to elicit reliable information to confirm diagnoses. Our data includes the percent of relatives with a past or current history of Tourette's disorder, transient tics, CMT, or multiple motor tics. Our category for CMT may differ from other reports which may exclude relatives with a history of one or more of the previous diagnoses. Most studies fail to specify inclusion and exclusion criteria for CMT. A family history of other movement disorders is not included since it is not significantly associated with any of our data. Fifty-eight patients (9.0%, not significantly different from expectations) had a family history of diverse movement disorders such as essential and senile tremor, focal, segmental or generalized dystonia, stereotypic movement disorder, Parkinson disease, and so on.

Relatives with Tourette or Tic Disorders

The genetic samples consist of 641 Tourette patients. Twenty-two adopted patients were not included because information was not available for the biological families. Three additional patients were excluded because family data were lacking. Table 4.9 tabulates the number and type of family member with Tourette's disorder and other tic disorders. Percentages are given only for relatives in the primary family because informants frequently cannot specify the exact number of relatives, or have lost contact with most of their relatives. As indicated in Table 4.9, 39 (1.5%) of 2,631 primary family members had Tourette's disorder, 245 (9.3%) had a tic disorder, and 284 (10.8%) had either a tic or Tourette's disorder. For both primary and secondary family members, 61 had Tourette's disorder, 434 had a tic disorder, and 495 had either one or the other disorder.

Siblings

Our data provide estimates for the chance of a sibling having tic disorders (Table 4.9). For example, the chance of a brother having Tourette's disorder

TABLE 4.9. *History of tic disorder in primary and other family members*

Family member	Total relatives N	Tourette's disorder N	Tourette's disorder %	Tic disorders N	Tic disorders %	TS or tic disorders N	TS or tic disorders %
Primary family members							
Parents							
Father	641	13	2.0	103	16.1	116	18.1
Mother	641	6	0.9	66	10.2	72	11.3
Total	1,282	19	1.5	170	12.3	189	14.7
Siblings[b]							
Brother	568	9	1.6	41	7.2	50	8.8
Sister	618	5	0.8	20	3.2	25	4.0
Total	1,186	14	1.2	61	5.1	75	6.3
Children[c]							
Son	78	5	6.4	8	10.3	13	16.7
Daughter	85	1	1.2	6	7.1	7	8.2
Total	163	6	3.7	14	8.6	20	12.3
Total	2,631	39	1.5	245	9.3	284	10.8
Other family members[a]							
Paternal grandfather	—	—	—	11	—	11	—
Paternal grandmother	—	—	—	8	—	8	—
Maternal grandfather	—	1	—	14	—	15	—
Maternal grandmother	—	1	—	15	—	16	—
Paternal uncle	—	2	—	19	—	21	—
Paternal aunt	—	—	—	19	—	19	—
Paternal cousin	—	4	—	17	—	21	—
Paternal great uncle	—	—	—	7	—	7	—
Paternal great aunt	—	—	—	2	—	2	—
Maternal uncle	—	4	—	19	—	23	—
Maternal aunt	—	—	—	11	—	11	—
Maternal cousin	—	7	—	33	—	40	—
Maternal great uncle	—	—	—	5	—	5	—
Maternal great aunt	—	2	—	6	—	8	—
Patient nephew	—	1	—	2	—	3	—
Patient niece	—	—	—	1	—	1	—
Total	—	22	—	189	—	211	—
Total	—	61	—	434	—	495	—

[a]Tic disorders include a history of chronic motor tic and transient tic disorder.
[b]Excludes 22 adopted patients and 3 patients with inadequate knowledge of their family history.
[c]Seventy-one patients had a total of 165 children; 2 adopted children excluded.
[d]Total number of relatives unknown.

is 1.6% and 7.2% for tics; the chance of a sister having Tourette's disorder is 0.8% for the disorder and 3.2% for tics.

These results were compared with available data in the literature. Similar percentages for siblings were reported in our sample and in the first three studies in Table 4.11 which include unselected consecutive patients. Percentages for the last three studies are higher than for our sample, possibly because of selection factors associated with volunteer samples. The highest percent-

TABLE 4.10. *Summary table of history of tic disorders in family members*[a]

Family member	Total relatives N	Tourette's disorder N	Tourette's disorder %	Tic disorders[b] N	Tic disorders[b] %	TS or tic disorders N	TS or tic disorders %
History of disorder in family[c,d]							
Primary family	641	35	5.5	207	32.3	227	35.4[e]
Other family members	641	15	2.3	64	10.0	74	11.5[e]
Total	641	50	7.8	271	42.3	301	47.0[e]
Number of individuals							
Primary family							
Parents	1,282	19	1.5	170	13.3	189	14.7[g]
Siblings	1,186	14	1.2	61	5.1	75	6.3[g]
Children[f]	163	6	3.7	14	8.6	20	12.3[g]
Total	2,631	39	1.5	245	9.3	284	10.9[g]
Other family members							
Paternal family[h]	—	6	27.3	83	43.9	89	42.2[g]
Maternal family[i]	—	15	71.4	103	55.4	118	57.0[g]
Patient family[j]	—	1	1.3	3	1.6	4	1.9[g]
Total	—	22	100.0	189	100.0	211	100.0[g]
Total	—	61	—	434	—	495	—
Sex of relative							
Primary family							
Males	—	27	69.2	153	62.4	180	63.4[g]
Females	—	12	30.8	92	37.6	104	36.6[g]
Other family members							
Males	—	16	72.7	105	55.6	121	57.3[g]
Females	—	6	27.3	84	44.4	90	42.7[g]
Total							
Males	—	43	70.5	258	59.4	301	60.8[g]
Females	—	18	29.5	176	40.6	194	39.2[g]

[a]Shapiro et al. (1965–1981).
[b]Tic disorders include a history of chronic motor tic and transient tic disorder.
[c]History of tic disorder in one or more members in a family.
[d]Excludes 22 adopted patients and 3 patients with inadequate knowledge of their family history.
[e]History of Tourette's or tic disorder in one or more members in a family.
[f]Excludes 2 adopted children.
[g]Total number of individuals with a history of a tic disorder.
[h]Includes paternal grandparents, aunts, uncles, cousins.
[i]Includes maternal grandparents, aunts, uncles, cousins.
[j]Includes nephew and niece.

ages are reported in a study of a small sample of patients primarily referred by the Tourette Syndrome Association (Pauls et al., 1984). All relatives in this study were interviewed, in contrast to other published studies in which patients or primary family members were interviewed for information about relatives. Higher percentages of Tourette's disorder and CMT were obtained from the interviewed relatives compared to the percentages reported for noninterviewed relatives (Pauls et al., 1981). Although a more conclusive study would compare the percentages elicited by interview of patients or informants with percentages obtained after interview of the relatives, with the use of a larger sample, more precise descriptions of the criteria for CMT and

TABLE 4.11. Studies citing siblings with Tourette and tic disorders[a]

Siblings	Current study (1965–1981)[b] (N = 1,186) %	Kondo and Nomura (1982)[b] (N = 49) %	Pauls et al. (1981)[b] (N = 86) %	Kidd et al. (1980)[c] (N = 99) %	Pauls and Kidd (1981)[c,d] (N = 185) %	Pauls et al. (1984)[c,e] (N = 44) %
Brother						
TS	1.6	—	—	—	2.7	6.8
CMT	7.2	—	—	—	8.6	9.1
Total	8.8	8.2	10.5	12.1	11.4	15.9
Sister						
TS	0.8	—	—	—	0.5	4.5
CMT	3.2	—	—	—	5.4	6.8
Total	4.0	0.0	5.8	6.1	5.9	11.4
Total						
TS	1.2	—	—	—	3.2	11.4
CMT	5.1	—	—	—	14.1	15.9
Total	6.3	8.2	16.3	18.2	17.3	27.3

[a]Tourette disorder: TS; chronic motor tic disorder: CMT.
[b]Unselected consecutive clinical patients.
[c]Tourette Syndrome Association volunteers.
[d]Combined sample of Kidd et al. (1980) and Pauls et al. (1981).
[e]Relatives interviewed.

reliability data, the results suggest that a family history method underestimates tic disorders in relatives.

An important limitation in all studies is that the age of siblings is not specified and many siblings may not be old enough to have reached the age of risk for Tourette's disorder or a tic disorder. The age of siblings should be included in future studies. A similar limitation applies to children at risk described in the next section.

Children

For 163 children of patients with Tourette's disorder, 3.7% had Tourette's disorder, 8.6% had a tic disorder, and 12.3% had either Tourette's or a tic disorder. The chances of a son having Tourette's disorder is 6.4% and for CMT 10.3%: The chances of a daughter having Tourette's disorder is 1.2% and for CMT 7.1% (Table 4.9). Data in the literature about the vulnerability of children of Tourette's disorder patients are not available. Future studies should use age-corrected samples of children, or study older children who have passed the vulnerable age period for the development of a tic disorder.

History of Tic Disorders in One or More Family Members

A history of Tourette's disorder was present in one or more primary family members for 5.5% of probands, a history of a tic disorder for 32.3%, and

35.4% for Tourette's disorder or a tic disorder (Table 4.10). The corresponding percentages for all family members is 7.8% for Tourette's disorder, 42.3% for tics, and 46.7% for tics or Tourette's disorder. The percentage of other family members with a history of Tourette's disorder or tics is significantly less than for primary family members, especially for tics. This might be due to decreased genetic loading, or to inadequate information about the extended family. The latter alternative is suggested by the results of the Pauls et al. (1984) study of interviewed relatives.

All published studies reporting genetic information in one or more primary family members are summarized in Table 4.12. The studies are grouped into four categories: (1) consecutive Tourette's disorder patients; (2) consecutive Oriental Tourette's disorder patients; (3) referred Tourette's disorder patients, primarily by the Tourette Syndrome Association (TSA); and (4) patients with tics. Category 1 and 2 are considered more representative of patient samples than are referred samples, which may include more severely afflicted patients, more of whom have ADD and other unspecified difficulties (Stefl, 1983). However, the percent of relatives with tic or Tourette's disorder in our questionnaire survey (TSA referred) sample did not differ from the percent reported in our interviewed sample (Table 4.12). It may be that TSA volunteers, who may be more severely afflicted, are more motivated to obtain information about other family members with tic disorders. The percent of relatives with Tourette's disorder or tics reported in Oriental and non-Oriental samples is not significantly different (see χ^2 comparisons in Table 4.12), but is significantly lower in the Oriental samples for tic disorder and total Tourette's disorder or tics, primarily because tics are reported less frequently in relatives. As expected, Tourette's disorder and total Tourette's disorder and tics are significantly more frequent in the referred TSA patient samples than in consecutive clinical Tourette's disorder patients, but the percent for tic disorder is not significantly different. This suggests that referred or volunteer samples report significantly more relatives with Tourette's disorder than clinical samples but similar percentages for relatives with tic disorders. Tic disorders tend to be reported similarly in all samples (Table 4.12). Whether these differences are meaningful or not requires further study. A conservative estimate, based on consecutive Tourette's disorder patient samples, of a history of Tourette's disorder in one or more primary family members is 7.0%, for tics 32%, and for either Tourette's disorder or tics 33%.

Relationship Between Tourette's Disorder and Tic Disorders

We previously suggested the likelihood that Tourette's disorder, CMT, or other tic disorders were similar disorders differing only on a continuum of duration, number, frequency, type, location, and severity of symptoms (Shapiro et al., 1978). This hypothesis has been given support by several family

TABLE 4.12. *Studies citing history of Tourette or tic disorder in one or more primary family members of probands with Tourette's disorder[a]*

	Total Tourette probands N	TS %	Diagnosis of relative	
			Tic disorder %	TS or tic disorder %
Studies				
1. Consecutive TS patients[b]				
Current study	641	5.5	32.3	35.4
Lucas and Rodin (1973)	21	—	—	4.8
Moldofsky et al. (1974)	15	—	—	66.7
Wassman et al. (1978)	14	—	—	35.7
Golden (1982)	75	21.3	32.0	40.0
Lucas et al. (1982)[c]	25	—	—	12.0
Asam (1982)	16	—	—	18.8
Erenberg et al. (1986)	200	—	—	37.0
Total	1,011	7.1	32.1	34.9
2. Consecutive Oriental TS patients[b]				
Kondo and Nomura (1982)	42	—	—	16.7
Lieh-Mak et al. (1982)[d]	15	—	13.3	13.3
Han-bai and Han-quin (1983)	19	5.3	—	5.3
Min (1983)	24	—	8.3	8.3
Total	100	5.3	12	12.0
Total consecutive patients	1,111	7.0	30.7	32.9
3. Selected referral of TS patients				
Eldridge et al. (1977)[e]	21	—	—	85.7
Nee et al (1980)[e,f]	50	32.0	32.0	64.0
Stefl (1983)[e]	397	12.4	31.0	43.3
Montgomery et al. (1982)[g]	15	—	—	60.0
Lees et al. (1984)[e]	53	—	—	45.3
Current questionnaire study	208	6.0	29.5	33.0
Total	744	13.3	29.9	43.5
4. Patients with Tics				
Zausmer (1954)[h]	96	—	—	31.3
Corbett et al. (1969)[i]	180	—	—	10.0
Total	276	—	—	17.4

Comparisons	TS			Tic disorder			TS or tic disorder		
	χ^2	df	$p=$	χ^2	df	$p=$	χ^2	df	$p=$
Sample 1 vs. 2 vs. 3	17.2	2	0.000	8.2	2	0.016	50.3	2	0.000
Sample 1 vs. 2	6.1	1	NS	8.2	1	0.004	19.0	1	0.000
Sample (1+2) vs. 3	17.6	1	0.000	0.1	1	NS	33.7	1	0.000
(Sample 1 vs. 3)	17.3	1	0.000	0.0	1	NS	23.5	1	0.000
(Sample 1 vs. 4)	—	—	—	—	—	—	15.4	1	0.000

[a]Tourette's disorder: TS.
[b]Consecutive clinical patients.
[c]Survey of enclosed community.
[d]Government records.
[e]Tourette Syndrome Association volunteers.
[f]Referrals to National Institutes of Health, Bethesda.
[g]Selected referrals.
[h]Patients described as having tics.
[i]Largely patients with tics, some TS.

studies (Kidd et al., 1980; Baron et al., 1981; Pauls et al., 1981; Comings and Comings, 1984; Price et al., 1985). However, these studies offer only indirect support for the tic disorder continuum hypothesis. A more definitive study requires concurrent comparison of patients in Tourette's disorder, CMT, and other tic disorder categories. Similarities and differences among tic disorders are discussed more fully in Chapter 10.

Sex Ratio of Relatives with Tic Disorders

As expected, and as previously reported by us (Shapiro et al., 1978), male relatives exceed female relatives for all relative categories: Tourette's disorder, tics and Tourette's disorder, or tics; fathers versus mothers, brothers versus sisters, sons versus daughters, total males versus total females in both primary family and other family members (Tables 4.9–4.12). Predominance of male relatives has also been reported in other studies (Kidd et al., 1980; Pauls et al., 1981; Baron et al., 1981; Price et al., 1985; Pauls et al., 1984) but not in two recent studies (Comings and Comings, 1984; Pauls et al., 1986a). These differences may be due to sampling differences. It is another indication of the necessity of establishing precise definitions and criteria for tics, Tourette's disorder and tic disorders, differential diagnosis for atypical non-tic movement disorders, associated symptoms, psychopathology, and other organic disorders to ensure meaningful future research on Tourette's disorder.

Higher Frequency of Tics Disorders in Families of Female Patients

We previously reported that families of female patients had a higher frequency of Tourette's disorder and tics than male patients (Shapiro et al., 1978). Similar results were reported by others (Kidd et al., 1980; Pauls et al., 1981; Baron et al., 1981; Pauls et al., 1984). This pattern is even more apparent in our current sample. The maternal compared with the paternal family included 71.4% versus 27.3% of relatives with a history of Tourette's disorder, 55.4% versus 43.9% with a history of a tic disorder, and 57.0% versus 42.2% with a history of Tourette's disorder or a tic disorder (Table 4.10).

Increased Risk of Tic Disorder to Siblings and Children Who Have a Sibling and Parents with Tic Disorders

Two studies provide evidence that there is an increased risk of another sibling developing a tic disorder if one sibling has Tourette's disorder and the parents have a tic disorder (Table 4.13).

The first study (Comings and Comings, 1984) demonstrated that Tourette's disorder in one parent, and especially Tourette's disorder or CMT in both

TABLE 4.13. Increased risk of tic disorder for siblings who have a sibling with Tourette's disorder and parents with tic disorders, and the risk of tic disorder for children of parents with tic disorders[a]

Studies and affected parents	Total N	% Risk in siblings		
		TS	CMT	Total
Comings and Comings (1984)[b]				
1. Neither parent affected	291	1.7	7.2	8.9
2. One parent affected with CMT	74	1.4	12.2	14.1
3. One parent with TS	36	8.3	13.9	22.2
4. Both parents with TS or CMT	12	25.0	16.7	41.7
5. One or both parents with TS or CMT	122	5.7	13.1	18.9
Total	413	2.9	9.0	11.9
Pauls et al. (1984)[b]				
6. Neither parent affected	18	0.0	5.6	5.6
7. One or both parents with TS or CMT	26	19.2	23.1	42.3
Total	44	11.3	13.6	25.0
		Percent risk in children		
Abe and Oda (1980)[c]				
8. Parents without tics	76	—	—	9.6
9. Parents with tics	177	—	—	19.7
Total	253	—	—	12.6

Comparisons	TS			CMT			Total		
	χ^2	df	$p=$	χ^2	df	$p=$	χ^2	df	$p=$
1,2,3,4	29.6	3	0.0000	5.2	4	NS	16.5	3	0.0000
4 vs. (1,2,3)	23.9	1	0.0000	—	—	NS	10.5	1	0.0012
3 vs. (1,2)	7.4	1	0.0067	—	—	NS	3.1	1	0.0236
2 vs. 1	0.0	1	NS	—	—	NS	1.4	1	NS
6 vs. 7	—	—	0.068[d]	—	—	NS[d]	7.2	1	0.007
8 vs. 9	—	—	—	—	—	—	4.9	1	0.026

[a]Tourette's disorder: TS; chronic motor tic: CMT.
[b]The effect on a sibling who has a sibling with TS and parents with tic disorders.
[c]The effect on children who have parents with tic disorders.
[d]Fisher Exact Test.

parents, significantly increased the risk of Tourette's disorder among siblings of patients, with a nonsignificant trend for CMT (see χ^2 analysis in Table 4.13). Pauls et al. (1984), in a study of interviewed relatives of Tourette's syndrome volunteers, reported a nonsignificant trend for a higher rate of Tourette's disorder and CMT in siblings if their sibling had Tourette's disorder and their parents had either Tourette's disorder or CMT. Abe and Oda (1980) reported significantly ($p < 0.03$) more tics in children of parents with tics compared with parents without tics (Table 4.13).

These preliminary studies suggest increased vulnerability for Tourette's disorder and CMT among siblings of patients with affected parents and for children of parents with tics. Larger samples are required and analyses should consider patient and parental sex, age at risk for samples, the diagnosis of Tourette's disorder or CMT and TTD among patients, parents, siblings, children, and other relatives. Interviews with family members are highly desirable. Such an analysis would provide more meaningful estimates of vulnerability of various family members.

Twinship

Study of twins provides additional and more definitive support for the importance of genetic factors in Tourette's disorder and CMT. Our twin data are independent of data on twins reported in the literature except for the study by Price et al. (1985) (Table 4.14). These data total 16 monozygotic (MZ), four same-sex dizygotic (DZ), and seven opposite-sex dizygotic twin pairs (χ^2 comparisons of the data in our sample with data in the literature are not significantly different). The largest series of MZ and same-sex dizygotic twins and the most thorough analysis of twin data is provided in the Price et al. (1985) study. It is based on 40 respondents to a mailed TSA questionnaire. This study is described separately because an unknown number of twin pairs overlap with our sample and other published reports. The distribution, however, for same-sex MZ twins in the Price at al. study and compared to other reports is not significantly different ($\chi^2 = 1.5$, df=2, NS). Limitations of this study include possible ascertainment bias because respondents were nonrandom TSA volunteers, an unknown number of twin pairs were young and could have developed Tourette's disorder or CMT subsequently, and possible diagnostic bias since the diagnosis for 38 subjects was by other physicians, confirmed by questionnaire and phone interviews, but not by personal interview. The lower ascertainment of DZ than MZ twins also suggests possible bias in ascertainment, since DZ twins are usually more frequent than MZ twins in twin studies (Price et al., 1985). A limitation for all twin studies is that determination of zygosity is based on physical similarity and the degree of difficulty telling twins apart in childhood, and not on genetic markers (Cohen et al., 1975).

The data in Table 4.14 suggest that concordance for Tourette's disorder and CMT in the combined group and Price study ranges from 77 to 87% for MZ twins and 23 to 25% for same-sex DZ twins. All seven opposite-sex DZ twins were discordant. These data provide considerable evidence for a genetic etiology for Tourette's disorder and CMT. However, the data also suggest heterogeneity, nonfamilial or nongenetic forms of Tourette's disorder and CMT, and that congenital, environmental, or developmental factors may cause tic disorders or be necessary for their expression of tic disorders.

Price et al. (1985) also reported family history data. The percent of first-

TABLE 4.14. Studies citing Tourette and tic disorders in monozygotic and dizygotic twins[a]

Twin type and study	Concordant for TS N	%	Concordant for CMT N	%	Discordant N	%	Total N
MZ (same sex)							
Current study[b,h]	7	70	2	20[j]	1	10	10
Other reports							
Ellison (1964)[c]	—	—	—	—	1	—	1
Escalar et al. (1972)[c]	1	—	—	—	—	—	1
Frost et al. (1976)[d]	—	—	1[i]	—	—	—	1
Wassman et al. (1978)	1	—	—	—	—	—	1
Jenkins and Ashby (1983)[c]	1	—	—	—	—	—	1
Waserman et al. (1983)	1	—	—	—	—	—	1
Total	4	67	1	17	1	17	6
Total	11	69	3	19	2	13	16
Price et al. (1985)[e]	16	53	7	23	7	23	30
DZ (same sex)							
Current study[h]	1	33[d]	—	0	2	67[c,d]	3
Other reports							
Bachman (1981)[c]	—	—	—	—	1	—	1
Total	1	25	—	0	3	75	4
Price et al. (1985)[f]	1	8	2	15	10	77	13
DZ (opposite sex)							
Current study[g,h]	—	—	—	—	7	100	7

[a]Monozygotic: MZ; Dizygotic: DZ; Tourette's disorder: TS; chronic motor tic: CMT.
[b]7 Males, 3 females.
[c]Male.
[d]Female.
[e]25 Male, 5 female.
[f]10 Female, 3 male.
[g]4 Male, 3 female.
[h]Twins described in Shapiro et al., 1978, also reported in Eldridge at al., 1977; Wassman et al., 1978; and Shapiro et al. (1965–1981).
[i]Both female twin pairs had CMT.
[j]Mother and MZ twin concordant for CMT.

degree relatives with Tourette's disorder and CMT was 1.5% and 15%, respectively, similar to our percentages of 1.9% and 12.2% (Table 4.9) and to the 2% and 16% reported by Pauls et al. (1981). These rates for Tourette's disorder or CMT were not significantly related to concordance, zygosity, sex of twin or relative. Of further interest were the significant correlations for age at onset for twins fully concordant for Tourette's disorder and for twins partially concordant (one twin with Tourette's disorder, the other with CMT), although, as noted by the authors, the results were not free of diagnostic or reporting bias. Moreover, although severity of tics was rated by informants during periods of greatest severity and subject to report bias, severity of motor (but not vocal or total motor and vocal tics) was significantly associated with fully concordant (both twins with Tourette's disorder) but not partially concordant (Tourette's disorder and CMT) pairs. The authors also report a significantly older age at onset in a small sample of concordant MZ pairs compared with discordant MZ pairs. No relationship was found between haloperidol responders and family history or concordance in MZ twins. They also report undefined obsessive-compulsive features in 83% of Tourette's disorder patients, a percentage which is inflated because many tic symptoms are classified as obsessive-compulsive symptoms. The retrospective results from this important study provide interesting heuristic hypotheses for future study and confirmation.

In addition, the authors, in a retrospective follow-up letter (Leckman et al., 1987), reported the birth weights for six of the seven MZ twin pairs who were discordant for Tourette's disorder. The birth weight was lower in the twin with Tourette's disorder compared to the twin without Tourette's. They speculate that the lower birth weight might reflect adverse intrauterine factors which led to Tourette's disorder in the twin with lower birth weight. This finding is related to the report by Pasamanick and Kawi (1956) that mothers of children with tics have more complications of pregnancy and parturition. Thus, perinatal events may contribute to the development of Tourette's disorder. This hypothesis will be evaluated by our data to be described later in this chapter.

Family History of Tic Disorders in Adopted (Nonbiological) Probands and in Nonadopted (Biological) Probands

Family history data are available for 22 adopted and 641 nonadopted patients with Tourette's disorder. The data gave us the opportunity of testing the hypothesis that if Tourette's disorder is heritable, a family history of tic disorders should be significantly less in the nonbiological families of the adopted probands than in the biological families of the nonadopted probands.

We compared the family histories for adopted and nonadopted probands in primary and total family members. None of the nonbiological primary family members or total family members of the adopted probands had a history of a tic disorder, whereas in the nonadopted biological families 227 primary family members and 301 total family members had a history of a tic disorder (Fisher Exact Test (2-tail), $p = 0.000$) (Table 4.15).

Information about the biological parents is available for only two of the adopted probands; a father of one and a grandfather of another had a tic disorder.

The finding that none of the nonbiological families of adopted probands had a history of a tic disorder is below expectations in the population: Perhaps this is due to the insensitivity of the family history method in eliciting data

TABLE 4.15 *History of tic disorders in one or more nonbiological relatives of adopted probands and biological relatives of nonadopted probands*

Samples	Family history of tic disorders	
	No	Yes
Primary family[a]		
Adopted probands, nonbiological relatives	22	0
Nonadopted, biological relatives	414	227
Total family members[a]		
Adopted probands, nonbiological relatives	22	0
Nonadopted, biological relatives	340	301

[a]Fisher Exact Test (2-Tail); $p = 0.000$.

about tics in the family. Nevertheless these preliminary results contribute additional evidence for genetic factors in Tourette's disorder and tic disorders (Table 4.10)

Genetic Markers

The identification of genetic markers for tic disorders is important to reduce heterogeneity and to derive concepts about etiology. Attempts to establish biological genetic markers for Tourette's disorder have been essentially unsuccessful. These include studies of HLA, B, C, and DR antigens (Arena et al., 1974; Comings et al., 1982a; Caine et al., 1985), the complement system (Arena et al., 1974), hypoxanthine guanine phosphoribosyltransferase (Van Woert et al., 1977; Johnson et al., 1977; Merrill et al., 1979), adenosine phosphoribosyltransferase (Merrill et al., 1979), plasma norepinephrine (Lake et al., 1977), dopamine-beta-hydroxylase (DBH) (Lake et al., 1977; Shapiro et al., 1984), erythrocyte catechol-*o*-methyltransferase (COMT) (Lake et al., 1977; Shapiro et al., 1984), platelet monoamine oxidase (MAO), COMT in fibroblasts (Giller et al., 1980), and cerebrospinal acetylcholinesterase (Singer et al., 1984). In our study, platelet MAO and plasma amine oxidase (PAO) were significantly higher in untreated Tourette's disorder patients with and without ADD compared with controls (Shapiro et al., 1984). In a small subsample of seven untreated Tourette's disorder patients with ADD, platelet MAO and PAO was significantly higher than in the controls but not for patients with TS-alone, and COMT was significantly lower and DBH significantly higher for the TS+ADD group compared with TS-alone patients and controls. Although carefully controlled, the results require replication. Choline in red blood cell but not plasma was reported as higher in Tourette's disorder patients in a controlled study (Hanin et al., 1979) and in Tourette's disorder patients compared with nonbiological relatives or controls (Comings et al., 1982b). An XYY karyotype has been reported in a single Tourette's disorder patient (Mersky, 1974). Also described are two brothers with Tourette's disorder and tuberous sclerosis, and a father with tuberous sclerosis (Matthews, 1981). These positive findings require replication and adequate control of many subtle variables.

Correlates of a Family History of Tourette and Tic Disorders

A family history of Tourette's disorder, tics and other movement disorders was correlated with 54 variables described in Table A.1. Significant variables are summarized in Table 4.16. Based on our general hypothesis that Tourette's disorder is a genetic or congenital organic CNS disorder that is unassociated with other factors (such as those reflected by our variables), we did not expect meaningful differences between patients with and without a family history of tics or Tourette's disorder. Our expectations were essentially confirmed. The amount of variance accounted for by most of the variables is small, and the number of significant variables is close to chance expectations. T-tests yielded similar probability levels.

The reason for the increase in the family history of Tourette's disorder over time is not readily apparent. Unexpectedly, a family history of Tourette's disorder and tics is uncorrelated ($r = -0.01$), suggesting that Tourette's disorder and tics are not genetically related, the small number of 50 (7.8%) relatives who had a history of Tourette's disorder was too small to detect a relationship, the tendency for family members is to report either Tourette's disorder or tics, but not both, or that family members with mild symptoms or CMT disorder may not have been identified. Interviews with the relatives would be necessary to confirm this. A family history of Tourette's disorder is significantly associated with less severe Tourette's disorder, less frequent tics of the limbs, fewer total cumulative symptoms, and younger age at onset of Tourette's disorder. Even more meaningful is the finding that family history is not significantly associated with patient sex, birth history, sibling status, maturational milestones, medical history, obsessive-compulsive symptoms, neurological and EEG abnormalities, and the diagnosis of ADD and obsessive compulsive disorder. Our expectations were also confirmed by the summary SRA (Table 4.16) which selected few, not very meaningful variables, that accounted for very little variance in the dependent variables.

The finding that ADD is not significantly associated with a positive family history of Tourette's disorder confirms our belief that these disorders are unrelated. Some investigators suggest that ADD or the symptoms of ADD precede and represent a form of Tourette's disorder (Mahler et al., 1945; Cohen et al., 1982) and that Tourette's disorder and ADD are genetically related (Comings and Comings, 1984). Further evidence that they are unrelated was provided by

TABLE 4.16. *Patient variables significantly correlated with a family history of Tourette's disorder, tic disorder, either Tourette's disorder or a tic disorder, and nontic disorders*[a]

Variables for patients with TS	Family history			
	TS	Tics	TS or tics	Non-tic
Demography				
Year evaluated	0.15[c]	0.03	0.08[d]	−0.04
Social class	−0.01	−0.09[d]	−0.10[e]	0.01
Past History				
Sat-walk-talk FS	−0.08[d]	0.01	−0.01	−0.05
Head trauma	−0.04	−0.01	−0.02	0.10[e]
Illness Variables				
Age at onset of TS	−0.07[f]	−0.11[e]	−0.12[e]	−0.02
Symptoms				
History of arm tics	−0.08[d]	−0.04	−0.04	0.05
History of leg tics	−0.11[e]	−0.01	−0.04	0.03
Echophilia	−0.04	−0.04	−0.04	0.09[d]
Total current tics	−0.10[e]	0.01	−0.03	0.02
Total cumulative tics	−0.07[f]	0.01	−0.04	0.08[d]
Fluctuation of tics	−0.05	−0.09[d]	−0.11[e]	0.04
Severity of TS	−0.10[e]	−0.06	−0.09[d]	0.04
Other variables[b]				
Family history of TS	—	−0.01	—	−0.01
Obsessive-Compulsive-like symptoms FS	0.02	0.06	0.06	0.05
Obsessive-Compulsive personality FS	0.02	0.02	0.02	0.06

Variables	Summary stepwise multiple regression analysis		
	r	R^2	Parameter estimate
Family history of TS			
Year evaluated	0.15[c]	0.02	0.02[e]
History of leg tics	−0.11[e]	0.03	−0.05[d]
Adjusted R[e]		0.03[c]	
Family history of tics			
Age at onset of TS	−0.11[e]	0.01	−0.02[e]
History of torso tics	0.10[e]	0.02	0.11[e]
Fluctuation of tics	−0.09[d]	0.03	−0.27[d]
Year of evaluation	−0.09[d]	0.04	−0.04[d]
Adjusted R[e]		0.04[c]	
Family history of TS or tics			
Fluctuation of tics	−0.11[e]	0.02	−0.29[e]
Age at onset of TS	−0.12[g]	0.03	−0.02[d]
Adjusted R[e]		0.03[c]	

[a]See Table A.1 for list of 54 variables; only significant variables included in table. Tic disorders include family history of chronic motor tic and transient tic disorders. $N = 641$; two-tailed test; variables at $p < 0.01$ are considered significant.
[b]Other nonsignificant variables included for general interest.
[c]$p < 0.0001$.
[d]$p < 0.05$.
[e]$p < 0.01$.
[f]$p < 0.10$.
[g]$p < 0.001$.

a recent genetic analysis indicating that Tourette's disorder and ADD are independent and not genetically related (Pauls et al. 1986a). Our results also indicate no significant association between positive family history of Tourette's disorder, tics, and obsessive-compulsive disorder, although others report a higher frequency of obsessive-compulsive disorder and obsessive-compulsive symptoms in Tourette's disorder patients and their families. (Yariyura-Tobias et al., 1981; Nee et al., 1980; Cohen et al., 1980, 1982; Montgomery et al., 1982; Grad et al., 1984; Comings and Comings, 1984; Pauls et al., 1986b). Our clinical impression and the results of our analysis is that the frequency of obsessive-compulsive symptoms and disorder is not greater than expected in the population. The reason for the discrepancy between studies is probably due to the absence of precise criteria differentiating obsessive-compulsive disorder, obsessive-compulsive symptoms, obsessive-compulsive-like symptoms, or impulsions and complex Tourette's disorder symptoms. These issues are discussed more fully in Chapter 6.

Summary and Conclusion

Analysis of these data suggest the following conclusions: Tourette's disorder and CMT are similar disorders, and are familial. More males than females are affected with both Tourette's disorder and CMT. Most studies report that Tourette's disorder and CMT occur more frequently in male than female relatives, but the risks to relatives of affected females are higher than to relatives of affected males. A family history of Tourette's disorder is reported more frequently in selected referrals or volunteer samples than in consecutive clinical patients. A family history of Tourette's disorder is unrelated to a family history of tics. A family history of Tourette's disorder but not a family history of tics is associated with less severe Tourette's disorder. A family history of Tourette's disorder or tics is unrelated to obsessive-compulsive disorder, obsessive-compulsive symptoms, compulsive personality disorder, ADD, and a past history of complex coprolalic and echophilic tics. The percentage of affected family members is higher in samples in which relatives are interviewed than in samples in which family history is obtained from patients. The percent of family members with a history of Tourette's disorder, tic disorder, or either Tourette's or tic disorder, in one or more family member is approximately 5%, 32%, and 35%, respectively, for primary family members and 8%, 42%, and 47%, respectively, for all family members. Transmission of Tourette's disorder or CMT in identical (MZ) twins is approximately 77 to 87%, approximately 25% in same-sex fraternal (DZ) twins, and is less frequent in opposite-sex fraternal (DZ) twins. The likelihood of Tourette's disorder or CMT is approximately 9% for a brother, 5% for a sister, 8% for a son, and 4% for a daughter. The mode of inheritance is still unknown but evidence for an autosomal dominant mode is increasing.

BIRTH HISTORY

The following factors are examined in this section: parents' age at birth, birth weight, history of abortions, pregnancy, and perinatal complications. All birth history variables were correlated with 54 variables (Table A.1). There were no meaningful correlations. The results for our sample are compared with available data in the literature (Table 4.17). They include a study by Kondo and Nomura (1982) of birth factors for 42 Tourette's disorder patients who were compared with 43 patients with Duchenne dystrophy, studies by Han-bai and Han-quin (1983) and Lees et al. (1984).

Parents' Age at Birth

Mothers' age at birth averaged 27.3 years (SD = 5.4, median = 27, range 16–45). Fathers' age at birth averaged 31.1 (SD = 6.6, median = 30, range 16–55). The distribution is similar to expectations in the general population.

Birth Weight

Increased vulnerability to brain damage in premature youngsters may be greater than in a child of normal weight (Wender, 1971). Birth weight for 128 patients available in the 1965 to 1974 sample averaged 7.2 pounds (SD = 1.2, median = 7.3, range 4.0–11.1) and was within the range for the general population. Birth weight data were not examined for the subsequent sample.

History of Abortions

For the total sample, 30.3% had a history of one or more pre, post, spontaneous, and induced abortions which is similar to the 30.4% reported for the 1965 to 1974 sample (Table 4.17). The percent for 42 Japanese mothers was 16.7% for spontaneous abortions and 59.5% for induced abortions. The total was higher than for our sample, but there was no significant difference between Tourette's disorder patients and patients with Duchenne dystrophy (Kondo and Nomura, 1982). These results are within expectations for the population.

Pregnancy Complications

Pregnancy complications for 135 Tourette's disorder patients in the 1965 to 1974 sample were rated in detail as follows: Each of the following rated one point: birth weight > 2.00 to 2.25 kg; mild immaturity (36 < 38 weeks); mild

TABLE 4.17. Birth history[a]

Variables	Current study (1965–1981) %	Other studies %
Prolonged labor		
None	96.4	
10–19 hr	0.2	
20–29 hr	1.0	
30–39 hr	1.0	
40–49 hr	1.1	
72 hr	0.5	
Birth procedure		
Gas anesthesia	50.5	
Spinal anesthesia	15.7	
Local anesthesia	6.7	
Natural labor	13.2	
Induced labor	12.5	5.7[b]
Other	1.4	
Unknown	—	
Pregnancy complications		
None	75.3	71.4[c]
Toxemia	2.1	4.8[c]
Infection during 1st trimester	1.7	
Accident	1.9	
Drug use during pregnancy	6.2	19.0[c]
Severe nausea & vomiting	5.4	4.8[c]
Birth complications		
None	77.1	61.9[c],75.6[b],72.2[d]
Prolonged labor	3.0	1.9[b]
Prolapsed umbilical cord	1.3	14.3[c],5.7[b]
Caesarean	5.1	4.8[c],3.8[b]
Breech delivery	4.9	9.5[c]
Other	8.7	
Total complications	23.0	38.1[c],24.5[b],27.8[d]
Abortions (prebirth)		
None	78.9	
1	15.3	
2	4.0	
3–6	1.9	
Total abortions	21.0	
Abortions (postbirth)		
None	548	86.6
1	59	9.3
2	21	3.3
3–4	5	0.8
Total abortions	85	13.4

TABLE 4.17. (Continued)

Variables	Current study (1965–1981) %	Other studies %
Total abortions		
None	438	69.7
1	118	18.8
2	47	7.5
3	14	2.2
4–10	11	1.8
Total abortions	190	30.3

Parents age (years)	Mean	Range
Mother	27.3 (± 5.4)	16–45
Father	31.1 (± 6.6)	16–55

[a] $N = 666$.
[b] Lees et al. (1984).
[c] Kondo and Nomura (1982).
[d] Han-bai and Han-quin (1983).

postmaturity (42 < 44 weeks); Hb% ever < 60; hospital admission for pyelitis; cardiac disease necessitating restriction of activity; moderate essential hypertension or toxemia (diastolic blood pressure 100 or more with or without albuminuria); antepartum hemorrhage (at > 28 weeks) of any kind. Each of the following rated two points: birth weight 2.00 kg or less; severe immaturity (< 36 weeks); severe postmaturity (> 44 weeks); severe essential hypertension or toxemia (diastolic blood pressure 110 or more with or without albuminuria). The following rated three points: eclampsia (diastolic blood pressure 90 or more and fits with no past history of epilepsy). The results for our sample were similar to expectations in the population.

For the total sample, 24.7% were rated as having one or more of the pregnancy complications listed in Table 4.17. The percent was similar to the percent found by Kondo and Nomura (1982) and was not significantly different from the Duchenne dystrophy control group.

Birth Complications

Birth complications for 137 Tourette's disorder patients in the 1965 to 1974 sample were rated as follows: Each of the following rated one point: total duration of first and second stages of labor for primiparas < 3 hr or > 48 hr; for multiparas < 1½ hr or > 36 hr; spontaneous breech delivery; assisted breech with or without forceps to aftercoming head; midcavity or high forceps for any reason other than those specified above and below; intrapartum hemorrhage; shoulder, face, or brow presentation; caesarean section. Each of the following rated two points: vertex with manual rotation and forceps delivery; internal version and breech extraction; low forceps for fetal distress; prolapsed cord. Hospital or birth certificate data were examined for 33 patients in the 1965 to 1974 sample and were compared with information provided by informants. A comparison of these data indicated that most of the reports of prolonged labor by mothers were inaccurate. Statements such as "born with cord around the neck" were unverifiable. The mother's specification of the use of forceps as a complication of delivery was usually described in the hospital records as low forceps delivery and was not a scorable complication of delivery. These observations about the unreliability of mothers remembering birth and delivery complications are in agreement with other reports (Wenar, 1963). Because of the unreliability of birth certificates and hospital records, these data were not systematically analyzed subsequently. The results of the above analysis, however, did not deviate from estimates in the population.

Birth complications were rated as present or absent for the total sample (Table 4.17). For the total sample, 32.0% had one or more birth complications. The percent is in the range reported by others: 24.5% by Lees et al. (1984), 27.8% by Han-bai and Han-quin (1983), 33% by Mahler et al (1945), and 38.1% by Kondo and Nomura (1982). The latter percent for Tourette's disorder patients was not significantly different from the Duchenne dystrophy control group. Length of labor and birth procedure for our sample were within the normal range (Table 4.17). Birth history has also been reported as not significant by Jagger et al. (1982) and Min (1983).

Perinatal Abnormalities

Total perinatal abnormalities are reported in 20% (Corbett et al., 1969) and 33.3% (Pasamanick and Kawi, 1956) of patients with tics. In patients with Tourette's disorder they are reported as 33.3% (Lieh-Mak et al., 1982), and not significant by Jagger et al. (1982), Min (1983), and Kondo and Nomura (1982). Two of the studies used a control group. Pasamanick and Kawi (1956) blindly rated birth certificates and hospital records for 51 tic and 51 matched subjects. Information about pregnancy and delivery included number of pregnancies, number alive, stillbirth, premature, length of labor, complications of pregnancy and labor, operative procedure, birth weight, and neonatal course. Abnormalities in the patients were present in 33.3% compared with 17.5% for the controls ($p < 0.05$). A limitation of this study was use of a clinical sample of patients with tics. Kondo and Nomura (1982) rated major maternal diseases before pregnancy, total live births, spontaneous and induced abortions, stillbirths, disordered pregnancies and deliveries, and total perinatal disorders. There was no significant difference between 42 Tourette's disorder patients and a control group of 43 patients with Duchenne dystrophy.

The relationship of pregnancy or delivery complications to neurological damage is poorly understood and inconclusively associated with hyperactivity (Rapoport et al., 1974), minimal brain dysfunction (Wender, 1971), cognitive impairment (Quay and Werry, 1972), and so on. Whatever the relationship is between perinatal complications and subsequent brain damage, its relationship to Tourette's disorder is even more inconclusive. If birth complications can cause brain damage or predispose children to psychopathology, these factors are implicated in only a small number of Tourette's disorder patients.

Since the percentage of Tourette's disorder patients with scorable perinatal hazards or abnormalities is negligible, it can be concluded that the data of this study do not support the association of perinatal abnormalities with Tourette's disorder. The failure to obtain any indications of abnormal perinatal factors in our sample does not support the Pasamanick and Kawi (1956) concept of a relationship between these factors and tics.

Birth Order

The potential relationship of birth order to physiological and psychological factors has obvious face validity, and has been related to epidemiological variables (MacFarlane et al., 1954) and specific medical disorders such as Briquet's syndrome (Morrison, 1983), neurosis (Norton, 1952), and homosexuality (Hare et al., 1979; Slater, 1962). Young mothers may have a more difficult first labor leading to fetal distress, and congenital abnormalities and chromosomal abnormalities may occur in children born to older mothers. Children of different sibling rank may be treated differently and may have different experiences than their siblings. Parental demands may be stricter for firstborn and more permissive for later children. Family dynamics and parents themselves may change over time affecting children differently. The relationship of birth order to Tourette's disorder might provide insights about etiology and also be of general interest.

Ordinal birth order for our sample is contrasted with results from only one available study in the literature (Lucas et al., 1982). The distributions for the two samples were not significantly different ($\chi^2 = 6.8$, df=1, NS) (Table 4.18). The percent of firstborn children versus others was not significantly different ($\chi^2 = 4.3$, df=6, NS) for studies 1 to 8, which included a random sample in an epidemiological study (MacFarlane et al., 1954) (Table 4.19).

Birth order status (only, oldest, middle, and youngest child) for our sample is contrasted with results from other published studies (Table 4.19). Although there is some variability among the studies, the distributions are not significantly different for studies 1, 3, 4 ($\chi^2 = 11.1$, df=6, $p = 0.09$) and only Mahler

TABLE 4.18. Ordinal birth order[a]

Variables	Current study (1965–1981)		Lucas (1982)	
	N	%	N	%
Ordinal birth order				
First	328	49.3	12	48.0
Second	205	30.8	5	20.0
Third	76	11.4	2	8.0
Fourth	34	5.1	2	8.0
Fifth	13	2.0	3	12.0
Sixth–Ninth	9	1.4	—	—
Total	665	100.0	24	100.0

[a] Shapiro vs. Lucas, firstborn vs. others, $\chi^2(1) = 6.8$, NS.

(1949) had a significantly different distribution ($\chi^2 = 21.9$, df=3, $p = 0.0001$). In an analysis of birth order in Japanese children (no data presented), birth order was not significantly related to Tourette's disorder (Kondo and Nomura, 1982), and Lucas et al. (1967) concluded that birth order was not significantly associated with Tourette's disorder.

Limitations of these studies as well as this analysis are the absence of many interacting variables required to adequately analyze birth order (Slater, 1962; Bytheway, 1974; Price and Hare, 1969; Morrison, 1983). These include age of parents, sex and age differences between siblings, social class differences, and use of an appropriate control group. Within these limitations, our data indicate that perinatal factors, parents' age at birth, and social class variables do not seem to be related to Tourette's disorder.

Although the available data do not rule out a possible relationship of birth order to Tourette's disorder, it does not seem very likely. A definitive conclusion requires additional analyses.

MEDICAL HISTORY

Childhood Illnesses

The possible association between childhood illness and tics has to be considered because of the occasional association of tic-like or other movement disorders with scarlet fever, rheumatic fever, chorea, encephalitis, and head trauma. Childhood illnesses which were common in the past, such as ear infections, German measles, measles, whooping cough, and mumps, are now rare. A history of streptococcal-induced infections, leading to rheumatic fever, rheumatoid arthritis, rheumatic heart disease, scarlet fever, chorea (Sydenham's chorea), and glomerulonephrosis were reported by a small number

TABLE 4.19. Birth order

Studies	Sample description	Total sample N	First-born[a] %	Only child[b] %	Oldest child[b] %	Middle child[b] %	Youngest child[b] %
1. Current study (1965–1981)	TS	659	49.8	11.5	38.2	34.1	16.1
2. Mahler (1949)	Most TS	33	60.6	33.3	30.3	9.1	24.2
3. Zausmer (1954)	Tics	96	53.1	11.5	41.7	24.0	22.9
4. Lucas et al. (1967); Challas et al. (1967)	TS	26	42.3	19.2	23.1	26.9	30.6
5. Min (1983)	TS, MT[c]	24	41.7	—	—	25.0	33.3
6. Debray-Ritzen and Dubois (1980)	TS, MT, tics	93	—	22.6	—	—	—
7. Lucas et al. (1982)	TS	25	48.0	—	—	—	—
8. MacFarlane et al. (1954)	Epidemiology	116	44.8	—	—	—	—

[a] Firstborn studies (1–8), $\chi^2(6) = 4.3$, NS.
[b] Only, oldest, middle, and youngest studies (1,3,4) $\chi^2(6) = 11.1, p = 0.09$.
[c] MT = motor tic.

of patients in the past, but not recently. Comparison of the frequency of these illnesses for early samples were within estimates for the population (Table 4.20). The veritable absence of childhood illnesses in recent samples and the lack of a relationship between these illnesses and the onset of tics strongly supports the view that they are not etiologically associated with tics or Tourette's disorder. An infection such as a slow virus occurring at some time in childhood is unlikely in our opinion, but possible.

The frequency of selected illnesses and head trauma for Tourette's disorder patients was compared with their frequency in a sample of patients with other movement disorders (Table 4.20). None of the comparisons were significantly different and the frequency of these illnesses was similar to expectations in the population.

Thirty percent of patients had a history of allergies (Table 4.20), not significantly different from the comparison samples. The percent reporting allergies may be much higher than the true prevalence; since many patients and physicians misinterpret vocal tics (sniffing, throat clearing, and coughing tics), and swollen nose (caused by touching, rubbing, or hitting tics) as allergic symptoms. Exacerbation of tic symptoms during periods of increased allergic symptoms and the results of allergic desensitization are often taken as evidence that Tourette's disorder has an allergic etiology. Lanier (1985) pointed out that an antigen-antibody response has not been demonstrated in Tourette's disorder, that the genetics of Tourette's disorder and allergy differ (predominance of males in Tourette's disorder and possible slight excess of females in allergies), that effective drugs for the treatment of allergies (antihistamines, antiserotonins, antiprostaglandins, and corticosteroids) are not useful for the treat-

TABLE 4.20. Medical history[a]

Variables	Tourette's disorder[b] %	Other tic disorders[c] %	Stereotypic movement disorder[d] %
Scarlet fever	6.4	7.8	0.0
Rheumatic fever	1.4	1.3	0.0
Chorea	0.3	1.3	0.0
Head injury	20.3	16.9	27.6
Concussion	4.1	7.8	3.5
Unconscious	4.5	2.6	3.5
Convulsion	4.7	2.6	6.9
Epilepsy	1.1	0.0	0.0
Allergy	30.1	29.9	24.1

[a] None of the chi-square comparisons for the listed medical illnesses and the three samples and between male and female TS patients is significant.
[b] $N = 666$.
[c] Other tic disorders include transient tic and chronic motor tic disorders; $N = 77$.
[d] $N = 29$.

ment of Tourette's disorder, that drugs useful for the treatment of the disorder (haloperidol, pimozide, etc.) are ineffective for the treatment of allergies, and concluded that current evidence does not support an association of allergies with Tourette's disorder.

Other alternative etiological factors and treatment for Tourette's disorder popularized in recent years, include holistic medicine, orthomolecular or megavitamin therapy (popularized by Williams, Hopper, Osmond, Cott, Yariyura-Tobias, and Donaldson), trace elements, artificial colors and dyes in foods as a cause of illness (Feingold), sensitivity to sugar in foods, and allergic response to various antigens (Mandell). Golden (1984) and a consensus panel of the medical board of the TSA (1985) concluded that there is no scientific evidence to support an etiologic role for any of these factors or for the effectiveness of the treatments derived from them. For many years an allergic explanation for Tourette's disorder, or the association of allergies with Tourette's disorder, has been mentioned frequently in the Tourette's disorder lay media and many patients have been treated unsuccessfully with desensitization procedures.

Despite anecdotal reports, there is no evidence in our opinion that medical illnesses cause or contribute to the development of Tourette's disorder.

Adult Illness

We have recorded all adult illnesses in patients with Tourette's disorder. Our data do not indicate that medical illnesses precede the onset of Tourette's disorder, nor are these patients predisposed to develop any particular medical illness.

SOCIAL CLASS

Social class is based on a weighted combination of occupational and educational status (Hollingshead and Redlich, 1958). The scale yields a linear measure from I (highest social class) to V (lowest social class). For patients under 21 and women who were housewives, ratings of social class were based on the head of the household.

Our sample veered toward higher social clases: 42.4% were college educated or had graduate professional training, 41.6% were business managers or higher executives, and 40.6% were in higher social classes (Table 4.21). Since 1981 it is our impression that the number of patients from lower social classes has increased, probably due to increased knowledge about Tourette's disorder.

TABLE 4.21. Social class variables[a]

Variables	%
Education	
Graduate professional training	21.7
College graduate	20.7
Partial college	16.5
High school graduate	28.6
Partial high school	6.9
Junior high school	3.5
Less than 7 years school	2.0
Occupation	
Higher executive	21.0
Business manager	20.6
Administrator	15.8
Clerical	18.0
Skilled manual	13.8
Semi-skilled	4.1
Unskilled	4.7
Housewife	1.9
Social class[b]	
I. High	19.5
II.	21.1
III. Middle	24.1
IV.	28.5
V. Low	6.8

[a] Hollingshead and Redlich (1958); $N = 666$.
[b] $N = 615$.

TABLE 4.22. *Marital status and children*[a]

Variables	% or N
Marital Status[b]	
Never married	50.9%
Married	35.6%
Separated or divorced	8.6%
Widow	0.5%
Divorced, remarried	0.9%
Widow, remarried	3.6%
Length of Marriage[c]	
Less than 1 year	7.3%
1–4 years	20.2%
5–12 years	29.4%
13–20 years	22.0%
> 20 years	21.1%
Children[d]	
Number of biological children	163
Number of adopted children	2

	Males		Females	
Marital status[e]	N	%	N	%
Never married	24	50.0	7	28.0
Married	21	43.8	10	40.0
Divorced	3	6.2	8	32.0

[a] Only adults over 25 years of age.
[b] $N = 222$.
[c] $N = 109$.
[d] $N = 71$.
[e] Data from 1965–1974 sample of 114 patients (A. K. Shapiro et al., 1978); $N = 73$.

MARITAL STATUS

The distribution of marital status of patients over 21 years was not significantly different from that reported in two epidemiological studies (Jagger et al., 1982; Stefl, 1983) ($\chi^2 = 4.0$, df=3, NS) (Table 4.22).

In our previous sample (1965–1974) of 73 patients over 21 years of age, there was a tendency for more males (50%) than females (28%) to be single ($p < 0.08$) and for significantly more females (32%) to be divorced than males (6.2%) ($p < 0.02$) (Table 4.22). The results suggest that females have slightly less difficulty marrying than do males, but that once married, have more difficulty staying married. These results are unrelated to the severity of Tourette's disorder. For the sample of 148 patients evaluated between 1975 and 1981, the percent of unmarried patients decreased slightly to 55.4%, divorced patients decreased to 5.4%, and married patients stayed about the same, 39.2% ($\chi^2 = 7.0$, df=2, $p < 0.03$) (Table 4.22). The main difference between the samples is the increase of single patients which is associated with a decrease in divorced patients ($\chi^2 = 7.0$, df=1, $p < 0.009$). Male and female marital status was not analyzed for the total sample. This analysis, as well as the occupational and psychosocial functioning of patients, and the effect of other variables such as the severity and treatment of Tourette's disorder, the relationship to associated diagnoses of ADD, etc., would contribute important information about the effect of Tourette's disorder on functioning and to the management and avoidance of subsequent impairment.

ORGANIC STIGMATA

The etiology of tic and Tourette disorders has been and continues to be perplexing. An organic hypothesis was stimulated by the effectiveness of haloperidol and its theoretical relationship to neurotransmitter systems, the ineffectiveness of psychological treatment, absence of specific or general psychopathology, and the higher than expected frequency of organic stigmata in patients. For the initial sample of 34 patients we reported higher than expected percentages of organic stigmata (neurological, EEG results, and psychological test abnormalities, non-right-handedness, learning or perceptual disorder, and attention deficit disorder) in a series of papers published between 1972 and 1974. These results were confirmed in our study of 145 patients described in 1978 (Shapiro et al., 1978) and in other studies (Table 4.24).

The higher than expected frequency of organic stigmata was interpreted as strongly supporting an organic etiology for Tourette's disorder. Based on the analysis of our larger current sample, we concluded that there was good evidence to question this conclusion. In this section, we carefully re-evaluate the evidence.

Maturational Milestones

The average age for selected maturational milestones for the total sample is essentially within expectations, similar to the findings reported by others (Jagger et al., 1982; Min, 1983) and implied by the absence of deviations reported in the literature (Table 4.23).

Handedness

Nondominant handedness (left or ambidexterous) has been reported as more frequent in younger children, males, patients with manic depressive and schizoaffective disorders, not excessive in patients with neurotic and personality disorders (Hecaen and Ajuriaguerra, 1964; Annett, 1970; Lishman and McMeekan, 1976), and is thought to be a possible correlate of organic impair-

TABLE 4.23. Maturational milestones[a]

Description	Age			
	Mean	SD	Median	Range
Sat unsupported	0.54	0.10	0.6	0.2–1.1
Walked by self	1.11	0.20	1.2	0.6–2.0
Talked first words	1.42	0.63	1.5	0.3–8.0
Bladder trained	2.20	0.81	2.0	0.8–12.0
Bowel trained	2.21	0.72	2.0	0.8–11.0

[a] $N = 666$.

ment. Hand preference was evaluated by questioning patients to determine if they used their right or left hand exclusively for writing, eating, throwing a ball, striking, and using tools. They were classified as either right or left handed or as ambidexterous if they used either hand or alternated hands when performing the above functions.

Although the frequency of left handedness varies from 1 to 30% in studies, the most likely estimate in the general population is 5 to 10% (Hecaen and Ajuriaguerra, 1964; Annett, 1970). For our total sample left handedness was 14.7% and ambidexterity 7.1%, totalling 21.8% (Table 4.30). The distribution is not significantly different for our 1965 to 1974 sample of 114 patients compared with our subsequent sample of 552 patients. The stability of these percentages is supported by nonsignificant differences for age and sex. The results suggest slight excess of nondominant handedness, and possible nonlocalizing sign of neurological abnormality among patients with Tourette's disorder, but this finding requires confirmation with more reliable and valid methods of determining handedness (Annett, 1970).

Retrospective analysis correlating nondominant handedness versus right handedness with 54 variables in the List of Variables (Table A.1) resulted in essentially chance findings. There was no relationship to age, sex, family history of tic disorders, severity of Tourette's disorder, IQ, and neurological and EEG abnormalities. However, there was a nonsignificant trend ($\chi^2 = 3.5$, df=1, $p < 0.06$) for nondominant handedness for patients with ADD (27%), compared with patients without ADD (20%) (Table 4.29). Although nonsignificant the trend indicates the possible importance of separating patients with TS+ADD and TS-alone.

Attention Deficit Disorder

Review of Literature

There was a higher than expected number of Tourette's disorder patients with organic stigmata in the first 27 patients evaluated between 1965 and 1971.

Abnormalities were found on neurological examinations, EEG recordings, psychological testing, psychological evaluations, and development (Shapiro et al., 1972). Prior to DSM-III (American Psychiatric Association, 1980), the term minimal brain dysfunction (MBD) was used to describe children of average intelligence with learning or behavioral disabilities associated with central nervous system deviations such as perception, conceptualization, language, memory, attention, impulse control, hyperactivity, and motor function (Clements and Peters, 1962; Clements, 1966). Many of our initial patients were described as "irritable, impulsive, never at rest, into everything, and having short attention spans, and other symptoms of MBD. . . hyperactivity, distractibility, excitability perceptual problems and so on" (Shapiro et al., 1978). The diagnosis was based on extensive interviews of patients, parents, and other informants, and records obtained from pediatricians, schools, neurologists, psychologists, and other professionals. The records and clinical interviews were independently reviewed by two of us (A.K.S., E.S.). Patients were classified as having MBD only if there was agreement in the independent evaluations. We reported MBD in 30% in 1972 (Shapiro et al., 1972b), 41% in 1973 (Shapiro et al., 1973c,d) and 56 to 62% in 1978 (Shapiro et al., 1978).

Previously Mahler et al. (1945) reported that most of her patients had symptoms characteristic of MBD. In two reviews, MBD symptoms were reported in 42% (Kelman, 1965) and 12% of patients (Fernando, 1967).

Although it was obvious to us at the time that the reliability for the diagnosis of MBD had not been established (Werry, 1968, Quay and Werry, 1972), we were bound by the diagnostic conventions of the time. We described our data as preliminary and requiring replication. However, the high percentage of patients with ADD, together with the higher percentage for other organic stigmata, was cited as evidence for an organic CNS etiology for Tourette's disorder (Shapiro et al., 1978). Seven subsequent papers were largely confirmatory, reporting MBD, hyperactivity, or ADD in a range of 10 to 67%, averaging 34% (Table 4.24).

Subsequent reports in the literature are consistent with our early results of higher than expected ADD in Tourette's disorder patients (Table 4.24). The percent for ADD averages 43% in four clinical studies. ADD is reported as 10% by Golden (1982), 29% by Min (1983), 54% by Comings and Comings (1984), and 67% by Moldofsky et al. (1974). Two epidemiologic studies, based on reports by patients, reported lower percentages of 25 to 26% (Jagger et al., 1982; Stefl, 1983).

Current Results for Attention Deficit Disorder

The diagnosis of ADD in our current sample is based on DSM-III (American Psychiatric Association 1980) criteria and required agreement by A.K.S. and E.S. as described in Chapter 2. The percent of patients with ADD was

TABLE 4.24. Studies citing organic central nervous system stigmata in patients with Tourette's disorder

Study	Attention deficit disorder %	Neurological abnormality %	EEG[a] abnormality %	Learning or perceptual disorder %	Left or ambidexterous handedness %	Overall organicity %	Bender-Gestalt test %	IQ[b] N	Discrepancy score[c] %
Mahler et al. (1945) (N = ?)	Most	—	—	—	—	—	—	—	—
Kelman (1965) (N = 19–65)	42	—	42	—	—	—	—	106	—
Feild et al. (1966) (N = 7)	—	—	86	—	—	—	—	Normal	—
Fernando (1967) (N = 65)	12	—	25	—	—	—	—	—	—
Lucas et al. (1967) (N = 13–15)	—	—	27	60	—	62	—	104	—
Challas et al. (1967) (N = 15)	—	—	—	—	—	—	—	—	—
Corbett et al. (1969) (N = 144)	—	—	—	—	—	—	—	99	—
Morphew and Sim (1969) (N = 32)	—	89	86	—	—	—	—	Normal	—
Fisarova (1972) (N = 27)	—	—	—	—	—	—	—	—	—
Shapiro et al. (1972a) (N = 27–34)	30	—	—	22	35	—	—	—	—
Shapiro et al. (1972b)	—	—	—	—	—	—	—	104	—
Lucas and Rodin (1973) (N = 18)	—	—	56	—	—	—	—	—	—
Shapiro et al. (1973a) (N = 21–34)	41	64	50	—	35	50–77	80	—	50

Study									
Sweet et al. (1973) (N = 22)	—	55	85	—	35	77	—	103	—
Shapiro et al. (1973b) (N = 34)	—	54	50	—	35	77	—	103	50
Shapiro et al. (1974) (N = 30–34)	—	54	50	—	—	77	83	104	50
Moldofsky et al. (1974) (N = 15)	67	—	—	—	—	—	—	—	—
Golden (1977a) (N = 15)	—	53	70	—	23	—	—	—	—
Shapiro et al. (1978) (N = 50–145)	56–62	57	—	—	—	68	42	106	50
Golden (1982) (N = 809)	10	27	—	30	—	40	—	106	—
Bergen et al. (1982) (N = 38)	—	11	34	—	—	—	—	—	—
Jagger et al. (1982) (N = 62–75)	25	—	19	19	17	—	—	Normal	—
Stefl (1983) (N = 280–296)	26	—	—	31	—	—	—	—	—
Han-bai and Han-quin (1983) (N = 13–19)	—	0	31	—	0	—	—	—	—
Min (1983) (N = 20–24)	29	29	60	13	5	—	—	—	—
Comings and Comings (1984) (N = 250)	54	—	—	—	—	—	—	—	—
Volkmar et al. (1984)	—	—	—	—	—	—	—	—	—
Lees et al. (1984) (N = 53)	—	—	15	—	11	—	—	100	—
Current study (N = 170–666)	25	24	36	16	22	—	37	98–103	21–39

[a] Studies reporting EEG abnormalities included only if another organic abnormality was reported; see Chapter 7 for all EEG studies.
[b] WAIS or WISC.
[c] Verbal-Performance WAIS or WISC IQ Difference Score above 14.

51% from 1965 to 1974, 21% from 1975 to 1978, and 16% from 1979 to 1981 (Table 4.1). For the total sample of 666 patients, 19.7% had TS+ADD+H and 5.4% had TS+ADD−H, or a total of 25.1% with any form of ADD.

It is clear from our results and the large range of 10 to 67% with TS+ADD reported in the literature (Table 4.24) that sampling characteristics influence the percentage of patients with TS+ADD, and that the association of ADD with Tourette's disorder has to be re-evaluated. Studies that include many ADD patients may yield data associated with ADD rather than Tourette's disorder, thus contributing to the problem of heterogeneity in tic disorders. What are the potential factors associated with the percent of ADD patients in samples and how does the presence of ADD influence results?

Problems Associated with the Percent of Patients with Attention Deficit Disorder Reported in Studies of Tourette's Disorder

Diagnosis of Attention Deficit Disorder

It is commonly acknowledged that the reliability and validity for the diagnosis of ADD is inadequate. This problem is reflected in the different diagnostic labels that are used to characterize this syndrome: defective moral control (Still, 1902; Bloom, 1984), minimal brain damage (Struass and Lehtinen, 1947), minimal brain dysfunction (Bax and MacKeith, 1963), hyperkinetic child syndrome (Stewart et al., 1966; Donnelly and Rapoport, 1985) or reaction of childhood (DSM-II, American Psychiatric Association, 1968), attention deficit disorder, with and without hyperactivity, attention deficit disorder, residual type for adults (DSM-III, American Psychiatric Association, 1980), and attention deficit hyperactivity disorder (DSM-III-R, American Psychiatric Association, 1987). There is increased consensus that ADD is not a homogeneous syndrome (Rodin et al., 1963; Weiss and Hechtman, 1979; Rutter, 1982; Lahey et al., 1984; Donnelly and Rapoport, 1985). Statistical and factor analyses have not been able to demonstrate that ADD is a homogeneous syndrome (Werry, 1968; Rodin et al., 1963; Rutter, 1982; McGee et al., 1985). There is controversy about whether ADD is associated with brain damage, neurological and EEG abnormalities, learning disorders, conduct disorders, aggression, oppositional behavior and other psychopathology, is a genetic illness, normally varies in the population, or is a continuous or discontinuous condition (Werry and Champaign, 1968; Ross and Ross, 1982; Rutter, 1982, 1983; Bloomingdale, 1984; Conners, 1985a, b; Shaffer et al., 1985). Moreover, the symptomatology changes with maturation and age (Weiss and Hechtman, 1979), the diagnosis is easier to make in childhood than in adolescence (*Psychopharmacology Bulletin*, 1985) and is especially difficult in adulthood (Wender et al., 1981, 1985). The problem in adulthood is further compounded by the disappearance of the symptoms of hyperactivity in approximately 66% of adults. These problems are reflected in our data.

Whereas the diagnosis of TS+ADD was made in 33% of our patients 16 years or younger, only 15% of patients over 16 years of age ($p = 0.0014$) had this diagnosis (Table 4.5).

Prevalence of Attention Deficit Disorder

Another problem is the wide range for estimates of the life-time prevalence of ADD in the population. The range has been reported to be between 0.8 to 20% (Bosco and Robin, 1980; Rutter, 1982; Bloomingdale, 1984; Shaywitz et al., 1984). Studies of Tourette's disorder patients report a much higher percentage of patients with TS+ADD. For five studies totalling 471 patients published between 1978 and 1984, TS+ADD is reported in 46% (range 10-67%) (Table 4.24) (Moldofsky et al., 1974; Shapiro et al., 1978; Golden, 1982; Min, 1983; Comings and Comings, 1984). On the other hand, Golden (1982) reports only 10%, and only 17% had TS+ADD in our sample evaluated between 1979 and 1981 (Table 4.1). These percentages are close to expectations in the population. Reports of a higher than expected percentage of ADD may be due to ascertainment bias. There is a greater likelihood that patients with two illnesses will more likely come to the attention of a physician and be diagnosed (Pauls et al., 1986a). In addition, because the symptoms of ADD begin earlier than Tourette's disorder, are disruptive and associated with greater severity of Tourette's disorder, ADD patients are likely to be evaluated earlier. Moreover, many patients with mild Tourette's disorder symptoms with ADD do not seek treatment and are less likely to be identified.

Sex Ratio in Attention Deficit and Tic Disorders

The male to female sex ratio for ADD has been estimated in a range of 4–10:1 (Weiss and Hechtman, 1979; Sandoval et al., 1980; Bloomingdale, 1984). As discussed previously the sex ratio for Tourette's disorder appears to be lowest for patients with mild tic symptoms and highest for those with more severe tics. The male to female ratio averages 1.17:1 in epidemiology tic studies, 1.50:1 in clinical studies of nonspecific tics, 2.63:1 in literature of Tourette's disorder reviews, 3.02:1 in Tourette's disorder questionnaire studies, and 3.90:1 in clinical studies of Tourette's disorder (Table 4.3). This pattern suggests that the male to female ratio increases with the severity of the tics or that the male to female ratio is higher for Tourette's disorder than for other tic disorders. Another factor is the concomitant diagnosis of ADD which may increase the sex ratio and the severity of Tourette's disorder (Table 4.2). The influence of ADD on increasing the male to female sex ratio was supported in a number of analyses. For eleven Tourette's disorder studies, the correlation of the male to female ratio with percent of patients with ADD, was 0.72 ($p = 0.01$), explaining approximately 52% of the variance (Table

4.3). The sex ratio for our total sample was 3.22:1 which is significantly lower ($p < 0.05$) than the average of 4.22:1 for other clinical studies of Tourette's disorder, in part because our sample has fewer ADD patients (Table 4.3). Moreover, the sex ratio dropped to 2.8:1 for Tourette's disorder patients without ADD, compared to 5.7:1 for Tourette's disorder patients with ADD ($p = 0.0016$) (Table 4.4). This relationship was strengthened when we compared our data with the data reported by Comings and Comings (1984). Although they reported a higher male to female ratio of 4.1:1 compared to our ratio of 3.2:1, the ratio for the Tourette's disorder group without ADD was similar for both samples (2.8:1 and 3.0:1, respectively) and was also similar for the Tourette's disorder group with ADD (5.7:1 and 5.8:1, respectively) (Table 4.4). Further support for the relationship between sex ratio and ADD is a comparison of mild and severe ADD (Comings and Comings, 1984). The sex ratio for severe ADD was 19.3:1 compared with 3.4:1 for mild ADD ($p < 0.0033$) (Table 4.4). Finally, in the younger TS+ADD group (16 years or less) in whom the diagnosis of ADD may be more valid, the sex ratio was 8.0:1 for TS+ADD compared to 2.9 for the TS-alone group ($p = 0.003$) (Table 4.5).

Several conclusions are incontrovertible: Sex ratios reported in studies of Tourette's disorder are highly correlated with the percent of patients with ADD, and high sex ratios imply that the samples include many patients with ADD. However, the higher male to female ratio cannot be attributed solely to ADD, since the ratio is higher than expected (2.8–3.0:1) in Tourette's disorder samples without ADD. Further analysis is warranted excluding patients with other organic CNS disorders that have a higher male to female ratio, such as learning disorders, pervasive developmental disorder, etc. Severity of Tourette's disorder, although unrelated to sex ratio ($r = 0.00$, NS), might interact with ADD and other variables. The variability in sex ratio reported in different types of studies and patient categories is perplexing and should be clarified. The results have important implications for the problems of homogeneity and heterogeneity for tic disorders.

Age and Diagnosis of Attention Deficit Disorder

As previously discussed, the diagnosis of ADD is more difficult to make in adults than children. ADD was diagnosed in 33% of patients 16 years or younger and in 15% of patients over 16 years of age ($\chi^2 = 9.96$, df=1, $p = 0.0014$) (Table 4.5).

Sample Changes over Time Associated with Attention Deficit Disorder

The change in the percent of patients with ADD in our samples has been described previously. Between 1965 and 1974, ADD was diagnosed in 51.2% of our sample, in 21.4% between 1975 and 1978, and 16.4% between 1979 and 1981 ($p = 0.0000$) (Table 4.1). The correlation of ADD with year of evaluation is $r = -0.20$ ($p = 0.0014$), which explains 4% of the variance for change in diagnosis over time. A further indication of variability for the diagnosis of ADD is the significant increase in the diagnosis of ADD from 24.9% for patients evaluated between 1965 and 1981, compared with 42.4% for those evaluated between 1981 and 1985 ($\chi^2 = 28.8$, df=1, $p = 0.0000$) (Tables 4.3, 4.4).

As previously discussed, this may be due to the severity of the illness in patients with Tourette's disorder now being referred to us, fewer patients with mild symptoms, and an increase in patients with more severe symptoms and diverse complications including ADD.

Private Versus Clinic Patients and Diagnosis of Attention Deficit Disorder

In recent years, concurrent with referral of more severe patients, we noted an increase in the number of referrals from state hospitals, residential treatment centers, and patients in lower socioeconomic classes. These patients have many more problems in general, including ADD. For example, in 1984, 68% of clinic patients had ADD compared to 32% of private patients ($\chi^2 = 6.7$, df=1, $p = 0.0099$) (Table 4.25). Perhaps some of the increase can be explained by our offer of free treatment to patients participating in several recent grant-supported large scale studies of drugs, which tended to attract patients with more severe Tourette's disorder, problems, and ADD. Thus, the percent of Tourette's disorder patients with ADD, and the usual secondary consequences of having ADD, is associated with the source of referral and place of evaluation.

Increased Severity of Tourette's Disorder with Attention Deficit Disorder and Hyperactivity

Our clinical impression throughout the years was that Tourette's disorder is more severe in patients with TS+ADD and especially those with hyperactivity.

TABLE 4.25. *Relationship of private and clinic patients to diagnoses of Tourette and attention deficit disorders*[a]

Diagnosis	Total		Private patients		Clinic patients	
	N	%	N	%	N	%
TS-alone	34	50.8	25	64.1	9	32.1
TS+ADD	33	49.3	14	35.9	19	67.9
Total	67	100.0	39	100.0	28	100.0

[a] $\chi^2 = 6.7$, df=1, $p = 0.0099$.

TABLE 4.26. *Significant correlations of severity of tic variables with attention deficit disorder and hyperactivity*[a]

Severity variables	TS+ADD[b]	Hyperactivity FS[c]	Conners Hyperactivity Index[d]
Severity of tics	0.24[e]	0.23[e]	0.24[e]
Age at onset of TS	−0.16[e]	−0.17[f]	−0.19[f]
Complex tics	0.09[g]	0.20[f]	0.23[e]
Coprolalia	0.23[e]	0.23[e]	0.26[e]
Copropraxia	0.06	0.18[f]	0.21[e]
Echophilia	0.04	0.21[f]	0.22[e]
Number current tics	0.02	0.20[f]	0.22[e]
Number cumulative tics	0.09[h]	0.32[e]	0.34[e]
Attention deficit disorder	—	0.49[e]	0.47[e]
Hyperactivity FS	0.49[e]	—	0.94[e]
Conners Hyperactivity Index	0.47[e]	0.94[e]	—

[a] Other variables (see variables 33–47, Table A.1) not included in the table were not significant.
[b] $N = 666$.
[c] $N = 318$.
[d] $N = 318$.
[e] $p < 0.0001$.
[f] $p < 0.001$.
[g] $p < 0.01$.
[h] $p < 0.05$.

To evaluate this hypothesis, variables reflecting severity of Tourette's disorder symptoms (variables 33–37, Table A.1) were correlated with TS+ADD versus TS-alone, the Conners Hyperactivity Index and Hyperactivity FS.

The results consistently support the hypothesis. TS+ADD and measures of hyperactivity [(which are correlated 0.47–0.49 ($p = 0.0001$)] account for 5 to 6% of the variance in ratings of Tourette's disorder severity and 12% for total number of tics. Other analyses (Table 4.27) suggest that increased severity of Tourette's syndrome is associated with both the TS+ADD+H and TS+ADD−H groups, but that other indices of severity are further increased by ADD patients with hyperactivity (TS+ADD+H).

A possible method of dissecting the effect of hyperactivity on severity is to treat patients with TS+ADD+H and TS+ADD−H with stimulants. Treatment with stimulants at an appropriate nontoxic dosage, which does not increase tics and decreases hyperactivity, should decrease severity of Tourette's disorder in the TS+ADD+H group but not in the TS+ADD−H group, if it is caused by hyperactivity or general arousal. If the severity of Tourette's disorder does not decrease more in the TS+ADD+H group than in the TS+ADD−H group, it would imply that general arousal associated with hyperactivity does not increase the severity of Tourette's disorder. Finally, if the severity decreases in both the TS+ADD+H and TS+ADD−H groups, it would suggest that other features of ADD (inattention, impulsivity, etc.) are the cause of increased severity.

The first interpretation is supported by three uncontrolled clinical studies that reported improvement of Tourette's disorder in approximately one-third of ADD patients treated with stimulants, although the change could have been due to spontaneous or other factors (Shapiro et al., 1981; Comings and Comings, 1984; Erenberg, 1985). A possible indirect indication that hyperactivity may not be the major factor derives from our procedures for treating patients with TS+ADD+H (see Chapter 12). We first titrate the dose of haloperidol to achieve maximum benefit on tics, which does not reduce hyperactivity, and then carefully titrate the dose of a stimulant for control of the hyperactivity. Although hyperactivity decreases, there is no increase in tics, unless the appropriate dosage is exceeded. A more direct test of the hypothesis would be to use the stimulant alone, before using haloperidol, but this has not been done. Hyperactivity alone, therefore, may not be an adequate explanation for the increased level of severity for patients with ADD+H. Other possible explanations include less ability to control, minimize, or reduce symptoms because of decreased ego resources, less motivation, preoccupation with other problems, and greater CNS involvement. Whatever the relationship between TS-alone, TS+ADD+H, and TS+ADD−H, these data explain a significant amount of the variability reported in studies of ADD associated with Tourette's disorder, the severity of Tourette's, the presence of other associated organic stigmata and psychopathology. They highlight the problem of heterogeneity among tic disorders and the importance of describing data separately for patients with TS-alone, TS+ADD+H, and TS+ADD−H.

Comparison of Patients with Tourette's Disorder Alone and Tourette's Disorder with Attention Deficit Disorder

Based on our clinical impression that there are important differences between patients with TS-alone, TS+ADD+H, and TS+ADD−H, we developed five hypotheses prior to analyzing our data. Retrospective analyses were done for heuristic purposes. Variables were compared for the three diagnostic groups utilizing ANOVA and Duncan Multiple Range Tests for continuous variables and chi-square and partitioning tests for categorical variables (Table 4.27). Occasional references are made to previous analyses. Hypotheses are largely related to differences between the total ADD (TS+ADD) group (with and without hyperactivity) and the TS-alone group. The results for each of the hypotheses are presented first followed by the retrospective analysis.

Hypothesis I

The expectation was that the percent of patients with the diagnosis of ADD would vary significantly over the years. More specifically, the percent of patients with ADD would be highest for patients evaluated between 1965 and

TABLE 4.27. Comparison of variables for patients with Tourette's disorder with attention deficit disorder and hyperactivity,[a] Tourette's disorder with attention deficit disorder without hyperactivity,[b] and Tourette's disorder without attention deficit disorder or hyperactivity[c]

Hypotheses and variables	Sample N	Mean or %			χ^2 or F[d] $p<$	Duncan or χ^e ($p<$)[e]		
		ADD+H	ADD−H	TS		ADD+H vs. ADD−H	ADD+H vs. TS	ADD−H vs. TS
Hypothesis I: Decrease of ADD sample over time								
1965–1974	121	40.5%	10.7%	48.8%				
1975–1978	313	15.7	5.8	78.6%				
1979–1981	232	14.2%	2.2%	83.6%				
Total	666	19.7%	5.4%	74.9%	0.0001	—	0.0001	0.0001
Hypothesis II: ADD overrepresented in sample								
Previous consultation FS	666	3.4	3.4	3.2	0.001	—	0.05	0.05
Previous diagnosis of TS	666	48.9%	47.2%	34.9%	0.01	—	—	—
Previous consultation or Rx	666	93.9%	97.%	85.2%	0.01	0.05	0.05	—
Duration of illness FS	666	9.9	13.5	14.8	0.0001	—	0.05	—
Years from onset to diagnosis	666	7.6	11.0	12.2	0.001	—	0.05	—
Durationn of illness	666	8.8	12.1	13.1	0.001	—	0.05	—
Age at first diagnosis of TS	666	13.3	17.3	19.1	0.0001	0.05	0.05	—
Age at first consultation	666	10.7	13.7	15.1	0.0001	0.05	0.05	—
Age at current evaluation	666	14.7	15.5	19.7	0.0001	—	0.05	0.05
Sex (percent males)	666	84.7%	86.1%	73.4	0.01	—	—	—
Hypothesis III: TS more severe in ADD sample								
Severity of TS symptoms	666	3.0	2.8	2.5	0.0001	—	0.05	0.05
Age at onset for TS	666	5.8	6.3	6.9	0.0001	—	0.05	—
Age at onset of motor tics	666	6.1	6.2	7.1	0.001	—	0.05	—
Age at onset of vocal tics	666	7.8	9.2	9.6	0.0001	—	0.05	—
Age at onset of coprolalia	209	10.3	9.2	12.0	0.10	—	—	—
TS onset to coprolalia (years)	209	4.7	4.6	5.7	—	—	—	—
Lifetime prevalence of tics:								
Face	666	90.8%	100.0%	93.2%	—	—	—	—
Head	666	90.1%	83.9%	91.6%	—	—	—	—

Arms	666	69.5%	66.7%	68.5%	—	—	—
Legs	666	42.0%	36.1%	40.5%	—	—	—
Torso	666	45.0%	47.2%	46.9%	—	—	—
Complex	666	77.1%	72.2%	65.9%	0.05	—	0.01
Vocal sounds	666	100.0%	96.9%	98.1%	—	—	—
Coprolalia	666	44.3%	41.7%	28.1%	0.001	—	0.0001
Mental coprolalia	666	5.3%	8.3%	3.2%	—	—	—
Copropraxia	666	16.0%	16.7%	11.6%	—	—	—
Echolalia	666	37.4%	28.6%	31.7%	—	—	—
Total number of current tics	666	7.0	8.2	6.9	—	—	—
Total number of cumulative tics	666	17.2	17.3	15.2	0.10	—	—
Hypothesis IV: More organic stigmata in ADD sample							
Neurological							
Normal	270	44.0%	69.2%	80.6%	0.0001	0.10	.0001
Borderline abnormality	91	41.8%	30.8%	17.1%			
Definite abnormality	19	14.3%	0.0%	2.3%			
Electroencephalogram							
Total Sample							
Normal	199	51.7	50.0	66.7	0.06ᶠ	—	—
Borderline abnormality	52	20.7	21.4	13.3			
Definite abnormality	74	27.6	28.6	20.0			
Sample less than 17 years of age							
Normal	114	45.7	43.8	63.0	0.01	—	0.05ᶠ
Borderline abnormality	29	24.3	6.3	9.2			
Definite abnormality	62	30.0	50.0	27.7			
Maturational milestones							
Age sat-walk-talk FS	666	3.1	3.4	3.0	0.001	0.05	—
Age sat	666	0.5	0.6	0.5	0.01	0.05	—
Age walked	666	1.1	1.2	1.1	0.02	0.05	—
Age talked	666	1.5	1.6	1.4	0.05	—	—
Age bladder-bowel trained FS	666	5.1	4.7	4.2	0.0001	—	0.05
Age bladder trained	666	2.5	2.3	2.1	0.0001	—	0.05
Age bowel trained	666	2.5	2.4	2.1	0.0001	—	0.05
Handedness							
Right vs. other handedness	666	74.0%	72.2%	80.0%	—	—	—

(continued)

TABLE 4.27. (Continued)

Hypotheses and variables	Sample N	Mean or %			χ^2 or F [d] $p<$	Duncan or χ^2 ($p<$) [e]		
		ADD+H	ADD−H	TS		ADD+H vs. ADD−H	ADD+H vs. TS	ADD−H vs. TS
Psychological Tests								
Bender-Gestalt Test	170	64.0%	60.9%	27.8%	0.0001	—	0.05	0.05
WISC								
Information	67	9.5	9.4	11.3	—	—	—	—
Comprehension	67	9.9	9.3	10.2	—	—	—	—
Arithmetic	67	9.4	8.7	11.6	0.01	—	0.05	0.05
Similarities	67	10.8	10.6	11.4	—	—	—	—
Vocabulary	67	10.2	10.1	11.4	—	—	—	—
Digit span	42	10.4	9.0	10.5	—	—	—	—
Picture completion	63	9.1	7.1	10.6	0.05	—	—	0.05
Picture arrangement	63	9.9	9.3	11.4	0.10	—	—	0.05
Block design	63	9.7	8.0	11.8	0.05	—	—	0.05
Object assembly	63	9.1	8.2	11.1	0.05	—	—	0.05
Coding or maze	63	8.5	8.2	10.2	—	—	—	—
Verbal IQ	131	99.3	95.9	107.1	0.05	—	—	0.05
Performance IQ	131	94.5	83.5	104.3	0.0001	0.05	0.05	0.05
Full scale IQ	131	96.8	89.1	106.3	0.001	—	0.05	0.05
VIQ-PIQ Discrepancy Score	131	13.8	15.1	13.3	—	—	—	—
Hypothesis V: More behavior problems and less assets in ADD sample								
Behavior Problems								
Hyperactivity FS	318	2.3	1.4	1.1	0.0001	0.05	0.05	0.05
Constant fidgeting	318	2.3	1.5	1.5	0.0001	0.05	0.05	—
Inattentive, distractible	318	2.4	1.5	0.8	0.0001	0.05	0.05	0.05
Restless, overactive	318	2.5	1.4	1.3	0.0001	0.05	0.05	—
Short attention span	318	2.3	1.5	0.8	0.0001	0.05	0.05	0.05
Excitable, impulsive	318	2.4	1.4	1.3	0.0001	0.05	0.05	—
Disturb other children	318	1.8	1.1	0.5	0.0001	0.05	0.05	0.05
Learning disorder FS	318	1.5	1.2	0.4	0.0001	—	0.05	0.05
Academic disabilities	384	1.9	1.5	0.5	0.0001	0.05	0.05	0.05
Reading disabilities	385	1.2	0.9	0.3	0.0001	—	0.05	0.05

	N							
Anger-moodiness FS	318	1.7	1.1	0.9	0.0001	0.05	—	—
Unpredictable, explosive temper	318	1.7	1.0	0.8	0.0001	0.05	—	—
Explosive anger	318	1.7	1.1	1.0	0.0001	0.05	—	—
Mood changes	318	1.7	1.1	0.9	0.0001	0.05	—	—
Destructive acts	318	1.0	0.8	0.4	0.0001	0.05	0.05	0.05
Easily frustrated	318	2.3	2.0	0.8	0.0001	—	—	—
Cries often and easily	318	1.4	1.0	0.8	0.0001	0.05	—	—
Inhibition FS	317	0.9	0.9	0.7	—	—	—	—
Difficulty expressing anger	317	0.8	0.7	0.6	—	—	—	—
Difficulty expressing emotion	317	0.9	0.9	0.7	—	—	—	—
Conners Parent Hyperactivity	318	20.8	13.5	10.0	0.0001	0.05	0.05	—
Obsessive-compulsive-like symptoms FS	317	0.8	0.8	0.7	—	—	—	—
Compulsive personality FS	317	1.1	1.2	1.2	—	—	—	—
Assets and abilities								
Coordination abilities FS	397	1.9	1.9	2.4	0.0001	—	0.05	0.05
Coordination	397	1.7	1.8	2.5	0.0001	—	0.05	0.05
Athletic ability	397	1.9	1.9	2.4	0.001	—	0.05	0.05
Mechanical ability	397	2.0	2.0	2.3	0.05	—	—	—
Intellectual-psychosocial FS	397	2.0	2.0	2.5	0.0001	—	0.05	0.05
Intelligence	397	2.4	2.3	2.7	0.01	—	—	0.05
School achievement	397	2.0	1.8	2.6	—	—	0.05	0.05
Verbal ability	397	2.5	2.5	2.7	—	—	—	—
Mathematical ability	397	1.5	1.8	2.4	0.0001	—	0.05	0.05
Emotional maturity	397	1.4	1.5	2.1	0.0001	—	0.05	0.05
Retrospective Analysis								
Demography								
Social class	666	2.9	2.8	2.8	—	—	—	—
Genetics (family history of:)								
Tourette's disorder	641	7.4%	0.0%	8.4%	—	—	—	—
Tic disorder	641	44.6%	52.9%	40.6	—	—	—	—
TS or tic disorder	641	49.6%	52.9%	45.5%	—	—	—	—
Other movement disorder	641	13.2%	5.9%	8.4	—	—	—	—
Birth history								
Parents' age at birth FS	666	26.8	29.2	27.2	—	—	—	—
Mothers' abortions	666	0.5	0.5	0.5	—	0.05	—	—
Pregnancy complications	666	35.9%	19.4%	20.4%	0.001	0.05	—	—

(continued)

TABLE 4.27. (Continued)

Hypotheses and variables	Sample N	Mean or % ADD+H	Mean or % ADD−H	Mean or % TS	χ^2 or F^d $p<$	Duncan or χ^2 ($p<$)[e] ADD+H vs. ADD−H	Duncan or χ^2 ($p<$)[e] ADD+H vs. TS	Duncan or χ^2 ($p<$)[e] ADD−H vs. TS
Birth complications	666	28.2%	20.0%	21.0%	—	—	—	—
Length of labor	666	2.2	0.1	1.3	—	—	—	—
Birth order	666	2.5	2.7	2.5	—	—	—	—
Clinical course								
Waxing and waning of severity	666	98.5%	97.2%	91.2%	—	—	—	—
Fluctuation of tics	666	95.4%	97.2%	95.3%	—	—	—	—
Periods of remission	666	23.8%	31.3%	28.5%	—	—	—	—
Length of remission	666	0.5	0.7	0.7	—	—	—	—
Years from onset to coprolalia	198	4.7	3.2	5.3	—	—	—	—
Effect of stimuli on tics[g]								
Interpersonal stimuli FS	394	3.4	3.3	3.3	—	—	—	—
Lectures, church, temple	372	4.3	3.5	3.5	0.01	0.05	0.05	—
School or work	360	4.1	4.1	3.5	0.001	—	0.05	0.05
Passive stimuli FS	394	4.2	3.9	3.9	—	—	—	—
Movies	371	5.2	4.9	4.6	0.01	—	0.05	—
Nonanxious absorption FS	394	3.2	3.0	3.0	—	—	—	—
Anxiety-fatigue FS	394	3.8	3.7	3.6	—	—	—	—
Pleasurable anticipation	394	5.2	4.9	4.6	0.001	—	0.05	—
Seasonable stimuli FS	394	4.1	3.9	3.8	0.01	—	0.05	—
Spring	336	4.4	4.1	4.0	0.002	0.05	—	—
Autumn	338	4.3	4.3	4.1	0.10	0.05	—	—

[a] ADD+H; $N = 131$.
[b] ADD−H; $N = 36$.
[c] TS; $N = 499$.
[d] F (ANOVA) for means; χ^2 (chi-square) for percents.
[e] Two-tailed tests used except where noted; df = 4 for partitioned χ^2; Duncan Extended Range Tests, $p < 0.05$.
[f] One-tailed test.
[g] Other variables (see variables 55–59, a–f, Table A.1) not included if not significant.

1974, lowest for patients evaluated between 1975 and 1981, and be increased subsequently. This expectation was confirmed: 51.2% of patients evaluated between 1965 and 1974 had ADD compared with 21.1% in the period 1975 to 1978, and 16.4% in the period 1979 to 1981 ($p = 0.0000$) (Table 4.27), and 42.4% for patients evaluated between 1981 and 1985 ($p = 0.0000$) (Table 4.4).

Hypothesis II

The expectation was that the percent of patients with ADD would be overrepresented in our sample of Tourette's disorder patients. Based on the higher than expected frequency of ADD in Tourette's disorder patients and the variability of the diagnosis for ADD in our sample and in published studies, we reasoned that patients with two illnesses (TS and ADD) are more likely to be diagnosed as having Tourette's disorder than if they only had TS-alone. Moreover, the symptoms of ADD which usually begin earlier than the symptoms of Tourette's disorder, are disruptive and lead to early referral, evaluation, diagnosis, management, and treatment. The symptoms of Tourette's disorder may be observed and diagnosed either at the initial evaluation or subsequently. This possibility is especially important and distinctly possible since only approximately 30% of Tourette's disorder and CMT patients seek evaluation for their symptoms (Pauls et al., 1984; Caine, 1985). Our expectations were that our data would provide indirect support for the hypothesis: TS+ADD compared with TS-alone patients would have an earlier onset of Tourette's disorder, more consultations for tics prior to our evaluation, a younger age at initial consultation for tics, more frequent diagnosis of Tourette's disorder prior to our evaluation, diagnosis of Tourette's disorder at a younger age, shorter duration between onset and diagnosis of Tourette's disorder, younger age at our evaluation, and shorter duration of illness. Our expectations were confirmed for all variables (Table 4.27).

Hypothesis III

Our hypothesis was that Tourette's syndrome patients with ADD had more severe disease than those with TS-alone. The hypothesis was evaluated by postulating that TS+ADD patients would have greater severity and an earlier age at onset of Tourette's disorder symptoms, earlier age at onset for muscular, vocal, and coprophilic tics, more lifetime or cumulative tics of all types, and more total current and cumulative symptoms. Almost all expectations were confirmed by the ANOVA's (Table 4.27) and correlations (Table 4.28). Tourette's disorder symptoms are significantly more severe for both the TS+ADD+H and TS+ADD−H groups. The trend for all tic types to be more frequent in the ADD groups are in the expected direction and might have reached significance if the groups were equated for age, since the ADD group was significantly younger and had less time available to develop these tics.

Hypothesis IV

We hypothesized that the TS+ADD group, compared with the TS-alone group, would have significantly more abnormalities on the neurological and EEG examinations, psychological tests (Bender-Gestalt Test, Wechsler Intelligence Scale for Children), delayed maturational milestones, and more frequent left handedness or ambidexterity. These expectations were confirmed (Table 4.27). This finding confirms our impression and conclusion that the ADD group accounts for a significant amount of the variance for organic findings reported in Tourette's disorder patients. Since the ADD group may be artifactually overrepresented in Tourette's disorder samples, TS-alone and TS+ADD groups should be studied separately.

Hypothesis V

Our expectation was that psychological adjustment and amount of psychopathology in patients with TS-alone is essentially no different from what would be found in the population, and that increased psychopathology and behavioral symptoms reported in the literature (Cohen et al., 1982; Leckman et al., 1983) is characteristic of or associated with patients who had TS+ADD. This expectation was confirmed in a comparison of the three groups on 26 of 33 behavioral variables (Table 4.27).

Retrospective Analysis

The retrospective analysis for the variables listed in Table 4.27 are for the most part not significantly different for the TS-alone and TS+ADD groups. As expected the male to female ratio is higher for the TS+ADD groups. Pregnancy complications were significantly greater for the TS+ADD+H than the TS-alone group. Family history of Tourette's disorder, tic and other movement disorders and features of the clinical course of Tourette's disorder were not significantly different. An interesting retrospective finding was the effect of stimuli on symptoms. The effect of stimuli on symptoms is rated on a six-point scale as 1: disappear, 2: marked decrease, 3: slight decrease, 4: no change, 5: slight increase, and 6: marked increase. Mean scores for Stimuli-Induced Factor Scores were highest for the TS+ADD+H group and lowest for the TS-alone group, suggesting decreased ability of the TS+ADD+H group to inhibit tics. It is well known that pleasurable anticipation usually increases symptoms in patients with Tourette's disorder. Symptoms were increased in the three groups, but significantly more in the TS+ADD+H group. Listening to a lecture or sermon decreased symptoms for the TS-alone and TS+ADD−H groups as expected, but symptoms significantly increased for the TS+ADD+H group. Similarly, symptoms are usually less noticeable in school or at work than in other settings (at home, alone, etc.). Symptoms decreased for the TS-alone group, but increased significantly for the TS+ADD−H and TS+ADD+H groups. These results suggest that patients with TS-alone can inhibit their symptoms somewhat better at lectures, school, and work, whereas the reverse is true for patients with TS+ADD+H and TS+ADD−H. Pleasurable anticipation increases symptoms in all patients, but significantly more so in the TS+ADD+H group. This pattern would increase psychosocial difficulties for patients with TS+ADD+H and result in negative reactions from others. The effect of other situational stimuli items on symptoms are not significantly different among the groups (see variables 55–59, a–f, Table A.1).

Stepwise Regression Analysis

A stepwise regression analysis (SRA) provided a final test of the hypothesis. We hypothesized that the SRA for the dependent variable TS+ADD versus TS-alone would select demographic and illness variables associated with referral and sample characteristics and variables associated with CNS dysfunction, and that only CNS dysfunction variables would account for significant variance in the final SRA. Our hypotheses were confirmed (Table 4.28).

Neurological, Electroencephalographic, and Psychological Test Abnormalities

To complete this section about patient characteristics, organic factors suggesting CNS impairment are summarized in Table 4.29. Consistent with our hypothesis, these organic factors are significantly higher for the TS+ADD group than for the TS-alone group. Each factor is discussed in detail elsewhere: neurological and EEG abnormalities in Chapter 7 and psychological test abnormalities in Chapter 6.

Conclusion

These results strongly indicate that studies of Tourette's disorder are confounded by the presence of TS+ADD patients in samples and that many

TABLE 4.28. *Attention deficit disorder; stepwise regression analysis*

Variables	r	R^2	Parameter estimate
Demography			
Year evaluated	−0.17[a]	0.03	−0.03[a]
Age	−0.17[a]	0.06	−0.01[a]
Male vs. female	0.12[b]	0.07	0.11[b]
Genetics			
—	—	—	—
Medical			
Bladder-bowel trained FS	0.23[a]	0.05	−0.12[c]
Pregnancy complications	0.13[c]	0.07	0.07[a]
Neurological			
Neurological abnormality	0.32[a]	0.10	0.26[a]
Behavior			
Learning disorder FS	0.50[a]	0.25	0.15[a]
Hyperactivity FS	0.49[a]	0.33	0.15[a]
Coordination FS	−0.25[a]	0.36	−0.08[b]
Illness variables			
Duration of illness FS	−0.16[a]	0.02	−0.01[c]
Previous diagnosis-consultation FS	0.15[a]	0.04	0.09[c]
Symptoms			
Severity of TS	0.24[a]	0.06	0.11[a]
Age at onset of TS	−0.16[a]	0.09	−0.03[a]
Summary SRA			
Hyperactivity FS	0.49[a]	0.30	0.16[a]
Learning disorder FS	0.50[a]	0.40	0.15[a]
Neurological abnormality	0.32[a]	0.46	0.18[c]
Pregnancy complications	0.13[c]	0.47	0.13[d]
Coordination FS	−0.25[a]	0.48	−0.07[d]
Adjusted R^2		0.47	

[a] $p < 0.0001$.
[b] $p < 0.01$.
[c] $p < 0.001$.
[d] $p < 0.05$.

published reports describe characteristics associated with ADD rather than Tourette's disorder. This confusion will perpetuate the problem of heterogeneity and impede further understanding of Tourette's disorder unless future research on Tourette's disorder controls for this variable.

SITUATIONAL EVENTS PRECEDING THE ONSET OF TOURETTE'S DISORDER

Situational events are frequently cited as precipitants of Tourette's disorder. Such events were recorded on the MDQ and evaluated during the clinical

TABLE 4.29. *Organic factors in patients with Tourette's disorder*

Variables	Total N	Total %	TS+ADD %	TS−alone %
Handedness				
Right	517	77.6	72.5	80.0
Left or ambidexterous	149	22.4	27.5	20.0
Total	666	100.0	100.0	100.0
Attention Deficit Disorder				
TS-alone	499	74.9		
TS+ADD+H	131	19.7		
TS+ADD−H	36	5.4		
Total	666	100.0		
Neurological Abnormality				
Normal	270	71.1	49.6	80.6
Borderline abnormality	91	23.9	39.3	17.1
Definite abnormality	19	5.0	11.1	2.3
Total	380	100.0	100.0	100.0
Electroencephalogram				
Normal	199	61.2	51.3	66.7
Borderline abnormality	52	16.0	20.9	13.3
Definite abnormality	74	22.8	27.8	20.0
Total	325	100.0	100.0	100.0
Bender-Gestalt Test ($N = 170$)				
Normal	88	51.8	36.7	72.2
Borderline abnormality	20	11.8	13.3	9.7
Definite abnormality	62	36.5	50.0	18.1
Total	170	100.0	100.0	
WISC and WAIS Verbal-Performance Discrepancy Score				
Below 15	100	59.9	52.4	71.9
15 and over	67	40.1	47.6	28.1
Total	131	100.0	100.0	100.0

Comparison	χ^2	df	p
Handedness	7.5	1	0.061
Neurological	48.3	2	0.000
EEG	7.5	1	0.024
Bender-Gestalt Test	22.2	2	0.000
Discrepancy Score	6.2	1	0.013

interview (Table 4.30). Situational events cited by 23% of the sample are too wide ranging to support the concept of a specific relationship of situational factors to the onset of Tourette's disorder.

Moreover, it is likely that any sample of individuals would cite similar premorbid events prior to the onset of any illness, including organic diseases such as homologous serum jaundice; in other words, they are random chance events. A definitive evaluation of the importance of these premorbid events

TABLE 4.30. *Situational factors preceding onset of Tourette's disorder*

Factors	%	N
None	77.0	513
Infection	4.7	31
Infection, death of family member	0.2	1
Infection, separation from family member		
Infection, accident, surgery	0.3	2
Allergy injections	0.3	2
Surgery	1.7	11
Surgery, infection	0.5	3
Surgery, divorce in the family	0.2	1
Surgery, accident	0.2	1
Divorce in family	1.5	10
Divorce in family, death of family member	0.3	2
Divorce in family, separation from family member	1.1	7
Divorce in family, death of family member, birth of sibling, accident	0.2	1
Divorce in family, birth of own child	0.2	1
Death of family member	3.5	23
Death of family member, divorce	0.3	2
Death of family member, separation from family member	0.2	1
Death of family member, birth of sibling	0.5	3
Death of family member, accident	0.2	1
Death of family member, surgery, accident	0.3	2
Separation from family member	2.0	13
Separation from family member, birth of sibling	0.2	1
Father's hospitalization, death of friend	0.5	3
Birth of sibling	1.5	10
Birth of sibling, accident	0.2	1
Accident	2.4	16
Skip grade in school	0.2	1
Entered class for intellectually gifted	0.2	1
Move to new neighborhood	0.3	2

to the onset of Tourette's disorder requires comparison with a medical-illness control group. However, since 77% of the sample did not cite premorbid events, and the cited events were so wide ranging, we are of the opinion that there is no relevant association between premorbid events and Tourette's disorder.

5

Signs, Symptoms, and Clinical Course

The signs, symptoms, and clinical course for 666 Tourette's disorder patients are described in this chapter and compared to data in the literature. Because the sample is larger than our previous samples and those reported by other investigators, the results provide a firm basis for describing Tourette's disorder. They also contribute to the development of reliable criteria for the diagnosis and differential diagnosis of tic disorders, and to clarifying of the problem of heterogeneity for tic disorders.

Features of the present illness, such as age at onset and duration of illness are described, followed by detailed description of the initial and subsequent signs and symptoms, clinical course, and other associated features. Although signs refer to objective evidence of a disease which is perceptible to a physician, and symptoms refer to change in a bodily or mental state, or subjective evidence of a disease perceived by a patient, we use the term symptoms to refer to both signs and symptoms. The data are presented in tables of means, standard deviations, medians and ranges, or both, based on the appropriateness of the description. Financial limitations precluded analyses controlling for factors such as sex, attention deficit disorder (ADD), age and duration of illness, and the results are described largely for the total sample. Whenever possible, we have indicated how these factors and other variables affect the results.

PATIENT CHARACTERISTICS

Age at Onset

The mean age at onset of tics is 6.7 years, with a median of 6 and range of 1 to 17 years (Table 5.1), not significantly different from our previous sample (Table 5.2) (Shapiro et al., 1978). The range has increased from 2 to 13

TABLE 5.1. *Age at onset of Tourette's disorder*

Age (years)	N	%	Cumulative %
1	1	0.2	0.2
2	22	3.3	3.5
3	60	9.1	12.6
4	87	13.2	25.7
5	84	12.7	38.4
6	91	13.8	52.2
7	81	12.3	64.4
8	73	11.0	75.5
9	57	8.6	84.1
10	46	7.0	91.1
11	17	2.6	93.6
12	19	2.9	96.5
13	12	1.8	98.3
14	6	0.9	99.2
15	3	0.5	99.7
16	1	0.2	99.8
17	1	0.2	100.0
Unknown	5	—	—
Total	666	100.0	—

years to 1 to 17 years. Over 90% of our sample developed tics by age 10, similar to two other reports which estimated that 80 to 95% of patients developed tics by age 10 (Torup, 1962; Erenberg et al., 1986); Tourette's disorder developed in 99.2% by age 14. The age at onset of Tourette's disorder, however, has been reported as beginning at age 35 in two male patients (Aranetta et al., 1979; Marneros, 1984). The age at onset was not significantly different for males and females in our sample.

However, informants frequently under- or overestimate the age at onset (Shapiro et al., 1978). Detailed questioning during the clinical interview and data obtained from medical records usually elicit a younger age at onset for tics compared to responses to questionnaires. For example, in our previous study, the reported age at onset was significantly older in questionnaires completed by patients compared to data obtained by interview (Shapiro et al., 1978). This finding was confirmed in a comparison of the age at onset in two samples studied between 1972 and 1979: responses of 208 patients who completed a questionnaire and responses of 496 patients who were interviewed. The mean age at onset for the questionnaire sample was significantly older (7.7 years) compared to the interviewed sample (6.9 years) (Table 5.2) (1-tailed t-test = 1.8, df-698, $p = 0.03$). Studies in the literature cite a mean age at onset that varies from 6.1 to 9.2 years, with a range of 1 to 19 years (Table 5.2).

The age at onset is a potentially important variable for study of Tourette's

TABLE 5.2. *Studies citing age at onset of Tourette and tic disorders*

Studies	N	Mean	SD	Median	Range
TS					
Tourette (1885)	9	9.2	—	—	6–16
Eisenberg et al. (1959)	7	6.1	—	—	4–8
Feild et al. (1966)	7	6.4	—	—	4–13
Challas et al. (1967)	11	7.1	—	—	4–10
Lucas et al. (1967)	15	6.6	—	—	4–10
Morphew and Sim. (1969)	5	8.6	—	—	2–15
Abuzzahab et al. (1971)	7	8.6	—	—	5–13
Fisarova (1972)	27	—	—	—	3–10
Moldofsky et al. (1974)	15	8.1	—	—	5–13
Shapiro et al. (1978)	114	7.0	2.7	7.5	2–13
Gonce and Dugas (1981)	27	7.0	—	—	4–12
Nee et al. (1980)	50	7.0	—	—	2–13
Lucas et al. (1982)	25	—	—	8.0	1–19
Golden and Hood 1982	80	6.5	3.0	6.0	2–13
Nomura and Segawa (1982)	97	—	—	—	2–15
Asam (1982)	16	8.0	—	—	4–14
Min (1983)	24	8.1	2.8	—	5–16
Han-bai and Han-quin (1983)	19	8.0	—	—	4–12
Comings and Comings (1985)	250	6.9	3.0	—	—
Lees et al. (1984)	53	7.0	2.8	—	7–16
Montgomery et al. (1982)	15	7.3	—	—	5–12
Erenberg et al. (1986)	200	6.3	—	—	—
Current study[a]	661	6.7	2.8	6.0	1–17
TS survey					
Jagger et al. (1982)	75	7.0	—	—	2–16
Stefl (1983, 1984)	431	7.4	—	—	1–16
Current study[b]	208	7.7	6.9	—	—
Zausmer (1954)	96	—	—	—	3–12
Corbett et al. (1969)	116	7.3	2.7	—	2–16
Negishi (1983)	29	7.0	—	—	—

[a]Consecutive clinical patients from 1965 to 1981.
[b]Questionnaire survey from 1972 to 1979.

disorder. The extreme variability is perplexing, difficult to interpret, and contributes complexity to conducting and interpreting the results of studies. Are there differences between patients who develop Tourette's disorder below the age of 5 years (our youngest patient was 1 year old) and those who develop Tourette's disorder after 13 years of age (our oldest patient was 17 years of age)? Is age a potential source of heterogeneity? Does the wide range for the onset of Tourette's disorder (1–19 years of age) indicate that Tourette's disorder is not a developmental disorder? Or, is there an organic CNS vulnerability or potential that requires an environmental factor for the development of this disorder?

For possible insights stepwise regression analysis (SRA) was done to account for variability of age at onset of TS (Table 5.3). Our impression was that TS+ADD patients would have a younger age at onset.

TABLE 5.3. *Summary stepwise regression analyses for dependent variables: Age at onset of Tourette's disorder, history of complex coprolalia, copropraxic, and echophilic tics*

Variables	T	R^2	Parameter estimate
Age at onset of TS			
Age	0.30^a	0.08	1.01^a
Duration of illness FS	0.16^a	0.69	-0.99^a
Attention deficit disorder	-0.16^a	0.70	-0.75^a
Copropraxia	-0.12^b	0.72	-1.23^a
Remission of symptoms FS	-0.19^a	0.73	-0.23^b
Adjusted R^2		0.52^a	
Complex tics			
Attention deficit disorder	0.09^b	0.03	0.09
Number of cumulative tics	0.41^a	0.20	0.02^a
Learning disorder FS	0.20^c	0.22	0.06^d
Adjusted R^2		0.21^a	
Coprolalia			
Number of cumulative tics	0.21^a	0.26	0.26^a
Mental coprolalia	0.21^a	0.32	0.06^a
Previous diagnosis or consultation FS		0.36	0.04^c
History of leg tics	0.11^b	0.39	-0.03^b
Severity of TS	0.46^a	0.42	0.03^b
Number of current tics	0.24^a	0.44	-0.02^d
Adjusted R^2		0.43^a	
Copropraxia			
Number of cumulative tics	0.37^a	0.19	0.01^a
Coprolalia	0.26^a	0.22	0.19^c
Bladder-bowel trained FS	0.09^d	0.24	0.03^d
Adjusted R^2		0.23^a	
Echophilia			
Number of cumulative tics	0.42^a	0.18	0.02^a
Severity of TS	0.25^a	0.18	0.05^b
Adjusted R^2		0.18^a	

[a] $p < 0.0001$.
[b] $p < 0.01$.
[c] $p < 0.001$.
[d] $p < 0.05$.

Most of the variance is accounted for by age and duration of illness; patients with an older age at onset have a shorter duration of illness than those with a younger age at onset. As expected TS+ADD was associated with a younger age at onset. The finding that more copropraxia and remissions are associated with younger age at onset is probably related to the increased possibility of developing copropraxia and remissions with a longer duration of illness. All variables accounted for unique variance in the dependent variable. Similarly, although not selected by the summary SRA, a family history of Tourette's disorder is associated with a younger age at onset, or, conversely, a family history of Tourette's disorder is not associated with an older age at onset ($r =$

0.11, $p < 0.01$). The correlation of several other variables suggest that organic factors are associated with the onset of Tourette's disorder at a younger age (bladder-bowel trained FS, $r = -0.19$, $p < 0.0001$; pregnancy complications, $r = -0.14$, $p < 0.001$; and hyperactivity FS, $r = -0.17$, $p < 0.01$).

Although the results do not provide an answer to any of our questions, they do suggest that the age of onset of Tourette's disorder be considered as a covariate in future studies.

Characteristics of Present Illness

Characteristics of the present illness are summarized in Table 5.4.

The means are consistently higher than the medians because patients with a longer duration of illness inflate the mean values. Therefore, median values may be a better approximation. For the total sample, the median age at onset of Tourette's disorder is 6 years of age. The first consultation occurred 3 years later at 9 years, but Tourette's disorder was not diagnosed until 4 more years had elapsed. The median number of years between onset and diagnosis was 7 years. The median age at our initial consultation was 14, with a range of from 4 to 69 years (average age 18.9 years, SD = 12.0), and the median duration of illness was 8 years, with a range of 0 to 62 years (average 12.2 years, SD = 11.5).

Some progress towards diagnosing Tourette's disorder at an earlier age has been made over the years, however. Comparing our first sample of 121 patients evaluated between 1965 and 1974 with 232 patients evaluated between 1979 and 1981, years from the onset of Tourette's disorder to diagnosis significantly decreased from 14.4 years to 10.0 years ($p = 0.0025$); age at first diagnosis significantly decreased from 17 years to 14.3 years ($p = 0.0281$); duration of illness significantly decreased from 15.8 years to 10.9 years ($p = 0.0006$); and age at evaluation significantly decreased from 22.6 years to 17.4 years ($p = 0.002$) (Table 4.1). However, there are no changes between sample 2 (1975–1978) and sample 3 (1979–1981) (Table 4.1); a repeat sample, evaluated between 1981 and 1985, has not been analyzed. It is obvious that much remains to be done to educate professionals about the recognition and diagnoses of Tourette's disorder.

TABLE 5.4. *Characteristics of present illness*

Variables	Mean	SD	Median	Range
Age at onset of TS	6.7	2.8	6	1–17
Age at first consultation	10.5	6.4	9	2–49
Age at diagnosis of TS	17.9	12.1	13	4–69
Years from onset to diagnosis	11.2	11.7	7	0–62
Duration of illness	12.2	11.5	8	0–62
Age at current evaluation	18.9	12.0	14	4–69

We discuss elsewhere our impression that reports of a higher than expected frequency of patients with TS+ADD+H is due to ascertainment bias, that is, patients with two illnesses are more likely to seek help than those with one illness; the symptoms of ADD+H occur earlier than those of Tourette's disorder; Tourette's disorder is more severe in patients with TS+ADD+H who often are referred at a younger age because of considerable interpersonal, familial, and scholastic problems. Correlations were used to evaluate our impression. The dependent variable is consultation or diagnosis for Tourette's disorder factor score (FS). This variable, derived from factor analysis, is the sum of the age at the first consultation and the age at the first diagnosis of Tourette's disorder. Age at first consultation or diagnosis of Tourette's disorder, FS is inversely correlated with TS+ADD ($r = -0.20$, $p < 0.0001$), hyperactivity FS ($r = -0.26$, $p < 0.001$), and learning disorders FS ($r = -0.19$, $p < 0.0005$). Thus, patients with ADD+H, hyperactivity, and learning disorders are more likely to have sought consultation and to be diagnosed at a younger age than patients without these disabilities.

SYMPTOMATOLOGY

The initial symptoms are presented in detail to sensitize clinicians to the possibility of incipient Tourette's disorder. A detailed description is also provided for the cumulative lifetime prevalence of symptoms, age at onset, persistence or disappearance of symptoms, complexity, variability, distribution, and clinical course. By examining the results of this large data set, we hope to identify the irreducible criteria necessary for the diagnosis and differential diagnosis of Tourette's disorder and to provide data that may help to clarify the problem of potential heterogeneity among tic disorders.

A major difficulty, however, is the unreliability of patient reports about age, type, and severity of original and subsequent symptoms and clinical course. Details are frequently confused, distorted, condensed, and omitted. We see this when current histories are compared with previous records, and patient responses are compared with data from other family members. Many informants date the age at onset to a period when symptoms are severe or chronic, often forgetting earlier, milder symptoms. Children have considerable amnesia for early symptoms and often deny having tics, while older patients frequently remember later symptoms as first symptoms and forget previously prominent symptoms. The older patient tends to blend symptoms together leading to an approximate history. Inaccuracies, omissions, commissions, and errors in evaluation were also found in the general medical and psychiatric histories. Another source contributing to unreliable data in questionnaires is the inclusion by patients of many nontic symptoms, such as mannerisms, habits, stereotypic movements, behavioral, personality, tempermental characteristics, and diverse psychopathology. There is a strong tendency in patients, families, and even physicians to explain all difficulties as due to Tourette's disorder, as well as the patient's need to be all inclusive. Data from epidemiologic studies that use questionnaires have similar problems. Not only are such studies subject to questionnaire response bias, but volunteers tend to be more severely afflicted with Tourette's disorder, ADD, psychopathology, and other problems. These issues are discussed more fully in other chapters and the problems associated with questionnaire surveys are discussed later in this chapter (Table 5.25).

In an effort to minimize these problems we utilize a semistructured interview schedule based on the Movement Disorder Questionnaire (MDQ) when interviewing patients and family members, and collect all previous medical, psychiatric, neurological, psychological, and school records. Although this approach is not optimal, the large data base yields a good approximation of patient symptomatology.

Initial Symptoms

Symptoms appearing within the first week after onset are recorded as initial symptoms (Table 5.5). Initial symptoms are categorized as simple motor (brief, relatively single, or isolated muscular contractions), complex motor (a seemingly more complex or complicated movement involving a number of coordinated muscular movements), inarticulate sounds, coprophilia, and echophilia.

The initial or first symptom, like the syndrome itself, is quite variable. Initial symptoms total 82 different tics. Symptoms began as a single tic in approximately 50% of patients and with more than one tic in 50%. Eye tics are the most frequent initial symptom (36.6%). Other frequent tics in order of frequency include horizontal or vertical head tic (15.5%), throat clearing (4.4%), facial grimace (3.0%), shoulder shrug (3.0%), arm tic (2.7%), mouth tic (2.6%), and sniffing (2.1%). When classifying initial symptoms by body region, they are in order of frequency tics of the face (45.1%), head (19.8%), inarticulate sounds (17.0%), complex tics (7.1%), upper limbs (5.9%), torso (2.7%), lower limbs (1.1%), coprolalia (1.1%), and palilalia (0.2%).

The difficulty of diagnosing Tourette's disorder based on the occurrence of initial symptoms is obvious. Throat clearing (4.4%), sniffing (2.1%), and coughing (0.6%) are frequently and understandably misinterpreted as upper respiratory, sinus, or allergic disorders, and parents frequently consult allergists and otolaryngologists about these symptoms. Other symptoms, such as spitting and cursing, and especially some of the bizarre complex tics, are frequently misinterpreted as psychological in origin. The child is disciplined by washing the mouth with soap to curb the coprolalia. Eventually psychologic consultation and treatment is sought. These symptoms are especially

TABLE 5.5. *Initial symptoms*[a]

Type of tic	N	%
Simple motor		
Face		
Eye	241	36.6
Forehead	2	0.3
Lips	3	0.5
Tongue protrusion	4	0.6
Tongue, other	1	0.2
Mouth	17	2.6
Facial grimace	20	3.0
Nose	9	1.4
Head		
Neck (horizontal)	82	12.5
Neck (vertical)	25	3.0
Shoulder shrug	20	3.0
Whole head	3	0.5
Upper limbs		
Upper arm	2	0.3
Lower arm	4	0.6
Whole arm	18	2.7
Hands	15	2.3
Lower limbs		
Lower leg	1	0.2
Whole leg	5	0.8
Feet	1	0.2
Torso		
Upper back	1	0.2
Abdomen	8	1.2
Buttocks	1	0.2
Whole torso	7	1.1
Diaphragm	1	0.2
Total (24 simple tics)	491	74.6
Complex motor		
Jumping	9	1.4
Hopping	4	0.6
Bend over	4	0.6
Hit self	3	0.5
Touch self	3	0.5
Stamping	2	0.3
Squatting	2	0.3
Deep knee bends	2	0.3
Touch others	2	0.3
Smell objects	2	0.3
Touch objects	2	0.3
Other repetitive	2	0.3
Skipping	1	0.2
Dance-like movements	1	0.2
Reverse self while walking	1	0.2
Kiss objects	1	0.2
Lick self	1	0.2
Insert finger in throat	1	0.2
Wipe nose	1	0.2
Retrace steps, touch object	1	0.2

TABLE 5.5. *(Continued)*

Type of tic	N	%
Rub mouth	1	0.2
Press abdomen	1	0.2
Total (22 complex tics)	47	7.1
Inarticulate vocal sounds		
Throat clearing	29	4.4
Sniff	14	2.1
Grunt	12	1.8
High-pitched sound or squeak	10	1.5
Stuttering or stammering	10	1.5
Cough	4	0.6
Bark	3	0.5
Snort	3	0.5
Spitting	3	0.5
"Huh" sound	3	0.5
"Ah" sound	2	0.3
Yelp or scream	2	0.3
Other sound	2	0.3
Noisy breathing	1	0.2
Click or clack sound	1	0.2
"mm" sound	1	0.2
"Pft" sound	1	0.2
"Hiccup" sound	1	0.2
"Gurgling" sound	1	0.2
"Frog" sound	1	0.2
"Muttering" sound	1	0.2
"Hmp" sound	1	0.2
"Clucking" sound	1	0.2
"Cooing" sound	1	0.2
"Yahoo" sound	1	0.2
"Uh" sound	1	0.2
"Chu" sound	1	0.2
"Beep" sound	1	0.2
Total (28 sounds)	112	17.0
Coprolalia		
Cunt	3	0.5
Fuck	1	0.2
Shit	1	0.2
BM	1	0.2
Shut up	1	0.2
Total (5 coprolalia)	7	1.1
Palilalia		
Own last words	1	0.2
Total		
82 different symptoms	658	100.0

[a]$N = 658$.

confusing in children who have behavioral problems associated with attention deficit disorder, hyperactivity, learning disorders, mental deficiency, autism, conduct disorders, and so on.

A particularly striking example of these difficulties is illustrated in the history of an only, middle class, male child with severe symptoms who was first seen at the age of 11. The parents initially dated the onset of symptoms to age 6, but following detailed questioning, the mother recalled a traumatic experience when her son was 4 years old. She picked him up tenderly, cradled him in her lap and gazed lovingly into his eyes. He responded to her tender embrace with an obscenity, the word *fuck*. The mother, abashed, nonplussed, upset, wondered where he had picked up the obscenity and promptly pushed him off her lap. When the behavior persisted, she stopped picking him up. At age 5 he began to string a number of obscenities together. He was told to scream the obscenities in the bathroom where they belonged. Many tics appeared one year later, but the diagnosis of Tourette's disorder was not made until the child was 11 years old.

Some children use the terms *doody* or *cockey,* which are commonly interpreted as childhood scatology. However, if usage persists and occurs too frequently and inappropriately, especially if tics are present, the diagnosis of Tourette's disorder should be considered. Many initial symptoms are difficult to identify because they are blended into appropriate cultural, environmental, and psychological contexts. These include, stammering and stuttering tics, sniffing, throat clearing, coprophilia, and various complex tics.

For most patients the first symptom is a simple single tic. Some patients, however, suddenly erupt with multiple, severe, or bizarre symptoms. It is important for clinicians to identify early tic symptoms to avoid misdiagnosis and possible development of secondary psychopathology.

Studies citing initial symptoms of Tourette's disorder are summarized in Table 5.6. The trend for selected initial tics is roughly similar overall, although the amount of variability is considerable. This is understandable given the unreliability of patient reports and the different methods used to describe and categorize symptoms by clinicians and investigators. The development of a systematic method of recording symptoms and a glossary with defined criteria is essential for future studies. At present, we do not know if the type, frequency, and severity of initial symptoms are correlated with other variables such as clinical course, associated features, and so on. There is general clinical consensus, however, that they are uncorrelated with other variables and do not have prognostic significance. The second through fifth consecutive symptoms were also carefully tabulated (Table 5.7). These data did not result in any discernable pattern for the type, number, severity, and age at onset for muscular, vocal, and coprophilic tics. The most notable feature is the extensive range for the age of onset for these variables and the increased variability for the development of successive symptoms.

TABLE 5.6. Studies citing initial symptoms of Tourette's disorder

Tics	Current study[a] (1965–1981) %	Golden[b] (1977) %	Nomura and Segawa[c] (1982) %	Lieh-Mak et al.[d] (1982) %	Montgomery et al.[e] (1982) %	Min (1983)[f] %	Han-bai and Han-quin[g] (1983) %	Corbett et al.[h] (1969) %	Morphew and Sim[i] (1969) %	Kelman[j] (1965) %	Comings and Comings[k] (1984) %
Eye	36.6	53.3	33.0	20.0	46.7	37.5	—	—	7.0	—	48.0
Total facial	45.1	—	—	80.0	—	—	—	51.8	39.8	—	66.0
Head	19.7	13.3	—	—	20.0	20.8	—	10.4	4.7	—	—
Neck	16.0	—	—	—	—	—	—	—	—	—	—
Total face or head	64.9	—	—	—	—	—	68.4	—	—	82.4	—
Limbs	7.0	—	—	—	20.0	—	—	—	16.3	17.6	—
Vocal	17.0	26.7	10.0	6.7	13.3	16.7	47.5	11.6	7.0	—	32.0
Torso	2.7	—	—	—	—	4.2	—	—	—	—	—

[a] $N = 658$.
[b] $N = 15$.
[c] $N = 97$.
[d] $N = 15$.
[e] $N = 15$.
[f] $N = 24$.
[g] $N = 19$.
[h] Nonspecific tic sample; $N = 180$.
[i] Review of the literature; $N = 43$.
[j] Review of the literature; $N = 34$.
[k] $N = 250$.

TABLE 5.7. *Age of onset for initial symptoms*

Symptoms	N	Age of onset (years)			
		Mean	SD	Median	Range
First symptom	661	6.7	2.8	6	1–17
Second symptom	665	7.6	3.1	7	2–24
Third symptom	651	8.6	3.8	8	1–34
Fourth symptom	666	9.1	4.6	8	1–35
Muscular tics	661	6.9	2.9	7	1.2–18
Vocal tics	651	9.4	4.7	7	1.2–40
Coprophilic tics	209	11.8	5.8	10	3–36

Summary of Initial Symptoms

Up to 82 different symptoms may usher in Tourette's disorder. The initial symptom is a single tic in about half of the patients and multiple tics in the other half. The most frequent symptom for our sample is an eye tic (36.6%) followed by inarticulate vocal sounds (17.0%), head or neck tics (16.0%), complex motor tics (7.1%), upper limb tics (5.9%), throat clearing (4.4%), facial grimace (3.0%), shoulder shrugs (3.0%), mouth opening (2.6%), sniffing (2.1%), and less than 2% for other symptoms. Coprolalia was the initial symptom in seven (1.1%) patients. Many initial symptoms, especially sniffing, coughing, throat clearing, stammering, stuttering, and complex tics, are misdiagnosed. Subsequent clinical course is often necessary to make the diagnosis. An additional diagnostic problem is the variable clinical course for the disorder. Other tics may develop 1 to more than 35 years after the onset of initial symptoms. The symptoms may disappear completely within 1 year, or in approximately 8% of patients, by the age of 18. Temporary remissions, varying between 2 weeks and 7 years occur in 27% of patients, and veritably all patients having a waxing, waning, and fluctuating clinical course (Table 5.17). These differences contribute to the difficulty of studying whether Tourette's disorder and other tic disorders are heterogeneous or homogeneous disorders.

Cumulative Lifetime Prevalence of Symptoms

Tabulation of the cumulative past and present symptoms, frequently reported in the literature, is fraught with methodological difficulties. Obviously, older patients with a longer duration of illness have a greater chance of developing more symptoms during their lifetime than do younger patients. On the other hand, a more reliable, accurate, and inclusive history of the symptoms may be obtained for younger patients with a shorter duration of illness and a history of fewer symptoms. For this type of data to be truly meaningful, the cumulative lifetime history of symptoms should be age-corrected, as indicated later in this chapter.

Nevertheless, to provide information about our sample and for comparison with reports in the literature, the cumulative lifetime past and present symptoms are described. It is important to remember that the data are derived from a sample with the characteristics summarized in Table 5.4. The tables summarizing the cumulative lifetime history of symptoms records the percent of patients with a history of the symptom, the mean, standard deviation, median, and range for the age at onset of the symptom and the percent with persistence (the converse of remission) of the symptom when evaluated initially by our group. Because the means for age at onset of the symptoms are consistently higher than the medians, reflecting the disproportionate influence of patients with an older age of onset, the medians are cited in discussion of the results. It should also be noted that the range for the age at onset is quite extensive for all symptoms. The age at onset for an eye tic varies from 1 to 46 years, and so on. Therefore, the results represent only general central tendencies characterized by extensive variability. Criteria for defining and classifying tics are discussed in greater detail in Chapter 10.

Cumulative Simple Motor Tics

A simple motor tic is essentially a brief muscular contraction of one or a limited number of muscle groups. They are categorized into 26 anatomic areas (Table 5.8).

The most frequent simple motor tics, in descending order, are eye tics (80%), horizontal neck (69%), shoulder shrug (55%), vertical head (47%), whole arm (44%), facial grimace (36%), mouth opening movement (34%), hand or fingers (34%), leg (26%), lips (25%), whole torso (24%), and less than 20% for the remaining tic types. The most frequent body region is the face or head; 99.2% of patients have a history of tics in this region, followed by 68.6% for upper limb, 46.5% for torso, and 40.7% for lower limb (Table 5.15). The median age of onset varies from age 7 for eye tic to 13 for upper leg tic, with a range of 1 to 58 years for all simple motor tics.

Our results are compared with eight studies in the literature that described cumulative lifetime symptoms (Table 5.16). Considering the different ages and duration of illness for the various samples, the results for simple tics in the first four studies are remarkably similar.

Cumulative Complex Motor Tics

Complex motor tics are coordinated contractions of several muscle groups. They appear more complicated and purposeful than simple motor tics, they

TABLE 5.8. Lifetime simple motor tics[a]

Symptom	Past history of symptom		Age of onset				Persistance of symptoms %	Duration of symptoms					
	N	%	Mean	SD	Median	Range		1 Year %	2 Years %	5 Years %	10 Years %	15 Years %	
Head													
Eye	534	80.2	7.9	4.6	7	1–46	75.9	51	60	71	74	74	
Neck (horizontal)	457	68.6	9.6	4.9	9	1–42	78.2	25	34	47	62	64	
Neck (vertical)	314	47.2	10.4	4.8	10	3–33	81.9	14	19	30	45	47	
Facial grimace	239	35.9	10.1	5.3	9	3–36	71.7	10	18	24	29	30	
Mouth	28	4.2	12.5	5.8	9	3–34	80.3	9	14	22	28	30	
Lips	109	16.4	11.2	7.1	9	2–46	71.1	6	9	13	20	24	
Tongue protrusion	109	16.5	11.2	5.0	10	4–29	68.1	3	4	8	11	14	
Nose	101	15.2	9.8	5.5	9	3–46	75.7	5	7	11	14	18	
Forehead	88	13.2	12.0	7.7	10	2–46	70.1	4	5	9	14	18	
Tongue, other	28	4.2	12.5	8.0	9.5	3–36	67.7	1	1	2	3	4	
Upper limbs													
Shoulders	367	55.1	10.1	5.5	9	3–52	73.9	15	23	35	44	45	
Whole arm	290	43.5	11.2	6.6	10	3–58	79.9	10	15	26	40	47	
Hands	228	34.2	11.4	6.4	10	1–56	80.2	8	11	18	27	32	
Upper arms	127	19.1	12.3	6.4	11	4–49	76.3	3	5	9	16	20	
Lower arms	103	15.5	11.4	5.3	10	3–30	72.9	3	4	8	13	16	
Lower limbs													
Whole leg	176	26.4	12.1	7.3	10	4–56	73.9	5	8	14	24	26	
Feet	95	14.3	13.5	8.2	11	2–56	72.6	2	4	7	12	16	
Upper leg	66	9.9	14.7	8.1	13	4–56	75.0	1	1	4	11	12	
Lower leg	57	8.6	14.5	10.7	11	4–56	77.8	2	2	4	8	10	
Torso													
Whole torso	160	24.0	11.3	5.9	10	4–54	72.9	5	5	12	17	18	
Abdomen	129	19.4	13.7	9.3	11	4–58	75.2	2	4	8	16	19	
Thorax	69	10.4	13.9	9.2	12	5–54	75.3	1	1	4	12	11	
Diaphragm	54	8.1	12.4	6.4	10	4–34	70.7	1	2	4	7	7	
Buttocks	33	5.0	15.0	10.0	12	5–54	76.9	1	1	2	5	8	
Upper back	26	3.9	13.1	6.9	10.5	6–30	66.7	1	<1	1	4	5	
Lower back	14	2.1	14.4	7.0	13	3–26	73.3	<1	<1	1	2	3	

[a] N = 666.

are experienced as and appear to be involuntary or unintended and a thing in themselves rather than done for some purpose. For the total sample, 456 (68.5%) patients had one or more of 54 complex tics listed in Table 5.9.

The most frequent complex tics, in descending order, are hitting self (21.6%), jumping (19.8%), touching self (13.2%) and others (11.4%), smelling hands (11.8%) and objects (10.9%), and less than 10% for each of the remaining 48 complex motor tics. Similar to our findings for simple motor tics, the range for age at onset is quite extensive. The earliest median age at onset is for smelling objects, licking self, kissing objects, and kneeling (median 8 years), followed by bending over, kissing others, and licking others (median 9 years). The range for the onset of complex motor tics is from 2 to 57 years. These results could not be compared with other published reports because none of them described complex tics in adequate detail. Our nomenclature for complex tics is arbitrary and there is a need for precise names, definitions, and criteria for complex motor tics, as well as for other types of tics (see Chapter 10).

Many of these symptoms, such as repetitively touching one's self or others without provocation, sudden hopping, skipping, jumping, stamping, squatting, kneeling, flexing trunk, deep-knee bends, retracing steps, twirling, and other odd movements are very disturbing to patients, their families, friends, and strangers. Patients report that people stare at them, if not openly then surreptitiously, and frequently move away or advise their children to avoid them. Police officers may interpret the movements as drug-induced and patients have been arrested. Teachers, friends, physicians, psychologists, and psychotherapists all too frequently interpret these and other symptoms as an indication of serious psychopathology. Moreover, many of these symptoms are categorized and interpreted erroneously as compulsions (Nee et al., 1980; Jagger et al., 1982; DSM-III, American Psychiatric Association, 1980; Cummings and Frankel, 1985), which has resulted, in our opinion, in spurious theorizing about a common etiology for obsessive compulsive disorder and Tourette's disorder (see Chapters 6 and 10).

Copropraxia includes socially unacceptable, commonly obscene gestures, such as pointing in the direction of or touching one's own or another person's breasts or genitalia, giving the finger or an elbow gesture, masturbatory movements, and so on. Although copropraxia can be classified as a type of coprophilia, it can also be considered a subtype of a complex motor tic or a complex copropraxic motor tic. Similarly, echopraxia, imitation of the movement of another person, could be considered a complex echopraxic motor tic. The rationale for including these symptoms in the complex motor tic category is discussed more fully in Chapter 10.

We hypothesize that complex tics are essentially another form of tic and are unrelated to other Tourette's disorder characteristics, such as obsessive compulsive disorder (OCD), obsessive-compulsive-like symptoms, and history of Tourette's disorder or tics in the family, except for being more frequent in patients with TS+ADD.

TABLE 5.9. *Lifetime complex motor tics*[a]

Symptom	Past history of symptom		Age of onset				Persistence of Symptoms %	Duration of illness				
	N	%	Mean	SD	Median	Range		1 Year %	2 Years %	5 Years %	10 Years %	15 Years %
Hit self	144	21.6	12.7	6.9	11	2–57	76.1	2	5	9	17	21
Jumping	132	19.8	11.4	5.9	10	3–45	73.8	4	6	12	14	14
Touch self	88	13.2	12.9	7.3	11	3–36	78.4	2	2	5	10	13
Smell hands	79	11.8	11.1	5.1	10	2–29	72.5	2	3	6	7	8
Touch others	76	11.4	11.1	4.3	10	3–22	71.6	1	2	4	5	7
Smell objects	73	10.9	9.3	4.3	8	2–30	73.1	2	4	8	9	7
Stamping	60	9.0	11.5	5.9	10	3–30	68.8	1	2	4	5	5
Bite mouth	55	8.3	13.4	7.2	11	2–40	76.8	1	1	4	6	8
Skipping	53	8.0	12.6	7.1	11	5–45	73.8	1	2	4	7	7
Dance-like movement	50	7.5	11.4	5.9	10	4–34	74.1	1	2	3	5	7
Kicking	49	7.4	10.7	5.8	10	3–32	71.7	1	2	5	5	5
Hopping	49	7.4	10.6	4.6	10	4–30	52.9	1	2	4	8	9
Squatting	48	7.2	10.4	4.5	10	4–30	53.8	1	2	4	5	7
Bending over	35	5.3	9.8	3.6	9	3–17	41.7	2	1	4	4	4

Behavior											
Retrace steps	34	5.1	12.3	5.2	12	6–26	54.3	1	2	5	7
Turning	32	4.8	12.3	7.9	10	3–34	59.4	1	3	4	5
Deep knee-bends	29	4.4	10.1	4.9	10	3–24	51.7	1	3	4	3
Lick self	27	4.1	8.8	3.9	8	3–22	51.9	1	1	2	3
Throw objects	26	3.9	11.5	6.5	10	3–33	76.9	1	2	2	3
Lick objects	25	3.8	10.5	5.0	10	3–23	56.0	1	1	3	4
Insert finger in throat	19	2.9	12.4	5.6	11	4–24	55.0	<1	1	2	2
Reverse-self walking	19	2.9	12.7	5.5	12	6–26	73.7	<1	1	3	4
Kiss others	19	2.9	9.3	2.4	9	4–14	78.9	<1	1	1	2
Kiss objects	17	2.6	10.0	3.6	8	7–20	76.5	<1	1	2	2
Smell others	11	1.7	11.0	4.1	11	2–17	91.7	<1	<1	1	2
Lick others	10	1.5	9.5	3.8	9	4–15	90.0	0	<1	<1	1
Kiss self	7	1.1	13.6	6.2	13	7–26	71.4	0	0	1	
Kneeling	6	0.9	9.2	2.0	8	8–13	57.1	<1	<1	1	1
Other[b]	58	8.7	11.4	6.4	10	2–34	77.9	2	4	6	9

[a] $N = 666$.
[b] Other: quick-step, double-stepping, pawing ground, step retracing and object touching, cross feet while walking, kick buttocks, brushing floor, touching the ground, heel clicking, hit objects, biting, hit others, chewing holes in objects, touching objects, bite fingers and arms, blow on hands, nose-wiping, nose-pulling, mouth-rubbing, dusting things, hair-twisting, toe-tapping, invert lower eyelids, body-rolling, pressing abdomen. $N = 26$.

The summary SRA (Table 5.3) comfirmed our expectation that patients with TS+ADD have more complex tics. The number of cumulative tics is another measure of Tourette's disorder severity ($r = 0.40, p = 0.0001$). Inclusion of the learning disorder FS suggests that other organic CNS factors may be related to complex tics. Especially noteworthy is the absence of significant correlation between complex tics and a history of tic or Tourette's disorders in the family, and with any measure suggesting obsessive-compulsive-like symptoms or OCD. The latter finding confirms our hypothesis that complex tics should be categorized as tic symptoms and not as obsessive-compulsive symptoms. The failure to differentiate these symptom categories in studies and reports in the literature has contributed to considerable confusion about the clinical phenomenology and management of patients, and questionable concepts about the etiology of both Tourette's disorder and OCD.

Cumulative Inarticulate Vocal Tics

Simple vocal tics include diverse and difficult to classify inarticulate noises, stuttering and stammering sounds, and emphasizing part of or a whole word or phrase in a sentence while speaking. Complex vocal tics include palilalia, echolalia, and coprolalia. Patients (98.5%) had one or more of the 77 vocal tics listed in Table 5.10.

Vocal tics are also quite variable. Many of them are difficult to describe or categorize and the pattern for each patient is distinctive. They are classified as symptoms of Tourette's disorder because they are involuntary or unintended, are an end in themselves rather than done for a purpose, coexist with other Tourette's disorder symptoms, spontaneously wax, wane, and fluctuate over time, and respond to the same medications that are effective for motor tics.

The most frequent simple vocal tics are throat clearing (56.6%), grunts (45.6%), high-pitched sounds (squeals, shrieks, yelps, crying-out) (33.3%), sniffing (33.0%), coughing (25.2%), screams (21.2%), snorting (20.0%), and 67 other vocal tics accounting for less than 20%. Vocal symptoms such as throat clearing, sniffing, coughing, snorting, expiratory and inspiratory hissing, and noisy breathing are often misdiagnosed, especially early in the illness, as allergic symptoms. Stuttering, stammering, and word garbling symptoms (13.4%), which do not resemble classic stuttering (Ludlow et al., 1982), may occur *de novo* or be associated with thoracic, abdominal, or diaphragmatic muscular contractions. Word accentuation (10.8%) is characterized by sudden increase in the loudness, change of pitch or clarity of a word or phrase during normal talking. It is frequently associated with thoracic, abdominal, or diaphragmatic tics, and possibly may occur *de novo*. These tics may be so frequent and intense that normal speech is impaired and unintelligible.

Since the criteria for the diagnosis of Tourette's disorder included one or more vocal symptom, all patients had vocal symptoms. These are classified as inarticulate or simple vocal tics or complex vocal tics which included echolalia, palilalia, coprolalia, and other involuntary words. The most frequent vocal symptoms is an inarticulate sound which was present in 98.5% of patients. The remainder had complex vocal tics. Simple vocal tics in studies are summarized in Table 5.16.

Cumulative Echophilia

Echophilia is defined as involuntary repetition or echoing of sounds, words, phrases, sentences, or movements. Echophilia can be categorized as complex vocal tics (echolalia, palilalia, mental echolalia or palilalia, and other types of echoing of words), and complex motor tics (echopraxia). The common element is the repetition or echoing of stimuli in the environment. A history of echophilia is present in 32.7% of our sample (Table 5.15).

Echolalia

Echolalia, present in 17.6% of patients, is defined as involuntary repetition of the last word, phrase, sentence, or sound of another person or sound in the environment (Table 5.11). The most frequent echolalic symptom is repeating the last word spoken by another person. Repetition of a phrase or a sentence is somewhat less frequent. Least frequent is repetition of the sound of another person, animal, automobile, train, and other noises in the environment. Some patients ejaculatively echo automobile horns, screeching brakes, and barking dogs. Occasional patients, less than 1.0%, describe symptoms which are referred to as mental echolalia: an unspoken repetition in the mind of the patient of the last word, phrase, sentence, or sound of another person or sound in the environment. Echolalia tends to occur intermittently and randomly and less regularly in response to certain sounds, words, or concepts.

Tourette (Gilles de la Tourette, 1885) concluded that all patients with Tourette's disorder had echolalia because he erroneously included the disorders of latah, myriachit, and the jumping Frenchmen in the syndrome. This error was corrected by Charcot, as reported by Melotti (1885), confirmed by the data in our sample and by other studies in the literature (Table 5.16).

Palilalia

Palilalia, present in 17.4% of patients, is defined as involuntary repetition of one's own last sound, word, phrase, or sentence. A less frequent type of palilalia, which is referred to as mental palilalia, is defined as the mental echoing of internally generated verbal stimuli to one's self, without overt vocalization. Other forms, reported in single patients, include repeating the

TABLE 5.10. Lifetime simple vocal tics[a]

Symptom	Past history of symptom		Age of onset				Persistence of symptoms %	Duration of symptoms				
	N	%	Mean	SD	Median	Range		1 Year %	2 Years %	5 Years %	10 Years %	15 Years %
Throat clearing	377	56.6	10.7	5.8	8	3–45	75.2	11	18	27	34	39
Grunt	304	45.6	11.2	5.9	10	3–55	76.0	9	12	25	40	43
High-pitched	222	33.3	11.3	5.8	10	3–43	72.9	6	8	16	22	24
Sniff	220	33.0	11.7	6.7	10	3–49	78.8	6	8	15	24	25
Cough	168	25.2	11.9	5.5	10	3–30	74.0	3	5	10	16	23
Scream	141	21.2	12.6	7.4	10	3–51	81.6	3	4	6	11	15
Snort	133	20.0	11.1	5.0	10	1–30	77.2	2	3	8	14	14
Shout	132	19.8	12.1	5.0	11	3–28	85.9	2	4	6	14	14
Bark	127	19.1	12.1	6.0	11	4–44	77.2	3	4	10	16	16
Humming	119	17.9	12.1	6.7	10	5–46	74.8	2	3	6	16	16
Spitting	117	17.6	12.8	7.4	10	4–48	69.2	0	3	7	11	13
Expiratory hiss	96	14.4	12.7	6.9	10	5–40	74.3	2	3	6	8	11
Clicking noise	91	13.7	12.9	6.8	11	2–40	74.3	2	3	6	12	12
Stuttering or stammering	89	13.4	9.9	5.6	9	2–32	70.8	4	6	9	11	10
Word accentuation	72	10.8	13.4	6.4	12	5–32	79.5	<1	1	3	6	9

Sound	N	%	Mean	SD	Median	Range	%					
Inspiratory hiss	63	9.5	12.2	6.2	11	4–36	70.1	1	2	3	5	6
Whistling	57	8.6	13.4	6.2	12	4–30	76.9	1	1	2	5	6
Noisy breathing	49	7.4	12.2	5.3	11	5–30	85.0	1	1	3	4	6
Ow sound	48	7.2	12.5	5.0	11.5	6–26	86.3	<1	<1	2	4	4
Tsk sound	48	7.2	12.2	4.8	11	5–28	73.6	1	1	3	5	5
Sucking	39	5.9	13.8	7.2	12	5–34	82.7	<1	1	1	1	2
Pft sound	38	5.7	14.5	8.0	12.5	5–45	72.5	<1	1	1	4	5
Hiccup sound	38	5.7	12.7	5.8	12	4–28	79.5	<1	1	3	4	5
Moaning sound	34	5.1	12.9	5.4	11.5	5–29	72.5	1	1	1	2	3
Gasping sound	32	4.8	12.4	5.6	10	6–24	73.5	<1	1	2	3	4
Blowing sound	30	4.5	13.8	10.7	10	5–48	83.7	1	1	3	3	4
Sucking sound	17	2.5	11.2	5.8	11	5–25	52.9	1	1	1	3	4
Ouch sound	11	1.6	11.1	4.0	11	5–18	90.1	0	0	0	1	0
Gurgling sound	8	1.2	9.9	3.7	9	6–15	50.0	<1	<1	<1	2	2
Bronx cheer	4	0.6	16.8	8.2	18	7–24	80.0	0	0	0	0	0
Other[b]	147	21.3	10–14	5.1	9–12	4–41	53.6	5	7	13	14	14

[a] $N = 666$.
[b] Other: ye, ee, eek, yoo, yahoo, er, eh, eh-eh, uh, whoo, hoot, ulp, uck, ump, urp, up, yuk, bop, huh, hmp, hey-ha, ugh, dah, phew, sh, pst, ptah, dip-dip, ch, cha, tut, liz, swallowing, gulping, groaning, growling, gaging, gigging, clucking, crowing, duck, frog, beep, burp, belch, muttering, breathing, teeth snapping. $N = 47$.

TABLE 5.11. Lifetime complex vocal and motor tics: Echophilia[a]

Symptom	Past history of symptom		Age of Onset				Persistence of Symptoms %	Duration of Symptoms				
	N	%	Mean	SD	Median	Range		1 Year %	2 Years %	5 Years %	10 Years %	15 Years %
Echo symptoms												
Echolalia	117	17.6	13.5	6.9	12	3–48	81.0	1	2	5	8	9
Palilalia	116	17.4	12.8	6.1	12	3–40	81.6	<1	2	5	9	11
Echokinesis	56	8.4	13.1	6.5	11	3–31	82.6	1	1	2	5	6
Other												
Other[b]	31	4.7	12.7	6.2	11.5	4–28	78.9	1	1	2	2	5

[a] N = 666.
[b] Other: mental echoing, repeat beginning of own sentence, add "2" to word endings, garbled speech, pull out hair, counting; N = 6.

beginning of a sentence, adding the word "too" to word endings, adding garbled sounds to words, and mentally repeating numbers.

Mental echoing

Ten patients describe symptoms difficult to classify, which we refer to as mental echoing. Mental echoing is defined as the unexpressed preoccupation or fixation on a word, phrase, sentence, or concept heard in conversation or observed in the environment, or that is internally stimulated in the absence of external stimuli. Mental echoing may interfere with concentration and full involvement in conversation or other mental activity. The preoccupation generally is unnoticed by others but may be interpreted as not paying attention, abstracted, bored, or phased out. Patients exert great effort to stop these thoughts, but they intrude over and over again as if they were controlled by a powerful internal force. The pattern or mechanism resembles a spontaneously generated, randomly appearing, circular or reverberating fixation which we term a *fixated reverberating circuit symptom*. These episodes may be infrequent, occur intermittently, and last for minutes or hours. For example, the word *knee* inadvertently came up in conversation and the patient repetitively returned to the thought of his knee. No other content was associated with the thought and it prevented the patient's full participation in conversation. Many other random words would set this off. Tourette (1885) describes a similar phenomena when he discusses patient number 11. Several other patients report the sudden intrusion of images, thoughts, or vague paranoid feelings that prevented full participation in work or conversation. They describe a vague feeling of danger such as being observed by an employer, friend, relative, stranger, monster, or extraterrestrial. These thoughts differ from those described by paranoid patients. Situational stimuli and psychodynamic factors are not apparent; they seem to appear *de novo*. Another patient had a series of continually changing intrusive polymorphous images and thoughts, such of women moving their bowels which caused him discomfort when eating in a restaurant if women were present, vivid oedipal fantasies, images of plunging a knife into his groin at the moment of orgasm, continual perseveration over words and concepts while reading, and so on. Normal individuals may experience similar thoughts, feelings, or fantasies, but they occur occasionally, momentarily, and fleetingly. In Tourette's disorder patients, however, the thoughts catch and repetitively echo in the person's mind. Similar symptoms occur in patients with severe forms of schizophrenia, and borderline and obsessive compulsive disorders. The fantasies in these patients, however, are persistent, prolonged, elaborated, systematized, and often psychodynamic factors are present. In contrast, Tourette's disorder patients are in contact with reality and recognize that the symptoms are unreal; psychodynamic factors are not associated with the symptoms, and they are unsystematized, unelaborated, impermanent, and the content tends to randomly fluctuate. Their occurrence in only ten patients makes it difficult to assess if they are more frequent than expected in samples without Tourette's disorder.

These symptoms were very striking when first observed. As we described previously (Shapiro et al., 1978), these patients were comprehensively and intensively evaluated by many psychiatrists, psychologists, and neurologists. The results of the evaluations did not support a psychodynamic, psychological, or neurophysiological basis for what ordinarily would be considered severe polymorphous perverse psychopathology. In fact, other indications of psychosocial pathology were absent in these patients. All of them have been followed for over 15 years; they are functioning very adequately, all are married, several with families, some are professionals, and others are businessmen. We have observed similar symptoms in many of our psychiatric patients. They seem to be an uncommon manifestation of Tourette's disorder. We evaluated the response to neuroleptics in only three patients. Neuroleptics reduced the more obvious motor and vocal tics in all three patients, but decreased the polymorphous symptoms only slightly in one, had no effect on them in one, and increased them in one. The results are, therefore, inconclusive.

The symptoms of these patients resemble those described in confessions of a tiqueur (Meige and Feindel, 1907). The patient had typical Tourette's disorder but, in addition, had a melange of continuing changing polymorphous symptoms that consumed him. The tiqueur described his symptoms vividly, insightfully, and with a detached sense of wonderment and humor, although with appropriate concern. He was obviously intelligent, cultured, articulate, and was a successful businessman, married and raised a family. Oliver Sacks eloquently focused attention on several of these patients whom he refers to as "Super Tourettes" (Sacks, 1987). Although these patients are rare, further study of this interesting group of patients is highly desirable.

Cumulative Echokinesis

Echokinesis, present in 8.4% of patients, is defined as the involuntary repetition, imitation, or echoing of a movement observed in another person (Table 5.11). It can result in imitation, or be experienced as an impulse which can be resisted. Patients with such symptoms avoid looking at another person with unusual movements, such as a facial grimace or other mannerism, because they are often impelled to copy the movement. Children watching a cowboy on television drawing a gun from his holster may feel a need to repeat the rapid movement. Echoing may take the form of increased symptoms (motor and vocal). Others note the return of a symptom a day or two before or after a visit to the doctor. Their memory has been jogged. An echokinetic response to a specific stimuli almost never persists, although the general tendency to echokinesis for random stimuli does persist if echokinesis is present. The percent of patients with echokinesis is rarely reported in the literature.

Correlates of Echophilia

The expectation, that echophilia would be significantly associated with severity of Tourette's disorder was confirmed. The SRA selected two variables (number of cumulative tics and severity of Tourette's disorder) which accounted for 18% of the variance for echophilia (Table 5.3). It would be of interest in future studies to analyze the relationship of different types of echophilia to each other and to other variables.

Coprophilia

Cumulative Coprophilia

Coprophilia is defined as involuntary, socially unacceptable, commonly obscene, sounds, words, phrases, concepts, or gestures. Coprophilia can take the form of a complex articulated vocal tic such as coprolalia, or as a complex motor tic such as copropraxia. Coprolalia has become somewhat of a misnomer in Tourette's disorder literature. Although it is commonly thought of as an obscenity, essentially it is a symptom that expresses something that is socially unacceptable. Since obscene words and gestures are indigenous in all cultures, it is understandable that most coprophilia includes common, four-letter type words and obscene gestures. However, coprophilia can be racial slurs, religious improprieties, political innuendoes, derogatory remarks, use of another person's name, or any other method of expressing something socially unacceptable or forbidden. Sometimes coprolalia takes the form of a neutral word that substitutes for or protects against socially unacceptable words or impulses. The range of coprophilic symptoms in our sample is summarized in Table 5.12.

Coprolalia

One hundred and one different coprolalic words or phrases were used by 213 (32.0%) patients (Table 5.12). Common four-letter words were used more frequently than obscene phrases or other types of socially unacceptable words or phrases. In addition to the seven most frequent words, 82 other types of coprolalia are grouped in an arbitrary classification consisting of male or female anatomy, racial, religious, and other categories, but could as easily be classified psychoanalytically as oral, anal, phallic, oedipal, etc.

Types of coprolalia

It is apparent that coprolalia can include socially unacceptable words or phrases other than common four-letter obscenities. Some of the listed words

TABLE 5.12. Lifetime complex vocal tics: Coprolalia[a]

Symptom	Past history of symptom N	%	Age of Onset Mean	SD	Median	Range	Persistence of symptoms %	Duration of symptom 1 Year %	2 Years %	5 Years %	10 Years %	15 Years %
Coprolalia[b]												
Fuck	163	24.5	11.8	5.4	11	3–36	69.9	3	5	10	17	21
Shit	114	17.1	12.3	5.5	11	4–33	76.1	2	2	6	12	14
Mother-fucker	42	6.3	14.5	6.9	12	6–36	86.0	1	1	2	4	5
Cunt	39	5.9	15.1	6.7	14	4–36	82.1	1	1	1	4	7
Prick	34	5.1	15.4	6.9	13	4–36	73.5	<1	<1	1	4	7
Cocksucker	34	5.1	14.8	7.4	12	4–36	91.2	1	1	2	4	6
Cockey	9	1.3	10.4	7.5	8	5–30	88.9	<1	<1	<1	1	1
Other[c]	155	20.0	11.6–12.0	4.6–5.7	11	4–33	74.3	1	3	5	13	16
Mental Coprolalia												
Other[d]	24	3.6	13.6	1.2	12.5	6–28	69.2	<1	1	1	4	5

[a]$N = 666$.
[b]$N = 213$.
[c]Others: $N = 94$. Male anatomy: penis, prick, dick, cock, balls, groin. Female anatomy: cunt, pussy, breast, boobs, knockers, dugs, nobs, tits. GI, excrement: shit, bull shit, shit on a monkey, shit fucker, bowel movement, crap, crap on a banana, cockey, doody, poo-poo, pookey-piss, I'm a poopie, you're a poopie, piss, piss-shit, butthole, bitch-ass, ass, asshole, fart-tart. Racial: nigger, nigger-damn, wop, cheap Jew bastard. Religious: hell, Jesus Christ. Parental: hold it dad, wait dad, mother, fuck you daddy. Homosexual: homosexual, gay, queer, faggot, I am or you are gay. Copulatory: fuck, fuck-shit, mother-fucker, mother-fucking, fuck-you-daddy, fuck god, fuck it bitch, fuck-a-doo, puck-puck, fugadoo, fucking bitch, fucking ass, fucking shit, fucker-damn, fucker-nigger-shit, oh man fuck, lousy-fucking-stinking bastards. Oral: suck, suck dick, suck it off, I sucked you, blow-job, cocksucker. Masturbatory: jerk off, jack it off. Other Sexual: whore, whore master, discharge, scum boy. Interpersonal: stupid, shut-up, pig, dummy, dumbell, you're weird, damn, goddamn, bastard, bitch son of a bitch, SOB.
[d]Other: $N = 24$. Fuck, fucking-shitting-niggereeo, nigger, mike, mother fucker, bastard, bitch, faggot, hair, oh cat, dorkey, shit, shit head, asshole, suck, gook, sugar foot, well cheap bums, your mom, mama, help, neat.

are in the racial, religious, and parental categories. Words and phrases such as "hold it dad. . . . wait dad. . . . mother. . . . hell. . . . Jesus Christ" could be considered responses to echophilic or other internal stimuli; they occur in conjunction with more obvious coprolalia, are experienced by the patient as coprolalia or as substitutes for coprolalia. The use of a common word such as *mother* may substitute for an unacceptable phrase like *mother-fucker*. Sometimes a patient may repetitively repeat the name of a previous mate in the presence of the current spouse. Although coprolalia increases with anger and tension, it also increases with pleasurable anticipation, such as going to the circus, and with nonspecific arousal and occurs sporadically without apparent stimuli in neutral situations. A patient, with a politically liberal orientation, erupted with racial epithets totally out of character with his usual behavior. Another patient would frequently erupt with long phrases such as "fuck you, you mother-fucking, cocksucker, cunt" or other combinations. Although the long phrases increased with anger or nonspecific tension, they also occurred in an ejaculatory, seemingly random fashion and without apparent stimuli. Coprolalia is expressed in a louder tone or pitch than is used in normal conversation, and interrupts the flow but not the rhythm of normal speech. Some patients inhibit the most extreme expressions by verbalizing the first part of the word, such as "fuh" for "fuck" or "kuh" for "cunt." Others can suppress their coprolalia by substituting neutral words, copropraxia, or mental coprolalia.

Effects of coprolalia

Although all of the symptoms of Tourette's disorder are disruptive, coprolalia is by far the most disconcerting, socially unacceptable, and disturbing symptom. Children are punished by parents, disciplined by teachers, ostracized by classmates, and shunned by strangers. Parents often relate with guilt that they punished, spanked, or washed the child's mouth with soap. Coprolalia often leads to withdrawal and isolation. One intelligent and otherwise well-adjusted patient related that because of the coprolalia he did not attend church, go to the movies, or keep his windows open in the summer, and would only work at night cleaning offices. Another patient with very severe coprolalia, who successfully worked, married, and raised a family, was particularly upset when his teen-aged daughters refused to bring their friends home and considered having a lobotomy. Several patients and families were forced to move repeatedly because of their own or their child's coprolalia. As the symptoms of Tourette's disorder unfold, patients have increasing thoughts of themselves as bizarre. With the onset of cursing they become more convinced that they may, in fact, be *crazy*.

Pitfalls in identifying coprolalia

Pitfalls include the mistaken belief that coprolalia is necessary for the diagnosis of Tourette's disorder, the difficulty of differentiating coprolalia from the normal use of obscenities, the interaction of coprolalia with psychosocial stimuli, and the variability for the age at onset, severity, and remission of coprolalia.

Many patients are able to intentionally or voluntarily inhibit, suppress, or substitute other symptoms for coprolalia. Suppressing coprolalia usually increases tension and other symptoms, ultimately cannot be inhibited, and frequently breaks through with a compensatory increase in severity. Patients may excuse themselves, go to a place where they can be alone, such as the nearest lavatory, and explosively release the coprolalia, after which they return to the social situation for a period of time. This type of *lavatory coprolalia* is so frequent that we term it a *presumptive sign of Tourette's disorder*.

Coprolalia, similar to other Tourette's disorder symptoms, almost always decreases in school, at work, and with strangers, and increases at home, with the family, when alone, and especially with tiredness in the evening. Because coprolalia increases at home and with the family, it is often interpreted as dynamically determined and having a psychological origin. This pattern, however, is characteristic of most Tourette's disorder symptoms. Patients tire of constantly inhibiting their symptoms, and, ultimately, although not intentionally or purposefully, tend to more readily release them at home. The pattern is somewhat similar to people displaying better manners outside than in their own home. It is not unusual, therefore, for outsiders to observe fewer and less severe coprophilia.

Symptoms are usually more frequent and intense before reaching the clinician's office and in the waiting room. They usually decrease once the patient is with the clinician who observes fewer symptoms than most other observers. Any suggestion or encouragement to relax and let out the symptoms does not work. Patients often remark that it is not their intention to inhibit the symptoms, but that something keeps them from ticing. Perhaps the constant pressure to inhibit the symptoms with strangers has become conditioned and they cannot undo the inhibition. An analogous situation would be to request that a person have no inhibitions in a social situation, behave the way they might at home, display bad manners while eating, express irritability and anger, dress scantily, and so on. Most would have difficulty doing so. Coprolalia, as other symptoms, easier to inhibit initially is more difficult to inhibit over time. It may increase with the clinician after he becomes less of a stranger.

Unfortunately, encouraging or bribing patients to inhibit coprophilic symptoms is fruitless and frustrating to both patients and families. Suggestions by parents of clinician about plausible methods of inhibiting or substituting less unacceptable symptoms for coprophilia are also ineffective. All patients, without encouragement or advice, experiment with different methods of controlling or reducing their symptoms. Coprophilia will not become a habit if it is not inhibited. Patients will readily give up coprophilic and other Tourette's disorder symptoms, if possible, and do so without symptom substitution after successful drug treatment. We advise families to ignore coprophilia in the home, and to provide a protective atmosphere in which these symptoms can be expressed without inhibition. Some family members, especially siblings, may have difficulty accepting this. However, since the patient can do very little about it, the problem should be fully discussed with other family members. Sometimes counseling is necessary.

On the other hand, differentiating involuntary coprolalia from intentional use of obscenities, can be difficult. Children sometimes use obscenities intentionally or voluntarily to express anger, irritation, or to act out against parents, and blame the obscenities on Tourette's disorder. However, coprophilic symptoms occur randomly and sporadically throughout the day, although situational stimuli may increase or decrease their frequency. They do not occur only with anger and frustration. If they do, parental injunctions, discussion, and other appropriate behavioral management are indicated.

One can also be misled about the diagnosis of Tourette's disorder if coprolalia is required for the diagnosis. Although coprolalia is pathognomonic, it is not essential for the diagnosis. Only five of Tourette's (1885) patients had coprolalia. As we discussed in our previous publications, there was a dramatic underdiagnosis of Tourette's disorder because clinicians relied on erroneous diagnostic criteria promulgated as far back as Meige and Feindel (1907) and established by the time Ferenczi (1921) wrote about Tourette's disorder. Erroneous diagnostic criteria were still cited as late as 1972 in *Merck's Manual,* probably the most widely used compendium of medical disorders in the United States. Current estimates of the lifetime prevalence of coprolalia have decreased markedly and other factors indicate that coprolalia is not an essential feature for the diagnosis of Tourette's disorder, nor should treatment be delayed until its appearance.

Frequency and persistence of coprolalia

Coprolalia was present in 56% of the original nine patients described by Tourettes (1885), similar to the 55% reported in our earlier sample of 114 patients (Shapiro et al., 1978) and to other early published reports (Moldofsky et al., 1974; Abuzzahab and Anderson, 1974) (Table 5.16). The percent of patients with coprolalia, however, has decreased significantly since that time, as indicated by the significant negative correlation between percent with coprolalia and year of evaluation ($r = 0.21$, df-664, $p < 0.0001$). Only 32% of our total sample of 666 patients have a history of coprolalia. The percent increases to 37.4% if copropraxia and mental coprolalia are included. These percentages are consistent with recent reports in the literature which vary from 21% to 37% (Table 5.16). The decrease in coprophilia might be related to the younger age of patients in recent samples who may, as they get older, develop coprolalia. An even more significant factor is that early samples comprised more severely afflicted patients. As Table 5.3 indicates, severity of Tourette's disorder correlates significantly with a history of coprolalia ($r = 0.46$, df-664, $p = 0.000$), and a more frequent diagnosis of TS+ADD, which also correlates significantly with a history of coprolalia ($r = 0.15$, df-664, $p = 0.0002$).

Copropraxia

Copropraxia is defined as an involuntary, socially unacceptable, commonly obscene, complex motor tic. This symptom was present at some time during the illness in 12.8% of our sample. Copropraxia commonly takes the form of an obscene gesture, and in our sample included touching or pointing toward one's own genital area (7.7%) or the genital area of another person (0.5%), obscene finger gesture (6.5%), masturbatory movements (2.4%), and sudden looking at one's own or another person's genital area (0.1%) (Table 5.13). Other types include an obscene elbow gesture and pointing toward or touching the buttocks or anus. The percentage of copropraxia reported in other samples is 11% (Golden, 1982) and 3% (Comings and Comings, 1984) (Table 5.16). The range for the age at onset and percent persistence or disappearance of copropraxia is similar to the range for coprolalia. As with coprolalia and other symptoms, most patients attempt to obfuscate or minimize the impact of the symptom by substituting other symptoms or partially expressing the symptom, such as touching an object, partially pointing, or saying "good" instead of making the gesture (explained by the patient as "good, I didn't do it"). Despite these attempts, copropraxia may appear in the most embarrassing circumstances such as giving the finger or making an elbow gesture when passing a policeman or when admonished by a teacher. It is sometimes difficult to decide whether other symptoms should be classified as copropraxia, such as spitting (occurring in 17.6%) and the too vigorous poking or squeezing of others, especially while expressing affection and love during coitus.

Mental Coprolalia

Mental coprolalia is defined as the unspoken, involuntary, sudden intrusion of socially unacceptable, commonly obscene, sounds, words, phrases, sentences or thoughts. Mental coprolalia, present in 3.6% of our patients, included 24 different words or phrases listed in Table 5.12. Coprolalia occasionally can be converted into mental coprolalia in social situations, but openly expressed with friends or family, and not infrequently only when alone.

Age at Onset for Coprophilia

In our sample only 32% of patients had a history of coprolalia, and 38% had a history of any type of coprophilia. Although the median age at onset for

TABLE 5.13. *Lifetime complex motor tics: Copropraxia*

Symptom	Past history of symptom N	%	Age at onset Mean	SD	Median	Range	Persistence of symptoms %	Duration of symptom 1 Year %	2 Years %	5 Years %	10 Years %	15 Years %
Copropraxia[a]												
Touch own genitals	51	7.7	11.2	6.6	10	1–29	82.4	1	2	3	4	5
Obscene finger gesture	43	6.5	12.1	6.4	10	5–36	76.1	<1	1	2	2	4
Masturbatory movements	16	2.4	10.5	4.8	11	1–21	82.4	<1	1	1	2	2
Touch others' genitals	10	0.5	10.0	3.9	9	4–17	90.9	0	0	1	<1	0
Look at crotch	1	0.1	23.0	—	—	—	100.0	—	—	—	—	—

[a] $N = 85$.

specific coprolalic words or phrases varied from 8 to 12 years of age, the range for any coprolalia varied from 1 to 36 years of age (Tables 5.12, 5.13). Moreover, although coprophilia was an initial symptom in 1.1% of patients (Table 5.5), it developed 4 years after the onset of Tourette's disorder in 51.9% of patients and from 7.5 to 25 years after the onset of Tourette's disorder in 20.7% of patients (Table 5.14). Given these observations and the recent consensual conclusion that coprophilia is only one but not an essential symptom of Tourette's disorder, it is not very persuasive that the diagnosis of Tourette's disorder should require the presence of coprophilia, and certainly indefensible that patients without coprophilia should not be treated with drugs known to be effective for Tourette's disorder.

Clinical Course of Coprophilia

In addition, because coprophilia may disappear after being present for a variable period of time, reliable estimates of the likelihood of the remission of coprophilia requires that patients be followed throughout their lives. Our data are limited to the percent of patients who had a history of coprophilia, and the percent in whom coprophilia subsequently remitted at the time of their initial evaluation. Nine to 30% of diverse coprophilic symptoms present sometime in the past had remitted at the time of their initial evaluation (Table 5.12). A better approximation of the course for coprophilia is available for the first 114 patients who were evaluated more thoroughly and completely than were subsequent patients. Sixty-three (55.3%) of 114 patients developed coprolalia. Coprolalia remitted in 12 (19%) of these patients, which is consistent with the 9 to 30% for the total sample.

Relationship of Coprophilia to Other Variables

Analysis of the data for the first 114 patients indicates that coprolalia is unrelated to the age at onset for Tourette's disorder. Moreover, spontaneous

TABLE 5.14. Development of coprophilia after onset of Tourette's disorder[a]

Years after onset of TS	N	%	Cumulative %
Initial symptom	23	11.1	11.1
0.5–1.5	25	12.0	23.7
2.0–4.0	60	28.8	51.9
4.5–7.0	57	27.4	79.3
7.5–25.0	43	20.7	100.0

[a]$N = 208$.

remission of coprolalia is unrelated to the age at onset of Tourette's disorder and coprolalia and to the years between the onset of Tourette's disorder and the development of coprolalia. Theoretical issues and the disruptive effect of coprophilia on patients warrants more detailed analysis in order to predict the development and natural course of patients with coprolalia.

Our expectations were confirmed that coprolalia would be associated with the year of evaluation ($r = -0.21, p < 0.0001$), previous diagnosis or consultation FS ($r = 0.21, p < 0.0001$), TS+ADD ($r = 0.23, p < 0.001$), neurological abnormalities ($r = 0.15, p < 0.01$), hyperactivity FS ($r = 0.23, p < 0.0001$) and severity of Tourette's disorder ($r = 0.46, p < 0.0001$), and would not be associated with genetic variables, medical history variables, and behavioral variables, including obsessive-compulsive symptoms (OCS), obsessive compulsive disorder (OCD), and compulsive personality disorder (CPD) variables. Coprolalia was less strongly associated with copropraxia than expected ($r = 0.26, p = 0.0001$), only 7% of the variance was shared, leaving most of the variance unaccounted for. Final SRAs for both coprolalia and copropraxia selected variables largely reflecting severity of Tourette's disorder symptoms (Table 5.3).

Puzzle of Coprophilia

Coprophilia is one of the more fascinating and puzzling symptoms of Tourette's disorder. In nonmedical literature, coprophilia has been labeled as the *Foulmouth syndrome, Cursing Sickness,* and *Curse of Tourette's syndrome,* although most Tourette patients do not have coprophilia. Professionals as well as lay people are intrigued by it, and it is the most difficult symptom to explain neurophysiologically. What is the explanation for this symptom? Although a meaningful explanation is not possible because there is little substantive information available, three possible explanations have been proposed. First, coprophilia is an organic symptom similar to other symptoms of Tourette's disorder; a second, coprophilia is a symptom expressing an unconscious conflict which reflects a psychological etiology for Tourette's disorder. A final possibility is that coprophilia is a psychophysiological symptom caused by an interaction of central nervous system and psychological factors in susceptible individuals.

Coprophilia as an Organic Symptom

First, let us consider the possibility that coprophilia, together with other symptoms of Tourette's disorder, is caused by an abnormality in the central nervous system. Several clinical observations support this possibility.

Basal ganglia

Klazomania is a rare sequela of encephalitis lethargica. Patients suddenly develop an oculogyric crisis associated with an organic mental syndrome. During this period patients writhe, shake, repetitively shout, and exhibit echolalia and coprolalia (Benedek, 1925; Wohlfart et al., 1961). All of these symptoms promptly disappear when the oculogyric crisis terminates. Patients do not use coprolalic words at other times. Klazomania, once considered a psychologic condition, is now generally accepted as having an organic etiology. Thus, we have a clear example that coprolalia can occur with a known organic illness with demonstrable pathology. It is also possibly significant that the illness includes a disturbance in the basal ganglia. Other disorders with basal ganglia disturbance and coprolalia include Sydenham's chorea and hemiballismus (Marti-Masso and Obeso, 1985).

Central nervous system

Coprolalia can also occur in patients after cerebrovascular accidents (CVA). These patients always have accompanying organic mental changes, and characteristically do not use obscenities prior to the CVA. In patients suffering from nonfluent aphasia after CVA, a coprolalic word is substituted for a forgotten one. Aphasics, frequently while struggling for a word erupt with an involuntary coprolalic word, not in frustration, but as if a pathway has been short-circuited. The audiogram, as in Tourette's disorder, has the appearance of a scream rather than a word (Van Lancker, 1975, and *personal communication*). Copropraxia occurs occasionally in senile patients. For example, I was requested to do a consultation on an 86-year-old woman who was threatened with expulsion from a nursing home because of intolerable behavior. She had led an exemplary life prior to her illness and was known never to have used obscenities. Her behavior in the nursing home consisted of repetitive and intractable grabbing for and touching the penises of patients. Fortunately, low dosages of phenelzine and thioridazine completely controlled the copropraxia. However, this type of organic copropraxia has a different clinical appearance from the copropraxia observed in Tourette's disorder. Copropraxia in Tourette's disorder patients is sudden, brief, and ejaculatory, and is not characterized by prolonged, patterned, or co-ordinated behavior. Similar reservations hold for the coprophilia (obscene words or gestures, touching, playing with, or smearing feces) that occurs in organically impaired senile, autistic, or other brain-damaged individuals. The etiology for these types of coprophilia may be different but related in some way.

Thalamus

Although not directly related to the pathophysiology of coprophilia, indirect evidence suggests that the thalamus may play a role in the generation of

Tourette-like symptoms. Schaltenbrand (1975a,b) reported phonation and speech evoked by bipolar electrical stimulation through a stereotaxic needle in the thalamus of patients with motor disorders or intractable pain. Stimulation of the ventral-oral anterior nucleus of the thalamus evoked monosyllabic yells and exclamations of surprise, fright or pain, and repetition of syllables similar to palilalia with or without contralateral head or arm movements. Coughing, swallowing, and clicking were elicited by stimulation at the borders of the centromedian and the internal ventro-caudal nucleus, whereas silencing or slowing of speech occurred with stimulation of the ventral-oral nucleus. Shaltenbrand postulates that these complicated activities are not organized primarily in the thalamus but are regulated by a "thalamic clock." Cautious interpretation of this data is necessary because spread of current may lead to false conclusions about localization in deep stimulation of the brain (Laursen, 1963). Coprophilia was not elicited by the procedure and one can only speculate with van Lanker (1975) about the relationship of these symptoms and coprolalia to brain structure.

Psychological Etiology for Coprophilia

The extensive literature suggesting a psychological etiology for Tourette's disorder and coprophilia has been reviewed in Chapter 1. Psychoanalytic concepts included displaced unconscious muscular eroticism toward the father (Sadger, 1914), defense against autopleasurable thumb-sucking (Oberndorf, 1916), narcissistic onanism (Ferenczi, 1921), anal sadism (Abraham, 1927), inhibited aggression (Mahler et al., 1945), and obsessive-compulsive neurosis or psychosis. Some suggest that the choice of an unacceptable symptom such as coprolalia reveals an unconscious, but consciously disowned conflict, a major failure of the ego's reality testing and an underlying psychosis. Others linked the etiology to schizophrenia (Woodrow, 1974), familial psychodynamics (Bruch and Thum, 1968), learned contingencies (Shapiro, 1976a), and other psychodynamic or psychosocial conflicts.

All of these psychological concepts are suppositions derived from isolated clinical observations or are based on theoretical speculation. There are no controlled studies supporting a psychological etiology for coprophilia. Moreover, no study has demonstrated that particular psychologic conflicts, characteristics, traits, or events are associated with or cause coprophilia. In addition, behavioral symptoms are not selected by summary SRAs for both coprolalia and copropraxia (Table 5.3). The reason for increased coprophilia in patients with TS+ADD ($r = 0.15$, df-664, $p = 0.0002$) (see also Table 4.27) may be due to increased susceptibility of patients with nonspecific central nervous system dysfunction. Our clinical experience is that coprophilia appears *de novo*, unpredictably, and without discernible external stimuli or internal psychological conflict. The symptoms are just as likely to occur in a well adjusted as in a poorly adjusted individual. The occurrence, as well as disappearance, cannot be predicted. Moreover, coprophilia occurs transculturally at a fairly consistent percentage (Table 5.16). Patients experience the symptom as involuntary and completely ego alien. Unlike a compulsion it is an end in itself, similar to a sneeze. Whereas psychological treatment has little effect on coprophilia, neuroleptics such as haloperidol often completely suppress it. Moreover, there is no symptom substitution as one would expect if coprophilia were a psychological symptom.

In our opinion, there is no evidence currently that psychosocial factors are etiologically related to or associated with coprophilia.

Psychophysiological Etiology for Coprophilia

There is an unfortunate tendency in medicine to attribute psychophysiological (previously called psychosomatic) etiologies for symptoms or disorders for which the pathophysiology is unknown and the psychopathology cannot be demonstrated (Shapiro, 1960, 1964, 1978; Shapiro and Shapiro, 1985a). A dual etiology is often invoked as an explanation for coprophilia as well as Tourette's disorder (Eldridge et al., 1977; Cohen et al., 1982; Friedhoff, 1982; Leckman et al., 1982b). The theory postulates an interaction between an organic susceptibility and psychopathology for the symptom to be expressed. Although this hypothesis is possible, it has not yet been demonstrated. Moreover, postulating a dual etiology does not appear to us to be parsimonious.

Impaired inhibition of impulses as a cause of coprophilia

The most specific concept of a dual or psychophysiological cause of coprolalia postulates an impairment of inhibition that permits the release of words, ideas, desires, wishes, and other impulses that are normally inhibited by individuals. The concept was first proposed by Trousseau (1873) who said of the obscenities: "Sometimes a patient is driven to utter aloud what he would conceal." Freud (1966) characterized coprolalia as a mental phenomenon and attributed the behavior to the patient's psyche. Coprolalia was explained as a perception by patients that they were unable to repress a particular sound, leading to fear of losing control not only of sounds but for words as well, and ultimately resulting in the feared coming true. The mechanism, described as a counter-will, was illustrated by a non-Tourette's-disorder patient whose need to keep from saying a name was reversed into saying the name aloud. Similarly, obscene words are secrets everyone knows and are compelled to acknowledge to each other. Similar concepts, which essentially postulate impaired inhibition of impulses, have been proposed by others (Eldridge et al., 1977; Cohen et al., 1982).

The concept may have derived from clinical observation of a unique and small group of Tourette's disorder patients with unusual problems. Some of these patients are well known to clinicians and have been evaluated and written about extensively (Sacks, 1987). A good example of an unusual and atypical patient with Tourette's disorder is the extended description of a patient by Meige and Feindel (1907). Some patients are preoccupied with the fear that they will blurt out that which they wish to suppress. Most of the time the fear that the patient will not be able to suppress the coprolalia is a real fear, and therefore not an obsession, compulsion, or other psychological-motivated symptom. Some patients report increased coprophilia when thinking about coprophilia, however, it appears to us to be an echoing type of Tourette's disorder symptom. Although these patients are rare, they attract disproportionate clinical interest.

Although this concept is poetically attractive, it is unparsimonious and unsupported by the clinical phenomenology. Impaired inhibition of impulses appears plausible since the mechanism can be observed neurophysiologically in ballismic and other neurological disorders, and clinically in psychiatric patients with poor impulse control. It is the mirror image of the proposed mechanism that is not in accord with clinical observation. The mechanism postulates that patients have wishes, desires, or impulses to express coprophilia. It also implies that such impulses are stronger in patients with coprophilia than in patients without coprophilia. If this is so, it follows that one should be able to detect clinically and experimentally greater impulsivity, stronger urges, less ego strength, and more general psychopathology in patients with coprophilia than in those without it. However, these traits are not more characteristic of Tourette's disorder patients with coprophilia than patients without coprophilia (Table 5.3) and are not more frequent than expected in the population. Samuel Johnson was consciously offended by profanity as are many Tourette's disorder patients who have coprophilia. Based on our social and clinical experience with Tourette's disorder patients, and our studies, impulsivity, aggressivity, the proclivity for intentionally using dirty words, and other psychopathology are no greater among Tourette's disorder patients than they would be in a random selection of patients without coprophilia or Tourette's disorder. Moreover, clinicians who have had experience with many Tourette's disorder patients can cite many individuals who have few or no problems in these areas and function quite well. How can the dual concept of increased impulses interacting with impaired inhibition explain coprophilia in these patients? One would have to postulate an unconscious mechanism which, according to psychoanalytic theory, is not consciously available to patients, although possibly discernible to a specially trained individual after listening to the patients' free associations for many years. Our conclusion is that psychophysiological mechanisms do not adequately explain the phenomenology of coprophilia.

Aberrant Stimulation of Neurons as an Explanation for Coprophilia

The pathogenesis of coprophilia is currently unknown. We can only hypothesize a particular mechanism. Our hypothesis is that coprophilia, as well as all Tourette's disorder symptoms, are due to neuroanatomic, neurotransmitter, or other neuropathology leading to a short-circuiting of neuronal pathways, and that the particular Tourette's disorder symptom is determined by the location of the pathophysiology. Coprophilia and other Tourette's disorder symptoms are thought to be somewhat analogous to epilepsy: An aberrant stimulus (excessive discharge or shortcircuiting) in various sites of the central nervous system, of varying intensity and spread, can produce generalized or focal movement, noises, auras, feelings, and behavior. The mechanism is most plausible for the motor symptoms and possibly for inarticulate vocal symptoms because potential neuroanatomic loci for these symptoms have been demonstrated, but least plausible for coprophilia and echophilia since anatomic or functional centers have not been demonstrated for these symptoms. We postulate that there is a functional neurological system that stores socially unacceptable or obscene sounds, words, sentences, concepts, or motor acts that because of aberrant stimulation, excessive discharge, or short-circuiting produces these difficult to understand symptoms.

Summary of Cumulative Lifetime Symptoms

Cumulative lifetime symptoms are categorized arbitrarily into anatomic regions or types of symptoms in Table 5.15.

The frequency of lifetime symptoms in descending order are tics of the face or head (99.2%), inarticulate vocal tics (98.5%), upper limb tics (68.6%), complex motor tics (68.5%), tics of the torso (46.5%), lower limb tics (40.7%), tics of both upper and lower limbs (73.6%), and complex vocal tics (coprophilia (37.4%), and echophilia (32.7%). The number of different symptoms totals 296. Approximately one-third of patients had two to ten symptoms, 44% had 11 to 30 symptoms, and the remainder had 31 to an incredible 60 symptoms during their lifetime. The number and diversity of symptoms accords Tourette's disorder the dubious distinction of having the greatest number of symptoms of any medical illness.

Studies in the literature citing the frequency of lifetime symptoms are summarized in Table 5.16. The reported ranges for various symptom categories are generally similar except for an increased percentage with coprolalia reported in early studies, and a smaller percentage of complex tics reported in one study. It is important to note again that the reported percentages require correction for the age of patients, duration of illness, and diagnosis of ADD.

TABLE 5.15. *Summary of Cumulative Lifetime Symptoms*[a]

Symptoms	Number of different symptoms	Number of patients	Percent of patients
Simple Motor			
Face	8	620	93.1
Head, neck	2	606	91.0
Total	10	661	99.2
Upper limb	5	453	68.6
Lower limb	4	271	40.7
Total	9	490	73.6
Torso	7	310	46.5
Total	26	666	100.0
Complex movements			
Total	54	456	68.5
Inarticulate vocal sounds			
Total	77	656	98.5
Echophilia			
Total	9	218	32.7
Coprophilia			
Coprolalia	101	213	32.0
Mental coprolalia	24	26	3.9
Copropraxia	5	85	12.8
Total	130	218	37.4
Total	279	666	100.0
Cumulative lifetime symptoms			
2–10 symptoms	—	216	32.4
11–20 symptoms	—	295	44.3
21–30 symptoms	—	114	17.1
31–40 symptoms	—	23	3.5
41–50 symptoms	—	10	1.5
51–60 symptoms	—	8	1.2

[a] $N = 666$.

SAMPLING PROBLEMS IN STUDIES OF TOURETTE'S DISORDER

The development of consensual agreement about the frequency of initial symptoms, developmental course, and cumulative lifetime symptoms has been hindered by the different methods used by investigators to describe, categorize, and tabulate Tourette's disorder symptoms. Moreover, the reported cumulative symptoms are not corrected for age, duration of illness, and the diagnosis of ADD, all of which are associated with higher frequencies for most cumulative symptoms. Several solutions to the problem are essential. Criteria for describing and categorizing symptoms should be developed by a consensus panel of experts so that all investigators and clinicians in future studies will use a standard method for reporting symptoms. Factor analytic methods should be used to reduce the large number of discrete symptoms into relevant categories.

TABLE 5.16. Studies citing cumulative lifetime regional symptoms

Symptom	Current study[a] (1965–1981) %	Comings and Comings[b] (1984) %	Golden[c] (1982) %	Nomura and Segawa[d] (1982) %	Lees et al.[e] (1984) %	Han-bai and Han-quin[f] (1983) %	Moldofsky et al.[g] (1974) %	Jagger et al.[h] (1982) %	Abuzzahab et al.[i] (1974) %	Min[j] (1983) %
Head or face										
Eye	80	56	73	>75	—	58	—	—	31	—
Neck	69	63	—	—	89	—	100	—	53	—
Facial grimace	36	29	—	—	—	—	—	—	—	—
Total	99	82	>90	>90	>94	84	100	>95	92	—
Limbs										
Upper	69	>32	—	a 70	51	84	87	83	78	—
Lower	41	21	—	a 40	40	58	73	61	54	—
Total	74	—	53	>70	—	—	—	—	—	—
Torso										
Total	47	—	45	250	41	53	80	61	—	—
Complex										
Total	59	21–24	—	—	—	—	—	—	—	—
Inarticulate sounds										
Total	99	96	—	>70	—	90	100	—	65	83

	$^a N=666$	$^b N=250$	$^c N=80$	$^d N=97$	$^e N=50$	$^f N=19$	$^g N=19$	$^h N=75$	$^i N=43$	$^j N=24$
Coprophilia	32	33	31	4–23	—	21	60	37	58	38
Coprolalia	13	3	11	—	—	—	—	—	—	—
Coproproxia	—	—	—	—	—	—	—	—	—	—
Total	37	—	—	—	—	—	—	—	—	—
Echophilia	18	—	19	—	—	16	7	—	23	—
Echolalia	17	—	20	—	—	—	—	—	—	13
Palilalia	8	—	1	—	—	—	—	—	—	—
Echokinesis	—	—	—	—	—	—	—	—	—	—
Total	33	—	—	—	—	—	—	—	—	—

$^a N = 666.$
$^b N = 250.$
$^c N = 80.$
$^d N = 97.$
$^e N = 50.$
$^f N = 19.$
$^g N = 19.$
$^h N = 75.$
$^i N = 43.$
$^j N = 24.$

Variables Affecting Reports of Lifetime Symptoms

Sources of variability for cumulative lifetime symptoms include the duration of illness, age of patients, the number of patients with TS+ADD in samples, and the reliability and validity of measurement.

Effect of Duration of Illness

Previously reported cumulative lifetime symptoms were derived from small samples with a wide range for age at onset and duration of illness. Obviously more symptoms are likely to develop the longer the illness persists. We, therefore, tabulated the cumulative lifetime symptoms reported at initial onset, and after 1, 2, 5, 10, 15, 21, and 30 years after the onset of Tourette's disorder. Age is adequately reflected by duration of illness since these variables are highly correlated ($r = 0.97$, $p < 0.0001$). Since the analysis indicated that the percent of symptoms did not increase significantly after a 15-year duration of illness (either staying the same or increasing only 1%), the results are summarized for 1, 2, 5, 10, and 15 years duration of illness (Tables 5.8–5.13).

The results strongly confirmed our expectation that the percent of cumulative lifetime symptoms increase with duration of illness and age. The percent for all symptoms progressively increases up to 15 years duration of illness, and by a smaller percentage, usually 1%, for some symptoms with over 21 and 30 years duration of illness. Some symptoms do not substantially increase after 5 years, symptoms such as eye blinking, kicking, bending over, throwing objects, kissing others, sucking and blowing sounds, and touching the genitals of others. The percents for some symptoms level off after 10 years, and for others continue to increase up to 15 years. Duration of illness is weakly but consistently correlated with a past history of tics of the head ($r = 0.08$, $p < 0.05$), arm ($r = 0.12$, $p < 0.01$), leg ($r = 0.17$, $p < 0.0001$), torso ($r = 0.07$, $p < 0.10$), inarticulate sounds ($r = 0.06$, $p < 0.10$), copropraxia ($r = 0.08$, $p < 0.05$), number of current tics ($r = 0.13$, $p < 0.001$) and number of cumulative tics ($r = 0.08$, $p < 0.05$).

These results are a better estimate than heretofore available of the lifetime prevalence of reported symptoms in Tourette's disorder and will provide clinicians and patients with an estimate of the likelihood of developing various symptoms over time. The duration of illness listed in the tables, from 1 to 15 years, added to the age at onset for Tourette's disorder, provides a basis for estimating the likelihood of having or developing a symptom during childhood, adolescence, or adulthood.

However, even these results have to be modified because of the possible effect of other variables.

Effect of Attention Deficit Disorder and Hyperactivity

We noted previously that complex and coprolalic tics are not associated with duration of illness. This finding may be due to the TS+ADD group who have significantly more complex, coprolalic, and total number of tics (Table 4.27) and who are significantly younger (Tables 4.5, 4.27) than the TS-alone group. The expected increase of these tics over time may be artifactually decreased by the younger age and shorter duration of illness in the TS+ADD group.

Our clinical impression that patients with TS+ADD+H have more tics than TS-alone patients tends to be confirmed. TS+ADD patients have higher mean scores than TS-alone patients on ten of 13 regional tics, although only complex tics ($p < 0.01$) and coprolalia ($p < 0.0001$) are significantly higher (Table 4.27). The hyperactivity FS, which correlates 0.49 ($p < 0.0001$) with TS+ADD, is positively correlated with complex tics ($r = 0.20$, $p < 0.001$), coprolalia ($r = 0.23$, $p < 0.0001$), copropraxia ($r = 0.23$, $p < 0.0001$) and number of cumulative tics ($r = 0.23$, $p < 0.0001$). The results, therefore, confirm our impression that patients with TS+ADD+H have more tics, especially complex tics, coprolalia, and total number of cumulative tics than patients with TS-alone.

Effect of Measurement

Other potential factors that may interfere in unknown ways with the reliable recording of cumulative lifetime prevalence of tics include unreliable histories given by patients or informants, different duration of illness, amnesia for early symptoms by older patients, and the different methods of classifying symptoms by clinicians and investigators. The development of reliable criteria for classifying the signs and symptoms of Tourette's disorder will increase immeasurably our ability to report reliable data.

CLINICAL COURSE

The clinical course of Tourette's disorder is characterized by change in frequency, location, type, intensity, and general overall severity of tics, unpredictable temporary or permanent remissions, and indeterminate prognosis (Table 5.17).

Spontaneous Fluctuation of Symptoms

We noted as early as 1970 that the clinical course for Tourette's disorder was characterized by spontaneous changes in type and location of tics. A

TABLE 5.17. *Spontaneous fluctuation, waxing and waning, and remission of symptoms*[a]

Variables	%
Spontaneous fluctuation or change in type of tic	95.9
Spontaneous waxing, or waning, or change in severity of tics	97.1
Spontaneous remission of tics for 1 or more weeks[c]	27.2
Length of remission	
<1 month	25.6
1–< 6 months	41.7
6–< 12 months	12.8
1–< 2 years	13.3
2–< 5 years	2.8
5–< 7 years	2.2
<7 years[b]	1.7

[a]$N = 666$.
[b]For the first 50 consecutive patients who were carefully followed up to the present time, three (7.9%) patients have had complete remissions, two for 19 years, and one for 15 years.
[c]$N = 181$.

particular tic or any tic could last from several weeks to years, disappear permanently, or unpredictably return. These observations were confirmed in a larger subsequent sample (Shapiro et al., 1978) and became generally accepted as one criterion for the diagnosis of Tourette's disorder. Although fluctuation of symptoms is not included as a criterion for Tourette's disorder in DSM-III (American Psychiatric Association, 1980), it will be included in DSM-III-R (American Psychiatric Association, 1987). Fluctuation of symptoms is present in 95.6% percent of patients in our sample (Table 5.17). Symptoms tend to fluctuate generally over 3-month periods, although the range can vary from 2 weeks to years in children and adolescents, and over much longer periods in adults.

Spontaneous Waxing and Waning of the Severity of Symptoms

The general overall severity of symptoms spontaneously changed, or waxed and waned over time in 97.1% of our patients (Table 5.17). Although precise or reliable measurement of severity by clinicians or judges is not always easy, ratings of change in severity by patients appears to have considerable face validity. Severity ratings usually include a combination and interaction of the frequency, strength, vigor, or loudness of one or all tics, the impact on others and their reaction to the tics and the patient's subjective sensitivity to the tics.

Severity of symptoms varies over time in a range of 2 weeks to 6 months, but more usually over 3-month periods in children and adolescents, and over much longer periods in adults. Symptoms may wax, wane, or fluctuate in tandem or independently in unpredictable ways. Spontaneous change in the severity of symptoms was noted by us prior to 1970, confirmed in a larger sample (Shapiro et al., 1978), included as a criterion in DSM-III (American Psychiatric Association, 1980), and will be included in DSM-III-R (American Psychiatric Association, 1987).

Spontaneous Remission of Symptoms

It is general clinical experience that most childhood tics spontaneously and permanently remit within a year. However, in patients whose tics last more than a year (Tourette's disorder or CMT), infrequent, spontaneous remissions usually of short duration occur and, although less frequent, can be permanent. Precise determination of the frequency of spontaneous permanent remission of all symptoms is difficult to assess because of sample ascertainment problems. Patients with mild symptoms often do not come to the attention of clinicians, and subsequent remissions may not be identified in these patients. Former patients are often lost to follow-up and those whose symptoms remit are more likely to discontinue treatment and not be identified. The age of patients, duration of illness, and length of follow-up varies markedly in studies and contributes additional problems of assessment. Remissions occurring at a later time may not be identified, and patients in remission may experience a return of symptoms in the future. A report by Klawans and Barr (1985) illustrates this observation. They describe four Tourette's disorder patients who had complete remissions in adolescence but return of symptoms after age 60. Another problem is the inclusion of patients in studies who have many different types of tic disorders such as transient tic disorder (TTD), chronic motor tic (CMT), chronic multiple motor tics, Tourette's disorder, atypical tic, and many non-tic movement disorders. Despite these limitations, a discussion of remissions is important to patients, clinicians, and investigators. Although there is considerable overlap in the type of tic conditions reported in the literature, those largely characterized as general tic disorders are discussed initially, followed by a discussion of studies of Tourette's disorder.

Spontaneous Remission in Tic Disorders

There are only four published studies of general tic disorders (Table 6.18). These comprehensive clinical studies provide a general discussion of these disorders, patient prognosis, and estimates of spontaneous remission. The major limitation of these studies, all published before 1970, is that DSM-III criteria for tic and Tourette's disorders were not available, and it is difficult to determine how many patients would be classifed today as having TTD, CMT, or Tourette's disorder. This is illustrated in a paper by Corbett (1976) in which between 10 to 30% of his previous sample (Corbett et al., 1969) were reclassified as having Tourette's disorder. Another limitation is that some studies specify the criteria for spontaneous remission as a tic-free period of 1 year (Zausmer, 1954; Torup, 1962) while others do not specify the length of the remission (Boncour, 1930; Corbett et al., 1969). The importance of duration of follow-up is supported by a significant relationship between the duration of follow-up and frequency of spontaneous remission in two of the studies ($p < 0.05$, Zausmer; $p < 0.02$, Corbett), although there was no relationship between these variables in our sample ($r = 0.06$, NS). Within these limitations, the data suggest that complete spontaneous remissions, lasting a year or more, are likely to occur at some time during the course of the illness in 24 to 65% of patients. Predictive factors for spontaneous remission, which may be a reflection of a tendency to improve in general, include female sex and duration of follow-up ($p < 0.05$) but no relationship to intelligence, age at onset, duration of illness before treatment, age at follow-up (Zausmer, 1954); better prognosis in children whose parents had tics only in childhood compared to parents who had tics during adulthood, but no relationship to sex (Torup, 1962); better prognosis in children with age at onset between 6 and 8 years of age compared to less than 6 or more than 8 years of age and length of follow-up ($p < 0.02$); and poorer prognosis for patients with coprolalia and tics of the limbs and lower body (Corbett et al., 1969). Two authors observed that tics tended to decrease at puberty (Zausmer, 1954; Torup, 1962). Because the studies were conducted before the use of haloperidol, they may be more useful in assessing the likelihood of spontaneous remissions without treatment. Remission of symptoms, an indication of improvement, was thought to be unrelated to psychotherapeutic or other nonspecific treatment.

Spontaneous Remission in Tourette's Disorder

There are many individual case reports in the literature describing spontaneous remission of symptoms in individuals with Tourette's disorder (Creak and Gutman, 1935; Abuzzahab and Anderson, 1974; Fernando, 1976; Lieh-Mak et al., 1982; Asam, 1982). The tendency to have periods of spontaneous remission of symptoms is supported by the data for our sample (Table 5.17). Complete remission of all symptoms was reported by 27.2% of our patients for variable periods of time. Some remissions lasted 1 week, most (67%) lasted less than 6 months, and only 6.7% lasted more than 2 years. We previously reported that four (5%) of 80 consecutive patients, age range 6 to 67 years, had a spontaneous remission when evaluated an average of 2.9 years (range 7 months to 8.5 years) after their initial evaluation (Shapiro et al., 1978). One of these patients subsequently had a return of symptoms. A better

TABLE 5.18. Studies citing clinical course for Tourette and tic disorders

Study	Sample size	Age at follow-up	Years of follow-up	Diagnosis treatment	Remission %	Remission Years	Improved	No change or worse
Tics (TS)								
Bonheim (1930)	31	—	2–3	Tics[a]	61%	?	36%	3%
Zausmer (1954)	41	—	1.5–11	Tics[a]	24%[e]	1	51%	24%
Torup (1962)	209	5–30	>1	Tics[a]	50%[f]	1	46%	6%
Corbett et al. (1969, 1976)	28	—	<2	Tics, TS	32%	?	64%	4%
	22	—	3–7	Tics, TS	27%	?	68%	5%
	23	—	>8	Tics, TS	65%	?	26%	9%
	73	6–29	2–28	Tics, TS[b]	41%[g]	?	53%	6%
Tourette's disorder								
Lucas (1967)	15	14–27	1–15	TS[c]	6%	?	88%	6%
Jenkins et al. (1976)	13	13–37	8–33	TS[d]	8%	5	—	—
Shapiro et al. (1978)	50	20–85	13–20	TS[d]	8%	15–19	—	—

[a] Nonspecific psychotherapy.
[b] Psychotherapy, behavior therapy, abreaction, CO_2.
[c] Psychotherapy and medication.
[d] Haloperidol.
[e] More improvement reported for longer duration of follow-up ($p < 0.05$) and for females ($p < 0.05$), tendency for tics to clear at puberty.
[f] Improvement unrelated to sex.
[g] More improvement reported with longer duration of follow-up ($p < 0.02$) and in patients with age of onset between 6 and 8 years of age, prognosis good in general, trend for less favorable prognosis for patients with coprolalia, tics of the limbs and lower body.

estimate for remission includes the first 50 consecutive patients that we evaluated between 1965 and 1971 who have been followed from 15 to 20 years. As indicated in Table 5.18, three (7.9%) patients, who ranged in age from 20 to 85 years, had remissions lasting from 15 to 20 years. The first patient with onset at age 8 of severe Tourette's disorder, had a complete remission at age 11 which has persisted for 19 years (Shapiro and Shapiro, 1968; case 5 in Shapiro et al., 1978). The second patient with onset at age 5.5, with subsequent severe symptoms, had a complete remission at age 8 which has been maintained for the past 15 years until the current age of 33 (case 7 in Shapiro et al., 1978). The final patient, with mild symptoms, had a complete remission at age 18 which has persisted for 15 years up to the current age of 33. Approximately 5 to 8% of subsequent patients had a spontaneous remission, but were followed for a briefer period of time. Unfortunately, we have not been able to follow up all patients.

Meaningful conclusions about the likelihood of a permanent remission is not possible from a review of the literature because sample characteristics and follow-up periods varied from study to study. The tic-free duration was not specified in one report (Lucas, 1967), the tic-free period without medication was 5 years in the second study (Jenkins et al., 1976) and our patient sample was followed for 15 to 20 years. Despite the sparsity of the data, two conclusions are possible: It is less likely for patients with Tourette's disorder to have a temporary and especially a permanent spontaneous remission compared to patients with general tic disorders, and the percentage chance of a permanent remission for clinically identified Tourette's disorder patients is probably approximately 8%. However, we cannot be sure that this percentage is valid. It is possible that individuals with mild Tourette's disorders, who may be underrepresented in patient samples, have a higher rate of spontaneous remission. The possibility of symptom exacerbation after a prolonged period of remission is illustrated in a report of four Tourette's disorder patients who had remissions before age 20, and a return of symptoms after the age of 60 (Klawans and Barr, 1985).

Factors Associated with Spontaneous Waxing, Waning, Fluctuation, and Remission of Symptoms

Most patients initially attribute spontaneous changes to psychological or situational events, but eventually conclude that they are spontaneous and only artifactually associated with stimuli. A small percentage (3–4%), however, describe their clinical course as stable and without spontaneous changes. Several factors are associated with the absence of these changes. Very young children at the onset of symptoms and patients with very mild symptoms that do not cause psychosocial distress tend to be less observant about symptom changes. Patients who use defense mechanisms such as suppression, repression, and denial are also less observant about the change of symptoms. However, we could not explain the absence of symptom fluctuation in a small group of patients. Their symptoms were not particularly mild, they were good observers, and the history was confirmed by other informants. Tics in these patients were more vigorous than the usual tics in Tourette's disorder patients. They did not have vocal tics, or if they were present, they were secondary to a strong diaphragmatic, abdominal, or generalized torso tic. Their symptoms did not wax, wane, and fluctuate, and their response to haloperidol was inadequate. The classification for these patients, CMT in DSM-III (American Psychiatric Association, 1980), will be included in the general category of CMT in DSM-III-R (American Psychiatric Association, 1987) but will not be specifically identified (See Chapter 10). However, recognizing that almost all patients report spontaneous changes in either type, location, frequency, intensity, or severity of tics over time, we recommend inclusion of this criterion for tics and Tourette's disorder. If waxing, waning, and fluctuation are not present, the diagnosis should be atypical tic disorder (see Chapter 10).

We do not know the cause of or have the ability to predict spontaneous waxing, waning, fluctuation, and temporary or permanent remission of symptoms. These changes are somewhat similar to the spontaneous changes frequently observed in rheumatoid arthritis. It is possible that these symptomatic changes in Tourette's disorder are caused by currently unknown metabolic shifts in the body.

For possible insights about the correlates of spontaneous remissions, an SRA was done using 54 variables (Table A.1). Because remission of symptoms usually occur before 17 years of age, only patients 17 years or younger were included in the analysis. Only two variables were selected from the seven variable categories: social class ($r = -0.16$, $p < 0.01$) and Tourette's disorder severity ($r = -0.12$, $p < 0.05$). Only social class, accounting for 2% of the variance in remission of symptoms FS, was selected by the summary SRA (Table 5.3). The results suggest that spontaneous remissions are more likely to occur in patients in higher social classes who tend to have less severe symptoms, or are less likely to occur in lower social class patients, who tend to have more severe symptoms ($r = 0.30$, $p < 0.0001$). These retrospective results require replication. However, the small amount of variance suggests that remissions, like the etiology of Tourette's disorder itself, is associated with unknown neuroanatomic, neurophysiological, or neurochemical factors.

Possible Complications

Infrequent complications include orthopedic disorders (Goetz et al., 1982), blindness caused by an eye hitting tic, excoriation or bruises caused by picking, hitting, or rubbing tics, self injury from complex motor tics such as biting or hitting self, temperomandibular injury from jaw clenching and teeth grinding tics, maceration of the lips from licking tics, and suicide. Withdrawal, interference with psychosocial and vocational functioning, and depression may occur in predisposed individuals, especially those with severe forms of the disorder.

SEVERITY OF SYMPTOMS

The severity of symptoms was rated on the Shapiro Tourette's Disorder Severity Scale (TS-Sev) (Table A.2). As described in Chapters 2 and 13, TS-Sev was rated by the clinician conducting the initial evaluation (usually A.K.S.). Another clinician (E.S.), independently reviewed the record and rated the TS-Sev Scale. Ratings initially done by E.S. were independently rated by A.K.S. Differences of opinion were resolved by discussion and consensus. The high reliability and validity of the TS-Sev Scale is discussed in Chapter 13.

Fifty-one percent of patients were rated mild or very mild, 34% were rated as having moderate severity, and 15% were rated as marked, severe, or very severe (Table 5.19). Our impression that the severity of symptoms had decreased over time was confirmed (Table 4.1). The average severity rating was 3.4 for 121 patients evaluated between 1965 and 1974, decreased to 2.6 for 313 patients evaluated between 1975 and 1978, and to 2.3 for 232 patients evaluated between 1979 and 1981 [$F(2,660) = 61.4$, $p = 0.0001$; Duncan Multiple Range Test $p < 0.05$ for all comparisons]. A comparison of ratings on the TS-Sev Scale for our previous sample of 114 patients evaluated between 1965 and 1974 (Shapiro et al., 1978) with the 551 patients evaluated between 1975 and 1981, indicates an increase in mild severity from 23% to 56%, a decrease in marked severity from 33% to 10%, and a decrease in severe ratings from 11% to 5%. Patients rated as moderate remained approximately the same, 34%, for both time periods.

These results underscore the variability in severity of Tourette's disorder evaluated by clinicians and reported in studies. The decrease in severity of

TABLE 5.19. *Ratings of severity of Tourette's disorder*[a]

TS Severity Scale	%	Cumulative %
1. Very mild	4.8	4.8
2. Mild	46.2	51.1
3. Moderate	33.6	84.6
4. Marked	10.1	94.7
5. Severe	4.4	99.1
6. Very severe	0.9	100.0

[a] $N = 666$.

Tourette's disorder in patients is generally acknowledged by clinicians and investigators (Butler, 1985).

Our expectations that severity of Tourette's disorder would decrease with age and duration of illness were not confirmed. Severity of Tourette's disorder significantly increased in our sample after the age of 13, after a 2-year duration of illness and remained stable subsequently (Table 5.20). In retrospect, however, it must be remembered that it is highly likely that the majority of patients who seek evaluation and are reported in studies in all clinical conditions (Cohen and Cohen, 1984), are probably more severely afflicted than those who do not identify themselves as patients, and therefore do not come to the attention of clinicians. In fact, specialists and researchers probably attract patients with more severe symptoms. Our impression is that the severity of Tourette's disorder is predominantly mild in the population, especially if patients with CMT are included. Patients with mild symptoms are less likely to seek clinical evaluation and treatment and are, therefore, less likely to be identified. Thus, severity of Tourette's disorder in clinical samples may be higher than in nonclinical samples and not appear to vary with age. The data, therefore, do not reflect changes over time in individual patients.

Our *a priori* expectations about the correlates of Tourette's disorder severity were largely confirmed. We anticipated that Tourette's disorder severity would be less severe in recent samples ($r = -0.37, p < 0.0001$), associated with more previous diagnosis-consultation FS ($r = 0.24, p < 0.0001$) would be more severe in patients with ADD ($r = 0.24, p < 0.0001$), neurological abnormalities ($r = 0.13, p < 0.01$), EEG abnormalities ($r = 0.09, p < 0.10$),

TABLE 5.20. *Relationship of the severity of Tourette's disorder and duration of illness*

	Rating of TS severity		
Patient status	N	Mean	SD
Duration of illness[a]			
1 year	34	2.38	0.85
>1–2 years	152	2.49	0.80
>2–5 years	196	2.73	1.06
>5–10 years	90	2.85	1.12
>10–15 years	72	2.72	0.83
>15–21 years	69	2.64	0.82
>21 years	53	2.66	0.88
Total	666	2.66	0.95
Age of patients[b]			
4–13 years	303	2.56	1.00
>13–21 years	156	2.73	1.08
>21 years	207	2.75	0.89

[a]$F(6/659) = 2.18, p = 0.04$
[b]$F(2/663) = 2.79, p = 0.06$

hyperactivity FS ($r = 0.23$, $p < 0.0001$), learning disorders FS ($r = 0.16$, $p < 0.01$) and would be associated with increased regional tics [confirmed for history of tics involving the arm ($r = 0.19$, $p < 0.0001$), leg ($r = 0.21$, $p < 0.0001$), torso ($r = 0.19$, $p < 0.0001$), complex tics ($r = 0.19$, $p < 0.0001$), coprolalia ($r = 0.46$, $p < 0.0001$), copropraxia ($r = 0.13$, $p < 0.001$), echophilia ($r = 0.25$, $p < 0.0001$), number of current symptoms ($r = 0.34$, $p < 0.0001$), number of cumulative symptoms ($r = 0.40$, $p < 0.0001$), and less remissions of symptom FS ($r = 0.12$, $p < 0.001$)]. Unanticipated was the significant correlation of Tourette's disorder severity with anger-moodiness FS ($r = 0.22$, $p < 0.0001$), obsessive-compulsive-like symptoms FS ($r = 0.15$, $p < 0.01$), social class (more severe in lower compared with higher social classes, $r = 0.17$, $p < 0.0001$), an inverse correlation with coordination abilities FS ($r = -0.13$, $p < 0.01$) and intellectual and psychosocial FS ($r = 0.20$, $p < 0.0001$). Our expectations are also confirmed by the SRA (Table 5.21).

TABLE 5.21. *Severity of Tourette's disorder: Stepwise regression analysis*

Variables	Simple r	R^2	Parameter estimate
Demography			
Year evaluated	−0.37[a]	0.14	−0.10[a]
Social class (1 = high, 5 = low)	0.17[a]	0.16[a]	0.11[a]
Genetics			
Family TS	−0.10[b]	0.01[b]	−0.34[b]
Medical			
Epilepsy	0.08[c]	0.01[c]	0.78[c]
Neurological			
Attention deficit disorder	0.24[a]	0.02[b]	0.39[b]
Behavior			
Hyperactivity FS	0.23[a]	0.05	0.17[b]
Intellectual-psychosocial FS	−0.20[a]	0.06[a]	−0.16[c]
Illness variables			
Previous diagnosis-consultation FS	0.24[a]	0.06[a]	0.34[a]
Symptoms			
Coprolalia	0.46[a]	0.22	0.79[a]
Number current tics	0.34[a]	0.27	0.03[a]
Echophilia	0.25[a]	0.28	0.20[b]
Age at onset of TS	0.06	0.28	0.03[b]
Leg tics	0.21[a]	0.29[a]	0.15[c]
Summary SRA			
Year evaluated	−0.37[a]	0.01	−0.02[c]
Coprolalia	0.46[a]	0.14	0.53[a]
Number current tics	0.34[a]	0.20	0.03[b]
Echophilia	0.25[a]	0.23	0.28[b]
Attention deficit disorder	0.24[a]	0.25	0.27[b]
Social class	0.17[a]	0.27	0.08[c]
History of leg tics	0.21[a]	0.28	0.19[c]
Adjusted R^2		0.27[a]	

[a] $p < 0.0001$.
[b] $p < 0.01$.
[c] $p < 0.05$.

SIGNS, SYMPTOMS, AND CLINICAL COURSE

The reason for the selection of social class and leg tics by the summary SRA is not readily apparent and requires replication. Leg tics, however, were reported by Corbett et al. (1969) to be associated with poor prognosis in patients with tic disorders and was one of the variables included in the SRA for coprolalia (Table 5.3). These results also provide evidence for the construct validity of the TS-Sev Scale (see Chapter 13). Noteworthy is the negative relationship between severity of Tourette's disorder and family history of Tourette's disorder ($r = -0.10$, $p < 0.10$) and the absence of a relationship with age at onset of Tourette's disorder.

STIMULI-INDUCED CHANGES IN SEVERITY OF SYMPTOMS

All experienced clinicians are aware that stimuli and situational factors affect the frequency, intensity, and overall severity of symptoms. However, inexperienced clinicians may be inclined to interpret these changes psychologically and interpret increased symptoms at home with the family as indicating family conflict. Family members, and patients, too, are often perplexed by these changes. Accordingly, in 1977, we decided that it would be helpful to collect data about the effect of various stimuli on symptoms. Other stimuli added after 1981 are not included in the analysis. Patients or parents rated the effect of the stimuli using the following scale: 6, increase markedly; 5, increase slightly; 4, no change; 3, decrease slightly; 2, decrease markedly; and 0, disappearance of tics. The mean ratings and period change of symptoms are summarized in Table 5.22. The results for 20 different stimuli recorded for 394 patients are summarized in Table 5.22. Factor analysis of the 20 items yielded five factors with respectable reliabilities (Table A.1). Data analysis includes the five factors and 20 items. Table 5.22 lists the percent increase or decrease of tics on a six-point scale for each of the stimulus items. The means are recorded for each factor score (see Table A.1 for other data about these scales). A score of 4 signifies that the stimulus has no effect on tics. Scores higher than 4 signify increased tics and scores lower than 4 signify decreased tics. The mean scores for the five-factor scales change appropriately with the content of scale items. Thus, the mean score of 4.5 for the anxiety-fatigue FS indicates increased tics in response to anxiety, pleasurable anticipation, etc. The low score of 3.0 for the interpersonal stimuli FS reflects decreased tics when under public scrutiny, and the score of 3.1 for the nonanxious absorption stimuli FS reflects decreased tics when absorbed in a nonanxious activity or situation. Two-tailed chi-square analyses were conducted for the 20 variables comparing increase versus no change vs decrease of symptoms.

Effect of Specific Stimuli on Tics

Our *a priori* expectations were confirmed. Symptoms significantly increased with anxiety, pleasurable anticipation, and with the family, and decreased

TABLE 5.22. Stimuli-induced changes in severity of Tourette's disorder[a]

Stimulus variables	Mean	Disappear	% Change in tic symptoms					Decrease vs. no change vs. $p(\chi^2) =$ [b]
			Decrease markedly	Decrease slightly	No change	Increase slightly	Increase markedly	
Interpersonal stimuli FS	3.0							
With family	4.6	0.0	2.9	5.5	37.5	36.2	18.0	0.0000
Driving in an automobile	4.0	2.0	9.1	15.4	44.9	18.9	9.8	0.0004
Lectures, church, temple	3.7	5.4	15.7	18.9	38.9	12.1	8.9	0.0000
In school or at work	3.6	1.1	17.1	28.7	33.9	11.1	8.1	0.0000
In the presence of strangers	3.2	3.1	28.2	35.1	22.5	6.2	4.9	0.0000
While sleeping	2.0	97.2	2.0	0.8	0.0	0.0	0.0	0.0000
Passive stimuli FS	3.9							
Reading	3.7	4.9	15.0	16.9	42.0	10.9	10.4	0.0000
Watching movies	4.0	3.5	11.0	16.6	38.1	15.7	15.1	NS
Watching television	4.1	2.6	9.4	15.6	40.3	13.8	18.4	0.0083
Nonanxious absorption stimuli FS	3.0							
While repairing an object	3.2	6.9	24.7	34.1	26.1	4.4	3.8	0.0000
Nonanxious absorption in a task	2.9	10.2	29.9	27.5	28.3	2.2	1.9	0.0000
Anxiety-fatigue FS	4.5							
Anxiety	5.6	0.0	0.3	0.8	6.7	23.5	68.8	0.0000
Pleasurable anticipation	4.7	2.1	4.7	6.1	23.4	38.4	25.3	0.0000
Evening[c]	4.6	0.3	2.2	6.3	43.3	24.7	23.3	0.0000
Afternoon[c]	4.3	0.6	2.0	5.4	61.4	22.8	7.9	0.0000
Morning[c]	3.5	3.0	18.4	20.2	48.2	5.0	4.2	0.0000
Seasonal stimuli FS[d]	3.9							
Summer	3.8	3.1	8.5	10.3	70.4	4.3	3.4	0.0000
Autumn	4.1	0.6	2.0	3.2	80.1	7.5	6.6	0.0000
Winter	4.1	0.6	1.7	2.9	78.7	7.8	8.3	0.0000
Spring	4.1	0.0	2.0	6.1	80.8	6.4	4.7	0.0000

[a]$N = 394$.
[b]All χ^2 analyses compared increase vs. no change vs. decrease-disappear of tic symptoms.
[c]Diurnal variation: total, $(p(\chi^2, df-6) = 0.0000$; morning vs. afternoon and evening, and afternoon vs. evening, p s$(\chi^2, df-2) = 0.0000$.
[d]Seasonal variation: total, $p(\chi^2, df-0.0000$; summer vs. other, $p(\chi^2, df-2) = 0.0000$; spring vs. autumn and winter, $p(\chi^2, df-2) = 0.0669$; autumn vs. winter $p(\chi^2, df-2) = $ NS.

significantly while sleeping, in the presence of strangers, while repairing an object, during nonanxious absorption in a task, and when in school, work, or attending lectures. No predictions were made for other variables, although they were all significantly different except for watching movies. Although there is considerable variability in the distributions, four overall patterns were discernible.

Effect of Sleep on Symptoms

Standing by itself is the disappearance of symptoms in 97% of patients during sleep, and a decrease of symptoms in the remaining 3%. It is possible that tics occur more frequently during sleep than reported. In fact, Barabas et al. (1984a) reported that Tourette's disorder patients while asleep had significantly more tics than a control group. However, criteria for differentiating tics from common myoclonic jerks during sleep were not specified. More importantly, tics during sleep were infrequently reported in the Tourette's disorder group, and generally are not observed clinically (Min, 1983). The marked decrease of tics during sleep indicates that cortical connections are necessary for the full expression of tics.

Stimuli-Induced Decrease of Tics

For most patients, symptoms diminish in the presence of strangers, while in school, at work, attending lectures, or at church. The underlying factor seems to be conscious, volitional, or intentional inhibition of symptoms so that they are less obvious to strangers. The inhibition may become partially automatic, a kind of subliminal inhibition that does not require active inhibition. The degree of success varies from patient to patient; some are able to inhibit symptoms for minutes to hours, some for as long as 8 hr. The ability to inhibit symptoms, however, usually decreases with time in these settings. Patients have different methods of controlling their symptoms. Some substitute an inapparent finger movement for a gross arm jerk, for example. Many express their symptoms surreptitiously. Others explosively release their symptoms in the lavatory. All patients can inhibit their symptoms when asked to do so, although the length of time can vary from 10 sec to hours. Volitional or intentional inhibition of symptoms can help differentiate Tourette's disorder from Sydenham's chorea (St. Vitus dance), myoclonus, myoclonic dystonia paroxysmal myoclonic dystonia with vocalizations, and diverse dystonic, atypical, and other movement disorders. This inhibitory ability allows patients to perform most motor functions. For example, parents may be afraid to allow their children to drive because of a vigorous head tic, and patients may be denied a driving license unless a physician attests to their ability to drive safely. In reality, patients inhibit their head-jerking while driving, releasing the symptom when it is safe to do so. One 6 feet, 7 inches tall, patient, with a vigorous arm-flailing tic, frightened fellow workers who feared he would lose control of the very large tools used in his work as a bus mechanic. However, he never had arm-flailing while holding a wrench. This ability is aptly demonstrated in the range of occupations of our patients. Some are surgeons, ophthalmologists, neurosurgeons, actors, singers, musicians, baseball, football, and basketball players who require a high degree of motor control. Rarely do their tics interfere with motor function because they can always be inhibited temporarily. However, a small percentage of patients have tics while writing which interferes with note-taking in school. A rare, potentially dangerous symptom which cannot be completely inhibited is hitting the eye with fingers, fists, or kitchen utensils, ultimately causing eye damage or blinding. Such symptoms constitute a medical emergency and should be treated vigorously with medication.

A more complicated mechanism for inhibiting tics may be involved in the symptom decrease observed during an initial office visit. Vocal symptoms are often very loud in the waiting room, but they decrease markedly and occasionally disappear completely in the doctor's office. Patients relate that they do not want to inhibit their symptoms and are not doing so consciously. In fact, they would prefer that the doctor see them. It is possible that since patients are conditioned to inhibit symptoms with strangers, they generalize to the doctor who, at least initially, is a stranger. This and other observations about the effect of stimuli on symptoms, as well as the choice and change of symptom, suggests that complicated behavioral interactions are involved which should be studied further.

Symptoms also consistently decrease while the patient is repairing an object or making a model, diorama, or is otherwise nonanxiously absorbed in a task, often without conscious inhibition. Even more dramatic, is the complete absence of all symptoms during sexual orgasm, although symptom change is variable during arousal and after orgasm. The results can be summarized as indicating that the stimuli most often associated with decreased tics include, in order of frequency: sleeping, nonanxious absorption in a task, the presence of strangers, repairing an object or making a model or diorama, morning hours, in school, at work, at lectures, church, or temple, and reading (Table 5.22).

Stimuli-Induced Increase of Tics

Our expectations were confirmed that tics would increase with anxiety and arousal from stimuli such as stress, irritation, arguments, agitation, anger, aggression, and taking tests. Even pleasurable anticipation increases tics, such as going to the circus, anticipating a date, during athletic competition, attending a horse race, and other general everyday experiences. Children frequently have increased tics just before they return to school in September, or during the first week of school while they acclimate to the new setting. Stress-induced tics occur only during periods of manifest or subjectively experienced anxiety. The slight, but statistically significant, increase of tics while riding in an automobile and watching television was not predicted. Tics were not significantly different while watching movies, perhaps because strangers are present. On the other hand, walking through a busy supermarket or mall generally increase tics. Also confirmed was the expectation that tics increase with the family, which has been discussed previously.

Thus, tics are more likely to increase with the following stimuli, in order of frequency: anxiety, pleasurable anticipation, with the family, and in the evening and afternoon hours (Table 5.22).

Effect of Diurnal Variation on Symptoms

Our empirical observation was confirmed that the symptoms for many patients are least frequent in the morning, increase in the afternoon, and are most frequent in the evening ($ps = 0.0000$) (Table 5.22). Patients report having their usual symptoms in the morning, or have a burst of symptoms just before leaving the house which then subside. Symptoms increase in the afternoon and especially in the evening. Progressive increase of tics over the day may be due to increased fatigue which lessens the patient's ability and desire to inhibit symptoms. Added to this is the lessened need to inhibit symptoms in the evening because the patient is at home with his family who are aware of the symptoms. Symptoms generally increase even more when alone, but not always, and they occasionally decrease. Some patients inhibit their symptoms equally at home and with strangers, usually because of inordinate sensitivity about their symptoms, not even wanting the family to see the tics. Symptoms usually decrease during the hypnagogic period before falling asleep, but it is not invariant, and the vigor of some symptoms may hinder falling asleep. Although these patterns predominate, many individuals have their own particular diurnal pattern (Caine et al., 1982). Again, the interaction with psychological factors has not been adequately examined and warrants further study.

Seasonal Effect on Tics

Retrospective analysis indicated that symptoms decrease significantly in the summer ($p = 0.0000$), increase slightly in the spring compared to winter or autumn ($p < 0.10$), and that there is no difference between the winter and autumn seasons.

Effect of Other Stimuli on Tics

Seventeen other stimuli added to the MDQ since 1981 were not formally analyzed. Our clinical impression is that their effect on symptoms is inconsistent. Although antianxiety-sedative-hypnotic drugs decrease symptoms with sedation, the effect of most other drugs (alcohol, antidepressants, cocaine, marijuana, lysergic acid and other psychomimetics, stimulants) and that of cigarettes, coffee, tea, cola drinks, sugar, vitamins, minerals, and various foods are variable. Although Gilles de la Tourette and others recommended quiet seclusion, many patients report that tics decrease during and following vigorous exercise. However, they also report that the effect is transitory and no answer to their problem because the tics decrease at the expense of chronic tiredness or exhaustion.

Effect of Attention Deficit Disorder and Hyperactivity on Stimuli-Induced Change in Tics

Our clinical impression for many years is that patients with TS+ADD+H have more severe Tourette's disorder symptoms and have more difficulty controlling or inhibiting their symptoms. We therefore hypothesized that the latter group would have significantly more tics than the TS-alone group on the five factor scores reflecting tic response to stimuli.

Table 4.27 includes items making up factor scores (FS) that significantly differentiated the groups; those not listed are not significant (see Table A.1 for complete list of items). The results confirm our clinical impression that various stimuli provoke more tics in patients with TS+ADD+H than in patients with TS-alone. Mean scores for all items are higher for the TS+ADD+H group than the TS-alone group, and higher on all of the stimuli factor scores, although significantly higher only for the interpersonal stimuli FS, the anxiety-fatigue FS, and the season FS (Table 4.27). Scores for the TS+ADD without hyperactivity tend to fall between scores for the TS+ADD+H and TS-alone groups except for significantly increased tics in lectures, church, or temple for the TS+ADD+H group, compared to the TS+ADD without hyperactivity group and significantly more tics in school or at work for the TS+ADD−H group compared to the TS-alone group.

To further clarify the relationship of stimuli-induced change in tics to diagnostic groupings, we correlated five-factor scores and 20 items with TS+ADD (all ADD with and without hyperactivity) versus TS-alone and hyperactivity FS. Only significant correlations are included in Table 5.23. All correlations are in the positive direction, indicating that patients with TS+ADD and high hyperactivity FS have more tics in response to stimuli than patients with TS-alone and those with low hyperactivity scores. While both patients with TS+ADD and high hyperactivity scores have more tics on most of the stimulus variables, tics increase in hyperactive patients more than in patients with TS+ADD when in the presence of strangers, with nonanxious absorption, and in the evening.

The following general trends can be discerned in the data. Stimuli that are

TABLE 5.23. *Correlation of stimuli-induced change in tics for patients with Tourette's disorder, with attention deficit disorder vs. patients without attention deficit disorder, and scores on the hyperactivity FS*[a]

Stimulus variables	TS+ADD vs. TS-alone	Hyperactivity FS
Interpersonal stimuli FS	0.12[b]	0.18[c]
Lectures, church, temple	0.16[c]	0.19[d]
With strangers	0.02	0.12[b]
School or work	0.20[e]	0.17[c]
Passive stimuli	0.09	0.10
Reading	0.09	0.11
Movies	0.09	0.10
Nonanxious absorption stimuli FS	0.04	0.11
Repairing object	0.07	0.12[b]
Nonanxious absorption	0.01	0.09
Anxiety-fatigue stimuli FS	0.15[c]	0.14[c]
Anxiety	0.07	0.14[b]
Pleasureable anticipation	0.19[d]	0.14[c]
Evening	0.04	0.13[b]
Seasonal stimuli FS	0.16[c]	0.16[c]
Autumn	0.11[b]	0.05
Winter	0.08	0.15[c]

[a]Tourette's disorder without ADD, TS-alone; Tourette's disorder with ADD, TS+ADD; factor score, FS.
[b]$p < 0.05$.
[c]$p < 0.01$.
[d]$p < 0.001$.
[e]$p < 0.0001$.

associated with increased tics in patients with TS+ADD+H and decreased tics in patients with TS-alone include movies, lectures, church or temple, school or work, and winter and spring seasons. Stimuli associated with increased tics in all groups include anxiety, pleasurable anticipation, being with the family, in the afternoon and evening, and during the autumn and winter months. Stimuli associated with decreased tics in all groups include while with strangers, nonanxious absorption, repairing an object, or building a model or diorama, morning hours, and summer months.

The final analysis utilized SRA for each of five dependent stimuli-induced factor scores: interpersonal stimuli FS, passive stimuli FS, nonanxious absorption FS, anxiety-fatigue stimuli FS, and seasonal stimuli FS. Our expectations were that TS+ADD, hyperactivity, and other organic stigma variables would account for more of the variance than other variables (Table 5.24).

Our expectations were largely supported. Hyperactivity was selected by the SRAs for interpersonal stimuli FS and anxiety-fatigue stimuli FS, TS+ADD by the SRA for passive stimuli FS, and neurologic abnormalities (which is

TABLE 5.24. *Stimuli-induced factor scores: Stepwise regression analyses*

Stimulus variables	r	r²	Parameter estimate
Interpersonal stimuli FS			
Hyperactivity FS	0.18[a]	0.03	0.09[b]
Social class	0.12[c]	0.04[d]	0.05[b]
Passive stimuli FS			
Attention deficit disorder	0.09[c]	0.03[c]	0.36[c]
Nonanxious absorption stimuli FS	—	—	—
Anxiety-fatigue stimuli FS			
Hyperactivity	0.14[b]	0.08[a]	0.16[a]
Seasonal stimuli FS			
Neurological abnormality	0.30[d]	0.07	0.20[a]
Age at onset of TS	−0.14[b]	0.10[a]	−0.03[b]

[a] $p < 0.001$.
[b] $p < 0.01$.
[c] $p < 0.05$.
[d] $p < 0.0001$.

correlated with TS+ADD, $r = 0.32$, $p < 0.0001$, and the hyperactivity FS, $r = 0.17$, $p < 0.05$) was selected by the SRA for seasonal stimuli FS. Selection of social class by the SRA for the interpersonal stimuli FS may be related to interpersonal situations being more stressful to lower class patients. The SRA for the nonanxious absorption stimuli FS did not select any variable. The seasonal stimuli FS is a measure of increased tics in winter months compared to decreased tics in summer months, or the converse. The first variable selected by the SRA is neurological abnormality, which correlates ($r = 0.32$, $p < 0.0001$) with TS+ADD and ($r = 0.17$, $p < 0.05$) with the hyperactivity FS. A possible interpretation is that TS+ADD+H patients have less increase of tics in the summer when not in school. However, all results reported for stimuli-induced change of symptoms require replication.

Perhaps, the most useful aspect of this analysis is its implications for patients with TS+ADD. Already burdened by Tourette's disorder and TS+ADD, often with hyperactivity, certain situations apparently further exacerbate symptoms in the TS+ADD group. Whereas the TS-alone group is able to inhibit symptoms somewhat in school, at work, during lectures, or in church or temple, while watching movies or TV, and during the winter and spring seasons, these stimuli exacerbate tics in patients with TS+ADD and hyperactivity. However, because the analysis only considered mean scores and there was a range of reactions, management of these situational factors has to be individualized.

While tics are affected differentially by diverse stimuli, these effects are not specific to Tourette's disorder and occur in many movement disorders. Our conclusion is that stimuli-induced change in tics is an epiphenomenon and not intrinsically associated with the etiology of Tourette's disorder. The mechanism explaining the effect of stimuli on tics, which involve basic brain areas such as the basal ganglia interacting with cortical area of the CNS, is interesting neuropsychologically, neuroanatomically, and neurochemically.

Effect of Ovarian Cycle, Pregnancy, Birth Control Pills, and Intercourse on Tics

Menarche, pre-, during, and postmenstruation, birth control pills, and menopause have inconsistent effects on tics. Pregnancy, however, may be associated with decreased tics. Five of our patients had a moderate to marked decrease in tics during pregnancy. After delivery, tics returned to their former level in four, and decreased 99% in one patient with severe Tourette's disorder. Another unmarried patient had a marked increase of tics during pregnancy, but her status was complicated by an unwanted pregnancy. Fernando (1967) reported increased tics in the first trimester, disappearance of all tics after 5 months of pregnancy in one patient, and no change in two pregnant women; and Creak and Guttman (1935) reported decreased tics in an unmarried woman in the second half of pregnancy. Tics are variably affected prior to and subsequent to orgasm but always disappear during orgasm. On the basis of these observations, a more consistent study of possible neuroendocrine mechanisms during pregnancy is warranted.

NATURAL COURSE AND PROGNOSIS

Unfortunately, very little information is available about the natural course or prognosis for Tourette's disorder. Follow-up studies of adequate duration are difficult to conduct and are not supported by granting agencies. However, some facts are well established, and there is general consensus among clinicians about the natural course of Tourette's disorder for most patients. Other aspects of the natural course are unknown and require future study.

Natural Course of Tic and Tourette Disorders

It is now well established that the natural course for Tourette's disorder is not ominous, as once believed, and does not result in intellectual deterioration, psychosis, and chronic hospitalization (Fernando, 1967; Shapiro et al., 1978), and is much better than previously thought (Fernando, 1967; Lucas, 1967; Shapiro et al., 1978). Tourette's disorder is not associated with any physical or psychological illness, character trait, or type of personality. The prevalence of other disorders in patients with Tourette's disorder is no different from expectations in individuals without Tourette's disorder. The only possible association, not yet fully established, and possibly related to ascertainment problems, is a greater frequency of ADD among Tourette's disorder patients. The main effect of having Tourette's disorder, in our opinion, is on psychosocial functioning, which is very much related to the combined effects of severity interacting with the intellectual and ego resources of the individual. The symptoms may cause some patients to withdraw, and may shape personality development and traits in others. Ominous consequences of having Tourette's disorder, although infrequent, include blindness from hitting the eye from vigorous muscular tics, temporomandibular and orthopedic complications, excoriation and laceration of the oral cavity from oral-biting tics, and so on. The most unfortunate consequence, fortunately infrequent, are feelings of hopelessness, depression, and suicidal rumination which may eventually lead to suicide. The symptoms themselves usually do not interfere directly with physical activity and with most academic, vocational, or recreational activities. For example, patients known to us include a neurosurgeon, gastrointestinal surgeon, two ophthalmologists, three internists, five psychiatrists, two medical students, four psychologists, two social workers, two journalists, two photographers, five lawyers, five musicians, two reporters, a comedian, the president of a country, teachers, nurses, police officers, mechanics, businessmen, and so on.

Studies of prognosis are infrequent and difficult to conduct, and the conclusions are severely limited by diverse methodological shortcomings (Table 5.18). All of the cited are totally patient-oriented, thus excluding unidentified individuals who may have milder symptoms and, hence, possibly a better prognosis. This possibility is suggested by the better over-all course in the four studies of tics compared to the three studies of Tourette's disorder. For the tic studies, the age at follow-up is either not specified or the range is extensive, varying from 5 to 85 years of age, and the duration of follow-up is brief or includes a wide range varying from 1 to 28 years. Moreover, the criteria for complete remission of tics is not specified (Bonheim, 1930; Corbett et al., 1969; Lucas, 1967). The length of the remission varies from more than 1 year in two studies (Zausmer, 1954; Torup, 1962), to 5 years in one study of Tourette's disorder (Jenkins et al., 1976), and to 8 to 18 years in our study of Tourette's disorder. Criteria for and the reliability of measures for the evaluation of improvement were not specified or were inadequate in all of the studies except for one study of Tourette's disorder (Shapiro et al., 1978). Finally, none of the studies assessed the intraclass reliability for measurement of improvement.

Considerable data exist indicating the importance of these variables for the study of the natural course of tics and Tourette's disorder. As previously noted, 27.1% of our patients had one or more periods of spontaneous remission lasting from less than 1 month to 19 years. It would be expected, therefore, that approximately 27% of Tourette's disorder patients can have a spontaneous remission lasting possibly as long as 7 years by chance if follow-up is limited to 7 years (Table 5.17). Because our data indicate that spontaneous remissions lasting more than 7 years are permanent (within the limits of our follow-up), our results are confined to patients with a remission lasting more than 7 years. It should be remembered, however, that Tourette's disorder symptoms may return even after prolonged periods of remission, as demonstrated by several patients whose symptoms disappeared in adolescence and returned in older age (Klawans and Barr, 1985). Other difficulties inherent in evaluating clinical course at any one time are due to spontaneous changes that occur in veritably all patients: 97% of patients have a spontaneous variation in severity over time, 96% have changes in the type of symptom over time (Table 5.17), approximately one-third have spontaneous remission of previous coprolalia, and 9 to 58% of symptoms that were present in the past and were no longer present when evaluated by us. (Tables 5.8–5.13). Another indication that spontaneous changes and possibly placebo effects strongly contribute to the difficulties of evaluating improvement is based on the results of treatment of 20 patients with placebo for 6 weeks in a double-blind crossover study of pimozide (Shapiro et al., 1984; see Chapter 11 for details). Improvement was rated blindly by patients, judges, and the clinician on seven dependent variables. The percent of improved patients on placebo averaged 36% for all seven variables, with a range of 15 to 55% for individual variables. The overall data suggest that about 35% of patients would be expected to improve at any one point in time. Thus, meaningful improvement would probably have to exceed 35%.

Within the methodological limitations of the seven studies summarized in Table 5.18, the following conclusions can be considered. For patients with tics, 24 to 61% have complete remissions, 26 to 68% improve, and from 3 to 24% have no change or a worsening of tics. Complete remission in patients with Tourette's disorder is approximately 8%, much lower than for tics. Only one study reported improvement in 88% of Tourette's disorder patients, higher than for patients with tics, 6% having no change or worsening of symptoms similar to the range for tics (Lucas, 1967).

Another generalization about the natural course of Tourette's disorder is based entirely on our clinical experience over the past 22 years. Approximately 8% of Tourette's disorder patients are likely to have a complete and permanent remission, usually during puberty and occasionally during adolescence. Remissions in adulthood have not occurred in any of our patients and are probably highly unlikely. Of the remainder, the general course during latency, up to approximately age 13, and during adolescence is the same in approximately 65% of patients. Severity decreases, sometimes markedly, during adolescence in approximately 35% of patients. In adulthood, after 18 or 21 years of age, the severity, waxing, waning, and fluctuation of symptoms decrease. Other clinicians also report decreased tics at puberty, (Bonheim, 1930; Zausmer, 1954; Torup, 1962), decreased symptoms of Tourette's disorder in late adolescence (Lucas, 1967) or in late adolescence or early adulthood (Bockner, 1959; Heuscher, 1953; Erenberg et al., 1986). Occasional exacerbations occur, usually without significant external stimuli, but tend to be brief. Despite these generalizations, the natural course is highly variable. Occasional patients, with a history of very mild symptoms, develop severe symptoms in adulthood, usually in the twenties, occasionally in the early thirties. These clinical statements about the clinical course of Tourette's disorder were proposed and heuristically accepted by a consensus panel of experienced clinicians (Consensus Panel of the TSA, 1985).

Prognosis for Individuals with Tourette's Disorder

Despite the general trends, it is not possible to predict the clinical course in individual patients. If controlled studies confirm that clinical course cannot be predicted, it would substantiate our belief that changes in tic and Tourette's disorders are caused primarily by internal, not readily observable, metabolic or anatomic changes in the central nervous system.

DIFFERENCES BETWEEN QUESTIONNAIRE SURVEY AND CLINICAL SAMPLES

We previously discussed some of the difficulties associated with questionnaires responses. All of our patients complete a comprehensive questionnaire before their initial evaluation, which is then carefully reviewed by experienced clinicians. It was disappointing to find that the completed questionnaires were grossly inadequate, and that they could only serve as a screening instrument. Every question had to be reviewed and corrected. Informants would both underestimate and overestimate the age at onset for the first symptom and the age at which other symptoms developed or disappeared. Patients tended to break down a single symptom into many different symptoms. For example, a facial grimace was recorded as a single symptom, but also as a separate tic of the eyes, brows, forehead, mouth, cheeks, and head; a complex limb movement was often recorded as separate tics of the shoulder, upper or lower limb, hands or feet, and fingers or toes. Symptoms categorized by us as an individual, single sound, or a complex tic are invariably recorded by patients as multiple tics rather than as a discrete tic. Mannerisms, habits, obscenities, obsessions, compulsions, stereotypic movements, and behavioral symptoms frequently are misinterpreted as tics. Confusion by informants about the criteria and how to describe tics is understandable. In addition, new patients in their zeal to be complete tend to be overinclusive. Another factor contributing to the problem of using questionnaire survey data is that many individuals who volunteer to complete questionnaires tend to have a more severe form of Tourette's disorder. These problems led to our skepticism about the reliability and validity of data derived from questionnaires. We concluded that questionnaires have a useful function as a screening device but that reliable data about Tourette's disorder requires careful scrutiny of data and verification by experienced clinicians.

These observations have implications as well for questionnaire surveys reported in the literature. In the past, because only small samples were available for study, investigators resorted to the use of questionnaire surveys (Shapiro et al., 1978; Jagger et al., 1982; Stefl, 1983, 1984; Erenberg et al., 1986). Questionnaire samples solicited through the TSA, advertisements, or mail may be biased in many other ways. Respondents may include disproportionate numbers of severely afflicted Tourette's disorder patients, and patients with concomitant diagnoses such as ADD, stereotypic movement disorder, mental retardation, pervasive developmental or autistic disorder, schizophrenic, or other psychotic disorders and diverse psychopathology. Moreover, the reliability of the diagnosis of Tourette's disorder cannot be evaluated. For example, of 1,373 patients evaluated by us for a tic or Tourette's disorder, 87 (6.3%) had another type of movement disorder, and 49 (3.9%) had no movement disorder at all (Table 2.1). For 237 respondents to our questionnaire survey, 31 (13%) did not fulfill the criteria for Tourette's disorder. It is impossible to know how many others would or would not fulfill the criteria for Tourette's disorder if they had been individually evaluated.

These problems prompted us to compare the data from our questionnaire survey sample to the data from a clinically evaluated sample. To increase our sample size in our early studies, notices requesting completion of our Tourette's disorder questionnaire were periodically published in the TSA Newsletter. Between 1972 and 1979, 237 patients responded. Of these, 206 (86.9%) fulfilled criteria for the diagnosis of Tourette's disorder. The diagnosis was arrived at by evaluation of the questionnaires by two experienced clinicians (A.K.S. and E.S.). The diagnosis was made independently and differences of opinion were resolved by discussion. The comparison group included 500 patients who were clinically diagnosed as having Tourette's disorder during the same period of time. The two samples were compared utilizing the 54 variables in the list of variables (Table A.1), using 2-tailed t-tests for continuous variables and χ^2 for dichotomous variables. Only significant variables are listed in Table 5.25; variables not cited are not significant. This analysis is largely retrospective except for the expectation that questionnaire patients would have more symptoms, more severe Tourette's disorder, more behavioral deviations, and more organic CNS stigmata.

Confirmed predictions were that patients in the questionnaire sample, compared to those in the clinically evaluated sample, report more symptoms (number of cumulative tics, $p < 0.001$; number of current tics, $p < 0.01$), have more severe Tourette's disorder, $p < 0.0001$; and higher previous diagnosis-consultation FS, $p < 0.001$). The expectations that questionnaire patients would have more behavioral symptoms was not confirmed except for less coordination abilities FS ($p < 0.01$) and intellectual-psychosocial assets FS ($p < 0.05$); more symptoms in seven of 11 symptom types ($p < 0.05$–0.001);

TABLE 5.25. *Comparison of variables between questionnaire sample and clinical sample (1972–1979)*[a]

Variables	Questionnaire sample $\overline{X}$ or %	Clinical sample $\overline{X}$ or %	t or χ^2 $p =$
Demography			
Sex (males)	69.6%	76.6%	0.05
Social class	3.1	2.8	0.001
Genetic			
Family history of TS	6.0%	6.0%	NS
Family history of tics	29.5%	44.7%	0.001
Family history of TS or tics	33.0%	48.3%	0.001
Family history other movement disorders	3.5%	9.3%	0.01
Medical			
Parents' age at birth FS	28.0	29.2	0.01
Neurological			
Neurological abnormality rating	1.2	1.3	0.05
Behavior			
Coordination abilities FS	2.0	2.3	0.01
Intellectual-psychosical assets FS	2.2	2.4	0.05
Compulsive personality FS	0.7	1.2	0.01
Illness variables			
Previous diagnosis-consultation FS	3.7	3.3	0.001
Symptoms			
Upper limb	84.1%	71.4%	0.0004
Lower limb	59.9%	43.6%	0.0001
Torso	55.1%	48.4%	0.0004
Complex motor	78.7%	69.6%	0.0135
Coprolalia	55.1%	32.4%	0.0001
Mental coprolalia	6.3%	2.8%	0.0280
All coprophilia	60.4%	37.0%	0.0001
Echophilia	48.3%	33.8%	0.0001
Total number	21.0	16.4	0.0001
Current symptoms			
TS severity	3.4	2.7	0.0001
Total current symptoms	8.8	7.4	0.0024
Clinical course			
Spontaneous variation of severity	99.4%	97.4%	0.0398
Spontaneous change of symptoms	99.4%	95.6%	0.0008
Periods of remission	10.7%	23.3%	0.0001
Length of remission	0.3	0.6	0.0005
Years from onset of TS to coprolalia	5.0	5.5	NS

[a]Questionaire sample, $N = 206$; clinical sample, $N = 500$.

other retrospective significant differences included shorter remission of symptoms FS ($p < 0.01$); and less frequent history of tics in the family ($p < 0.05$), etc. The expectation of more organic CNS stigmata was not confirmed.

A possible explanation for the less frequent history of tics in family members is that relatives with mild tics may not be identified as easily as relatives with more severe forms of a tic disorder such as Tourette's disorder unless inquiry is made by the clinician. However, both samples reported that 6% of families had one or more family members with a history of Tourette's disorder, suggesting that questionnaire responses reliably report a history of Tourette's disorder in the family. The significantly lower social class for the questionnaire sample suggests, as discussed previously, that patients seen in private practice are from somewhat higher social classes. The absence of significant differences for other variables in the retrospective analysis suggests that questionnaire responses for these variables are reliably reported. These include birth history, sibling status, maturational milestones, and patient medical history.

The overall conclusion is that responses of volunteers to questionnaires have questionable reliability and validity. They may be useful for the assessment of socioeconomic and vocational problems, and to determine the need for treatment resources for a subset, but not for all Tourette's disorder patients.

6

Psychology, Psychopathology, and Neuropsychology

In the first section of this chapter we discuss the controversy about the relationship of psychopathology to Tourette's disorder. The history and data in the literature about the role of psychological factors in the genesis of Tourette's disorder and the psychopathological consequences of having Tourette's disorder are critically examined. Clinical opinions and studies in the literature are contrasted with the data from our studies. Our hypotheses are that CNS organic factors, behavioral problems, psychopathology, obsessive-compulsive symptoms, obsessive compulsive disorder, and attention deficit disorder (ADD) are not intrinsic to Tourette's disorder, that psychopathology is associated with a secondary diagnosis of ADD, and that psychopathology in Tourette's disorder patients without ADD is not more frequent than expected in the population.

In the second section, we review and critically evaluate psychological and neuropsychological studies and potential organic CNS factors that may be associated with Tourette's disorder, contrast these results with the results of our studies, and discuss their possible relationship to the etiology of Tourette's disorder.

PSYCHOPATHOLOGY

History of Psychopathology

As described in Chapter 1, Tourette's disorder was considered an organic, often hereditary, illness for many years after it was first described by Tourette in 1885 (Gilles de la Tourette, 1885). Tourette's early attitude about the mental state of the patient was initially optimistic, referring to it as excellent in all respects. He observed that the major disadvantage of the illness for the patient was related to the severity of the symptoms. In contrast, Guinon (1886) writing in the same period felt that these Tourette disorder patients almost always exhibited a state of mental instability characterized by countless phobias, arithromania, and agoraphobia. In 1899, Tourette, referring extensively to Guinon, revised his earlier thinking by focusing on the mental instability of patients and the nervous and mental disorders in the family background. However, the etiology according to nineteenth century neurologists was "neuropathic" antecedents, that is, mental instability such as alcoholism in another family member (Trousseau, 1873; Beard, 1886).

Psychological causation became increasingly popular after 1900. Psychoanalysts believed that tics were symbolic expressions of an underlying intrapsychic conflict, and Tourette's disorder was variously characterized as a neurosis resembling hysteria (Freud, 1966), displaced unconscious muscular eroticism towards the father (Sadger, 1914), a defense against autopleasurable thumb-sucking (Oberndorf, 1916), narcissistic onanism (Ferenczi, 1921), anal sadism (Abraham, 1927), inhibited aggression (Mahler et al., 1945), obsessive-compulsive neurosis or psychosis and other unconscious psychological conflicts (Shapiro et al., 1978). Others described Tourette's disorder patients as having schizophrenia, underlying psychosis, obsessive-compulsive neurosis or character traits, hysteria, inhibition of hostility, and poor prognoses both intellectually and psychologically (Ascher, 1948; Mesnikoff, 1959; Schneck, 1960; Dunlap, 1960; Bruch and Thum, 1968; Lindner and Stevens, 1967; Morphew and Sim, 1969). This period was one in which psychogenesis for symptoms of undetermined etiology was emphasized and overinterpreted (Shapiro 1959; 1960; 1970a,b; Shapiro et al., 1978; Shapiro and Shapiro, 1985a). Clinicians and theoreticians hypothesized etiology from interpretation of clinical phenomenology for many disorders including Tourette's disorder (Eisenberg et al., 1959). Tourette's disorder was especially subject to these tendencies because of its fluctuating clinical course, occasional remissions, and because most reports in the literature were limited to single case histories. Such clinical conditions are prone to the *post hoc, ergo propter hoc* logical fallacy, after the fact, therefore because of the fact. The predominant psychodynamic formulation from about 1945 to 1975 interpreted the tics and other symptoms as symbolic expressions of a massive unconscious conflict about the expression of hostility and aggression, resulting in reaction formation, obsessions, compulsions, and symptom substitution, and ultimately revealed an underlying psychotic process. Such concepts may have contributed to the erroneous and extensive belief that Tourette patients ultimately become psychotic and deteriorate intellectually.

In the 1960s, following the successful use of haloperidol to treat the symptoms of Tourette's disorder, data began to accumulate about pathophysiological, neurological, and genetic factors in patients with Tourette's disorder (Shapiro et al., 1978). The emphasis on underlying psychological mechanisms as etiologic to the disorder became less prominent, and many authors concluded that the etiology was a neurophysiological disorder of the central nervous system (CNS), probably of the basal ganglia (Mahler et al., 1945;

Mazur, 1953a,b; Balthazar, 1956; Rapoport, 1959; Bockner, 1959; Milman, 1960; Baker, 1962; Wechsler, 1952; MacDonald, 1963; Faux, 1966; Corbin, 1970; Snyder et al., 1970; Woodrow, 1974; and others) (see also Table 4.24).

It was apparent to us during the clinical evaluation and treatment of patients that psychological conflicts, defenses, ego status, and social functioning, family background, and dynamics were inadequate to explain the bizarre symptomatology. During this historic period of overemphasizing and overinterpreting a psychogenic origin for symptoms of undetermined etiology, there was a tendency to interpret the symptoms and then to infer etiology from the interpretation. Once these concepts entered the literature, busy clinicians accepted and imposed these formulations on patients (Shapiro, 1970a,b). With increased personal and clinical contact with Tourette's disorder patients, clinicians increasingly concluded, as we did, that the syndrome could not be attributed to a psychological etiology (Abuzzahab and Anderson, 1973; Challas et al., 1967; Eisenberg et al., 1959; Fernando, 1967; Feild et al., 1966; Kelman, 1965; Lucas et al., 1967; Mahler and Rangell, 1943; Moldofsky et al., 1971, 1974).

In the late 1970s, however, there was a resurgence of interest in the relationship of psychopathology to Tourette's disorder and recent clinical reports have suggested that a broad range of psychological symptoms are intrinsic to the disorder (Cohen et al., 1978, 1980, 1982, 1983; Comings and Comings, 1984). These authors conceive of Tourette's disorder as a neuropsychiatric disorder consisting of tic, behavioral, and psychological symptoms. Hyperkinesis and attentional difficulties are thought to precede the onset of tics, and the associated psychological symptomatology includes severe compulsions, irritability, intolerance of frustration, antagonistic behavior, strong sexual and aggressive urges, phobias, anxiety, and minor and major depression. They hypothesize that a disturbance in behavior is intrinsic to Tourette's disorder and suggest that present diagnostic criteria do not adequately portray the behavioral problems of Tourette's disorder patients, and that behavioral difficulties are more of a problem than the tics themselves. However, these retrospective clinical impressions have not been evaluated in a controlled or prospective study. Without an adequate control group it is impossible to determine if Tourette's disorder patients would differ on measures of psychopathology when compared with a non-Tourette's-disorder patient sample. Moreover, Tourette's disorder patients who refer themselves for clinical treatment and study may not constitute a random sample and may be more severely disturbed in general. We return to this issue later in this chapter.

Family Psychopathology

The major limitation of studies in the literature citing family psychopathology in patients with Tourette's disorder is that all are based on uncontrolled, retrospective clinical impressions (Table 6.1). Moreover, the diversity of the described psychopathology does not permit generalizations. Because at the time of our early studies there were numerous references to excessive mental illness and paranoid, dominant, and borderline characteristics in the family, we described and tabulated them in our previous book (Shapiro et al., 1978, Table 4.8, p. 94). Based on the intensive clinical evaluation of our first thirty consecutive patients we concluded that psychopathology in the family of Tourette's disorder patients was neither more specific nor more frequent than would be expected in the population (Shapiro et al., 1978). The current evidence fails to support the concept of family psychopathology in Tourette's disorder.

The evidence from our early studies supported a CNS etiology for Tourette's disorder based on the much higher than expected frequency of neurological and EEG abnormalities, minimal brain dysfunction, and left-handedness or ambidexterity, higher male to female ratio of 3 to 1, absence of specific or excessive psychopathology in families or patients, absence of specific psychological stimuli or trauma preceding the onset of Tourette's disorder, evidence of genetic transmission of Tourette's disorder, absence of response to psychological treatment, response to low dosages of haloperidol without symptom substitution, and emerging data about the relationship of the basal ganglia to parkinsonism, L-DOPA, dopamine, neuroleptics, tardive dyskinesia, and other movement disorders (Shapiro and Shapiro, 1968; Shapiro et al., 1972a,b; 1973a,d; 1978 Wayne et al., 1972; Sweet et al., 1973).

Patient Psychopathology

Studies of psychopathology are described chronologically and are separated into those primarily reporting general psychopathology, the relationship of psychopathology to ADD and to obsessive compulsive disorder.

General Psychopathology

Recent History of Psychopathology in Tourette's Disorder

In the introduction to this chapter we described our early clinical impression that psychopathology was not etiologic or intrinsic to Tourette's disorder and our hypothesis that Tourette's disorder is a CNS disorder. In 1972 we began to systematically study these issues (Shapiro et al., 1972a,b, 1973c, 1978; Shapiro et al., 1974). Evaluation of psychopathology and brain dysfunction was limited primarily to comprehensive psychometric and projective test procedures that were extensively used at the time and were part of our clinical intake procedure. Although we were aware at the same time that the reliability of these psychological tests had not been demonstrated, none of the alter-

TABLE 6.1. *Studies citing family psychopathology in Tourette's disorder*

Study	Diagnosis	Total patients	Family psychopathology
Bonheim (1930)	Tics CMT	47	46.8% Nervousness, mother > father, 4.3% psychosis, 2.1% schizophrenia
Zausmer (1954)	Tics	96	Neurosis in 32.3% of parents, 50% of families, anxiety in 52% of parents, 58% of families, psychopathic personality in 2% of parents, 13% of families, 12% psychosis, and 8% mental deficiency in families
Corbett et al. (1969)	Tics	179	Psychiatric treatment of a parent in 31% of tiquers, 19% in medical clinic, 6% dental clinic
Challas et al. (1967)	TS	11	Parental dominance 9%
Lucas et al. (1967)	TS	15	Three groups: excessive aggression, inhibited aggression, no disturbance
Morphew and Sim (1969)[a]	TS	43	Suicide 3, schizophrenia 1, various psychopathology in 77% of fathers and 63% of mothers
Abuzzahab and Anderson (1974)[a]	TS CMT	430	Neuroticism in 57%, but common problems not significantly associated with TS
Shapiro et al. (1978)	TS	114	History of mental illness 22% in primary family; moderate or marked tendencies in parents of paranoia 24%, dominance in 40%, borderline in 8%; but family psychopathology not significantly associated with TS
Nomura and Segawa (1979)	TS	37	No specific psychiatric disorder
Nee et al. (1980)	TS	50	Medical care for emotional problems in 52%, 52% alcoholism
Stefl (1983, 1984)[b]	TS	431	Alcohol problems 8%, drug problems 3%, marital problems 21%, obsessive compulsive behavior 33%, greater in family with a history of TS
Golden and Hood (1982)	TS	80	No significant family history of psychopathology
Min (1983)	TS CMT	24	No psychosis, psychiatric problems rare
Pauls et al. (1984)	TS CMT	32	25% of 122 first degree relatives had OCD

[a]Review of the literature.
[b]Questionnaire survey.

natives, including newly introduced neuropsychological tests, had yet demonstrated evidence of reliability and validity.

Our initial clinical study evaluated several hypotheses in the literature about the relationship of specific psychopathology to Tourette's disorder (Shapiro et al., 1972a). The subjects were 34 patients with Tourette's disorder who were evaluated psychiatrically (A.K.S.) and psychologically with a test battery consisting of the Wechsler Adult Intelligence Scale (WAIS) or the Wechsler Intelligence Scale for Children (WISC), Rorschach Test (RT), and Bender-Gestalt Test (BGT). In addition, Minnesota Multiphasic Personality Inventory (MMPI) scores were completed by 17 adult patients with Tourette's disorder. Two experienced psychologists independently rated the protocols for schizophrenia, underlying psychosis, obsessive-compulsiveness, inhibition of hostility, hysteria, somatization, and general adjustment. The overall results found few patients free of problems, but specific psychopathologic factors did not characterize patients with Tourette's disorder, and there was no support for the concept that psychopathology was related to the etiology of, or was a concomitant or characteristic of patients with Tourette's disorder. The study cited the difficulty of assessing how much of the psychopathology was caused by the illness and subtle organic CNS pathology.

A second measure of psychopathology used was the MMPI. The MMPI scores of Tourette's disorder patients were compared with scores for 305 psychiatric outpatients who had applied for outpatient psychiatric treatment at the Payne-Whitney Clinic, New York. Only the depression scale was in the pathological over-70 range for Tourette's patients compared to four scales in the over-70 range for the outpatients. The profiles indicated that patients with Tourette's disorder were less impaired than the average psychiatric outpatient and that the elevated depression scale may reflect the effect on patients of enduring a chronic illness. A serious shortcoming of this study, the absence of an independently and blindly assessed control group of patients, was corrected in a subsequent predictive controlled study.

The samples comprised 47 patients with Tourette's disorder and 48 randomly selected Payne-Whitney Clinic psychiatric outpatients who were matched for age, sex, and IQ. Psychological test measures were the WAIS or WISC, RT, and BGT. All protocols were blindly and independently rated by two experienced psychologists using a four-point rating scale (0: none, 1: mild, 2: moderate, 3: marked or severe) for the presence or absence of schizophrenia, other psychosis, underlying psychosis, obsessive-compulsive neurosis or traits, inhibition of hostility, hysteria, and general adjustment. Interpretation of protocols was based on extensively used criteria at the time (Klopfer and Kelly, 1946; Rapaport, 1946; Beck, 1949; Schafer, 1953; Goldfried et al., 1971). The results, comprehensively described previously (Shapiro et al., 1978), are summarized in Table 6.2.

Our expectations were confirmed that previously hypothesized psychopathology presumably associated with Tourette's disorder, such as schizophrenia,

TABLE 6.2. *Comparison of psychopathology between patients with Tourette's disorder and psychiatric outpatients blindly rated by two senior psychologists from projective psychological test protocols[a,b]*

Psychopathology	TS vs. control sample		Rater agreement %
	Psychologist A χ^2(df-3)	Psychologist B χ^2(df-3)	
Schizophrenia	3.1	0.9	87.4
Other psychosis	0.0	0.0	100.0
Underlying psychosis	4.4	0.9	11.5
Obsessive-compulsive	2.0	0.8	46.3
Inhibited hostility[c]	3.2	9.7[c]	30.5
Hysteria	3.1	0.8	44.2
General and maladjustment	0.8	1.3	41.0

[a] Patients with Tourette's disorder, $N = 47$; psychiatric outpatients, $N = 48$.
[b] Psychopathology ratings: 0, none; 1, mild; 2, moderate; 3, marked; or severe.
[c] $p = 0.02$, inhibition of hostility rated significantly higher for controls than TS subjects by psychologist B.

overt and underlying psychosis, obsessive-compulsive traits, inhibition of hostility, hysteria, and general maladjustment was not significantly greater in the Tourette's disorder than in the control group, and therefore not specifically associated with Tourette's disorder. All comparisons between the two samples were not significantly different except for lower ratings by one psychologist of inhibited hostility ($p = 0.02$) for the Tourette's sample. The results indicated that patients with Tourette's disorder did not differ from a nonselected group of psychiatric outpatients. We would not expect significant differences between the Tourette's disorder sample and a nonselected group of not too ill psychiatric outpatients with a low frequency of schizophrenia, other and underlying psychosis, obsessive compulsiveness, and hysteria. While inhibited hostility, however, was lower for the Tourette's disorder group, general maladjustment was similar for both the Tourette's disorder and psychiatric group. The latter finding was unexpected since our clinical impression was that patients with Tourette's disorder are better adjusted than psychiatric patients. Differences between the groups might have been obscured by the low agreement among raters (Table 6.2).

A more specific test of our expectation that Tourette's disorder patients were better adjusted than psychiatric patients was obtained with the MMPI. We compared the T scores for 65 Tourette's disorder subjects with the T scores of three outpatient samples who participated in other studies (256 anxious outpatients, 244 neurotic depressed outpatients, and 301 outpatients with mixed diagnoses) (Figure 6.1).

Scores for Tourette's disorder patients were significantly lower (most p values < 0.001) than for the three psychiatric outpatient samples on measures

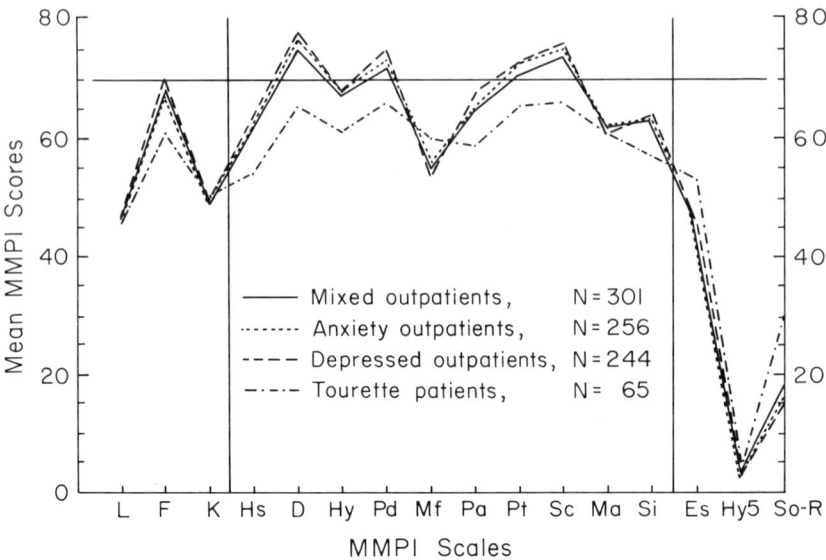

Fig. 6.1. T scores for Tourette's disorder patients compared with T scores for three outpatient samples.

of hysteria, depression, hypochondriasis, paranoia, psychasthenia, schizophrenia, social introversion, hypomania, impulsivity, anxiety, repression, dominance, and dependency, and the score for ego strength was significantly higher for the Tourette's disorder sample compared to the three other samples ($p < 0.001$) (Shapiro et al., 1978; Shapiro and Shapiro 1980b). This result suggests that Tourette's disorder patients have less psychopathology than a broad group of psychiatric outpatients and are not characterized by any specific psychopathology. Moreover, mean scores for all of the psychopathology variables on the MMPI were within the normal range, below a T score of 70 for Tourette's disorder patients.

These results provided substantial confirmation of the hypothesis that common psychopathological factors do not characterize patients with Tourette's disorder, and support for our clinical impressions that psychological factors were unrelated to the etiology of Tourette's disorder, were not intrinsic to the disorder, and that Tourette's disorder patients were less impaired than psychiatric patients.

Several shortcomings of this study should be noted. There was wide divergence between the ratings of the two psychologists on most of the projective test measures of psychopathology indicating that the ratings or tests were insensitive and unreliable measures of psychopathology. Although the MMPI results indicated that all measures of psychopathology are significantly less for Tourette's disorder patients than for the three psychiatric outpatients samples, the study provided no information about whether Tourette's disorder patients have more specific or general psychopathology than a matched, randomly selected, nonclinical sample. Nor did the study control for the presence or absence of ADD in the Tourette's disorder sample, a major problem in all studies, that is discussed later in this chapter.

It was our impression that following publication of these studies and after considerable initial resistance, an organic etiology for Tourette's disorder, without associated psychopathology, was accepted by most clinicians and investigators. However, there has been a recent resurgence of a belief that psychopathology is etiologically related to or is an inevitable consequence of Tourette's disorder.

Reports and Studies Citing Psychopathology

Most of the reports citing psychopathology up to 1986 are based on clinical impression, retrospective tabulation of patients and uncritical citation of these references in other papers (Table 6.3). Psychopathology, exclusive of obsessive compulsive disorder (OCD) or obsessive-compulsive symptoms (OCS), is mentioned in 20 uncontrolled reports (Table 6.3, studies 1–19,21) and four controlled studies (Table 6.3, studies 22,23,25,26).

Uncontrolled reports of psychopathology

The clinical impression that psychopathology is associated with Tourette's disorder has been most frequently articulated by Cohen, Leckman, and the group at the Yale Child Study Center. Although formal tabulation of results and controlled studies have not been done, the group has extensive clinical experience with Tourette's disorder. Tourette's disorder is conceived of as a neuropsychiatric disorder consisting of tics, and a broad range of behavioral and psychological symptoms which are thought to be intrinsic to Tourette's. Hyperkinesis and attentional difficulties are thought to precede the onset of tics and the disorder is associated with severe compulsions, obsessional thoughts, irritability, impulsivity, frustration intolerance, hyperactivity, antagonistic behavior, strong sexual and aggressive urges, phobias, anxiety, minor and major depression and behavior, and conduct and learning problems. The authors hypothesize that these problems are intrinsic to Tourette's disorder and suggest that present diagnostic criteria do not adequately portray the behavioral problems in Tourette's disorder (Cohen et al., 1978, 1980–1983; Leckman and Cohen, 1983; Leckman et al., 1985). Although we respect the clinical impressions of the authors, after carefully reviewing the symptoms described in the published case histories, our impression is that most of the patients studied by the authors have a secondary diagnosis of ADD, hyperactivity, and other CNS disorders which are not intrinsically associated with Tourette's disorder. The degree of reported psychopathology may be a

TABLE 6.3. *Clinical reports and studies citing psychopathology and obsessive-compulsive symptoms in Tourette's disorder*

Study	Sample	Psychopathology	OCS[a]
Uncontrolled clinical reports			
1. Feild et al. (1966)	15	Mental deterioration, schizophrenia or other serious personality disorders in 40%	—
2. Challas et al. (1967)	11	All anxious, hostile, inhibited; one parent punitive, the other indulgent; 36% first child	—
3. Shapiro et al. (1972a, 1973, 1974, 1978)	30–114	Psychopathology within expectations in the population except for ADD	OCS within expectations in the population
4. Moldofsky et al. (1974)	14	Hyperkinesis 67%, enuresis 33%, sleep disturbance 80%, stuttering 33%[b]	—
5. Golden (1977a,b, 1978a,b, 1979, 1982, 1984)	15	General good level of adjustment, no tic personality or common psychopathology, general adjustment similar to psychiatric outpatients possibly from illness or CNS abnormalities, many hyperactive	Compulsive touching objects, self or others[c] and sniffing, smelling, biting chewing[c]
6. Yaryura-Tobias et al. (1977)	55	Aggressive behavior 62%, self-mutilation 18%[b,c]	Urge to tic[c], OCS (not defined) alone 29% and with urge to tic 53%[c]
7. Cohen et al. (1978, 1980, 1982, 1983)	—	ADD 50–60%, serious school performance difficulties 30–40%, behavioral difficulties (irritability, frustration intolerance, attentional problems) are prodromal to onset of TS. Other problems include antagonistic behavior, strong sexual and aggressive urges, phobias, anxiety, depression and severe compulsions[b]	Severe compulsions[c], OCS 40%[c], attentional and compulsive disorders are part of underlying genetic diathesis for TS
8. Nomura and Segawa (1979)	97	No specific psychopathology, neurotic 4%	—
9. Debray-Ritzen and Dubois (1980)	93	ADD 18%, language disability 17%, enuresis 14%, encopresis 3%, sleeping difficulty 19%, behavior problem 0.8%, neurotic traits 20%, minor phobias 1%, no behavior problems 26%	—

Study	N		
10. Nee et al. (1980, 1982)	5	Impulsive antisocial behavior 26%, learning disabilities 40%, sleep disturbance 44%, self-destructive behavior 48%[c], inappropriate sexual activity[b,c]	OCS behavior (not defined) 68%[c], 90% over 21 years, most often touching[c]
11. Gonce et al. (1982)	80	No specific psychopathology, neurotic 4%	—
12. Lieh-Mak et al. (1982)	15	Poor social adjustment associated with EEG abnormality and low IQ scores[b]	—
13. Montgomery et al. (1982)	15	No psychiatric illness 26.7%, mentally defective 6.7%	—
14. Min (1983)	24	Abnormal development 50%, hyperactivity 29%, learning difficulties 13%, enuresis 8%, encoporesis 4%, stuttering 4%, impulsive, temper and competitive 54%, polite and shy personality 29%[b]	OC illness (not defined) 67% (27% mild, 40% moderate or severe) Obsessive and meticulous 17%, OCP obsessive trait 13%, OCD obsessive compulsive disorder (not defined) 4%.
15. Han-bai and Han-quin (1983)	19	No psychopathology 84%, mental retardation 5%	Obsessions (not defined) 11%
16. Butler (1985)	—	Most patients appear well adjusted	—
17. Lees et al. (1984)	53	High incidence of psychopathology	Compulsive touching self and others 61%[c], striking[c]
18. Comings and Comings (1985)	250	ADD with hyperactivity 54%, discipline problems 42%, exhibitionism 14% enuresis 36%[b]	OC behavior 45% in females and 29% in males: touching[c], smelling[c], mental[c], echolalia[c], palilalia[c]
19. Erenberg et al. (1986)	200	Over 50% learning problems and or ADD with or without hyperactivity (ADD 35%), learning problems 39%, adjustment reaction 10%, neurotic or psychotic 9%[b]	—
20. Current study	666	Psychopathology within expectations in the population for TS patients without ADD	OCS within expectations in the population.
Controlled studies			
21. Shapiro et al. (1978)	50	Schizophrenia, psychosis, inhibited hostility, hysteria, general adjustment not significantly higher than psychiatric OPD controls on projective tests	OCD and OCS not significantly higher than psychiatric OPD controls on projective tests.
22. Wilson et al. (1982)	—	More disturbance than in dissimilar sample of normal children and similar to children in special education classes (no control for ADD)[b]	—

(continued)

TABLE 6.3. (Continued)

Study	Sample	Psychopathology	OCS[a]
23. Frankel et al. (1986) Cummings et al. (1985)	63	—	52% of TS patients compared to 12% controls had high scores on an inventory interpreted as reflecting a diagnosis of OCD[c,d]
24. Grossman et al. (1986)	29	MMPI scale D, Pd, Pt, and Sc > 70 in female, paid volunteer TS subjects significantly higher than poorly described paid volunteer controls; retrospective study	—
25. Grad et al. (1984)	25	TS significantly higher than volunteer staff and friend controls: ADD+H 40%, oppositional disorder (6 of 9 with ADD+H) 40%, major depression 20%; no difference for other diagnoses; retrospective study[b]	OCD in 28% of TS compared to 8% for control subjects on DICA, higher OCS scores on CBCL and no difference on revised Leyton Inventory[c,d]
26. Current study	58	Psychopathology on the CBCL not significantly different between TS-alone and normal controls, and significantly lower than a TS+ADD+H group; prospective study	Obsessive-compulsive scale from the CBCL not significantly different between the TS-alone and normal controls, and both significantly lower than a TS+ADD+H group

[a]OCS = obsessive compulsive symptoms.
[b]Psychopathology may be due to high percentage of patients with ADD.
[c]One or more, usually all symptoms cited as compulsions are typical TS tics.
[d]Compulsive personality traits were cited as OCS.

function of ascertainment bias. The Yale Child Study Center is a tertiary major child psychiatric center and may attract patients who require hospitalization because they may be more severely afflicted with Tourette's disorder and have more severe psychopathology. Deviant sample characteristics for Yale Tourette's disorder patients are suggested by the very high ratio of males to females in their published studies: ten of 11 patients (Cohen et al., 1982), six of six patients (Leckman et al., 1982b), and 12 of 13 patients (Leckman et al., 1985). A male preponderance is frequent among patients with ADD. Another indication that the Yale samples are more severe than reported elsewhere are the diagnoses reported for 13 patients: 11 patients with ADD, six with specific developmental disorder, two with OCD, one with pervasive developmental disorder, and one with major depression (Leckman et al., 1985).

Another center with extensive experience with Tourette's disorder is the Department of Medical Genetics, at the City of Hope National Medical Center in California. D.E. Comings, a geneticist, and B.G. Comings, a social worker, used a clinical structured questionnaire to study 250 patients with Tourette's disorder, 54% of whom had ADD with hyperactivity (ADD+H) (Comings and Comings, 1985). A significant percent of these patients were described as having problems with discipline, anger, violence, enuresis, and exhibitionism. Only when assessing discipline problems did they separate the TS+ADD+H and TS-alone groups. Patients with TS+ADD+H had significantly more discipline problems than whose without ADD, although TS-alone patients had more discipline problems than expected but not as severe as reported for the TS+ADD+H group. Major shortcomings of this clinical report were the absence of a control group making it difficult to know if the percentages of Tourette's disorder patients with behavioral problems are significantly different from an appropriate control group, the reliance upon instruments without established reliability and validity, and the use of a single rater.

Of the 20 uncontrolled clinical reports summarized in Table 6.3, seven (35%) did not report excessive or specific psychopathology among Tourette's disorder patients (studies 3,5,8,11,15,16,20). Of the 13 (65%) studies reporting psychopathology, there are indications that the cited psychopathology is associated with ADD, hyperactivity, learning disorders and other CNS organic conditions in nine (69%) of the reports (studies 4,6,7,9,10,12,14,18,19). Moreover, the cited psychopathology is very diverse. The only possible generalization is that the tendency for ADD to be associated with Tourette's disorder is higher than expected.

Current Study. After studying the first 114 patients, and our conclusion that psychopathology was unassociated with Tourette's disorder, we did not intensively evaluate psychopathology in our patients. However, as a routine part of our ongoing study of Tourette's disorder, all past medical, psychiatric, psychological, and school records are reviewed and patients are evaluated using a screening semi-structured diagnostic interview. If psychopathology is

TABLE 6.4. *Gross clinical psychopathology in Tourette's disorder*[a]

Psychopathology or diagnostic disorders	N	%
Schizophrenic disorder	3	0.5
Borderline personality disorder	3	0.5
Obsessive-compulsive disorder	10	1.5
Conduct disorder	2	0.3
Mental retardation	2	0.3
Organic mental disorder	5	0.8
Attention deficit disorder with hyperactivity	109	16.4
with stereotypic movement disorder	11	1.7
with obsessive-compulsive disorder	6	0.9
with epilepsy	1	0.2
Attention deficit disorder without hyperactivity	27	4.1
with stereotypic movement disorder	3	0.5
with obsessive-compulsive disorder	2	0.3
Other Psychopathology[b]	51	7.7
Total gross psychopathology	235	35.3
No gross psychopathology	431	64.7

[a] $N = 666$.
[b] Includes diverse diagnostic categories such as neurotic, adjustment or personality disorders which were not specifically evaluated.

evident, a more thorough evaluation is done. Our conclusions are based on a clinical evaluation of gross or obvious psychopathology, and it does not include minor or not clinically meaningful symptoms, personality traits, or adjustment problems. The percentages for psychopathology are probably an underestimate, except for ADD, and are not strikingly different from expectations in the population (Table 6.4).

After careful review of the clinical reports cited in Table 6.3, we concluded that there is little support for the concept that psychopathology, except in patients with ADD, characterize patients with Tourette's disorder.

Controlled studies of psychopathology

Only six studies in the literature were controlled studies; the Grad et al. study (*unpublished*) was presented at the American Psychiatric Association meeting in Los Angeles in 1984 (Table 6.3, study 25); the results of our current study (Table 6.3, study 26) are described later in this chapter. The results of our predictive controlled study (Shapiro et al., 1978) and its limitations have been described previously (Table 6.3, study 21).

Wilson et al. (1982) (Table 6.3, study 22) attempted to identify and quantify psychopathology in 21 children with Tourette's disorder using the Behavior

Problem Checklist (BPC), the WISC, and the Wisconsin Card Sorting Test (WCST). The BPC scores for the 21 children with Tourette's disorder were compared to the scores of 102 problem children attending a special education class and a normative sample of 285 public school children. They concluded that the Tourette's disorder sample showed considerably more disturbance than children in general, and the nonspecific pattern of the scores were more like children in the special education class. They found a significant relationship between the total number of problems on the BPC, WISC Verbal IQ, and number of errors on the WCST. The finding that the scores of Tourette's disorder children were similar to those in a special education class suggests that the Tourette's group may have included many children with a diagnosis of ADD+H (not identified in the report), thus explaining the similarity between the two groups. Moreover, the BPC was completed by the parents of Tourette's disorder children while teachers completed the BPC for the normative sample. Hypotheses were not explicitly stated and the findings of this essentially retrospective study must be considered inconclusive.

Grossman et al. (1986) (Table 6.3, study 24) administered the MMPI to 29 Tourette's disorder patients and 29 controls. The controls were matched on age, sex, and social class variables but had higher IQ scores than Tourette's disorder subjects. Both Tourette's and control subjects were paid volunteers solicited by the Tourette Syndrome Association and through public notices. No information was provided about the severity of Tourette's disorder, the associated diagnosis of ADD, number of subjects on medication, and their motivation to participate in the study and other characteristics of the control group. Hypotheses were not explicitly stated prior to the analysis and the study is essentially a retrospective study. In a sophisticated statistical analysis, however, Tourette's disorder patients had significantly higher MMPI scores than control subjects on lie (L), validity (F), hypochondriasis (Hy), depression (D), psychopathic deviate (Pd), masculinity-femininity (Mf), psychasthenia (Pt), and schizophrenia (Scl). Other scores, including ego strength (ES), were not significantly different. However, scores for male Tourette's disorder subjects were above normal (70–80), on D, Pd, Mf, and Pt, and for both sexes on Sc. These results are different from those of our early study of 65 Tourette's disorder patients who were given the MMPI; in our study no score was in the pathological range above 70 (Shapiro et al., 1972a, 1974, 1978) (Fig. 6.1). Several factors may account for the higher scores on some of the variables for Tourette's disorder subjects in this study. The paid volunteer control group may have responded to items in a more socially desirable manner (SO-R) since they were nonpatients (no information was given about this measure). The Tourette's disorder sample may have included patients with ADD and other CNS pathology, patients requiring treatment with neuroleptics, and severely afflicted and impaired patients who may display help-seeking behavior by volunteering. These factors may have resulted in higher scores for male subjects, and contributed to positive responses to many MMPI items. For example, patients with Tourette's disorder would tend to answer yes to items 62, 103,

194, and 358, and having Tourette's disorder would influence the response to items 16, 32, 84, 351, and 356. Moreover, since hypotheses were not explicitly stated prior to the analysis, the study is essentially retrospective. Prospective studies using nonvolunteers, with adequate controls and methodology, are necessary to resolve the differences between the two MMPI studies.

A study with many noteworthy features was reported by Grad et al. (1984, *unpublished*) at a meeting of the American Psychiatric Association. The patients were evaluated with the Diagnostic Interview for Children and Adolescents (DICA), (with limited but adequate evaluation of reliability), a revised version of the Leyton Obsessional Scale for children (reliability and validity not evaluated), and the Achenbach Child Behavior Checklist (CBCL). Twenty-five Tourette's disorder children were compared with 25 controls who were matched on age, sex, social class, and school achievement variables. Tourette's disorder subjects compared to controls were diagnosed on the DICA as having significantly ($p < 0.05$) more ADD+H (10 versus 0) oppositional disorder (9 versus 0), major depressive disorder (5 versus 1), and OCD (7 versus 2), but there were no significant differences for diagnoses of separation anxiety, conduct, overanxious, and avoidant disorders. Limitations of the study include failure to establish hypotheses prior to the study and not reporting the results for other measures. The study, therefore, is a retrospective study, and the significant findings may be due to chance. Moreover, six of the nine children diagnosed as having oppositional disorder also had a diagnosis of ADD, which is frequently associated with psychopathology such as oppositional traits. These results, therefore may be due to ADD+H. The diagnosis of OCD (see our discussion in a later section) may have included many tic symptoms which were erroneously categorized as OCS. Finally, it was highly likely that the control group was less disturbed than a random selection of children, since they were volunteers "from a group of friends and relatives of hospital personnel." These limitations, in our opinion, do not justify the conclusion that psychopathology is associated with Tourette's disorder.

Our hypothesis that psychopathology is primarily associated with a secondary diagnosis of ADD+H in Tourette's disorder patients has been given some support by the results of The Ohio Tourette Study (Stefl, 1983, 1984), a questionnaire and epidemiological study of 528 patients (82% response) with Tourette's disorder in Ohio. Many problems were reported: temper, obsessive-compulsiveness, self-abusive behavior, anxiety, mood swings, aggressivity, running away from home, lying, stealing, insomnia, sleepwalking, night terrors, and enuresis. Many of these problems were related to the age, sex, and income, as well as to the diagnoses of minimal brain dysfunction (MBD) and ADD+H. Except for bad dreams, sleepwalking, and enuresis, all of the problems listed above were significantly related to these diagnoses. Stefl concludes in the 1983 report (not cited in the 1984 publication) that "These findings appear to confirm the impressions of Shapiro and Shapiro that many behavioral symptoms associated with Tourette's disorder may be caused by ADD or MBD."

In our opinion the frequent reports of psychopathology in Tourette's disorder, often uncritically cited in both the lay and professional literature, are not supported by data in the reviewed clinical reports or controlled studies. Our opinion, however, represents a minority view among clinicians and investigators. There is a clear need for controlled studies to resolve the controversy about psychopathology in general and the relationship of ADD to both psychopathology and Tourette's disorder.

Relationship of Attention Deficit to Psychopathology

Our revised concepts about the relationship of ADD to Tourette's disorder are discussed in detail in Chapter 4. The high proportion of 30 to 62% of Tourette's disorder patients with MBD or ADD identified in our early studies suggested that MBD or ADD was associated with Tourette's disorder, and this association was cited as evidence of an organic CNS etiology for this disorder. In later samples, between 1979 and 1981, the percentage of patients with TS+ADD decreased to 16.4% (Table 4.1). The disparity between early and later estimates of ADD in patients with Tourette's disorder was attributed to ascertainment bias since patients with both Tourette's disorder and ADD are more likely to be diagnosed (see Chapter 4). As the percent of patients with TS+ADD declined, so did severity of Tourette's disorder (Table 4.1). These findings, it seemed to us, provided less evidence of an organic etiology for Tourette's disorder and suggested that the psychosocial functioning of these patients was related to the associated diagnosis of ADD.

We examined this relationship in our current sample. For the total sample of 666 patients with Tourette's disorder, 24.9% were diagnosed as having ADD+H or ADD−H using a semistructured interview based on DSM-III criteria. We compared the TS+ADD groups to the TS-alone group on 33 behavioral factor scores and items. Significant differences between the TS-alone and the TS+ADD groups were obtained on 27 of the 33 behavioral and asset variables indicating significantly more behavioral disturbance in the Tourette's disorder ADD+H group (Table 4.27).

Our results, as do the results of others, require replication using more reliable and valid measures of psychopathology. Nevertheless these findings, combined with our extensive clinical experience, suggested a strong association between psychopathology in patients with Tourette's disorder and a clinical diagnosis of ADD. DSM-III criteria for ADD+H include primary symptoms of inattention, impulsivity, and hyperactivity. The associated symptoms include obstinancy, stubborness, negativism, bossiness, bullying, increased mood liability, low frustration, temper outbursts, low self-esteem, and lack of response to discipline; and possible complications include school failure, conduct disorder, and antisocial personality disorder. Thus, the major behavioral characteristics said to be intrinsic to Tourette's disorder (Cohen et al., 1983) encompass the primary and associated symptoms of ADD+H. If the percentage of Tourette's disorder patients with ADD reported in studies of psychopathology is high, it may explain the increased reports of psychopathology in patients with Tourette's disorder. Unfortunately, this issue is not addressed in any of the clinical reports and studies of psychopathology.

Controlled Study of Psychopathology

Resurgence of the issue of psychopathology in Tourette's disorder prompted us to design a prospective controlled study to evaluate the relationship of psychopathology to Tourette's disorder (supported in part by a small grant from the TSA). By psychopathology we designate symptoms of behavioral disturbance or problems, and impaired social competence (school performance, social competence, and adaptive functioning).

The present study was designed to evaluate the hypothesis that psychopathology ascribed to patients with Tourette's disorder is associated with a secondary diagnosis of ADD+H and is not intrinsically related to Tourette's disorder.

Sample

All subjects were 6- to 11-year-old male subjects. The experimental sample included 30 patients with a diagnosis of Tourette's disorder alone (TS-alone) and 28 male patients with Tourette's disorder and attention deficit disorder with hyperactivity (TS+ADD+H). The control sample included a random sample of 300 normal male subjects, and 300 patients referred for mental health services in the past 6 months (referred sample).

The Tourette's disorder samples were drawn from consecutive new patients applying for evaluation over a 1-year period at the Tourette and Tic Laboratory and Clinic, Mount Sinai School of Medicine, and from the private practice of the co-investigator (A.K.S.). All patients applying for evaluation complete a Movement Disorder Questionnaire (MDQ), and an Achenbach Child Behavior Checklist (CBCL).

The control samples were supplied by Dr. Thomas Achenbach from an extensive data set used to develop the CBCL. The data consisted of raw scores on the CBCL, age, social class, and race variables.

Diagnoses

The diagnosis of Tourette's disorder was made using DSM-III criteria during the initial intake evaluation and was confirmed by the alternative co-investigator after a review of the record. The diagnosis of ADD+H was made using DSM-III criteria during the initial evaluation, fulfillment of DSM-III criteria for ADD+H derived from the ADD+H self-rating scale completed by the parents (ADD Rating Scale), and a score of 15 or more on the Conners

Parent Teacher Abbreviated Symptom Questionnaire (Conners Hyperactivity). Both forms are included in the MDQ.

Measures

Parents of the TS subjects completed the Movement Disorder Questionnaire (MDQ) and an Achenbach Child Behavior Checklist (CBCL) before the diagnostic evaluation. Either parent of the Normal and Referred Samples completed only the Achenbach Child Behavior Checklist.

Movement disorder questionnaire

This is a comprehensive questionnaire to elicit relevant demographic, family, prenatal, maturational, medical, neurological, psychological, psychiatric, academic, movement disorder, and treatment histories.

ADD confidence scale

In addition a confidence rating for ADD+H was assigned based on the following scale: 0 = no evidence of ADD+H; 1 = fulfillment of DSM-III criteria for ADD+H self-rating in the questionnaire and confirmed by the clinician during the interview of parents and observation of the child, and confirmed by the alternative co-investigator after review of the record; 2 = evidence of ADD+H from parents (number 1 above) plus confirmation from the Conners Abbreviated Parent-Teacher Questionnaire completed by parents, and neurological, psychiatric, neuropsychological, and school records and evaluations.

ADD rating scale

Sixteen items are designed to elicit a history of ADD+H. The criteria for ADD+H in DSM-III require the presence of the traits inattention, impulsivity, and hyperactivity. Symptoms are rated as not at all (0), just a little (1), pretty much (2), and very much (3). A diagnosis of ADD+H requires that three symptoms for inattention be rated pretty much or very much, at least three for impulsivity and two for hyperactivity. Ratings range from 0 to 48.

Conners hyperactivity

Ten items in the MDQ include the Conners Abbreviated Parent-Teacher Questionnaire. The scores range from 0 to 30; scores of 15 or above indicate hyperactivity.

Social class

The occupational scale was used to define social class according to the list of occupations used by Hollingshead and Redlich (1958). This method of evaluating social class was used by Achenbach for the normal and referred samples.

Child behavior checklist (CBCL)

The CBCL is a widely used standardized inventory for assessment of the behavioral and social functioning of children. The inventory comprises 113 behavioral problems and 20 social competence items with a parental option to add one physical and one behavioral item. The parent responds to the behavioral item as not true (0), somewhat or sometimes true (1), or very true or often true (2) for now or within the past 6 months. The 20 social competence items are scored on a three- or four-point scale.

Parents were also requested to have the teacher complete a Child Behavior Checklist (Teacher's Report) but only a small percentage of teacher's reports were returned. A separate report on these will be prepared in the future. The following scores were derived from the CBCL.

Total Behavior Problem Score (TBPS). The total score is the sum of the 113 listed items scored 0 to 2 converted to a T score. The item "nervous movements or twitches" was scored as a zero for both experimental and control subjects. Scores above 70 indicate pathology.

Behavior Problem Score Without Hyperactivity (H). The scores for the 11 items of the Hyperactivity Behavior Scale are subtracted from the total raw behavior problem score. The new BPS is labeled BPS−H. This score is used to contrast the two Tourette's disorder groups to determine how they differ with regard to non-hyperactive-type psychopathology.

Externalizing Score. The scores on 41 items are summed and converted to a T score to indicate the primary concentration of the child's problems.

Social Competence Score. Three scales make up the Social Competence Score; activities with six items pertaining to sport, nonsport, job and chore activities; social with six items pertaining to friendship organizations, and social behavior; school items about academic performance on reading, writing, spelling, arithmetic, and other facts about academic functioning. The scores for the three scales are summed and converted to a T Score. T Scores below 30 are considered to be in the pathological range.

CBCL Subscales. Nine subscales are derived from the CBCL: Hyperactive, aggressive, delinquent, uncommunicative, obsessive-compulsive, social withdrawal, depressed, somatic complaints, schizoid or anxious.

Shapiro TS Severity Scale

This scale is completed by the clinician during the initial evaluation of Tourette's disorder subjects and provides a measure of initial severity of tic symptoms. Patients and collaterals together with the physician rate the degree to which the tics are noticeable to others, elicit comments or curiosity, interfere with functioning, and cause patients to appear odd or bizarre. The ratings for four items are summed yielding a qualitative description of severity that varies from very mild to very severe.

Hypotheses

The main hypothesis is that psychopathology (defined as higher TBPS and lower Social Competence Scores) will be significantly lower for the TS-alone sample than for the TS+ADD+H and referred samples, will be significantly higher for the TS+ADD+H sample than the normal sample, and that psychopathology for the TS-alone sample will not be significantly different from the normal sample.

Moreover, we reasoned and hypothesized that if psychopathology is associated with TS+ADD+H, there should be a direct relationship between severity of psychopathology and the severity of ADD+H.

Data Analysis

Ratings for the TS Severity Scale, ADD Rating Scale, ADD Confidence Level, Conners Hyperactivity, and Duration of Illness were compared using one-way analysis of variance. Data for family history of Tourette's disorder and family history of tics were analyzed using chi-square tests for independence.

Univariate one-way analyses of variance (ANOVAs) were conducted examining each CBCL scale separately. The primary tests of hypotheses involving Total Behavioral Problem Scale and the Social Competence Scale were conducted using ANOVAs. Univariate one-way ANOVAs were also conducted on age and social class. Comparisons among means for each dependent variable were made using the Scheffe method of multiple comparisons with alpha = 0.01. It should be noted that slight differences in degrees of freedom of ANOVAs are due to missing data from some variables.

It is expected that severity of Tourette's disorder and duration of illness would not be associated with psychopathology. No predictions were made for the individual behavior scales but the expectation is that the TS-alone sample would not differ significantly from the normal sample and that both the TS-alone and normal sample would have significantly lower scores than the TS+ADD+H and referred sample on the following variables: delinquent, aggressive, and externalizing scales.

The hypothesis that the degree of psychopathology would be directly related to the degree of ADD+H was evaluated by correlating indices of ADD+H severity (ADD Rating Scale, ADD Confidence Level, and Conners Hyperactivity) with the previously described psychopathology variables.

Results

The results of the ANOVA indicated no significant differences between the TS-alone group and the TS+ADD+H group on age, duration of illness, and Tourette's disorder severity. There was a significant difference between the Tourette's disorder groups on the ADD Rating Scale and Conners Hyperactivity Score ($p < 0.0001$) (Table 6.5).

TABLE 6.5. *Comparison of mean scores on the Achenbach Child Behavior Checklist Scales for Children with Tourette's disorder without attention deficit disorder or hyperactivity, Tourette's disorder with attention deficit disorder and hyperactivity, Normal controls, and Referred controls*[a,b]

						Scheffe Extended Range Test[c]			
Variables	TS-alone	TS+ADD+H	Normal controls	Referred controls	F, T, or χ^2	TS-alone	TS+ADD+H	Normal controls	Referred controls
Sample characteristics									
Age[d]	9.0	8.7	8.5	8.5	1.0				
Social class[d,e]	69.2	57.9	40.9	38.8	33.7[f]				
Family history of:									
TS[g]	16.7%	17.9%	—	—	0.1				
Tics[g]	36.7	28.6	—	—	0.3				
TS or tics[g]	50.0	39.3	—	—	0.6				
Duration of illness[h]	3.4	3.4	—	—	0.0				
ADD rating scale[d,h,i]	9.6	28.6	—	—	102.3[f]				
Conners Hyperactivity[d,h,j]	7.2	19.8	—	—	116.5[f]				
TS severity[h]	3.0	3.5	—	—	1.1				
Test of hypotheses									
Total Behavior Problem Scale (TBPS)[k]	56.3	72.8	50.5	68.6	68.6[m]	A	B	A	B
Behavior Problem Scale without Hyperactivity (BPS-H)[l]	28.2	60.3	18.4	49.5	162.4[m]	A	B	A	B
Social Competence Scale[k]	48.6	35.8	50.1	36.7	85.0[m]	A	B	A	B

Retrospective analyses

Behavior Problem Scales[a]

Scale	Normal controls	TS-alone	TS+ADD+H	Referred	F				
Hyperactive	56.5	73.4	57.6	68.5	138.3[m]	A	B	A	C
Aggressive	58.7	74.8	57.3	68.7	114.8[m]	A	B	A	C
Delinquent	58.5	66.6	57.8	68.1	55.8[m]	A	B	A	B
Uncommunicative	61.0	69.3	57.8	67.9	81.9[m]	A	B	A	B
Obsessive-compulsive	57.3	67.8	57.4	65.2	88.3[m]	A	B	A	B
Social withdrawal	59.4	71.0	57.9	65.2	96.5[m]	A	B	A	B
Depressed	62.6	70.4	57.3	68.7	95.6[m]	A	BD	C	AD
Somatic complaints	61.3	63.0	57.8	61.6	20.5[m]	A	A	B	A
Schizoid or anxious	61.1	67.8	57.8	64.8	55.5[m]	AB	C	A	BC
Externalizing Scale	53.1	71.4	50.9	68.1	200.7[m]	A	B	A	B

[a] Achenbach Child Behavior Checklist Scales for Children: males 6–10 years of age; TS-alone: $N = 30$; TS+ADD+H: $N = 28$; normal controls: $N = 300$; referred controls: $N = 300$.
[b] Data for normal and referred control samples provided by T. A. Achenbach (Achenbach and Edelbrock, 1983); referred sample comprised children referred for evaluation to a mental health facility in the past 6 months.
[c] Scheffe multiple range test; letters A, B, C, and D represent homogeneous subsets; differences $p < 0.01$.
[d] Analysis of variance.
[e] Social class is defined by Hollingshead and Redich (1958), 9-step occupational scale.
[f] $p < 0.0001$.
[g] χ^2.
[h] T-test.
[i] Total score from the Attention Deficit Disorder Scale is a measure of the severity of ADD+H, which is the sum of ratings (not at all, 0; just a little, 1; pretty much, 2; very much, 3) for 16 criteria listed in DSM-III for the diagnosis of ADD+H.
[j] Conners Abbreviated Parent Questionaire.
[k] Analysis of covariance with occupational status as covariate.
[l] Total raw score on the Total Behavior Problem Scale from which Hyperactivity Scale items were subtracted.
[m] $p < 0.001$.

Family history of tics, Tourette's disorder, and tics and Tourette's disorder were not significantly different for the Tourette's disorder samples using chi-square analysis. The results of the univariate one-way ANOVA for social class was significant with the Tourette's disorder samples having a higher social class than the normal and referred samples ($p < 0.001$). Subsequent analyses were done covarying for social class.

The results presented in Table 6.5 indicate that the four samples were significantly different on Total Behavior Problem Scale ($p < 0.001$) and on the the Social Competence Scale ($p < 0.001$). Specific contrasts using the Scheffe multiple range significance level confirmed our prediction that the TS+ADD+H sample would have significantly higher Total Behavior Problem Scale score and lower Social Competence Scale more than the TS-alone group and the normal sample, but not from the referred sample, and that the TS-alone group scores would be similar to those for the normal sample but significantly different from the TS+ADD+H group and the referred sample.

In addition we examined the data to see if the BPS−H score accounted for the differences between the two Tourette's disorder samples on the TBPS. We subtracted the hyperactivity raw score from the raw score for TBPS. The

TABLE 6.6. *Correlation of indices of severity of attention deficit disorder with hyperactivity (ADD Rating Scale, ADD Confidence Level and Conners Hyperactivity) with psychopathology[a]*

Psychopathology	ADD Rating Scale	ADD Confidence Level	Conners Hyperactivity
Total Behavior Problem Scale (TBPS)	0.58[b]	0.68[b]	0.66[b]
Behavior Problem Scale Without Hyperactivity (BPS−H)	0.50[b]	0.61[b]	0.61[b]
Social Competence	−0.52[b]	−0.48[b]	−0.54[b]
Behavior Problem Scales			
Hyperactive	0.80[b]	0.85[b]	0.76[b]
Aggressive	0.58[b]	0.68[b]	0.71[b]
Delinquent	0.51[b]	0.58[b]	0.65[b]
Uncommunicative	0.34[c]	0.35[c]	0.40[c]
Obsessive-compulsive	0.52[b]	0.63[b]	0.52[b]
Social withdrawal	0.47[d]	0.60[b]	0.52[b]
Depressed	0.27[e]	0.37[c]	0.32[c]
Schizoid or anxious	0.21	0.34[c]	0.54[b]
Externalizing	0.69[b]	0.73[b]	0.79[b]

[a] $N = 58$.
[b] $p < 0.0001$.
[c] $p < 0.01$.
[d] $p < 0.001$.
[e] $p < 0.05$.

BPS-H was still significantly different ($p < 0.001$), indicating that the differences were not due only to the hyperactivity scale, but were related to other psychopathology.

Our hypothesis that severity of ADD+H would be associated with severity of psychopathology was confirmed by consistently high and significant correlations between indices of severity of ADD+H and severity of psychopathology (Table 7.6).

Although no predictions were made for the individual behavior scales our expectation that the TS-alone and normal samples would have lower scores than the TS+ADD+H and referred samples on delinquency, aggressivity, and externalizing were confirmed.

We also retrospectively examined the differences between the groups on the other behavior scales. There was a difference at the 0.001 level of significance between the TS-alone group and the normal sample on depression and somatic complaint scores. Scores on depression for the TS+ADD+H sample were significantly higher compared to the TS-alone, normal, and referred samples. The TS-alone, TS+ADD+H, and referred samples did not differ significantly from each other but did differ from the normal sample.

On all the other behavior scales, the TS-alone Sample did not differ significantly from the normal sample, but did differ significantly from the TS+ADD+H and referred sample.

Discussion

The major prediction of the study is that psychopathology in Tourette's disorder patients is accounted for by the associated diagnosis of ADD+H. On the overall measures of psychopathology, Tourette's disorder patients with ADD+H are most like the referred sample of 6- to 11-year-old male subjects, whereas patients with TS-alone are most like the normal sample and differ from the TS+ADD+H and referred samples.

The higher scores for both Tourette's disorder groups on depression and somatic complaints may be due to the effect of having a chronic illness. They may be a secondary response to the disorder. Patients with Tourette's are more likely to experience negative feedback from peers and others who often react to the symptoms with rejection, cruelty, and teasing. Tourette's disorder patients are likely to respond with feelings of low self-esteem and depression, especially as they recognize that the illness is chronic and will not go away. Certainly if the symptoms are severe, numerous somatic complaints including headaches, muscle pain, etc., may be frequent, making patients sensitive to and understandably more likely to complain about their somatic state.

Conclusion

The study confirms the hypothesis that psychopathology is not more frequent in 6- to 11-year-old male patients with TS-alone than in a matched sample of normal children. The importance of separating groups of subjects with Tourette's disorder based on the presence or absence of ADD+H is also confirmed by this study. Unless this is done, it is not possible to specify whether differences between patients are due to normal variability or to lumping together two heterogenous samples. Moreover, it would be most unfortunate to label all Tourette's patients as emotionally disturbed if this is true of only a specific subset of TS patients.

The results of this study require confirmation using patient samples of both sexes, with other age ranges and other dependent measures of psychopathology.

OBSESSIONS, COMPULSIONS, AND IMPULSIONS

To better understand the resurgence of interest in the relationship of OCD and OCS to Tourette's disorder, this section discusses their historic background, problems in study of OCS, OCD, and Tourette's disorder, reviews clinical reports and controlled studies in the literature, contrasts reports of OCS-OCD in Tourette's disorder with the frequency of these symptoms in a control sample, describes the results of our studies, proposes that some Tourette's disorder symptoms resembling OCS be referred to as impulsions and presents a heuristic schema for classifying OCD, OCS, impulsions, and other symptoms.

History

Tourette's disorder was often thought of as a psychosis before 1950 and as an obsessive-compulsive (neurotic or psychotic) syndrome from 1950 to 1970 (Abraham, 1927; Mahler et al., 1944; Mesnikoff, 1959; Asher, 1966; Shapiro et al., 1978) (see Introduction). The hegemony of these diagnoses are dramatically illustrated in the history of a patient evaluated by us in 1967 (Shapiro and Shapiro, 1971). It also illustrates the dangers of excessive, overelaborate, and premature theorizing as a substitute for careful clinical observation, which may then iatrogenically influence concepts about etiology and treatment.

The patient was evaluated at Johns Hopkins Hospital at the age of 30. The clinical projective test report read as follows:

> The interesting dichotomy between his pleasant social manner and the violent tic is reminiscent of some paranoid schizophrenics who, after replying to a question of an examiner, will turn their head and speak in foul and violent obscenities to their private companions. It gives the same impression of early splitting in the

personality and direct contact with the raw unconscious. Without treatment it might be predicted that the tic will increase and that while he will not become a withdrawn schizophrenic, he will certainly become more and more schizoid.

To the patient's statement that "there is hardly anything I would do—to get well," the psychologist responds, an interesting slip which reveals the unconscious hostile character of the symptomatology.

He has lost contact with his own internal aggressive, hostile, and power-driving impulses, with the result that they speak for him without his voluntary control. It is tempting to guess that he might be able, as so many stutterers are, to lose the tic at a movement of conscious rage or anger.

The patient is a deeply infantile and regressed personality who for many years has been unable to recognize or accept in any way his own hostile aggressive and power-striving impulses. These have been split off from the rest of the personality and apparently have a life of their own without his voluntary or conscious control. He cannot be said to be truly schizophrenic, although there are many schizoid features in the personality structure. Rather, he represents a case of arrested social-emotional development. There are some paranoid traces which seem to strenghten his constant checking, as a child might, upon the emotional climate and judgment of the world around him. There is something of a psychopathic streak in his revengeful protests, as though he were demonstrating to the world 'You see what they made of me.' The tic itself expresses all of these elements in a dramatic fashion without any awareness of the implications on his part.

The shift from psychotic to obsessive-compulsive etiology is illustrated by an evaluation of the patient 13 years later at age 43, in 1964, at the Payne Whitney Psychiatric clinic. The psychologist's report describes the patient as:

an anxious, basically passive individual, with easy tolerance of his passivity. It is only in this man's fantasy life—and symbolically in symptomatology—that his powerful craving for the virility of personality and freedom of instinctual expression with which he identifies his masculine ego ideal find expression. [Note how the psychological interpretation of the tic is the basis for interpretation of some of the test data, sic.] The patient's impulse life is both fearful and confusing to him . . . deeply insecure . . . he feels enormous anger and hostility toward the important people in his life . . . kept from expression these feelings . . . experiences considerable guilt . . . the patient's ego organization is quite rigid but fairly well integrated. His obsessive-compulsive controls are relatively effective, despite their failure to control his ejaculative cursing [which fits the Gilles de la Tourette's Syndrome]. This latter seems to offer both a means of releasing unacceptable hostility and a symbolic expression of the virility which the patient has not achieved in his personality development. It may also represent a mechanism through which his ego defenses have remained intact and by which he has avoided the emergence of a full psychotic process. The record suggests that he could easily develop a paranoid process . . . The diagnostic impression is 'chronic, psychoneurosis, obsessive-compulsive type, in association with Gilles de la Tourette's Syndrome . . . his mode of adjustment is primarily that of an obsessive-compulsive neurosis.'

The patient was described by the psychiatrist at discharge as follows:

He smiled often and related to the examiner in a boyish manner, not seeming to regard such obscene outbursts as relevant. The appearance of obscenities seemed to be related to superficial hostilities and showed some relationship to sex and authority figures. His obscenities sometimes appeared in situations in which they were peripherally appropriate (political arguments), but were mostly irrelevant or founded on superficial hostilities. He could not be made to appreciate the most obvious connections between his verbal productions and feelings." Diagnostic impression: "Obsessive-compulsive reaction, manifested by compulsive reaction, manifested by compulsive obscene outbursts with tics (Gilles de la Tourette's Syndrome).

The patient re-entered the Payne Whitney Psychiatric Clinic in 1967 at age 46 for treatment with haloperidol. The records were thoroughly reviewed and the patient was again comprehensively evaluated. The psychiatrist (A.K.S.) and the staff at a psychiatric conference could not confirm the diagnosis of obsessive compulsive syndrome, symptoms, or character, nor did a thorough review by psychologists (E.S. and another senior psychologist) of the clinical projective test records that were done 3 years earlier. In fact, neither did the psychologist, who originally administered, scored, and interpreted the clinical projective tests, characterize the patient as obsessive-compulsive when given the protocols to review blindly. The patient was treated successfully with haloperidol, achieving over 90% reduction of symptoms at a dosage of 2 mg/day over the past 20 years. Discontinuation of medication on several occasions resulted in return of severe pretreatment symptoms.

There were two main reasons for characterizing Tourette's disorder as an obsessive-compulsive syndrome, although the differences between compulsions and organic movements had been known for a long time (Benedek, 1925; Lewis, 1936). Tourette's disorder symptoms, repetitive movements, noises, and words superficially resemble compulsions, and psychoanalytic theory postulated an unconscious obsessive-compulsive conflict in Tourette's disorder. Thus, in the records of our early patients the symptoms were invariably described as compulsions, the psychodynamics and etiology as obsessive-compulsive conflicts, and the diagnosis as an obsessive-compulsive neurosis or psychosis.

Another reason was that the criteria were somewhat different in the past. OCD was classified in the 1952 version of DSM-I (DSM-I, American Psychiatric Association, 1952) as obsessive-compulsive reaction (OCD) and compulsive personality (CP), reflecting a Myerian orientation, and in the 1968 version of DSM-II (DSM-II, American Psychiatric Association, 1968) as obsessive-compulsive neurosis and obsessive-compulsive personality, reflecting a psychoanalytic or psychodynamic orientation. There was a tendency at the time, however, to psychodynamically link or interchangeably use criteria for both OCD and CP in psychiatric diagnosis and interpretation of clinical projective tests (Rapaport, 1946; Schafer, 1953).

The tendency to loosely characterize Tourette's disorder patients as obsessive-compulsive is reflected in older reviews of the literature which relied on these broad psychodynamic criteria: obsessional symptoms 8.8% (Kelman,

1965), mild obsessional tendencies 29% (Fernando, 1967), obsessional 34.9% (Morphew and Sim, 1969), obsessive compulsive neurotics 33% (Abuzzahab and Anderson, 1973). Despite the lack of clear diagnostic criteria these reviews are often uncritically cited in current literature as evidence of OCD in Tourette's disorder.

The distinction between involuntary tics and voluntary (now referred to as intended) compulsions was clarified by us in a series of papers published between 1968 and 1978 (Shapiro and Shapiro, 1968, 1971; Shapiro, 1970a,b,c; 1972;1973;1978). We concluded from our clinical experience and studies that OCS and CP did not characterize patients with Tourette's disorder. Our studies may have contributed to the decreased citation of Tourette's disorder as an obsessive-compulsive reaction, neurosis, psychosis, or personality disorder in more recent papers (see Tables 6.2, 6.3). However, the issue of OCS has resurfaced due to the ebb and flow of clinical investigations and in no small measure due to labeling of some tic symptoms as compulsions in the 1980 version of DSM-III (DSM-III, American Psychiatric Association, 1980).

A DSM-III Advisory Committee Member on Childhood and Adolescent Disorders was given the task of reviewing our book on Tourette's disorder (A.K. Shapiro et al., 1978) to develop a nomenclature for tic disorders. The recommendations were informally discussed by the Chairman of the Task Force and us (A.K.S. and E.S.) on several occasions. Although there was agreement about many of the criteria in DSM-III, there were also disagreements. In relation to OCS we disagreed with the inclusion of the statement in Associated Features for Tourette's disorder. "There may be other symptoms, such as . . . obsessive thoughts of doubting and compulsive impulses to touch things or to perform complicated movements such as squatting, deep knee bends, retracing steps and twirling when walking." We felt there was insufficient evidence for the statement and that the specified compulsive impulses were, in fact, tics. It led unfortunately to classifying tics as compulsions in many published papers, and ultimately to the concept that OCS is associated with Tourette's disorder. For example, in a survey of patients with Tourette's disorder (Jagger et al., 1982), symptoms classified under "Compulsive Actions" include "head-banging, kissing, touching objects, kicking, tapping, touching self or others, biting self, touching sexual organs, and mimicking others," all of which we would classify as typical tics and not OCS. In another often quoted paper, OCS behavior (not defined) is cited as occurring in 68% of Tourette's disorder patients (Nee et al., 1980). The erroneous classification of tics as OCS in this paper was recently acknowledged by the second author of the paper, Dr. Eric Caine, at a recent meeting (TSA Clinical Symposium, 1985). In fact, there is now general consensus that these symptoms should be classified as tics rather than compulsions (Consensus Meeting of the TSA, 1986).

Interest in study of OCS and OCD has increased recently, probably stimulated by the failure of psychoanalytic theory and therapy to adequately explain or treat the condition (Salzman and Thaler, 1981), the development of improved psychometric (Philpott, 1975; Berg et al., 1986) and biological procedures (Lieberman, 1984; Turner et al., 1985; Insel, 1984; Elkins et al., 1980), and reports of successful treatment with behavioral techniques (Rachman and Hodgson, 1980; Marks, 1981, Foa et al., 1983) and chlorimipramine and other drugs (Insel, 1984, Lieberman, 1984; Turner et al., 1985, Elkins et al., 1980). However, there is an unfortunate tendency to uncritically lump many different symptoms into the OCS category, without adequate criteria or measures, with superficial, uncritical quoting of papers and discussion using analogy, simile, metaphor, and often what appears to be free association resembling a former era in psychiatry which distorted and prevented progress in the study of Tourette's and many other disorders. For example, in papers proposing an organic etiology for OCD, the organic etiology of Tourette's disorder, and the high percentage of OCS erroneously reported in Tourette's disorder are cited as evidence that OCD has an organic etiology.

Problems in Study of Obsessive-Compulsive Symptoms in Tourette's Disorder

After reviewing current literature on OCS, OCD, and Tourette's disorder, it was striking how well our conclusions were mirrored in a seminal paper on OCD (then called obsessional illness) written 50 years ago by Lewis (1936). Lewis begins his paper by noting that he was "struck by the variety of problems" and the difficulty of stating them "for a topic as wide as obsessional illness," that it is "harder to state the problems clearly than to present the alleged solutions offered in the literature. Some of these solutions deal with problems that are indefinite and indeed unsubstantial; others are global; they cover so wide a field that it is difficult to examine them without examining the nature of man." Understanding requires "bold speculation, and the use of methods as yet unthought of or suspect" and recommends "Descartes rules— to doubt everything that is not clear, to avoid precipitancy, and to divide up every difficulty into as many parts as are possible and necessary for its better solution; also to proceed from the simplest and plainest facts," and concludes that OCD "has not usually been treated on such lines." Lewis also notes "that the obsessional experience is so widespread over psychic activity and so commonly found with other abnormal psychic states" that obsessional neurosis is an insecure category, and in the past was called psychasthenia by Janet, latent schizophrenia by Bleuler, and an affective psychosis by Stocker and Maudsley; that obsessional character traits occur in normal individuals, can be observed in many other psychiatric and CNS disorders, are frequently not associated with OCD and that a "subjective feeling of compulsion and resistance is important in OCD." He also discussed the differential features of many other symptoms that are frequently cited as OCS: impulsions, persistence, perseveration, stubborness, preoccupations, disagreeable ideas or affects, rituals, ceremonials, gluttony paranoia, phobias, delusions, stereotype and organic symptoms. He differentiated compulsions from tics, coprolalia, and organic CNS symptoms by noting that unwilled organic symptoms are viewed with detachment, that the "movements are the primary happening" . . . and "not the secondary happening, expressions of a resistance," which occurs in "almost all obsessional actions." The concepts of "resistance" and that the "movements are the primary happening" were absorbed in DSM-III and DSM-III-R, the latter specifying that compulsive "behavior is not an end in itself."

OCS-like symptoms continue to be extensively cited in schizophrenia, depression, manic depressive illness, neurosis, anxiety, phobic and panic disorders, hypochondria, organic brain disorder, posttraumatic stress syndrome, mental retardation, anorexia nervosa, epilepsy, myxedema, arteriosclerosis, head trauma, parkinsonism, and in normal persons (Benedek, 1925; Lewis, 1936; Insel, 1984; Weiner et al. 1976; Rasmussen and Tsuang, 1986). Patients can be classified as having obsessions, compulsions, obsessive slowness, impulsions, and compulsive personality, either alone or in various combinations (Rachman and Hodgson, 1980; Insel et al., 1985; Weiner et al., 1976; Rasmussen and Tsuang, 1986). Although DSM-II, III, and DSM-III-R classify OCD as an anxiety disorder, others believe that OCD should be classified as a separate entity (Insel et al., 1985; DSM-III-R meetings and correspondence of the Advisory Committee on Anxiety and Obsessive Compulsive Disorders, 1985, 1986). Problems in study of OCS are much more difficult than study of Tourette's disorder, and unfortunately papers linking OCS and TS ignore many problems extensively discussed in the OCD literature. It is generally recognized that problems of reliable and valid measurement, criteria, and diagnosis of OCS and OCD are difficult, vague, and unsatisfactory (Lieberman, 1984; Rasmussen and Tsuang, 1984, 1986; Rachman and Hodgson, 1980; Rachman and Desilva, 1978; Philpott, 1975; Pauls et al., 1986b; Insel, 1984; Berg et al., 1986; Turner et al., 1985; Weiner et al., 1976).

Review of Clinical Reports and Studies of Obsessive-Compulsive Symptoms and Disorder in Tourette's Disorder

Of 26 papers in the literature that discuss psychopathology in Tourette's disorder, OCS is mentioned by only 16 (62%), 12 are uncontrolled clinical reports, and 4 are somewhat controlled studies (Table 6.3). It is noteworthy that OCS or OCD is reported as higher than expected in Tourette's disorder in 11 papers and as within expectations in the population in four papers, all four negative reports authored by the current authors (A.K.S., E.S.) (Table 6.3, studies 1,20,21,26). We reported that the prevalence of OCS (not defined other than use of DSM-III criteria) based on nonblind clinical evaluations was within expectations in one population in two studies (Table 6.3, studies 3,20). For the nine clinical reports citing higher than expected OCS in Tourette's disorder, one was based on inclusion of tics as compulsions (Table 6.3, study 5); six did not define OCS and cited tics as evidence of OCS (Table 6.3, study 6,7,10,14,17,18); one did not define OCS and cited OCP as evidence of OCS (Table 6.3, study 14); one did not define OCS (Table 6.3, study 15). Moreover, it is perhaps relevant that nine (45%) of the 20 clinical reports about psychopathology did not cite OCS as a characteristic of Tourette's disorder.

Of four controlled studies, one (Table 6.3, study 21) used blind assessment and controls. The controls (psychiatric outpatients), however, were appropriate only to test the hypothesis about the specificity of OCS in Tourette's disorder but not for comparing Tourette's disorder patients with normal controls. In addition, the measures (clinical projective tests) were retrospectively deemed unreliable and invalid. This study has been described previously (Shapiro et al., 1972a, 1973c,d, 1974, 1978).

The Frankel et al. (1986) and the Cummings and Frankel (1985) study (Table 6.3, study 23) compared 63 Tourette's disorder patients with 11 OCD patients and 41 normal controls described as hospital personnel without a history of mental illness. Control subjects included 83% female subjects compared to 30% for Tourette's disorder subjects, who were all over 18 years, compared with 21% under 18 years for Tourette's disorder, and controls had more education. The dependent variable was a 40-item four-point scale modified from a version of the Leyton Obsessional Scale with added items. They report that 51.6% of Tourette's disorder patients exceeded a criterion score of 70 (not defined) compared with 12% for the normal controls ($p < 0.00005$). Limitations of the study include nonblind evaluations, absence of evidence for the reliability and validity of the new scale, inclusion of typical tic symptoms such as palilalia, echolalia, echokinesis, coprolalia, mental coprolalia, touching things and self (in 10 or 25% of the items) (items 7,8,13,14,20,21,25,29,38,40), inclusion of many (28%) compulsive personality trait items (items 4,5,9,10,11,28,30,33–37) and aggressivity (items 19,23,24,39). Although this study was noteworthy for use of a control group, failure to more fully describe how controls were recruited or selected and the use of volunteers, excluding those with a psychiatric history and different demographic characteristics, are major limitations of this study. The use of an inappropriate control group can unwittingly result in erroneous support or rejection of a hypothesis. Conceptual problems common in most reports and studies are illustrated by unwarranted reliance on DSM-III (see previous discussion about problems associated with the development of criteria in DSM-III), and the inappropriateness of diagnosing OCD from scale scores. In addition, DSM-III is misquoted as defining compulsions as involuntary. Obsessions in DSM-III are defined as " . . .ego-dystonic, i.e., they are not experienced as voluntarily produced . . . ," and compulsion is defined as " . . .performed according to certain rules. . . ." Nowhere does it state that obsessions and compulsions are involuntary. In fact, the voluntary nature of compulsions is made explicit in DSM-III-R (American Psychiatric Association, 1987): "Compulsions . . . purposeful, and intentional behavior that is performed according to certain rules . . . ," and "Obsessions . . . experienced as intrusive. . . ." Another major conceptual error, again common in the literature, is equating scale scores (without evidence of reliability and validity) to a diagnosis of OCD. The authors state, based on a criterion score exceeding 70 on the inventory, that patients had OCD. This score, without data about severity, resistance, interference, or the fulfillment of DSM-III-criteria for " . . . a significant source of distress . . . or interfere with social or role functioning," does not qualify as a basis for the diagnosis of OCD.

Some of the features of the study of OCS by Grad et al. (1984) (Table 6.3, study 25) have been described in the section on psychopathology. Twenty-five children were compared with an equal number of controls. Instruments included the DICA, a revised Leyton Obsessional Scale for Children, and the CBCL. Previously described limitations of this study include the use of a new version of the Leyton scale without adequate evidence of its reliability and validity which included many tics, compulsive personality, and aggressive items. In addition, the obsessive-compulsive scale in the CBCL is markedly inadequate, including items such as loud, brags, daydreams, strange behavior and ideas, confused, nightmares, anxious, overtired, sleeps little, can't sleep, stares blankly, walks and talks in sleep, excess talk and twitches. Also, the sample included 40% of children with TS+ADD+H. Given these problems, it is not unexpected that some measures of OCS were significantly higher in the Tourette's disorder than in the control sample. Moreover, the selection of the normal control group would veritably guarantee that the Tourette's disorder sample would have higher scores on most measures of psychopathology. The normal control group included volunteers who were children of professional colleagues and hospital personnel. Problems inherent in the use of volunteers have been discussed extensively in the literature. Experimental and control groups that are dissimilar are subject to differential social desirability and demand characteristics (Orne, 1962; Shapiro, 1971). An appropriate control group for a Tourette's disorder study should include patients matched for age, sex, ethnicity, social class, and a movement disorder like essential tremor, epilepsy or narcolepsy, a cosmetic disability like neurodermatosis or disfiguring facial hemangioma, or medical condition such as diabetes (Lasagna et al., 1954; Perlin et al., 1958; Pollin and Perlin, 1958; Richards, 1960; Esecorer et al., 1961; Orne, 1962; Rosenthal and Rosnow, 1975; Shapiro and Morris, 1978; Shapiro and Shapiro, 1984).

The fourth study, our previously described current study (Table 6.3, study 26) reported that ratings of the Obsessive-Compulsive Scale from the CBCL for the TS-alone and normal control groups were not significantly different but that the TS+ADD+H and referred sample scored significantly higher on the Obsessive-Compulsive Scale than both the TS-alone and normal samples (Table 6.5), and that the severity of ADD and hyperactivity correlated 0.52 to 0.63 ($p < 0.0001$) with the Obsessive-Compulsive Subscale of the CBCL. The major limitation of this study, similar to all others, is that the Obsessive-Compulsive Scale from the CBCL has not been externally validated.

Our interpretation of the reviewed data is that current evidence does not support the hypothesis that OCS or OCD is associated with Tourette's disorder. The most that can be said for the concept based on some clinical impressions and inadequately controlled studies is that it is a hypothesis that requires confirmation.

Obsessive-Compulsive Symptoms and Disorder in the Population Compared with the Results of the Current Study

These considerations lead to two important questions: What is the frequency of OCD and various types of OCS in the population? Several studies are available that provide partial answers to these questions. Our hypothesis is that the prevalence of OCD and OCS in Tourette's disorder is not significantly different from estimates in the population.

Obsessive Compulsive Disorder

Our diagnosis of OCD utilized a semi-structured interview designed to elicit DSM-III criteria. As described previously, the diagnosis of OCD was made at the initial evaluation by one of us (A.K.S. or E.S.). The alternative clinician reviewed the record independently, but not blindly. There were minor differences of opinion about some patients which were resolved by discussion. All diagnoses were done in 1981 to 1982 before publication of the results of the previously mentioned epidemiological studies. OCD was diagnosed in ten (1.5%) patients with TS-alone and eight (1.2%) in patients with TS+ADD (Table 6.4). These percentages are not significantly different from estimates of 1.3 and 2% in the population (Weissman et al., 1986; Robins et al., 1984; Reiger et al., 1984; Rasmussen and Tsuang, 1984). Obviously, limitations cited for previous clinical reports apply to our results.

Obsessive Compulsive Symptoms

Although the prevalence of OCD is low, nonclinical control samples have a high percentage of OCS. Most normal people are thought to have some symptoms resembling clinical obsessions and compulsions, but it is difficult to determine when to diagnose them as having a clinical disorder (Rachman and DeSilva, 1978; Hoogduin, 1986). At what quantitative or qualitative point, level or degree of distress, resistance, interference, and other proposed indices does OCS become a clinically diagnosed disorder?

For example, how would one classify two symptoms that I (A.K.S.) have had for 40 years. When speaking with someone, if the conversation is not too interesting to me or I am thinking of something else, I will tend to line up a part of the persons' body (top or sides of their head, shoulders, etc., with a horizontal or vertical object (walls, ceiling, bookcase, etc.) in the room. It is not readily noticeable to anyone except my wife. Also, while a passenger in an automobile, again if bored, I flick (tic-like) my index finger in the direction of every passing lamp post. There are no other OCSs except for mild and common compulsive traits characteristic of researchers. It is highly likely that if I had Tourette's disorder I would be labeled as having OCS and even possibly OCD in the previously described studies of OCS-OCD in Tourette's disorder. I was interested in this symptom and thoroughly explored its possible dynamic meaning during 4 years of psychoanalysis (many of us did this in the past). No particular interpretation was given by the analyst and it fell by the wayside as an unimportant symptom without precise dynamic meaning. Should the symptom be classified as a learned habit or mannerism, an impulsion, a minor compulsion, or a residual stereotype? My interpretation is that the symptom is a stereotypic movement that serves as a defense against residual symptoms of a minor ADD+H.

Since the question of OCS in Tourette's disorder has resurfaced, I continually ask colleagues, friends, relatives, neighbors, and whoever else will listen, whether they have obsessions or compulsions. Only one person (E.S.) denied any OCS. Another problem was noted by Cantwell (1984) who cites the uselessness of many common items in behavior scales, such as obsessive ideas, which are "always checked by parents" because "when we go to Toys 'R Us and we won't buy him a toy, he won't shut up."

Formal studies of OCS are infrequent. However, as part of a controlled study of OCD in children, Berg et al. (1986) using a revised version of the Leyton scale for children, tabulated OCSs in 28 adolescent controls (Table 6.5). OCS was surprisingly high: repeated thoughts and words 60%, worry about being clean enough 57%, have to do certain things 43%, checking taps, switches repeatedly 39%, checking doors, windows 39%, having to check several times 29%, need to count several times 25%, and so on. Compulsive personality or trait symptoms varied from 18% to 64% (Table 6.5). Most of these patients, if they had Tourette's disorder, would have been cited as having OCS or OCD in the reviews and studies listed in Table 6.3. In fact, these percentages are higher than the percentages reported in patients with Tourette's disorder and higher than the percentages reported for relatives of Tourette's disorder patients (Table 6.5).

To evaluate the frequency of common OCS in Tourette's disorder patients we tabulated selected OSC and CP items for 319 Tourette's disorder patients (mean age 18.1, range 4–68 years), for 28 normal controls (mean age 13.7,

TABLE 6.7. Obsessive-compulsive-like symptoms and compulsive traits in Tourette's disorder and comparison with a control sample

Item	Total TS sample[a]				TS sub-sample[b]	Control sample[c]	
	Not at all %	Just a little %	Pretty much %	Very much %	Total yes %	Items	Total yes %
Obsessive-compulsive-like symptoms							
Checking things that you know you have already done, like doors, switches, etc.	59	19	13	9	40	Checking taps, switches repeatedly; checking doors, windows; checking several times, have to	39 39 29
Counting things many times/or going through numbers in your head	65	20	10	5	25	Need to count several times	25
Touching things over and over again	80	10	5	4	17	Do certain things, have to	43[d]
Repetitive thoughts that you cannot turn off such as worry about germs, fear of accidents to loved ones, violence, etc.	53	19	16	13	43	Repeated thoughts or words; family members get hurt; worry about being clean enough	60 50 57

Compulsive (personality) symptoms							
Cleaning room or home more often than is needed to be sure it is clean	33	25	30	13	61	Making things extra clean; clothes always neat and clean; fussy about clean hands	36[d] 29[d] 25[e]
Even when doing something perfectly, feeling it is not done quite right	36	31	19	15	55	Lack of sureness, repetition; indecisive, a frequent problem; repetition until correct; redo papers to insure perfection	39 39 36 57
Having to keep things in a certain order, or getting dressed in a certain set pattern	49	22	18	12	39	Special places to put things; careful to have neat papers, doing things in an exact manner	46 50 18[f]
Saving things even though they are of little value, like boxes, newspapers, etc.	31	27	21	21	63	Hoarding in one's room	64

[a]Total TS sample: $N = 319$, mean age 18.1 (SD = 11.1), range 4–68.
[b]TS subsample: $N = 114$, mean age 13.5 (SD = 2.1), range 4–18.
[c]Control sample: $N = 28$, mean age 13.7 (SD = 1.9), range 4–18.
[d]$p < 0.01$.
[e]$p < 0.001$.
[f]$p < 0.05$.

range 4–18) from the Berg et al. study (1986), and a subsample of Tourette's disorder patients in the same age range as the Berg et al. study (mean age 13.5, range 4–18) (Table 6.7). Only items rated pretty much or very much are considered significant. Our interpretation of the data is that the frequency of OCS (which includes those diagnosed as having OCD) is roughly similar to expectations in the population. Moreover, except for the small number of patients in our study who were clinically diagnosed as fulfilling DSM-III criteria for OCD (2.7%), none of these patients rated the degree of interference or resistance as pretty or very much (data recorded but not analyzed because of nonsignificant ratings of these variables). In another study of OCS of 124 normal adults, only 20.2% did not have any obsessive thoughts, 25.8% had only obsessive thoughts, 11.3% had only impulses, and 42.7% had both obsessive thoughts and impulses (Rachman and Hodgson, 1980; Rachman and DeSilva, 1978). The symptoms of OCD, compared to these common normal obsessional thoughts, are less readily accepted by the individual, linger longer, provoke more tension and resistance, are more egodystonic, coexist with many other OCSs, usually include cognitive elaboration, and both obsessions and compulsions, and induce distress and interference with functioning.

It is unquestionably clear that studies of both OCS, OCD, and Tourette's disorder have very limited, if any, value if the clinical sample is not compared with an appropriate control sample, using reliable and valid measures and blind ratings. Since none of the studies in the literature have utilized these well-established and universally accepted criteria for an adequate study, it is possible, likely in our opinion, that the high percentages of OCD and OCS reported in the literature are spuriously high and characterized by type I errors.

Differential Features for Obsessive Compulsive Disorder, Obsessive-Compulsive Symptoms, Tourette Symptoms, Impulsions, and Other Movements

Revised Criteria for Obsessive Compulsive Disorder in DSM-III-R

Proposed diagnostic criteria for the diagnosis of OCD in DSM-III-R are similar to those in DSM-III. The criteria are described in the first column of Table 6.6. These criteria are used as a potential basis for differentiating symptoms for conditions listed in the top row. Other differentiating features described in the literature are listed at the end of the table.

Proposed Differential Features

The proposed similarity and differences among disorders is based on our interpretation of the data in the literature and our clinical experience. No doubt others would classify the data differently. It is proposed for heuristic purposes and as an indication that the tendency to "lump" all OCS-like symptoms into one category is untenable, and that separation or "splitting" of symptoms into different categories has heuristic value. In our opinion, the linkage of OCD or OCS and Tourette's disorder is highly questionable. We do not infer that the categories are inviolate. Indeed, we had to make many arbitrary decisions about how to categorize various features. It is likely that many of these issues will not be resolved until the pathophysiology of these disorders is established.

Obsessive Compulsive Disorder Versus Obsessive-Compulsive Symptoms

The main difference between OCD and OCS is criteria B in DSM-III-R. OCD requires marked distress and interference with functioning. Many compulsive symptoms may appear to be "an end in themselves," not be induced by a "dreaded event or situation," may be "connected in a realistic way with what it is designed to neutralize or prevent," may not be "clearly excessive," and for obsessions no attempt may be made "to ignore or suppress them or neutralize them with some other thought or action." Reliable data from controlled studies about the range or prevalence for OCS in normal and clinical samples are not available in the literature. References in the literature usually cite the relationship of Tourette's disorder to compulsions and rarely to obsessions (Table 6.3). Our clinical impression, similar to Hoogduin (1986), is that obsessive symptoms alone are less frequent than compulsions, that compulsions are almost always associated with obsessive thoughts, that obsessions occur alone only occasionally and only infrequently fulfill the criteria for OCD (in a recent tabulation of OCD symptoms, only 4.5% had only obsessions) (Rasmussen and Tsuang, 1986) and they do not occur among Tourette's disorder patients more frequently than expected in the population. There are also no data to indicate whether OCS and OCD should be conceived of as a continuum, differing only on a continuum of severity, or as a spectrum, such as some symptoms being continuous and others discontinuous.

Tourette Versus Obsessive-Compulsive Disorder and
Obsessive-Compulsive Symptoms

We have already discussed the erroneous classification of Tourette's disorder as OCD, in the past and the error of referring to many classical tic symptoms as OCS in DSM-III and in clinical reports and studies. This error has been rectified in DSM-III-R which does not classify complex movements such as "touching, squatting, deep knee bends, retracing steps and turning when walking" as compulsions. As indicated in Table 6.8, the only similarity between Tourette's disorder and both OCD and OCS is that the symptoms

TABLE 6.8. Comparison of DSM III-R criteria for obsessive-compulsive disorder with tic and other disorders, symptoms, and normal physiological functions[a]

DSM III-R criteria and other features	Obsessive-compulsive disorder	Obsessive-compulsive symptoms	Tic disorder (TS CMT TTD)[b]	TS impulsion	Sensory TS subtype SS[c]	Sensory TS subtype M[c]	Stereotypic movement disorder	Dystonic disorder[d]	Epileptic disorders	Sneezing, normal eye-blinking
Obsessive-compulsive disorder or neurosis (300.30) Either obsessions or compulsions: The essential feature is recurrent obsessions and compulsions sufficiently severe as to cause marked distress, be time-consuming, or significantly interfere with the individual's normal routine, occupational functioning, or with usual social activities or relationships with others.	+	—	—	—	—	—	—	—	—	—
Obsessions Persistent ideas, thoughts, impulses, or images that are experienced, at least initially, as intrusive and senseless or repugnant.	+	+	Infrequent[e]	?	—	—	—	—	—	—
For example, repeated impulses to kill a loved child, or recurrent blasphemous thoughts in a religious individual.	+	+ or −	Infrequent	—	—	—	—	—	—	—
The individual attempts to ignore or suppress them or to neutralize them with some other thought or action.	+	+ or −	Infrequent[e]	?	+ or −	−(+)	—	—	—	—

The individual recognizes that the obsessions are the product of his or her own mind and are not imposed from without (as in thought insertion).	+	+	+	+	+	+	+	+	+
The most common obsessions are repetitive thoughts of violence (killing one's child), contamination (becoming infected by shaking hands), and doubt (repeatedly wondering whether one has performed some action, such as having hurt someone in a traffic accident.	+	–	–	–	–	–	–	–	–
Compulsions									
Repetitive,	+	+	+	+	+	+	+	+	+
purposeful,	+	+	–	–	+	–	+	–	–
and intentional behaviors	+	+	–	+	–	–	+	–	–
that are performed in response to an obsession,	–	–	–	–	–	–	–	–	–
or according to certain rules	+	+	–	–	–	–	–	–	–
or in a stereotyped fashion.	+	+	+	+	+	+	+	+	+
The behavior is not an end in itself,	+ or –	–	+ or –	+ or –	+	+ or –	–	+	+
but is designed to neutralize or to prevent discomfort	+	+	+	+	–	+	–	–	–
or some dreaded event or situation.	+ or –	–	–	–	–	–	–	–	–
However, either the activity is not connected in a realistic way with what it is designed to neutralize or prevent, or it is clearly excessive.	+ or –	–	–	–	–	+ or –	–	–	–

(continued)

TABLE 6.8. (Continued)

DSM III-R criteria and other features	Obsessive-compulsive disorder	Obsessive-compulsive symptoms	Tic disorder (TS CMT TTD)[b]	TS impulsion	Sensory TS subtype SS[c]	Sensory TS subtype M[c]	Stereotypic movement disorder	Dystonic disorder[d]	Epileptic disorders	Sneezing, normal eye-blinking
The act is performed with a sense of subjective compulsion that is coupled with a desire to resist the compulsion (at least initially).	+	+ or −	−	−	−	−	+ or −	−	−	−
The individual recognizes that his or her behavior is excessive or unreasonable,	+	+ or −	−	+ or −	−	−	+ or −	−	−	−
and does not derive pleasure from carrying out the activity, although it provides a release of tension.	+	+ or −	+	+	+	+	−	+	+	+
The most common compulsions involve handwashing, counting, checking and touching	+	?	?	?	?	?	?	?	?	?
Tic disorders (307.20–307.23)										
A tic is an involuntary, sudden, rapid,	−	−	+	−	+	−	−	+	−	+
recurrent, nonrhythmic, stereotyped	−	−	+	−	+	−	+ or −	+ or −	+	+
motor movement or vocalization.	+	+	+	+	−	+	+ or −	+(−) / −(+)	+(−)	+(−) / −
The tic is experienced as irresistible but can be suppressed for varying periods of time.	+	+	+	+	+	+	+	+	−	+(−)

Other differential features										
Age of onset	>15	?	<15	<15	<15	<15	<7	Variable	Variable	Birth
Sex ratio	M = F	?	M > F	M > F	M > F	M > F	M > F	M > F	M = F	M = F
Genetics[g]	OCD < TS	?	TS > OCD	?	ST = TS	ST = TS	+	=, −	+	+
Prevalence	1.3–2%	?	47%[f]	?	?	?	?	Variable	100%	100%
IQ	Normal	Normal	Normal	Normal	Normal	Normal	Lower	Normal	Normal	Normal
Premorbid personality	Normal (Obsessional)	?	Normal	?	Normal	Normal	ADD	Normal	Normal	Normal
Symptoms										
Clonic, jerky	−	−	+	−	−	−	−(+)	−(+)	+	+
Tonic, prolonged	+	+	−	+	+	+(−)	+(−)	+	−	−
Common simple motor tics: eye, hands, shoulder, face, mouth, and hands	−	−	+	−	−	+	−(+)	+	−	(+)
Common complex motor tics: hit self, jumping, copropraxia, echopraxia, touching, smelling	−	−	+	−	−	−	+	−	−	−
Complex vocal tics: echolalia, palilalia, coprolalia	(+)	(+)	+	+	−	−	+	−	−	−
	−	−	+	−	−	−	−(+)	−	−	−
Ideational, associated dynamics	−	−	−	−	−	−	+	−	−	−
Sexual, aggressive, coprophilic themes	Common	+ or −	Coprophilia	No	No	No	No	No	No	No
Treatment										
Neuroleptics	−	?	?	(+)	+	+	−(+)	−	−	−
Antidepressants (chlorimipramine, etc.)	+	?	−	?	−	−	−	−	−	−
Behavioral therapies	+	?(+)	?	?	?	?	(+)	−	−	−

[a] + = Present, positive, yes; − = not present, negative, no; ? = unknown; (+) or (−) = somewhat positive or negative.
[b] TS = Tourette's disorder, CMT = chronic motor tic, TTD = transient tic disorder.
[c] SS = sensory stimulus or involuntary sensation; M = intended or voluntary movement.
[d] Dystonic disorders such as focal, segmental, or generalized dystonia.
[e] Mental echophilia and mental coprophilia are classified as tics.
[f] Refers only to obsessions or compulsions.
[g] Family history of TS 8%, tics 42%, TS or tics 47%.

are repetitive, stereotypic, not experienced as pleasurable although providing release of tension, attempts may be made to ignore, suppress, or neutralize symptoms, and are recognized as not imposed from outside as in thought insertion. In our opinion the linkage of OCD or OCS and Tourette's disorder is highly questionable, and can only be resolved be careful empirical study.

Fear about something bad happening is possibly the major factor that differentiates OCD from OCS and Tourette's disorder impulsions. In my clinical experience over the past 30 years (A.K.S.), I have evaluated or treated approximately 60 patients with OCD. All had a major fear component that unmercifully fueled their obsessions and compulsions leading to extreme discomfort and interference with functioning. In the list of most frequent obsessions in OCD, Rasmussen and Tsuang (1986) describe fear of contamination, fear of aggression, fear of sexual acting-out, need for symmetry or exactness to keep something bad from happening, somatic obsessions about something bad happening in the future. Only 4.5% have only obsessions, most also have compulsions, the most frequent being checking, cleaning, and counting. The symptoms in clinical patients with OCD are not minor habits that can be ignored; they grip the individual in ceaseless fear and preoccupation with methods of avoiding danger. Janet, too, according to Pitman (1987) referred to obsessions and compulsions as "ideas and impulses . . . that come to dominate the patient's mental life" and "usually involve forbidden thoughts and acts of a sacrilegious, violent, or sexual nature, that are often the ones most objectionable to the patient and most in contrast with what he wishes to do." How this group differs from those with obsessive slowness, which occurs infrequently (Rachman and Hodgson, 1980), benign infrequent, everyday OCS or impulsions in Tourette's disorder warrants empirical study.

We have the impression, from discussions with colleagues and careful reading of papers that variable criteria are used by different investigators for the diagnosis of OCD, OCS, impulsions, and tics. Many symptoms that we would classify as tics are cited as OCS or OCD by others (Table 6.3). Symptoms associated with compulsive personality disorder, such as difficulty expressing emotion, formal, stingy, perfectionism, preoccupation with details, stubborness, indecisiveness, more concern with work than relationships, and so on, are also cited as evidence of OCS (Table 6.3). Hoogduin (1986), in a sensitive clinical paper, cites the necessity of differentiating OCS and OCD from morbid preoccupations (ego syntonic concern about real problems causing distress), phobias (avoidant behavior associated with relief of distress), delusions (in which the content is ego syntonic), and brain damage (in which the OCS do not have intellectual content or intentional qualities and tend to be stereotypic and mechanical).

The clinical papers by Lewis (1936), Rachman and Hodgson (1980), and Hoogduin (1986) seem to us to capture the qualitative essence of OCD in clinical patients, whereas studies, frequently done by researchers without clinical experience, include isolated OCS symptoms, together with secondary symptoms of anxiety, depression, aggression, etc., which may include items from factor analyses, (see description of the Obsessive-Compulsive Scale in the CBCL as an example) and are more epiphenomena rather than the essence of OCD. Some of these difficulties are illustrated in an otherwise sophisticated paper by Pauls et al. (1986b). The authors begin their paper on "Gilles de la Tourette's Syndrome and Obsessive-Compulsive Disorder" by stating: "Gilles de la Tourette anecdotally reported an association between recurrent motor and phonic tics and obsessive-compulsive behaviors. He described a patient who suffered from tics and vocalizations as well as obsessive thoughts that 'tormented' her. He wrote that 'the more tormented she becomes by fear that she will say them again; and this obsession forces these words into her mind and to the tip of her tongue.' " However, our translation reads quite differently: "It is that the more they seem revolting by their vulgarity, the more she is tormented by the fear of mouthing them and that this preoccupation is precisely what puts them on the tip of her tongue when she cannot master it anymore." The statement, in fact, should not be attributed to Tourette since he is quoting the Marquise du Dampierre's explanation for her coprolalia, and the terms *obsessive-compulsive behavior*, *obsessive thoughts*, and *obsessions* are not used by either the Marquise or Tourette. These misquotations illustrate the different interpretations as well as the looseness and vague definitions for obsessions and compulsions that characterize much of the literature on OCD in Tourette's disorder.

Moreover, we would not classify as an obsession the Marquise's concern about erupting with involuntary coprolalia and suspect that the Marquise would concur that it is a real concern, which is "connected in a realistic way with what it is designed to neutralize or prevent" and is not clearly excessive (DSM-III-R). The authors also do not quote in their criteria for a compulsion the statement in DSM-III that "The behavior is not an end in itself, but is designed to produce or prevent some future event or situation." This characteristic is an important clinical criterion for differentiating a compulsion from a tic, since a tic is a thing in itself and a compulsion is done for a purpose, usually an intended action to prevent a dreaded future event. Omitting this characteristic may increase the number of patients cited as having OCD. In addition, in another publication describing the same study "Obsessional and compulsive symptoms" are described as "involuntary" (Pauls et al., 1986c). DSM-III describes an obsession as "they are experienced as voluntarily produced" and a compulsion as an "act" which is performed. DSM-III-R makes explicit that a compulsion is "intentional behavior." The lack of precise criteria for differentiating compulsions and tics could further increase the percentage of patients and relatives reported as having OCD.

A further indication of a very broad array of symptoms that would be classified by the authors as OCD is the description of three cases. In case A, thoughts of touching objects and person, a frequent Tourette's disorder symptom, is referred to as obsessional. Other symptoms, since they were done until they felt "just right" rather than to avoid a dreaded future event, would be classified by us as Tourette's disorder impulsions (see Chapter 10). We have cited many other studies which classify many typical Tourette's disorder symptoms as compulsions. If we are correct in our differentiation between Tourette's disorder symptoms and OCS, it would mean that many Tourette's disorder symptoms are being classified OCS, which would erroneously inflate the frequency of OCS, whereas, in fact, the cited OCSs are merely another way of describing Tourette's disorder symptoms.

In addition, the symptoms in case B are largely compulsive personality characteristics. Other sources of difficulty in this study include the use of TSA volunteers, no data about the reliability of diagnoses, and the failure to use a blindly evaluated control group to eliminate bias and to evaluate the frequency of OCS in the population.

If all of these sources of error were adequately controlled, we would predict that OCD and probably OCS would not be significantly higher, or only slightly but unimportantly higher in Tourette's disorder patients compared with an adequate control sample.

In our opinion all published studies have similar problems and shortcomings. We use the Paul et al. study (1986a–c) to illustrate these possible problems because it is an important and otherwise sophisticated study.

Impulsions

Stimulated by reports in the literature of OCS in Tourette's disorder, we began to collect responses to OCS items in our patients (see Chapter 2 for description and Table A.1 for list of items). Patients or informants rated items on a four-point scale. During the intake evaluation, these ratings were carefully reviewed and corrected because many responses included typical tic symptoms such as touching objects, self, or others, stereotypic movements, mannerisms, habits, and so on. Eight of the items are listed in Table 6.7. Ratings of "pretty much" or "very much" are considered significant. Although from 9 to 25% rated OCS (first four items in Table 6.7) as "pretty much" or "very much," these ratings are not significantly different from the control group for three of the items, and are actually significantly lower ($p < 0.01$) than the control group for "touching." Although the items are not exactly equivalent, four of 11 compulsive (personality) traits occur more frequently among Tourette's disorder than control subjects.

Initially, we were surprised that so many patients had OCS-like symptoms. However, as we conducted our informal survey, we were equally impressed with how many of our colleagues and friends had similar symptoms. Our impression that these symptoms are more common in the population than previously thought is supported by the frequency reported for the control sample (Table 6.7).

Secondly, as we evaluated patients, we concluded that the symptoms were phenomenologically different from tics and clinically different from the pathological symptoms characterizing psychiatric patients with OCD. Tourette's disorder patients describe symptoms such as repeatedly (two to eight times usually) opening and shutting light switches, turning television knobs on and off, checking doors, touching various objects or parts of their bodies, lining up the corners of a room and so on. Patients describe these symptoms as different from their tics because they are intended or voluntary acts, whereas their tics are involuntary. Subjectively, they have a need to repeat the act a certain number of times until a feeling of satisfaction is achieved, and they experience only mild discomfort if prevented from doing so. Resistance is mild and interference with functioning is unusual. Moreover, unlike compulsions associated with OCD, the behavior is not associated with or designed to neutralize or prevent a future dreaded event from occurring.

These symptoms that we refer to as impulsions do not fulfill the criteria for OCD in DSM-III or DSM-III-R. Some of the clinical features suggest to us that these obsessive-compulsive-like symptoms or impulsions may be associated with Tourette's disorder, and respond, unlike the symptoms of OCD, to treatment with neuroleptics. This possibility, however, has to be modified because their frequency in the population is unknown, and they may be no more frequent than that in the general population.

The failure to clarify the precise nature of these symptoms, the absence of criteria for their identification and the failure to differentiate them from classical compulsions and tics may be responsible for the high percentage of OCD reported in Tourette's disorder.

Thus, for clarity, to reduce the confusion in the literature about OCD, OCS, and obsessive-compulsive-like symptoms and for heuristic purposes, we propose that these obsessive-compulsive-like symptoms be referred to, as impulsions, as did Charcot and Tourette (1885); and Meige and Feindel (1907). We use the term as defined in the Hinsie and Campbell (1970) *Psychiatric Dictionary:* "A stimulus that sets the mind in action. The stimulus may originate in (1) the objective world, or (2) the subject himself: (a) his soma-within or any part of the body; (b) his psyche, its conscious or its unconscious part. In psychoanalysis, the term impulse most commonly refers to the instincts; a basic impulse is an instinct, the source of which is a 'somatic process in an organ or part of the body.' " It has also been defined as "an application of sudden force causing action" in the *Oxford English Dictionary* (1971) "an influence acting usually unexpectedly or temporarily on the mind or will and urging action" in *Webster's Dictionary* (1961).

PSYCHOMETRIC AND NEUROPSYCHOLOGICAL TESTING

Formal assessment techniques of brain behavior relationships in Tourette's disorder were largely confined in the past to the use of standard psychometric and projective test batteries. Neuropsychological assessment techniques were not commonly used. The standard assessment battery usually consisted of the WISC or the WAIS, the BGT, Rorschach Inkblot Test, Thematic Apperception Test, and other projective techniques. In 1965, when we began our studies of Tourette's disorder, we routinely administered these tests as part of our intake procedure as did most clinics. Although these tests were not designed primarily to measure brain dysfunction, some researchers believed they were sensitive to cerebral damage. In fact, Piotrowski (1937) had established ratings scales for projective tests to measure brain damage, and Wechsler (1944) looked at the differential scores among the subtests of the WAIS to study brain function. These tests were used because they provided us with the opportunity to compare our results with other studies that used a similiar battery to test patients with tics or Tourette's disorder. Later studies reviewed subsequently in this chapter replaced this battery with neuropsychological tests which are alleged to provide more specific indices of CNS impairment.

Psychometric Tests

Review of the Literature

Piotrowsky (1945) administered the Rorschach to 12 children with tics. The findings were generally descriptive, characterizing the children as being unable to integrate many experiences, and experiencing psychological insults with undesirable effects. The maturation process of these children varied considerably. Neurotic anxiety was marked, as was a general lag in individual initiative. Although Piotrowski had developed a number of "signs" that could be identified and used to diagnose brain lesions, his report was primarily clinical, possibly due to the overwhelming belief at that time that tics were a psychological manifestation and should be studied on a purely psychological basis (Piotrowski, 1937).

The first study to identify CNS correlates in children with Tourette's disorder was by Lucas et al. (1967). Fifteen children with Tourette's disorder were tested with an IQ Test, the BGT, and projective drawing tests. The range of intellectual functioning varied from 85 to 146. A mean IQ could not be calculated because not all patients were given the WISC. Five patients had no signs of encephalopathy, four patients were rated as having suggestive signs of encephalopathy, and four had definite signs such as poor motor control, directional confusion, rotation, size discrepancy, tremors, and poor impulse control. The projective drawings for this group were rigid, unanimated, and perseverative. The four subjects with suggestive signs showed poor utilization of space, poor planning, and immaturity. Thus, 53% of the sample had definite to highly suggestive signs of encephalopathy on the BGT. Handwriting was also grossly impaired. A further analysis was based on the severity and nature of the learning problems. Nine children (60%) were judged to have moderate to severe learning deficits. These deficits included distractability, low frustration tolerance, marked difficulty in conceptualization, and abstraction and difficulty in shifting. They were noted to have poor handwriting and to be clumsy and poorly coordinated. The psychological test findings and school functioning for some of the children showed definite evidence of mild brain damage. A close correlation was found between the ratings of encephalopathy and school difficulties. These children were characterized as having low frustration tolerance, distractibility, and poor impulse control, behaviors which are part of the diagnostic criteria for ADD. Therefore, it is possible that the CNS deficits and psychopathology might be related to the presence of ADD in these children. Descriptively, many of these children appear to fulfill the criteria for ADD, and as noted elsewhere, the presence of CNS deficits is highly associated with a secondary diagnosis of ADD.

A major limitation of the Lucas at al. (1967) study, the Corbett study (to be discussed subsequently), as well as our studies, was the use of tests that were not designed to identify brain damage or specific deficits associated with brain damage. In addition, except for our study, the results were not contrasted with a control sample. Nonetheless, they were important in demonstrating neurological correlates of Tourette's disorder and in stimulating research on CNS factors in these patients.

Corbett et al. (1969) reported a mean WISC IQ score of 94.4 (SD 17.5) for 82 children with tics, only some of whom had Tourette's disorder. These patients were attending the Maudsley Hospital of the Brixton Child Guidance Clinic. Some children were tested with the Stanford-Binet instead of the WISC. The mean converted score on the Binet for 62 children was 105.7 (SD 17.5). The mean IQ for the combined score was 98.8 (SD 18.2), not significantly different from the total clinic population. These scores are in agreement with our findings that the intelligence of children with tics and Tourette's disorder is in the average range. Patients were divided into a primary group of 18 subjects in whom the tics were the presenting complaint, and a secondary group in whom the tics were secondary to other complaints. The secondary group had a lower overall IQ score, Verbal IQ (VIQ) score, and Performance IQ (PIQ) score than the primary group, but all scores were within the average intellectual range. No significant differences were reported in either group between the VIQ and PIQ scores. A significantly higher coding subtest score was achieved by the primary group than by a control group. Habit disorders, such as disorders of defecation, speech, and gratification, were significantly higher in the tic group compared to a hospital sample; conduct disorders, such as temper and aggression, truanting and wandering, and fighting, were significantly higher in the hospital sample; neurotic and psychic symptoms, such as depression, were higher in the hospital group than among the tic patients, but obsessional symptoms and hypochondriasis were higher among the latter. Although obsessional symptoms were significantly more common in the tic group, the percentage was still comparatively low (only 12.5%). The increase of speech disorders in the tic group is not surprising since speech difficulties are a symptom found in some patients with tics (Wagner, 1970; Ludlow et al., 1982).

Ferrari et al. (1984) studied ten medication-free Tourette's disorder children of average intellectual functioning using a more extended battery. Fifty percent of the children had a 15-point discrepancy score between the VIQ-PIQ scores, and two children had a discrepancy score greater than 34 points. Low arithmetic scores were also recorded on the Wide Range Achievement Test (WRAT) and BGT scores were 23 months below expected levels. The authors concluded that the findings represent a dysfunction of visual-perceptual skills, which confirmed our results (Shapiro et al., 1978).

Our early studies were designed to test the hypothesis that Tourette's disorder was a CNS disorder, and as discussed in the first section of this chapter, to test commonly held beliefs about underlying psychological factors in Tourette's disorder. In our initial study we administered the WAIS or WISC, BGT, Rorschach, and MMPI to 30 patients with Tourette's disorder (Shapiro et al., 1972a, 1973c). The correlation between the ratings of two psychologists for organicity was 0.96 on the BGT, 0.87 for the Rorschach, and 1.00 for an overall rating of organicity using all the tests. Discrepancies between VIQs and PIQs were significantly higher in the Tourette's disorder sample than for a normal standardized population for the WAIS; 80% had mild to marked ratings of organicity on the BGT, and 76.7% (23 patients) had abnormalities on the overall rating of organicity.

Our initial study was replicated subsequently using blind evaluations and a control group. The sample consisted of 50 patients diagnosed as having Tourette's disorder and 50 psychiatric outpatients, matched for age, sex, and IQ (Shapiro et al., 1978). Two senior Ph.D. psychologists blindly rated the protocols using various measures of organicity and a third judge with extensive clinical experience in the rating of organicity, using clinical judgment alone, rated each record as organic or nonorganic. An overall rating of the degree of organicity based on the WAIS or WISC and BGT ratings was used. The results for all raters strongly supported the hypothesis that subjects with Tourette's disorder had more organic deficits than a matched group of psychiatric outpatients. In addition, 50% of the Tourette patients compared to 14.0% of the controls had a significant discrepancy of 15 points or more between VIQ and PIQ scores on the WAIS or WISC ($\chi^2 = 25$, df-3, $p = 0.0001$) (Table 6.10).

Current Study

After completion of the previously described studies we discontinued routine administration of projective tests. We did, however, collect and tabulate the results of projective tests done elsewhere. With time, the number of patients given these tests dwindled. Limitations of the current study include absence of blind ratings, evaluation of reliability, and the recognition that since these tests are given more frequently to patients with suspected ADD, learning disorders (LD) and other CNS damage, the patient sample would include a disproportionate number of such patients. For example, ADD or LD or both were present in 65% of patients given the BGT, and 82% given the WISC or WAIS. It would be expected, therefore, that these groups would elevate the scores for the total sample in contrast to scores achieved by a sample of TS-alone patients. We hypothesized that a high percentage of patients with ADD would artifactually elevate organic findings. We analyzed our results by separating the total sample into three samples: TS-alone, TS+ADD, and TS+ADD or LD. Our hypothesis was that the TS-alone group would have significantly lower indices of organicity than the TS+ADD group, and would not be significantly different from expectations in the population (see Table 6.10.)

Bender-Gestalt test

Ratings of the BGT for 165 subjects, summarized in Table 6.9, were again abnormal in 48% of the total sample, similar to the results for our first 50 patients. However, as expected, organic abnormalities were significantly higher in the TS+ADD group (63%) than for the TS-alone group (29%) ($\chi^2 = 3.7$, df-3, $p < 0.05$) (Table 6.9). For 56 with ratings on LD or ADD, 55% had organic signs on the BGT compared to 20% of the TS-alone group ($\chi^2 = 6.4$, df-2, $p < 0.05$).

TABLE 6.9. Bender-Gestalt Test Ratings

Study	Sample size N	Normal %	Borderline. abnormality %	Definite abnormality %
TS study (1965–1973)[a]				
TS sample	50	58	—	42
Control sample	50	84	—	16
TS study (1965–1981)[b]				
TS-alone	70	71	10	19
TS+ADD	95	37	14	50
Total	165	52	12	36
TS subsample[c]				
TS-alone	15	80	7	13
TS with ADD or LD[c]	56	45	7	48
Total	71	52	7	41

[a]$\chi^2 = 8.6$, df-1, $p < 0.02$.
[b]$\chi^2 = 3.7$, df-3, $p = 0.03$.
[c]TS subsample comprised 71 subjects who were both given the Bender-Gestalt Test and had ratings for learning disabilities (LD): $\chi^2 = 6.4$, df-2, $p < 0.05$.

Verbal-performance difference scores

Verbal-Performance Difference Scores (V-P), derived from the WISC and WAIS, which indicate CNS organic impairment, were available for 173 patients (Table 6.10). For the total sample, 40% had V-Ps of 15 or more points, slightly lower than the previous sample, but exceeding expectations of 12.5% in the population (Field, 1960). Similiar to the findings for the BGT, V-P scores equal to or over 15 were present in significantly fewer TS-alone (30%) than TS+ADD (47%) ($\chi^2 = 5.1$, df-1, $p = 0.024$). However, 30.1% with V-P scores exceeding > 15 in the TS-alone group is higher than the population estimate of 12.5%. Similar to the analysis for the BGT, 65 patients who had scores on the V-P and ratings for LD were dichotomized into those with ADD or LD and those with TS-alone (without ADD or LD). The V-P scores for the TS-alone group exceeded > 15 in only 10%, which is within population estimates ($\chi^2 = 0.1$, df-1, NS).

Wechsler intelligence scale for children

Analysis of the relationship of subtests on the WISC to diagnosis provides further support for our hypothesis. All subtests are negatively correlated with the diagnosis of TS-alone (or positively correlated with ADD), and scores for TS+ADD patients are significantly lower ($p < 0.10$–0.01) for 14 variables (Table 4.27).

TABLE 6.10. *Verbal-Performance Difference Scores*

Study	Sample size N	Verbal-Performance Difference Scores	
		<15%	≥15%
TS study (1965–1973)[a]			
TS sample	50	50	50
Control sample	50	86	14
TS study (1965–1981)[b]			
TS-alone	67	70	30
TS+ADD	106	53	47
Total	173	60	40
TS Subsample[c]			
TS-alone	10	90	10
TS+ADD+LD	55	64	36
Total	65	68	32
Standardization sample[d]	200	87	13

[a]$\chi^2 = 21.9$, df-2, $p = 0.0001$.
[b]$\chi^2 = 5.1$, df-2, $p = 0.024$.
[c]TS subsample comprised 65 subjects who were both given the Bender-Gestalt Test and had ratings for learning disabilities (LD): Fisher Exact Test $p = 0.097$
[d]Standardization sample (Field, 1960) compared with TS-alone (without ADD or LD) subsample, Fisher Exact Test, NS.

Conclusion

The importance of separating Tourette's disorder samples based on the presence or absence of ADD is particularly important when examining brain behavior relationships because children with ADD often have specific developmental disorders,, nonlocalized soft neurological signs, motor-perceptual dysfunctions, and EEG abnormalities. Academic difficulties are common and often result in school failure (DSM-III, American Psychiatric Association, 1980). Thus, consistent with all of our analyses, it is apparent that organic indices from psychometric tests are largely due to the Tourette's disorder group with ADD, LD, and possibly other CNS impairment. An important general question is whether some of the psychological test findings, and specifically which ones, are possibly related to Tourette's disorder samples without other indications of CNS impairment. If CNS impairment is associated with Tourette's disorder, it should be present in all patients. But potential specific CNS impairment in Tourette's disorder may be obscured by the results from patients with other CNS disorders which are not primarily associated with Tourette disorder. Future study warrants study of homogeneous Tourette's disorder patients and the use of more specific, reliable and valid psychological tests. The next section describes studies using recently introduced neuropsychological tests, with the potential for greater specificity of identifying neurological impairment.

Neuropsychological Tests

The development of test batteries to evaluate brain function in individual patients gave impetus to the study of CNS factors in Tourette's disorder. These batteries allegedly identify critical areas of brain dysfunction or damage (Reitan, 1975). The Halstead-Reitan Neuropsychological Battery (HRNB), for example, was designed for this purpose. The HRNB has been used to detect differences in neuropsychological functioning in patients with and without cerebral damage and to evaluate the differential effect of damage to the right and left hemispheres. The majority of studies to be discussed used the HRNB, the WRAT, Wechsler IQ tests (WISC or WAIS), the BGT, and other tests of motor and perceptual functioning.

Sand (1972) administered the HRNB to detect cerebral impairment in a single 9-year-old boy with Tourette's disorder. No indication of cerebral impairment was found and the subject performed well on tests that required motor, problem solving, and eye-hand coordination. Logue (1973) also tested a single 11-year-old boy with the HRNB. Test results indicated chronic diffuse cerebral dysfunction specifically in high level cognitive areas. Specific deficits were reported on the Category Test, Trail Making Test, and on Tactual

TABLE 6.11. CNS deficits in patients with tics and Tourette's disorder

Study	Battery	Patients	Ages (years)	IQ	Organic deficits
Lucas et al. (1967)	IQ, Bender, Projective drawing	15	11–29	Average	8/13 (Visuopractic)
Corbett et al. (1969)	IQ, Clinical interview	180	Maj < 18	Average range	No organicity except for V-P IQ discrepency
Wagner (1970)	WISC, Bender, Rorschach, DAP	1	9	Average range	
Shapiro et al. (1972a, 1973)	IQ, Bender, Rorschach	30	8–64	Average range	11/30 (Visuopractic)
Sand (1972)	WISC, Halstead-Reitan, WRAT, Bender-Gestalt	1	10	Average range	No significant organicity
Logue et al. (1973)	Reitan, Neuropsychological Battery	1	11	Borderline	Chronic diffuse organicity (visuopractic and memory)
Shapiro et al. (1978)	IQ, Bender, Rorschach, MMPI	50	6–64	Average range	25/50 (Visuopractic)
Thompson et al. (1979)	WAIS, Halstead-Reitan Neuropsychological Battery	4	7–34	Borderline to average range	3/4 (Visuopractic) 2/4 (Language)
Incagnoli and Kane (1982)	WISC, Halstead-Reitan, Bender-Gestalt, WRAT	13	10–13	Average range	2/13 (Visuopractic)
Sutherland et al. (1982)	WAIS, WISC, tests of speech lateralization, memory, visual perception, spatial orientation, frontal lobe, language	32	Most < 14	Average range	(Visuopractic, memory, language)
Hagins et al. (1982)	WISC-R, Woodcock Johnson, Learning Disorders Unit Neuropsychological Battery	10	7–13	Average range	(Visuopractic)
Joschko and Rourke (1982)	WISC, WRAT, Halstead-Reitan Neuropsychological Battery	3	8–10	Average Range	2/3 (Language and memory)
Plaisted et al. (1983)	Luria Nebraska Neuropsychological Battery	9	13–20	Average range	3/9 (Impaired visuopractic)
Bornstein et al. (1985)	WISC-R, Halstead-Reitan, WRAT, Peabody, Knox Cube, Groved Pegboard	7	9–15	Borderline to average range	V-P IQ Discrepancies (Visuopractic deficits)
Ferrari et al. (1984)	WISC-R, Bender, WRAT DAP, Piers-Harris	10	7–14	Average range	5/10 (Visuopractic)
Current study	IQ, Bender, V-P Difference Scores	173	6–64	Average range	50/106 with TS+ADD (Visuopractic)

Performance Test using the left hand. Also bilateral errors were made when the subject was asked to identify numbers written on the fingertips and finger agnosia with the left hand.

Incagnoli and Kane (1982, 1983) tested 13 male Tourette's disorder subjects between the ages of 10 and 13 using the WISC-R, BGT, WRAT, and HRNB. Four subjects had significant VIQ-PIQ difference scores. Scores on the WRAT indicated significant impairment of the arithmetic subtest. Visual-motor discrepancies scores showed significant impairment on visual-motor tasks involving the copy of designs. On the HRNB there was no evidence of generalized cerebral dysfunction. However, the scores of one child were in the brain-damaged range and another was classified as learning-disabled. They concluded that the overall pattern represented a dysfunction of nonconstructional visuopractic abilities. Although only a small number of the subjects in this study had cerebral impairment on the HRNB, specific disabilities were identified in the majority of the patients, specifically perceptual difficulties of a visuoconstructive type. No information was provided about the number of subjects with TS+ADD.

Joschko and Rourke (1982) attempted to demonstrate a specific pattern of deficits in the HRNB battery in three children with TS. Again the results indicated individual disabilities but none of the subjects had specific brain deficits. There was evidence of information-processing deficiencies in one subject who demonstrated problems in sustained attention, immediate auditory-verbal memory, verbal fluency, and phenomi-grapheme matching. Another child had a 24-point discrepancy between V-P IQ scores on the WISC-R but the neuropsychological test did not indicate brain impairment. Arithmetic scores on the WRAT were also depressed. Although conclusions cannot be drawn from the small sample size, the pattern of deficits in at least one subject was consistent with previous studies (Shapiro et al., 1978; Incagnoli and Kane, 1982).

Bornstein et al. (1985) administered the HRNB and other tests including the WISC-R and the WRAT to seven male patients with Tourette's disorder between the ages of 9 and 15. Many of the patients were described as being distractible, having poor concentration, and doing messy or incomplete homework, but only one patient had a diagnosis of ADD+H. The average IQ was lower than the group reported by Shapiro et al. (1978). Four of seven patients had at least a ten-point discrepancy between the V-P IQs, with three having a 15-point discrepancy, similar to the frquency reported by Shapiro et al. (1978). Abnormal scores were reported on several measures of the HRNB in more than half of the subjects: Category Test, Trail-Making Test (part b), Tactual Performance Test (Time), and fingertip writing (both hands). Only one subject obtained an impairment index indicating cerebral dysfunction. On the WRAT, low arithmetic scores were obtained by the majority of subjects, and impairment was found on tests that tapped nonverbal visual and/or motor skills. The pattern of nonverbal and visuospatial deficits according to the authors implicate the right cerebral hemisphere, or a diffuse subcortical disturbance, with behavioral deficits more consistent with the right than the left hemisphere. Although not totally confirming of right hemisphere dysfunction, the findings are consistent with other previously described reports.

Similar deficits were reported by Sutherland et al. (1982) using the Montreal Neurological Institute Battery. Thirty-two medicated Tourette's disorder patients were compared to 47 learning-disabled subjects and 30 schizophrenic subjects. Neuropsychological impairment was demonstrated in children and adults with Tourette's disorder compared to the control subjects: impaired performance IQ for subjects 9 years of age or older, deficits in memory and copying of visually presented nonverbal material, reduced verbal fluency, and short-term memory for stories.

Conclusion

Although by no means definitive, the weight of the evidence suggests that patients with Tourette's disorder have a wide variety of disabilities and that many of them perform poorly on tests which tap visual-perceptual abilities, suggesting possible right hemisphere involvement (Lucas et al., 1967; Logue et al., 1973; Shapiro et al., 1978; Thompson et al., 1979; Incagnoli and Kane, 1982; Sutherland et al., 1982; Harcherik et al., 1982; Bornstein et al., 1985; Ferrari et al., 1984). However, a significant number also have academic and learning disabilities without firm evidence of basic CNS pathology. Limitations of these studies include inadequate evidence for the reliability and validity of neuropsychologic tests, failure to specify whether patients were medicated, absence of appropriate control groups, and inclusion of an unknown number of subjects with ADD, LD, and other CNS impairment.

SPEECH AND LANGUAGE

Despite the presence of vocal tics, surprisingly few studies of speech and language development have been done. Frank (1978) conducted a psycholinguistic study of videotaped interviews of three Tourette subjects. Vocal tics occurred in the pauses and the length of pauses was greater than in normal speech. Patients tended to have tics before clauses and not within words. A similar finding on position of vocal tics was reported by Ludlow et al. (1982). Ludlow et al. (1982) tested 54 consecutive Tourette's disorder patients and 54 normal subjects matched for age and sex using measures of speech production or verbal fluency and the Neurosensory Center Comprehensive Examination for Aphasia. Tourette's disorder subjects spoke significantly less than controls and produced most of their tics while speaking at the beginning, end, or less frequently, during speech clause production. The groups differed in the type of vocal tics, with the Tourette's disorder subjects producing significantly more laryngeal than lingual tics. Neither the speech nor language component of Tourette patients appear to correlate with motor tic symptomatology. Vocal tics were characterized as nonverbal and verbal (jargon, coprolalia, word production, palilalia, and stereotypic phrases). Although normal subjects had nonverbal tics, only two had verbal tics, whereas 35% of Toruette's disorder subjects had verbal tics. The authors suggest that coprolalia involves both the cortical system, which provides control of the production of speech and language behavior, and an older system, which terminates in the cingulate gyrus (See Chapter 4 for other possible explanations).

CONCLUSION

The problem of neuroanatomic localization has important implications for the pathogenesis of Tourette's disorder. The neuropsychological studies reviewed in this chapter report equivocal fundings. Although the evidence suggests right hemisphere localization, there is some evidence of possible left hemisphere dysfunction. In addition, impairment of verbal fluency and speech implicate several areas of the brain. The findings also suggest that there is a subgroup of Tourette's patients who have neurological and behaviorial impairment. The heterogeneity of the findings makes it difficult to specify a particular neuroanatomical loci. Moreover, the results from all of the reviewed studies are confounded by inclusion of subjects with ADD, hyperactivity, learning, and other CNS disorders. Meaningful future research and progress requires study of a TS-alone group, as well as a separate group with CNS disorders.

7

Neurology

This chapter reviews the neurological data in the literature relevant to Tourette's disorder and describes the results of our current studies: post-mortem studies, review of tic-like symptoms associated with other disorders (genetic and familial syndromes, neurological disorders, dystonias, choreas, hyperekplexias, acquired CNS pathology, perinatal complications, developmental disorders, neuroleptic-induced movement disorder, and other disorders), the effect of treatment interventions (neurosurgery, pharmacotherapy), neurological examination, and studies of the electroencephalogram (EEG), evoked potentials, premovement potential, computerized axial tomography (CAT), position emission tomography (PET), and magnetic resonance imaging (MRI), and sleep and arousal studies.

POST-MORTEM STUDIES

Unfortunately, only three cases of Tourette's disorder, uncomplicated by other disorders known to be associated with CNS pathology, have been described in the literature (Richardson, 1982). Bing (1925) described a patient with multiple tics whose brain on gross examination revealed meningeal thickening, but microscopic examination was not performed. De Wulf and Van Bogaert (1940) reported negative gross and microscopic findings in a patient with Tourette's disorder. A well-documented patient with Tourette's disorder was reported by Clauss and Balthasar (1954) and Balthasar (1956). A male patient developed facial tics and continuous asymmetric choreic movements of the face, neck, and shoulders between 3 and 6 years of age. The movements remitted until the age of 10 years at which time the patient developed rapid abnormal movement of the head, limbs, and feet. Subsequent symptoms included movements of the face and tongue, vocal tics, and coprolalia. On autopsy, the brain had a normal appearance, but microscopic examination revealed mild meningitic inflammation, focal neuronal loss in the third and fifth cortical layers, and a small area of neuronal loss in the medial thalamus. The main finding, however, was an increase in the number of small neurons in the caudate and putamen. Because of its similarity to the histology of the normal early developing brain, Balthasar (1956) suggested that Tourette's disorder might be caused by a developmental arrest or anomaly of the corpus striatum. A fourth autopsy described a 9-year-old boy with severe mental retardation and hyperactivity who had multiple motor and vocal tics and nontic symptoms such as teeth-grinding, head-banging, rocking movements, and tongue-biting (Borak, 1969). Bilateral cryothalamotomies were done which led to some improvement of the tics, but not of the self-aggressive tendencies. One of two EEG's were abnormal, and a pneumoencephalogram showed marked dilation of the left lateral ventricle, rounding of the upper-lateral cornis, and slight dilation of the third ventricle. The post-mortem changes were extensive, and many of the findings were related to or consistent with the patient's mental retardation, previous infectious diseases, or to postoperative changes.

An additional post-mortem has been reported recently by Haber et al. (1986). A 57-year-old male with a diagnosis of St. Vitus' dance without evidence of rheumatic fever, had multiple psychiatric hospitalizations, and chronic hospitalizations for most of his life. He was treated with multiple neuroleptics such as haloperidol, thioridazine, perphenazine, methylphenidate. At age 52 he received electric convulsive treatment and surgery for hypernephroma which metastasized to the lungs and led to his death at age 57. He had a documented diagnosis of Tourette's disorder with motor, vocal, and coprolalic tics but no family history of tic disorder, although his father developed parkinsonism late in life. Post-mortem examination was performed on the left half of the brain. The external appearance of the brain was normal on gross examination. There was a focally destructive lesion in the inferior parietal gyrus and a 2-mm slit-like defect in the medial putamen. The temporal horn was enlarged. On microscopic examination, a lesion of the occipitotemporal gyrus consisted of gliosis of Sommer's sector of the hippocampus and a focal lesion in the subiculum. A large region of the superior head of the caudate was pale, vasculated, and cavitated. Multiple cavitated lesions were present in the cerebellar cortex, cerebral cortex, caudate, and putamen, which were attributed to emboli.

Immunohistochemical studies included determination of the distribution of enkephalin-like (ELI), dynorphin-like (DLI), and substance-P-like (SPI) immunoreactivity in the globus pallidus and subtantia nigra, where they are most highly concentrated in the normal brain, and the regional distribution of acetylcholinesterase (AChE). The result for the patient with Tourette's disorder was contrasted with a group of patients with Huntington's chorea. ELI, SPI, and AChE were normally distributed in all regions of the brain of the patient with Tourette's disorder, but DLI stained lighter and was totally absent in the globus pallidus. For patients with Huntington's chorea, ELI, SPI, and DLI stained lighter than normal in the basal ganglia, although some DLI was present in the globus pallidus. The authors suggest that diminished DLI might be specific for Tourette's disorder.

Several problems are associated with the interpretation of these results. The extensive pathology in the caudate and putamen, and changes in the globus pallidus might have been due to secondary infarction of these structures. The authors argue, however, that the lesions in the caudate and putamen were small and would not account for the loss of DLI, especially because of the normal distribution for ELI and SPI. Another problem is the history of extensive use of neuroleptic drugs which could have induced chronic changes in the brain. A third problem is that the multiple lesions could have been caused by embolic infarction, although an apparent source for the emboli was not found. Although a cardiac cause should be considered, the patient's cardiac history and status were not described and a general autopsy was not done. Basilar artery plaques were seen, but rheumatic heart disease was not eliminated as a possible source of the emboli. The patient might have had Sydenham's chorea as a child, having had a diagnosis of St. Vitus' dance and a history of many choreiform symptoms, which could alter the morphology and biochemistry of the brain.

Although the results are difficult to interpret because of the complicated clinical and treatment history and post-mortem findings, the absence of dynorphin-like immunoreactivity in the globus pallidus is interesting and warrants further study. Verification might include determination of peptide levels in the CSF and other neuropathological studies.

Autopsy studies are obviously very important for study of the anatomy and etiology of Tourette's disorder. Current techniques, not available in the past, include measurement of neurotransmitters in various brain areas. Although approximately a half-dozen brains have become available for study during the past 22 years, preparation was inadequate and the results were inconclusive. The paucity of post-mortem studies has led to many other, usually indirect, methods of studying the etiology of Tourette's disorder.

TIC-LIKE SYMPTOMS ASSOCIATED WITH OTHER DISORDERS

Numerous reports in the literature describe tic-like symptoms that are associated primarily or secondarily with diverse disorders. Because the movements in these patients appear to us as different from the classical tics of Tourette's disorder and since careful criteria for differentiating tics from other movements have not been established (see Chapter 10), we refer heuristically to the movements as tic-like symptoms rather than tics. Despite many differences between these disorders and Tourette's disorder, the similarity of some of the movements to tics warrant further study and may provide leads about the underlying neuropathology of Tourette's disorder.

Perinatal Complications and Developmental Disorders

Numerous examples can be found in the literature of types of motor, vocal complex, corprophilic, and echophilic symptoms that are linked to birth trauma, asphyxia, infections, and other perinatal complications (Baker, 1962; Weingarten, 1968; Marra et al., 1980; Golden and Greenhill, 1981; Burd and Kerbeshian, 1985; Kerbeshian and Burd, 1986) or idiopathic developmental disorders of infancy and early childhood (Barr et al., 1972; Realmuto and Main, 1982; Barabas and Matthews, 1983; Shaenboen et al., 1984) (Table 7.1). The diversity of the clinical reports indicates that they occur more frequently than generally assumed. These symptoms, usually stereotypic, or other atypical movements, differ from the classical tics of Tourette's disorder in many ways and are frequently associated with seizure disorders, behavior disorders, or obvious neurological dysfunction. We have evaluated many patients with these symptoms but in our opinion the symptoms do not resemble the tics observed in Tourette's disorder. Moreover, abnormal perinatal and developmental disorders are within the normal range for our sample (see Chapter 4, Table 4.14).

Genetic and Familial Syndromes

A small group of patients with known or assumed genetic abnormalities, frequently with other neurological disorders, physical anomalies, autism, mental deficiency, specific neurological and other organic symptoms, have motor or vocal tic-like symptoms (Merskey, 1974; Singh et al., 1982; Lewis and Bertorini, 1982; Kerbeshian et al., 1984 (Table 7.2).

Neurological Disorders

Numerous neurological disorders include motor or vocal tic-like symtoms which can be differentiated from Tourette's disorder clinically and etiologically (Table 7.3). For example, tics can occur in patients with myoclonic or choreic hyperkinesias. Some of these disorders are clearly distinguishable from Tourette's disorder based on age of onset, specific inheritance pattern or family history, predominance of an abnormal movement other than tics, associated neurological features, and laboratory or CAT scan findings.

Hallervorden-Spatz Disease

Hallervorden-Spatz Disease is a rare familial disorder that begins in childhood or adolescence. Although dystonic and occasionally bizarre posturing occur, associated rigidity and ataxia make the differential diagnosis from

TABLE 7.1. Tic-like symptoms associated with developmental disorders or perinatal insult

Study	Suspected etiology	Neurological status	Tic symptoms	Associated features
Baker (1962)	Birth trauma	Psychomotor retardation	Motor, vocal	Seizure disorder
Weingarten (1968)	Perinatal complications	Diffuse spasticity	Motor, vocal	Torticollis
Barr et al. (1972)	Idiopathic	Spasticity lower extremities, talipes equinovarus deformity, mental retardation	Facial motor, vocal coprolalia	—
Marra et al. (1980)	Premature birth	Left hemiparesis, spastic athetoid cerebral palsy	Complex and simple motor, vocal, compulsive behavior, coprolalia	Seizure disorder with focally irritative EEG, aggressive outbursts
Golden and Greenhill (1981)	Perinatal complications, congenital infection	Mental retardation, "soft signs" tremor, hyperreflexia	Simple and complex motor, vocal, coprolalia, echolalia	Psychosis, hyperactivity, aggressivity,
Realmuto and Main (1982)	Idiopathic	Pervasive developmental delay, right hyperreflexia bilateral extensor planter responses	Motor, vocal, echolalia	Moderate nonspecific diffuse EEG abnormality
Barabas and Matthews (1983)	Idiopathic	Pervasive developmental disorder	Simple motor, vocal	—
Shaenboen et al. (1984)	Colpocephaly	Psychomotor retardation	Motor, vocal	CT Scan: markedly enlarged occipital horns of lateral ventricles
Burd and Kerbeshian (1985)	Perinatal complications	Pervasive developmental delay, athetosis lower extremities, visual impairment	Simple and complex motor, vocal	Ganser syndrome, compulsive behavior

TABLE 7.2. *Tic-like symptoms associated with genetic or familial syndromes*

Study	Genetic abnormality or disorder	Syndromal features	Tic symptoms	Associated features
Merskey (1974)	XYY	—	Simple motor, vocal	Agressive behavior
Singh et al. (1982)	XXY and 9_p mosaicism	Multiple physical anomalies	Simple motor, vocal	Mental retardation
Lewis and Bartorini (1982)	Duchenne muscular dystrophy (X-linked recessive)	Muscular dystrophy	Motor, vocal	—
Kerbeshian et al. (1984)	Fragile X syndrome	Mental retardation, facial dysmorphism	Simple motor, vocal, coprolalia	Seizures, autistic features

Tourette's disorder a simple matter. Moreover, these patients may have leg wasting with pes cavus deformities, pigmentary retinal degeneration and optic atrophy, with multiple associated features which are not present in Tourette's disorder. CAT scanning may show caudate atrophy. Pathologically the disease is characterized by golden-brown discoloration of the medial segment of the globus pallidus, and to some extent of the red nucleus and substantia nigra. This discoloration is caused by the deposition of metals, especially iron, in the involved structures.

Wilson's Disease

Wilson's disease is an autosomal recessive disease caused by an inborn error of copper metabolism. It causes a wide range of abnormal movements, especially marked tremor localized in the arm when held in the outstretched position ("wing beating"). Rigidity and dystonia also occur. Spasms of laryngeal or pharyngeal muscles can produce bizarre vocalizations which can be confused with vocal tics. Other characteristics include neurologic signs, evidence of hepatic dysfunction, Kayser-Fleischer rings, and low levels of serum ceruloplasm with elevated urinary copper excretion. The disease causes widespread pathology, most conspicuously in the basal ganglia.

Hyperekplexias

The hyperekplexias are an infrequent group of heterogeneous disorders characterized by excessive startle reactions (Table 7.3). An unexpected auditory or tactile stimulus elicits excessive and sometimes violent motor reactions which frequently result in falls without loss of consciousness. Several geographically localized forms of the disorder have been described. The "jumping Frenchmen of Maine" is a form of hyperekplexia first described in French-Canadian lumberjacks (Beard, 1880; Stevens, 1964; Kunkle, 1967; Chapel, 1970; Saint-Hilaire et al., 1986). Some of these patients have symptoms of echolalia and echopraxia, features in common with Tourette's disorder but spontaneous tics are not present. Other forms include myriachit reported in Siberia (Hammond, 1884), and latah described in Malaysia and Indonesia (Aberle, 1952; Yap, 1952; Simons, 1980). These disorders, erroneously included within the rubric of Tourette's disorder by Gilles de la Tourette (Tourette, 1884, 1885), were correctly differentiated by Charcot (1885) shortly afterward (see Lees, 1985, for an excellent review of these disorders).

Other hyperekplexias

Other forms of hyperekplexia include a familial, autosomal dominant disorder associated with congenital hypertonia and nocturnal myoclonus (Suhren

TABLE 7.3. *Neurological disorders with tic-like symptoms*

Disease of syndrome	Age at onset	Associated features	Course	Predominant type of movements
Hallervorden-Spatz	Childhood–adolescence	May be associated with optic atrophy, club feet, retinitis pigmentosa, dysarthria, dementia, ataxia, emotional lability spasticity, autosomal recessive inheritance	Progressive to death in 5–20 years	Choreic, athetoid, myoclonic
Dystonia muscularum deformans	Childhood–adolescence	Autosomal recessive inheritance most common form, primarily among Ashkenazi Jews; a more benign autosomal dominant form also occurs	Variable course, often progressive but rare remissions	Dystonia
Sydenham's chorea	Childhood, usually 5–15 years	More common in females usually associated with rheumatic fever (carditis, elevated ASLO titers)	Usually self-limited	Choreiform
Huntington's chorea	Usually 30–50 years, but childhood forms are known	Autosomal dominant inheritance, dementia, caudate atrophy on CAT scan	Progressive to death 10–15 years after onset	Choreiform
Wilson's disease (hepatolenticular degeneration)	Usually 10–25 years	Kayser-Fleischer rings, liver dysfunction, inborn error of copper metabolism; autosomal recessive inheritance	Progression to death without chelating therapy	"Wing-beating" tremor, dystonia

Hyperekplexias (including latah, myriachit, jumping Frenchman of Maine)	Onset generally in childhood	Familial; may have generalized rigidity and autosomal dominant inheritance	Nonprogressive	Excessive startle response, may have echolalia, coprolalia, and forced obedience
Myoclonic disorders	Any age	Numerous etiologies, some familial, usually no vocalizations	Variable, depending on etiology	Myoclonus
Myoclonic dystonia	5–47 Years	Nonfamilial, no vocalizations	Nonprogressive	Torsion dystonia with myoclonic jerks
Paroxysmal myoclonic dystonia with vocalization	Childhood	Attentional, hyperactive and learning disorders; movements interfere with ongoing activity	Nonprogressive	Bursts of regular, repetitive clonic (less tonic) movements and vocalizations
"Tardive Tourette's syndromes"	Postantipsychotic medication use	May be precipitated by discontinuation or reduction in medication	May terminate after increase or decrease of dosage	Orofacial dyskinesias, choreoathetosis, tics, vocalization,
Neuroacanthocytosis	Third or fourth decade	Acanthocytosis, muscle wasting, parkinsonism, autosomal recessive inheritance	Variable	Orofacial-dyskinesia and limb chorea, tics, vocalization

et al, 1966; Andermann et al., 1980; Kurczynski, 1983), and a sporadic form of this disorder (Gastaut and Villeneuve, 1967) which becomes symptomatic in the second and third decades. The primary distinction from Tourette's disorder is that the symptoms are elicited by sudden stimuli.

Dystonia

Dystonia is a hyperkinesia characterized by increased and generally sustained contractions of antagonistic muscle groups. Pure dystonic posturing rarely resembles the fleeting movements of tics, but occasional confusion can occur if the dystonia is rhythmic or has superimposed jerks. The idiopathic dystonias of childhood are of two types, an autosomal recessive form which generally begins before adolescence and primarily occurs among Ashkenazi Jews, and an autosomal dominant form with later age of onset and unclear predilection. The typical dystonic nature of the symptoms and family history should clarify the differential diagnosis. These disorders should be differentiated from dystonic-like symptoms associated with the sensory tic subtype of Tourette's disorder (see Chapter 10).

Chorea

Choreic movements are brief, random, arrhythmic, jerky involuntary movements that are slower than myoclonic movements. Patients often attempt to incorporate the abnormal movements into ongoing normal activity in an effort to make them less noticeable. Patients often cannot maintain the tongue in a protruded position ("jack-in-the-box tongue") or maintain continuous pressure of the grasping hand ("milkmaid grip").

Sydenham's Chorea

Sydenham's chorea usually is a self-limited choreic syndrome, thought to be a manifestation of rheumatic fever. There is evidence that antibodies to antigens on the group A streptococcal membrane cross-react with structures in the basal ganglia, suggesting a possible etiology for this disorder. The movements of Sydenham's chorea are increased with voluntary actions and the symptoms are choreic and not stereotypic.

Huntington's Chorea

Huntington's Chorea is an autosomal dominant disorder which generally begins in mid-life but can occasionally occur in childhood. The latter group tends to have prominent rigidity which differentiates the disorder from Tourette's disorder. Other diagnostic clues include a change in personality and prominent dementia. The CAT scan may show the characteristic ventricular enlargement and atrophy of the caudate nucleus. On post-mortem examination, the cellular loss and gliosis affects the caudate and putamen, and may involve the cerebral cortex, thalmus and brainstem structures.

Neuroacanthocytosis

The acanthocytoses are categorized into three forms by Lees (1985). Bassen-Kornzweig disease has an autosomal recessive inheritance, and appears in early childhood with steatorrhea, retinitis pigmentosa, spinocerebellar degeneration, and opthalmoparesis. A second adult form has an autosomal dominant inheritance and symptoms of a progressive cerebellar and pyramidal syndrome. The third group (Levine et al., 1968; Lees, 1985; Spitz et al., 1985) is thought to be either an autosomal recessive or sporadic inherited disorder. Symptoms generally develop in the third or fourth decade of life and display heterogeneous neurological features such as ataxia, motor neuron disease, parkinsonism, weakness, dysarthria seizures, dementia, etc. The abnormal movements are largely choreiform (hence the alternative term, choreoathetosis) but may include tic-like movements, vocalizations, and echolalia. In two post-mortem examinations, the pathology involved the caudate and putamen in a manner resembling Huntington's disease.

Other Choreic Syndromes

Other choreic syndromes (chorea gravidarum, lupus-erythematosus-associated chorea, familial benign chorea, paroxysmal choreoathetosis) can be distinguished by the type of movement, family history, or associated signs, and only rarely are they confused with Tourette's disorder.

Myoclonus

Myoclonic forms of hyperkinesia, with multiple etiologies, are more difficult to differentiate from tics and Tourette's disorder (Marsden et al., 1982). The movements of myoclonus are brief, lightening-like, and may be unilateral or bilateral, rhythmic or dysrhythmic, synchronous or asynchronous, and elementary or complex (Feinberg et al., 1986). Myoclonus is often clearly familial (Lindenmulder, 1933; Daube and Peters, 1966; Mahloudji and Pikielny, 1967; Korten et al., 1974; Przuntek and Muhr, 1983), and is often associated with epilepsy, either as fragments of epilepsy in various pediatric disorders, or as a familial disease (Marsden et al., 1982). Many other symptomatic or secondary forms, with known etiologies, are described in the literature (Swanson, 1962; Marsden et al., 1982; Fahn et al., 1986). Myoclonic symptoms, in contrast to tics, are much more sensitive to stimuli and often interfere with ongoing or voluntary activities. Myoclonic symptoms are usually simple jerk-like tics, but often include complex motor sequences. Myoclonus is not suppressible even for brief periods, whereas tics can be inhibited for variable periods of time. Finally, vocal tics are not present in myoclonus but are frequent in tic disorders (Tables 7.3, 7.4).

Overlapping Syndromes

Other syndromes include an overlap of dystonic, myoclonic, and tic symptoms. Moreover, dystonic movements might be clonic or tic-like (Fahn and Eldridge, 1976). Davidenkow (1926) described two siblings with dystonic postures and superimposed jerks which he termed hereditary myoclonic dystonia. A similar combination of dystonia with superimposed myoclonus was described in a group of patients by Obeso et al. (1983). A subsequent report described a small group of patients who displayed rhythmic, stereotyped, bilaterally synchronous movements and vocalizations with tonic (dystonic) and myoclonic (tic-like) features (Feinberg et al., 1986); all patients also had ADD (Table 7.4).

Postinfectious, Toxic, and Traumatic Syndromes

Many tic-like symptoms have been reported extensively in encephalitis lethargica (Von Economo, 1931; Van Bogaert and Nyssen, 1925; Benedek, 1925; Weingarten, 1968; Wohlfart et al., 1961; Sacks, 1982). Dyskinesias and tics occurred occasionally in the acute and frequently in the postencephalitic phases of this disease. Some patients treated with L-DOPA for postencephalitic Parkinson's syndrome, have an exacerbation of motor and vocal tic-like symptoms (Sacks, 1982), which, however, in our opinion resemble chorea more than tics. The syndrome of klazomania, an occasional sequelae of postencephalitic patients, which is characterized by oculogyric crises, change in mental status, fits of shouting, echolalia, and coprolalia, bears some resemblance to the symptoms of Tourette's disorder (Benedek, 1925; Wohlfart et al., 1961). However, the pathology is reported to be in the midbrain, subthalamus, and hypothalamus (Adams and Victor, 1985), which has potential implications for Tourette's disorder. However, because this disease causes widespread CNS damage clinicopathological correlation is difficult.

One of the authors (T.E.F.) has personally observed a case of acquired immune deficiency syndrome (AIDS) without evidence of CNS infection, with dementia, choreiform and tic-like movements, and complex stereotypes such as touching fingers to tongue before touching objects. Post-mortem examination revealed widespread involvement of the CNS in cortical, subcorti-

TABLE 7.4. Comparison of five types of movement disorders

Characteristics	Dystonias	Myoclonus	Myoclonic dystonia	Tourette disorder	Paroxysmal myoclonic dystonia with vocalizations
Tonic contractions	+ + + + +[a]	+ / + +	+ + +[b]	+ +[c]	+ + + +
Abrupt contractions	+ / + +	+ + + +	+ + +	+ + + +	+ + + +
Rhythmic	+[d]	+	+ +	+	+ + + +
Bilateral symmetric	+	+	+	+	+ + + +
Stereotyped	+ / + +	+ / + +	Variable	+ + + +	+ + + +
Paroxysmal	+ / + +	+ + +	+ + +	+	+ + + +
Interference with voluntary movement	+ + + +	+ + + +		+ + +	+ + + +
Vocalization	+	+		+ + + +	+ + + +
Family history	May be familial	May be familial	Nonfamilial	With Gilles de la Tourette syndrome, 8%; with other tic disorders, 42%	Nonfamilial
Treatment response	Variable	Variable	Variable	Good response to haloperidol	Poor response to haloperidol

[a] + + + + +: Always present or clinically prominent.
[b] + + + +: Usually present or of moderate clinical importance.
[c] + +: occasionally present or plays minor clinical role.
[d] +: Rarely present or clinically insignificant.

cal, and brainstem loci consistent with diffuse LAV/HTL V-III related encephalitis (Navia et al., 1986).

Tic-like symptoms have been reported in single patients following head trauma (Fahn, 1982a), gasoline inhalation (Koranyi, 1977), carbon monoxide poisoning (Pulst et al., 1983), infections (Kondo and Kabasawa, 1978), and angiographic complications (Bleeker, 1978), but unfortunately without anatomic studies. The patient with carbon monoxide poisoning is described as developing subsequent motor, vocal, coprophilic, and echophilic tics. A CAT scan revealed diffuse cerebral pathology, and low-density lesions in the basal ganglia (Pulst et al., 1983). These clinical reports suggest a basal ganglia etiology for diverse tic-like symptoms that are possibly related to Tourette's disorder.

Neuroleptics

Numerous reports cite tic-like symptoms appearing after the use of neuroleptics in patients with schizophrenia or pervasive developmental disorder (Klawans et al., 1978; Fog et al., 1980; Deveaugh-Geiss, 1980; Singer, 1981; Seeman et al., 1981; Mueller and Aminoff, 1982; Klawans et al., 1982; Fog et al., 1982; Munetz et al., 1985). Tic-like symptoms might include motor tics, vocalizations, coprolalia, echolalia, and palilalia. The symptoms, occasionally termed "tardive Tourette syndrome," are described as including motor, vocal, coprophilic, and echophilic tics. However, the differential diagnosis between Tourette's disorder and tardive dyskinesia is frequently complicated, and usually requires prolonged evaluation and observation. Of the many patients referred to us with this diagnosis none were diagnosed as having tics characteristic of Tourette's disorder. The predominant symptoms resembled choreioform movements more than tics. Motor tics occurred infrequently and were an insignificant aspect of the movement disorder. Vocal tics were not brief or tic-like, but tended to be rhythmic, "mm," sighing or, gutteral sounds. Our personal experience makes us skeptical of this diagnosis. These observations, despite our reservation, have possible implications for understanding the pathophysiology of Tourette's disorder, and some authors believe they strengthen the argument for a dopaminergic disturbance in Tourette's disorder.

Other Disorders

The attempt to understand the etiology of Tourette's disorder has led to many clinical reports describing movements that variously resemble tics. We have examined many patients with other disorders and diverse movements, personally, by observing videotapes or in consultation. However, in our opinion, rarely do the symptoms resemble classical tics. For example, stimulants are

TABLE 7.5. *Tic-like symptoms associated with acquired CNS pathology*

Study	Suspected etiology	Site of pathology	Tic symptoms	Associated features
Von Economo (1917, 1931); Van Bogaert and Nyssen (1925); Weingarten (1968); Wohlfart et al. (1961); Sacks (1982); and others	Encephalitis lethargica	Primarily midbrain, subthalamus, hypothalamus; although pathology may be throughout CNS	Simple and complex motor and vocal tics, coprolalia, echolalia, echopraxia, palilalia	"Shouting fits," bizarre behavior, psychosis, Parkinson's syndrome, tics occasionally exacerbated with dopaminergic drugs
Koranyi (1977)	Gasoline inhalation	Presumed diffuse	Simple motor and vocal tics, coprolalia	Abnormal EEG: symmetric theta and theta bursts fronto-centrally
Bleeker (1978)	Postangliographic complications	No documented lesion site	Simple and complex vocal tics, palilalia	Emotional lability, amnestic syndrome
Kondo and Kabasawa (1978)	Postinfectious	Unknown	Simple motor and vocal tics, echopraxia	EEG: occasional asymmetric theta bursts prior to movements; elevated ASLO titers
Fahn (1982a)	Posttraumatic	Unknown	Complex motor tics	Some asymmetric distribution of tics
Pulst et al. (1983)	Carbon monoxide poisoning	Cortical atrophy, large ventricles and low density lesions in basal ganglia on CT scan	Simple and complex motor and vocal tics, coprolalia, echolalia, palilalia	Inappropriate sexual behavior

thought to induce tics in animals, and many studies have been done using symptoms of hyperactivity, hyperalertness, hyperdistractability, sniffing, turning, pawing, stereotype, etc., as a model for tics. Although the theoretical basis is compelling (stimulants increase catecholamines and excess catecholamines cause Tourette's disorder, symptoms induced in animals by high dosages of stimulants do not resemble tics. Many atypical movements diagnosed as Tourette's disorder have been interpreted by us as tardive dyskinesia, Huntington's chorea, stereotypic movements associated with schizophrenia, brain damage from senility and other causes, and atypical movements of unknown etiology. The association of some of these movement symptoms with tics may represent an underlying causal relationship, a random relationship, or the presence of two different disorders. The possibility of a common pathway for these disorders and Tourette's disorder, despite differences in symptoms and the clinical histories, warrants further study, but caution is needed before interpreting the symptoms and etiology as similar.

TREATMENT INTERVENTIONS

Neurosurgery

Seven patients with Tourette's disorder are reported as improved after neurosurgical procedures such as lesions in the frontal-thalamic white matter, dentate and various thalamic nuclei (Baker, 1962; Stevens, 1964; Cooper, 1969; Hassler and Dieckmann, 1970; Nadvornik et al., 1972). A common factor among these procedures is a lesion of thalamic nuclei (ventrolateral, rostral intralaminar, medial) or lesions which interupt thalamic input (dentato-thalamic) or output (thalamo-cortical). However, these clinical reports are inconclusive because of the small samples, absence of controls and inadequate follow-up evaluations. Organic central nervous system impairment, a serious liability of neurosurgical procedures, occurred in two patients evaluated by us.

Pharmacotherapy

The major hypothesis about the etiology of Tourette's disorder derives from the pharmacotherapy of Tourette's disorder. The most effective drugs—possibly the only effective drugs—are neuroleptics such as haloperidol, pimozide, fluphenazine, penfluridol, and others which reduce dopamine transmission. Other support frequently cited includes the increase of tics by stimulants and L-dopa, and reports of "tardive Tourette's disorder" after prolonged use of neuroleptics. The results of some studies of cerebrospinal fluid dopamine suggest that postsynaptic dopamine (D2) hypersensitivity in the basal ganglia

TABLE 7.6. *Neurosurgical interventions in Tourette's disorder*

Study	Patient symtoms	Neurosurgery	Result
Baker (1962)	Vocal and motor tics, seizure disorder (one patient)	Bimedial frontal leucotomy complicated by frontal abcess treated by aspiration	"Marked reduction in tics"
Stevens (1964)	Rhythmic head movements, arm and body jerks, coprolalia, echolalia, echopraxia (one patient)	Transorbital lobotomy	"Marked decrease in the frequency, duration and amplitude" of tics and coprolalia
Cooper (1969)	Multiple motor tics, vocal tics (one patient)	Ventrolateral nucleus of the thalmus, bilaterally (twice on left side)	Reduction in motor tics, 90%, complete relief from vocal tics
Hassler and Dieckmann (1970)	Case 1: motor tics, echolalia, coprolalia; case 2: motor and vocal tics, coprolalia, obsessive-compulsive; case 3: motor and vocal tics	Rostral intralaminar, median and ventral-oral internal nuclei	Improvement, 70–90, 100, and 70%, respectively
Nadvornik et al. (1972)	Myoclonic movements in the face and diaphragm with vocal tic (one patient)	Transtentorial bilateral dentatotomy	Movements decreased, bark-like sounds disappeared

ELECTROENCEPHALOGRAMS

Review of the Literature

We previously reviewed studies of EEGs in Tourette's disorder reported in the literature up to 1974 (Table 7.7) (Shapiro et al., 1978). Abnormal EEGs are reported more frequently in studies (62.8%) than in reviews (39.7%) ($\chi^2 = 17.3$, df-1, $p = 0.0000$). Studies done after 1974 report significantly less EEG abnormalities (36.0%) than earlier studies (62.8%) ($\chi^2 = 38$, df-1, $p = 0.0000$) (Table 7.7). However, the range of EEG abnormalities varies from 12.5 to 67%.

Obvious questions include: What are the reasons for the decreased percentage of EEG abnormalities, are the abnormalities significantly higher than expectations in the population, and do the abnormalities reflect the underlying pathophysiology of Tourette's disorder? Interpretation of studies in the literature are difficult because of the extensive range of reported abnormalities, age and type of patients, variable criteria for rating abnormalities, and absence of evidence of reliability for the ratings of blind procedures and of consistent types of abnormality. Nevertheless, the high percentages and extensive range of reported EEG abnormalities and the reason for the significant decrease over time require explanation. Our hypothesis is that the variability and decrease over time is due to the age of patients, the percentage of patients with ADD, other CNS impairment, and the number of patients being treated with drugs.

Some of these problems are illustrated by a blind evaluation study, that reported abnormal EEGs, mainly sharp waves and slowing, in 57% of 45 TS

TABLE 7.7. *EEG abnormalities cited in the literature*[a]

Study	Sample size N	Abnormal EEG %	EEG abnormality
Reviews			
Kelman (1965)	19	42.1	
Fernando (1967)	65	25.0	
Lucas and Rodin (1973)	46	50.0	
Abuzzahab and Anderson (1973)	102	44.1	
Total	232	39.7	
Studies (1959–1978)			
Eisenberg et al. (1959)	7	57.1	
Dolmierski and Kloss (1962)	2	100.0	

TABLE 7.7. *(Continued)*

Study	Sample size N	Abnormal EEG %	EEG abnormality
Guggenheim and Haynal (1964)	3	100.0	
Feild et al. (1966)	7	85.7	
Challas et al. (1967)	15	26.6	
Fernando (1967)	4	25.0	
Fisarova (1968)	5	100.0	
Fisarova (1972)	29	89.7	
Zawadzki (1972)	5	100.0	
Wayne et al. (1972)[b]	32	50.0	
Lucas and Rodin (1973)	18	55.6	
Shapiro et al. (1978)	79	47.0	
Total	164	62.8	
Studies (1981–1984)			
Hashimoto et al. (1981)	9	67.0	
Caparulo et al. (1981)	16	31.3	
Bergen et al. (1982)	38	34.2	Diffuse slowing and/or slow bursts common (12), patients with irritative features (2)
Krumholz et al. (1983)	40	12.5	Excess slowing (4), irritative (1)
Han-bai and Han-quin (1983)	13	30.8	Diminished alpha, excess theta or low-amplitude sharp waves.
Min (1983)	20	60.0	Slow wave (2), slow and sharp (5), focal abnormality (1), bilateral sharp waves and slowing (8), other (4)
Volkmar et al. (1984)	45	55.6	Sharp waves (9), slowing (4), sharp waves and slowing (8), other (4)
Barabas et al. (1984b)	35	20.0	Paroxysmal abnormality in 11%, nonfocal slowing 9%
Lees et al. (1984)	53	15.1	Spike and wave (1), focal sharp theta (2), mild diffuse theta (5)
Verma et al. (1986)	30	20.0	
Current study	325	38.8	Diffuse slowing (2), epileptiform (4),
Total	630	35.2	(see text)

[a]Studies 1959–1978 vs. 1981–1984; $\chi^2 = 43.5$, df-1, $p = 0.0000$.
[b]Sample included in Shapiro et al. (1978).

patients (Volkmar et al., 1984). However, the reliability of the ratings and the relationships to attention deficit disorder (ADD), neurological impairment, and drug treatment was not assessed. Some of these problems were addressed by Bergen et al. (1982) who reported that overall 34% (13 of 38 patients) had abnormal EEGs. The abnormalities were largely diffuse slow-wave abnormalities or slow-wave bursts. However, six of 13 patients with abnormal EEGs were taking haloperidol compared to three of 25 patients with normal EEGs ($p = 0.025$), and four of 13 patients with abnormal EEGs had minor neurological or psychomotor abnormalities compared to two patients with normal EEGs ($p = 0.078$). The authors stressed the importance of controlling for neurological abnormalities and the use of neuroleptics which can induce slowing of the EEG (Borenstein et al., 1962; Hollister et al., 1963; Kurtz, 1976). If the patients on drugs and with neurological abnormalities are excluded, only four (17.4%) of 23 patients had abnormal EEGs, which is within expectations. The authors concluded that the EEG does not significantly reflect the pathophysiological basis for Tourette's disorder.

Lower percent EEG abnormalities and an effect of medication was cited by Krumholz et al. (1983) who reported that 12.5% of 40 Tourette's disorder patients had EEG abnormalities, a percentage that is within normal expectations. Moreover, all five patients with abnormalities were receiving medication, including haloperidol, compared to eight of 35 in the group with normal EEGs. Of the EEGs in 35 unselected and unmedicated children with Tourette's disorder (average age 10.3, range 5.7–16.4 years) (relationship to ADD not described), four (11%) had paroxysmal and three (9%) had nonfocal slowing (Barabas et al., 1984d). These three studies report EEG abnormalities in a range expected in the population.

A recent study by Verma et al. (1986) described 30 Tourette's disorder patients, 7 to 40 years of age, who were drug-free, had normal neurological exams, normal intelligence (WISC-R IQ score ≥ 80), and no history of seizure disorder. No control was used for ADD, nor was the rater blind to diagnosis. EEGs were abnormal in six (20%) of patients, slowing in two (6.69%), and with epileptiform activity in four (13.3%) patients. Thirteen percent with epileptiform activity is comparable to the 14.7% of paroxysmal activity reported in normal children from 1 to 15 years of age (Eeg-Olofsson et al., 1971), but is higher than 4.9% reported for 16 to 21-year-old normal adolescents (Eeg-Olofsson, 1971). The overall abnormal rate of 20% is less than expected in normal children (32%) and similar to normal adolescents (23%) (Eeg-Olofsson, 1971).

The percent of abnormalities reported in the literature since 1975 averages 36% (Table 7.7). This percentage is grossly within expectations in the population (Eeg-Olofsson, 1971; Petersen and Eeg-Olofsson, 1971; Eeg-Olofsson et al. 1971). Moreover, the actual percentage may be lower if the ratios of children to adults, medicated patients, and those with ADD and other organic disorders are partialed from the total percentage of abnormal EEGs. These factors will be considered in analysis of the data of our current study.

Current Study

We previously reported EEG results for 79 consecutive patients who were blindly and independently rated ($r = 0.85$, $p < 0.001$) by two experienced electroencephalographers (Wayne et al., 1972; Sweet et al., 1973; Shapiro et al., 1978). Ratings of abnormality were based on features described by Stevens et al. (1968): 0, normal; 1, nonspecific or borderline abnormality (mild background disorganization, slight increase in theta slowing, excessive rapid beta activity, rare asynchronous delta, very rare sharp-wave activity, or more than expected asynchronous response to hyperventilation for the age of the patient); 2 to 3, significant abnormality (increasing degrees of disorganization, theta and delta slowing, significant paroxysmal activity such as sharp waves, spikes, spike and waves, or focal abnormalities). Our current sample has increased to 325 patients.

To help explain the considerable variability in EEG abnormalities reported among Tourette's disorder patients, the following factors are examined: variability of EEG abnormalities, decreased EEG abnormalities reported over time, and the effect of age, ADD, neurological abnormalities, and medication on EEG abnormalities. We then evaluate the hypothesis that if these factors are controlled, EEGs will not be significantly different in Tourette's disorder patients compared to population estimates.

Type of Electroencephalogram Abnormality

A subset of 91 abnormal EEG reports from our sample were available in sufficient detail for adequate review (TEF) to determine the type of abnormality. Some patients had more than one abnormality. The most common feature was background slowing or "disorganization" (59.3%). This was followed by sharp waves and/or spikes (38.5%) (unilateral 12.1%, bilateral 26.4%), and focal slowing (18.7%) (unilateral 9.9%, bilateral 8.8%, and slow burst 2.2%). For 17 patients on medication (12 on haloperidol, three on other neuroleptics, and three on other medications), 14 had slow wave abnormalities, and seven had sharp waves or spikes in addition to slowing. However, slow-wave abnormalities were present in 57 patients not on medication.

The nonspecific and variable features of the EEGs reported in the literature and in our review indicate that no general type of EEG is associated with Tourette's disorder and specific pathopathology cannot be inferred from currently available EEG studies. However, potential meaningful factors from EEGs may be obfuscated by the effect of age, diagnosis, and medication.

Decreased Electroencephalogram Abnormalities Reported Over Time

We previously cited a significant decrease in the percent of Tourette's disorder patients with abnormal EEGs reported in the literature ($p = 0.0000$) (Table 7.7). Our results support this trend (Table 7.8).

Total EEG abnormalities are significantly higher (46.8%) for the 1965 to 1974 sample than for the 1975 to 1981 sample (36.2%) ($p = 0.0000$), and the correlation coefficient comparing year of evaluation with abnormal EEGs is $-.015$, ($p = 0.005$). Decreased EEG abnormalities over time, as with neurological and organic central nervous system factors, which has been discussed previously, is at least partially due to the frequency of severe Tourette's disorder and of ADD in our earlier samples. Whatever the reason, the results indicate that the role of EEG abnormalities in Tourette's disorder requires reexamination.

Effect of Age on Electroencephalograms

The total percent of abnormal EEGs for the 1965 to 1974 sample is 46.8%, 25.3% with nonspecific abnormalities, and 21.5% with significant abnormalities (Table 7.8). However, the percent of abnormalities is significantly higher ($p = 0.02$) for the sample 16 years or younger (71.1%) than for the sample over 16 years (24.4%). Moreover, the percent of significant abnormalities is 4.9% in the sample over 16 years, which is within expectations for adults in the population. The sample studied between 1975 and 1981 have a significantly lower number of abnormal EEGs (36.2%) compared to the earlier group (46.8%) ($p = 0.0000$) (Table 7.8). The percentage of significant abnormalities in the over 16-year-old sample (14.6%), although

TABLE 7.8. *EEG ratings by year and age*

Sample	Sample size N	Normal %	Nonspecific abnormality %	Significant abnormality %	Total abnormal %	χ^2(df-1)	$p =$
1965–1974 sample							
16 Years or younger	38	28.9	31.6	39.5	71.1		
Over 16 years	41	75.6	19.5	4.9	24.4		
Total	79	53.2	25.3	21.5	46.8	7.8	0.02
1975–1981 sample							
16 Years or younger	150	62.7	8.7	28.7	37.3		
Over 16 years	96	65.6	19.8	14.6	34.3		
Total	246	63.8	13.0	23.2	36.2	51.9	0.0000
Total sample							
16 Years or younger	188	55.9	13.3	30.9	44.1		
Over 16 years	137	68.6	19.7	11.7	31.4		
Total	325	61.2	16.0	22.8	38.8	52.8	0.0000

χ^2 for total 1965–1974 sample vs. 1975–1981 sample; $\chi^2 = 80.1$, df-2, $p = 0.0000$.

TABLE 7.9. *Relationship of EEG ratings to age and attention deficit disorder*

Group	Sample size N	Normal %	Nonspecific abnormality %	Significant abnormality %	Total abnormal %	χ^2(df-1)	p =
Less than 17 years							
TS-alone	119	63.0	9.2	27.7	37.0		
TS + ADD	86	45.3	20.9	33.7	54.7		
Total	205	55.6	14.2	30.2	44.4	12.9	0.01
17 Years or older							
TS-alone	91	71.4	18.7	9.9	28.6		
TS + ADD	29	69.0	20.7	10.3	31.0		
Total	120	70.8	19.2	10.0	29.2	0.1	ns
All ages							
TS-alone	210	66.7	13.3	20.0	33.3		
TS + ADD	115	51.3	20.9	27.8	48.7		
Total	325	61.2	16.0	22.8	38.8	17.5	0.02

χ^2 for sample 17 years or younger vs. over 17 years; χ^2 = 17.7, df-2, p = 0.0001.

higher than in the earlier sample (4.9%), is again within expectations for adults. EEG abnormalities for the total sample of 325 patients is significantly higher for the 16 years or younger sample (44.1%) than for the over 16-year-old sample (31.4%) (p = 0.0000) (Table 7.8), and the percent of significant EEG abnormalities (11.7%) is within expectations for adults. Thus, age of patients, usually unrecorded in the literature, is required for more meaningful interpretation of EEG abnormalities in Tourette's disorder.

Effect of Attention Deficit Disorder on Electroencephalograms

The results for 315 patients are categorized by age as less than 17 years of age or 17 years or older, and by diagnosis as TS-alone or TS + ADD (Table 7.9).

Our expectations that abnormal EEGs would be higher in the TS + ADD group than in the TS-alone group is confirmed for the less than 17-year-old group (p = 0.001) and for the total sample (p = 0.001). Although abnormal EEGs are not significantly different for the two diagnostic groups in the 17 years or older group, significant abnormalities (12.7%) are within expectations for the population. The results suggest an interaction between age, diagnosis, and abnormal EEGs.

Relationship of Neurological Abnormalities to Electroencephalograms

Data were available for 281 patients who had both EEGs and neurological examinations. Our expectations were confirmed that neurological abnormalities would be associated with abnormal EEGs (p = 0.03) (Table 7.10).

TABLE 7.10. Relationship of neurological abnormalities to EEG ratings[a]

Neurological abnormality	Sample size N	Normal %	EEG abnormality		Total abnormal %
			Nonspecific abnormality %	Significant abnormality %	
Normal	190	64.7	10.5	24.7	35.2
Nonlocalizing	77	55.8	26.0	18.2	44.2
Definite	14	57.1	21.4	21.4	42.8
Total	281	61.9	15.3	22.8	38.1

[a] $\chi^2 = 10.7$, df-4, $p = 0.03$.

Effect of Medication on Electroencephalograms

Of the 79 patients in the 1965 to 1974 sample, eight patients were on haloperidol; EEGs were normal in four, one was definitely abnormal, and three had EEG findings consistent with the effect of haloperidol. For nine other patients on diverse drugs, the EEG was significantly abnormal in one patient and the remainder had EEG effects consistent with an effect of medication. The results, summarized in Table 7.11, confirm our expectation of a medication effect on EEGs. EEGs are significantly more abnormal for patients on drugs (76.5%) compared to patients not on drugs (38.7%) ($p = 0.0001$). The main effect of drugs is on nonspecific EEG abnormalities (64.7% compared to 14.5%) ($p = 0.006$).

Interrelationship Among Variables

The previous analyses strongly indicate complicated interrelationships among variables. The complexity is illustrated in the intercorrelations of year evaluated, age, ADD, EEG abnormality, and neurological abnormality (Table 7.12). The Bender-Gestalt Test was added as another widely used indicator of CNS impairment. Use of medication was not included because these data were not programmed for analysis.

The intercorrelations demonstrate low but significant relationships among some but not all variables. Moreover, other variables (see Table A.1) also may be related. To evaluate the interrelationship among all variables, stepwise regression analyses (SRAs) were done.

TABLE 7.11. *Relationship of medication to EEG ratings*[a]

Patients	Sample size N	Normal %	Nonspecific abnormality %	Significant abnormality %	Total abnormal %
Not on drugs	62	61.3	14.5	24.2	38.7
On drugs	17	23.5	64.7	11.8	76.5
Total	79	53.2	25.3	21.5	46.8

[a] $\chi^2 = 17.8$, df-1, $p = 0.0001$.

TABLE 7.12. *Intercorrelation of selected variables*

Variables	Year	Age	ADD	EEG	Neuro	Bender-Gestalt Test
Year evaluated	—					
Age	−0.13[a]	—				
ADD	−0.20[b]	−0.19[b]	—			
EEG abnormality	−0.15[c]	−0.16[c]	0.14[c]	—		
Neurological abnormality	−0.18[a]	−0.02	0.32[b]	0.02	—	
Bender-Gestalt Test abnormality	0.02	−0.01	0.35[b]	0.08	0.25[a]	—

[a] $p < 0.001$.
[b] $p < 0.0001$.
[c] $p < 0.01$.

Stepwise Regression Analyses

The previous analyses suggest the possibility that abnormal EEGs reported in Tourette's disorder may be an artifact of age, ADD, neurologic abnormality, and medication. We therefore hypothesized that EEG abnormality would be associated with younger age, diagnosis of ADD, or other CNS impairment (effect of medication not analyzed), and would not be associated with characteristic Tourette's disorder variables such as genetic factors and symptoms.

To test this hypothesis, and to retrospectively identify variables associated with abnormal EEGs for heuristic purposes, SRA was done using the procedure described in Chapter 2.

The results largely support our hypothesis (Table 7.13). Abnormal EEGs are associated with CNS impairment (epilepsy and history of head trauma), younger age, and year of evaluation. More echophilic and less complex tics, which contribute a smaller amount of significant unique variance, may be chance findings and require replication. Our interpretation of the EEG data supports our concept that abnormal EEGs are not associated with Tourette's

TABLE 7.13. *EEGs: Stepwise regression analysis*

Variables	Simple r	Multiple R^2	Parameter estimate
Demography			
Age	−0.16[a]	0.03	−0.04[b]
Year evaluated	−0.16[a]	0.06[b]	−0.01[a]
Genetics	—	—	—
Medical history			
History of epilepsy	0.19[c]	0.03	0.73[a]
History of head trauma	0.17[a]	0.06[b]	1.35[c]
Neurological	—	—	—
Behavior	—	—	—
Illness Variables			
Duration of illness FS	−0.15[a]	0.02[a]	−0.01[a]
Symptoms			
Echophilia	0.14[a]	0.02	0.25[a]
Complex tics	−0.13[d]	0.04	−0.25[a]
Inarticulate sounds	−0.13[d]	0.05[c]	−1.31[d]
Summary SRA			
History of epilepsy	0.19[c]	0.03	1.44[c]
Age	−0.16[a]	0.06	−0.02[b]
Year evaluated	−0.16[a]	0.10	−0.04[c]
History of head trauma	0.17[a]	0.13	−0.68[a]
Echophilia	0.14[a]	0.14	0.22[a]
Complex tics	−0.13[d]	0.16	−0.20[d]
Adjusted R^2	—	0.14[b]	—

[a] $p < 0.01$.
[b] $p < 0.0001$.
[c] $p < 0.001$.
[d] $p < 0.05$.

disorder if the following factors are controlled: age, ADD, epilepsy, head trauma, neurological and other CNS disorders, and medication. A more definitive evaluation of the hypothesis, described in the next section, requires the study of a group of age-controlled patients without ADD, epilepsy, and other obvious indications of CNS damage, and who are unmedicated.

Electroencephalograms in Unmedicated Tourette Patients Without Attention Deficit Disorder and Over 16 Years of Age

EEGs for 310 patients with adequate information about the diagnosis of ADD and use of medication were reviewed. For 78 TS-alone (non-ADD) and medication-free patients, 49 are 16 years or younger, and 29 are over 16 years of age (Table 7.14).

For the 16 years or younger Tourette's disorder group, although abnormal

TABLE 7.14. *EEGs in unmedicated Tourette patients without attention deficit disorder by age and study sample*

Sample	Sample size N	Normal %	Nonspecific abnormality %	Significant abnormality %	Total abnormal %	χ^2(df-1)	p =
16 Years or younger TS sample[a]							
1965–1974 sample	8	37.5	25.0	37.5	62.5	3.2	NS
1975–1981 sample	41	65.9	7.3	26.8	34.1		
Total	49	61.2	10.2	28.6	38.8		
Over 16 years TS sample[b]							
1965–1974 sample	16	62.5	31.3	6.3	37.5	3.2	NS
1975–1981 sample	13	69.2	15.4	14.3	30.8		
Total	29	65.5	24.1	10.3	34.5		
Total sample							
All ages for both samples	78	62.8	15.4	21.8	37.2		
Control sample							
16 Years or younger	743	67.5	—	—	32.4	6.6	0.01
Over 16 to 21 years	185	77.3	—	—	22.7		

[a]16 Years or younger vs. over 16 years sample: $\chi^2 = 5.1$, df-1, NS; 16 years or younger TS vs. control sample: $\chi^2 = 0.8$, df-1, NS.

[b]Over 16 to 68 years TS sample vs. over 16 to 21 year control sample: $\chi^2 = 1.9$, df-1, NS.

EEGs are higher in the earlier (62.5%) than in the later sample (34.1%), the difference is not significant. Similarly, for the over 16-year-old group, abnormal EEGs are not significantly different in the earlier (37.5%) than in the later (30.8%) sample. Moreover, total abnormal EEGs are not significantly different between the two age groups (38.8% versus 37.2%). Thus, for unmedicated, non-ADD Tourette's patients, EEGs are rated normal in 62.8%, nonspecific abnormality in 15.4%, and significant abnormality in 21.8%. The results also indicate that the decline in EEG abnormalities over time are largely due to a decrease in the number of patients with ADD over time.

These results were compared with a large sample of 743 children 16 years or younger and 185 adolescents over 16 to 21 years of age (Eeg-Olofsson, 1971; Petersen and Eeg-Olofsson, 1971; Eeg-Olofsson et al., 1971). EEGs were classified as normal or abnormal (which included both our nonspecific and significant abnormality groups). Although the frequency of abnormality was higher in the Tourette's disorder sample, all comparisons were not significantly different (16 years or younger Tourette's versus control sample, over 16- to 68-years-old Tourette's sample versus over 16- to 21-years-old control sample (Table 7.14). Moreover, the control sample only included patients over 16 to 21 years of age which would probably yield fewer abnormal EEGs than our adult sample which varied from over 16 to 68 years of age. In addition, the control sample excluded patients with perinatal complications, disordered development, head injury, CNS disease, family history of idiopathic convulsive disease, paroxysmal headache or abdominal pain, enuresis or encoporesis after the fourth year, tics, stuttering, night terrors, nail-biting, metabolic disease, conduct disorder, and developmental or mental disorders (Peterson and Eeg-Olofsson, 1971). These factors which were not excluded from the Tourette's disorder sample would further decrease the percentage of abnormal EEGs in this sample.

Limitations of these results include absence of standardized procedures for recording EEGs, blind ratings of the Tourette's disorder and control samples and indices of reliability for the ratings. These limitations may be offset by the large sample size, which is approximately equal to the total number of patients reported in 21 studies in the literature.

These results confirm our expectation that EEG abnormalities are essentially within normal expectations in the population, and support our conclusion that abnormal EEGs are unrelated to Tourette's disorder in non-ADD, unmedicated age-corrected Tourette's patients.

Clinical Use of Electroencephalograms in Tourette's Disorder

The results suggest that routine EEGs are not useful for study of the etiology, clinical diagnosis, or management of Tourette's disorder (Krumholtz et al., 1983, 1984), and in our opinion should not be obtained routinely, unless indicated by other factors in the differential diagnosis or for use in research.

NEUROLOGICAL EXAMINATION

Prior to the present study, neurological evaluations were reported by five investigators (Table 4.23). Neurological abnormalities in Tourette's disorder patients are reported in 89% (Fisarova, 1972), 54 to 64% (Shapiro et al., 1973a,b; 1974, 1978; Sweet et al., 1973), 27 to 53% (Golden, 1977a, 1982), 11% (Bergen et al., 1982), 0% (Han-bai and Han-quin, 1983), and 29% (Min, 1983).

Probably the most consistent and comprehensive evaluation of Tourette's disorder patients was done by our collaborator, Dr. R. Sweet. At the time Tourette's disorder was new to us and our examinations were extensive, detailed, and comprehensive. Dr. Sweet examined 70 consecutive Tourette's disorder patients, which have been described in great detail in previous publications (Sweet et al., 1973; Shapiro et al., 1978). Neurological evaluations were rated as: 1, normal; 2, borderline (soft or nonlocalizing signs); and 3, definite (or facial) abnormalities. Forty (57.1%) of the 70 patients had neurological deficits. Thirty-one patients had unilateral impairment of rapid alternating movements, pronator drift, hyperreflexia, increased tone, unilaterally decreased associated movements, or decrease in tone and check on one side. Seven patients had some degree of facial assymetry and six had choreioform movements. Other disturbances included poor coordination, mirror movements, release signs, and rotatory nystagmus. The percentage of patients with soft neurological signs (57.1%) was noted to be considerably higher than reported by Stevens et al. (1968) who found that 20% of 88 children without behavioral disturbances had at least one abnormality on neurological examination.

Subsequently, 327 additional patients were added to the sample for a total of 397 patients in our current sample. Neurological examinations were performed by either R. D. Sweet, A. K. Shapiro, and a small number of records from other neurologists, if sufficiently detailed to be useful. All the records were reviewed independently by A. K. S. and E. S. and rated on the previously described rating scale. A small number of differences were resolved by discussions between the two raters.

For 380 patients in our sample who had neurological examinations, 24% had borderline and 5% had definite neurological abnormalities (Table 4.30). However, similar to other analyses, the percent with neurological abnormalities has decreased significantly over time ($r = 0.18$, df-378, $p < 0.001$) and is signifcantly lower in the 1975 to 1981 sample (15%) than is the earlier sample (57.1%) ($\chi^2 = 49.2$, df-1, $p = 0.0000$). Moreover, neurological abnormalities are significantly higher for the TS + ADD+H group (56.1%) than for both the TS + ADD − H (30.8%), and TS-alone (19.4%) groups (ANOVA, $p = 0.0001$) (Table 4.27), and significantly correlated with the diagnosis of TS + ADD+H versus other diagnoses ($r = 0.36$, df-378, $p = 0.001$).

These data should be interpreted cautiously. Most of the neurological abnormalities are classified as "borderline," "soft," or "nonlocalizing." They include a broad group of subtle neurological, neuromotor, neurosensory, or neurocognitive abnormalities. The use of the prefix "soft" designates in a general fashion that no fixed structural lesion underlies the abnormality. Their clinical importance is the possibility that they may indicate CNS factors (Shaffer et al., 1985) that account for their presence. Borderline abnormalities have been referred to as equivocal (Kennard, 1960), soft signs (Bender, 1956) and more recently as nonfocal (Shapiro et al., 1978) or nonlocalizing (DSM-III-R). These abnormalities are related to maturational development (Shapiro and Perry, 1976), to children under 8 years of age (Shapiro et al., 1978) decrease with age (Peters et al., 1975) and thought to be significant after the age of 8 years (Kinsbourne, 1973; Hart et al., 1974). Although several studies have demonstrated that neurological abnormalities can be rated reliably (Rutter et al., 1970; Werry et al., 1972) the concept of nonlocalizing signs has been criticized (Ingram, 1973; Barlow, 1974; Schmitt, 1975). Further complexity is apparent from the results of a large and well controlled study in which nonlocalizing neurological signs were not significantly associated with ADD (Shapiro et al., 1978; Shaffer et al., 1983).

In addition, the results are derived from different clinicians using different neurological tests, they were not compared with a blindly evaluated control group, and their reliability was not assessed. These shortcomings also characterize all published reports (Table 4.24), which tend to report a higher than expected percentage of neurological abnormalities than expected in the population.

Moreover, referral bias probably contributes to the increased percent of abnormalities reported in the literature. Patients with diverse neurological dysfunction are more likely to be given a neurological examination, and increased neurological abnormalities are reported in minimal brain dysfunction, hyperactive syndrome (Clements, 1966; Shapiro et al., 1978), learning disabilities (Peters et al., 1975; Shapiro et al., 1978), and schizophrenia (Quitkin et al., 1976; Shapiro et al., 1978). Samples with high percentages of these and other organic conditions are more likely to include patients who have been evaluated neurologically, thus increasing the likelihood of identifying neurological abnormalities. Tourette's disorder patients without organic conditions are less likely to be evaluated neurologically, thus reducing the possible identification of neurological abnormalities. The percentage of neurological abnormalities reported in Tourette's disorder, therefore, may be artifactually elevated.

Similar to our hypothesis about EEG abnormalities, we hypothesized that neurological abnormalities would be associated with other CNS impairment and would not be associated with other variables characterizing Tourette's disorder. Our expectations were confirmed by the results of the SRA (Table 7.15).

Variables selected by the SRA for three of the category groups (medical, neurological, and behavioral history) and the final summary SRA are characterized by CNS organic impairment.

These results contribute support for our concept that although Tourette's disorder is an organic disorder of the CNS, it is not primarily associated with neurological or behavioral sequelae.

EVOKED POTENTIALS

Stimulus evoked response or evoked potential (EP) is a computer averaging technique of potentials elicited in a time-locked relationship to a stimulus. The stimuli include auditory evoked potentials (AEP), visual evoked potentials (VEP), and somatosensory evoked potentials (SEP).

Auditory Evoked Potential

A study of AEPs in a patient with Tourette's disorder, with and without haloperidol, were reported as demonstrating significantly shorter P_2 (150–320 msec) and N_2 (220–380 msec) latencies compared to a normal control group matched on age and sex (Surwillo, 1981). Corresponding amplitudes were reduced, but disappeared after therapy with haloperidol. The short latency response of the AEP, possibly representing events in the brainstem, were

TABLE 7.15. *Neurological examination: Stepwise regression analysis*

Variables	Simple r	Multiple R^2	Parameter Estimate
Demography			
Year evaluated	0.32[a]	0.03	−0.03[b]
Genetics	—	—	—
Medical history			
Age bladder-bowel trained FS	0.14[c]	0.02	0.05[c]
Mothers' abortions	0.12[d]	0.03[c]	0.08[d]
Neurological			
ADD	0.32[a]	0.15[b]	—
Behavior			
Coordination FS	−0.26[a]	0.07	−0.15[c]
Learning disorder FS	0.26[b]	0.09[b]	0.09[d]
Illness Variables	—	—	—
Symptoms			
Coprolalia	0.15[c]	0.02	0.16[d]
Number current tics	−0.11[d]	0.05	−0.02[b]
TS severity	0.13[c]	0.06	0.08[d]
Age of TS onset	−0.10[d]	0.07[b]	−0.02[d]
Summary SRA			
ADD	−0.32[a]	0.15	0.38[a]
Age bladder-bowel FS	0.14[c]	0.20	0.10[b]
Adjusted R^2	—	0.19[a]	—

[a] $p < 0.0001$.
[b] $p < 0.001$.
[c] $p < 0.01$.
[d] $p < 0.05$.

reported as not significantly different in controls compared to ten Tourette's disorder patients not on medication and seven on medication (Krumholz et al., 1983).

The late components of the AEP at a latency of 80 to 400 msec, potentials elicited by tasks requiring attention to an auditory stimulus, or discrimination of task-relevant from nontask relevant stimuli, were studied in six Tourette's disorder patients on and off medication (pimozide or clonidine) who were compared with a normal control group (Van de Wetering et al., 1985). Numerous differences in the late components of the AEP between 80 to 280 mg. were reported for medicated and unmedicated patients and controls. The amplitude of the N_1 component with a peak latency in the range of 170 to 200 msec was smaller in patients before medication than in the controls and returned toward normal with medication. This component has been regarded as related to selective attention (Hillyard et al., 1978). Four of the subjects in this study had school difficulties, and the authors suggest that some of their findings may be related to attention deficits.

Visual Evoked Potential

VEPs were studied in five Tourette's disorder patients on haloperidol, five patients not receiving medication, and 12 normal, age- and sex-matched controls (Domino et al., 1982). Latencies were prolonged in waves IV (110–130 msec), V (120–180 msec), and VI (150–206 msec) in patients receiving medication. Latencies in drug-free Tourette's disorder patients did not differ from controls. Amplitudes for wave IV were significantly smaller or larger than controls in the drug-free and treated groups, respectively. The authors interpreted the results as partly due to drug effects and abnormal dopaminergic transmission in Tourette's disorder.

Somatosensory Evoked Potential

SEPs were reported in only one study, and reported as normal in three Tourette's disorder patients (Obeso et al., 1982).

Effect of Dopamine-Blocking Drugs on Evoked Potentials

Several studies indicate that the latency of EPs is increased by dopamine-blocking drugs: Increased latency of the VEP in rats treated with alpha-methylparatyrosine and haloperidol (Dyer, 1981; Onofrj and Bodis-Wollner, 1982), increased latency and diminished amplitude in the SEP in schizophrenic patients treated with haloperidol (Saletu et al., 1971), in adult subjects (Bodis-Wollner et al., 1980), and in children (Saletu, 1977).

Conclusion

It is unclear from the available studies whether EPs in Tourette's disorder differ from controls. Conclusions about EPs in Tourette's require the study of larger samples matched with control subjects and controlled for medication, the presence of ADD, hyperactivity, learning, and other disorders.

BEREITSCHAFTS (PREMOVEMENT) POTENTIAL

Our conclusion after carefully observing and studying our first patient in 1965, and confirmed by hundreds of subsequent patients, was that the essential feature of the motor and vocal tics is involuntary or unintended physiological responses to unknown CNS stimuli. Clinically, tics resemble normal eye-blinks which are "a thing in themselves" (DSM-III-R) like myokymia, myoclonus during sleep, or a sneeze. This concept, initially resisted, is generally accepted by most, but not all, investigators and clinicians. Heretofore, the conclusion that tics were involuntary was based only on descriptions of the tics by patients and clinical observations.

The Bereitschafts or premovement potential (BP) (Kornhuber and Deecke, 1965; Rothenberger and Kemmerling, 1982) is a negative brain potential considered to be a readiness or premovement potential, which appears 500 to 1,500 msec prior to the initiation of a voluntary or intended muscle movement (Rothenberger and Kemmerling, 1982). It has its highest amplitude in central and parietal derivations and can be recorded by EEGs prior to voluntary muscle movements. The BP provided a means for evaluating the hypothesis that tics are involuntary. This important study was done by Obeso et al. (1981, 1982) in Tourette's disorder. Using computerized back averaging techniques, the BP of Tourette's disorder patients was recorded before involuntary or unintended motor tics and before volitional or intended imitation of the tics. The results clearly demonstrated that BPs were not present prior to a tic, but preceded volitional imitation of the tic. These results provide the first physiological evidence that tics are involuntary, provide a physiologic method to distinguish involuntary from intended movements, and suggests a noncortical origin for tics. The study should be replicated and extended to include study of inarticulate vocal sounds, coprolalia, copropraxia, echolalia, palilalia, and impulsions.

COMPUTERIZED AXIAL TOMOGRAPHY, POSITRON EMISSION TOMOGRAPHY, AND MAGNETIC RESONANCE IMAGING

Computerized Axial Tomography

CAT scan abnormalities, such as ventricular enlargement or asymmetrics, have been reported in 38% of 16 patients with Tourette's disorder, approximately half with attentional disorders and poor school performance (Caparulo et al., 1981). However, a subsequent report, with better methodology, more rigorous criteria of abnormality, and control groups, failed to demonstrate abnormalities in a group of 19 patients with Tourette's disorder (Harcherik et al., 1985), and CAT scans have been reported as normal in two clinical studies of five (Min, 1983) and 53 patients (Lees et al., 1984).

Positive Emission Tomography

PET utilizes intravenously injected molecules (most commonly glucose) tagged with radioisotopes to derive a two-dimensional picture of brain metabolism and neurochemistry. Only one study of five drug-free Tourette's disorder patients has been reported (Chase et al., 1984). The results, considered tentative and preliminary by the authors, included no difference in overall cerebral glucose metabolism, 16% increase of glucose utilization in the basal ganglia, an inverse relationship between severity of vocal tics, and the metabolic rate of the middle and inferior frontal lobes and postcentral gyrus, and coprolalia was inversely correlated with left parasalvian hypometabolism.

Magnetic Resonance Imaging

Studies utilizing MRI, sometimes referred to as NMR, have not yet been reported in the literature. Several investigators have informed us that the results in approximately 12 Tourette's disorder patients were negative.

SLEEP AND AROUSAL DISTURBANCE

Sleep

Clinical reports of disturbed sleep in Tourette's disorder patients cover a wide range: 12% sleep disturbance (not defined) in 12 patients (Moldofsky et al., 1974); 44% sleep disturbance (not defined) in 50 Tourette's patients (Nee et al., 1980).; 27% of 15 patients (one each: sleepwalking, talking in sleep, restless sleep, night-awakening) (Glaze et al., 1983); 17.5% of 57 patients with somnambulism (not defined) (Barabas et al., 1984b); and 27% of 57 patients (nightmares, 6; difficulty falling asleep, 3; night awakening, 3; talking in sleep, rocking during sleep, 1), and past but not present history of somnambulism (Erenberg, 1985). However, sleep disturbance have not been noted in most studies reviewed by us, and clinically they do not appear to us to be more frequent than expected in the population. Some of the discrepancy might be due to age (older patients having less sleep disorders), ADD, and other asociated diagnoses. Confirmation requires control for these factors, adequate criteria, and appropriate control groups.

Arousal

On the other hand, sleep studies suggest the possibility of a higher frequency of sleep disturbance than clinical reports. Mendelson et al. (1980) reported a 30% decrease in delta sleep (stages 3 and 4 combined) in six Tourette's disorder patients off medication (duration not stated) compared with normal controls. Sleep latency, efficiency, and total sleep did not differ from controls. Intermittent awakenings were more frequent, but not significantly more frequent in Tourette's disorder patients than controls. Decreased delta returned to normal values when patients were given haloperidol. Increased awakenings ($p < 0.01$) decreased REM ($p < 0.01$) were confirmed in a preliminary study by Glaze et al. (1983). Stage 3/4 delta sleep, however, was increased ($p < 0.01$). They also report normal awake EEGs in 11 patients, sleep disturbance (enuresis, somnambulism, frequent awakenings) in six of the patients, 10- to 20-sec episodes of intense arousal and disorientation (rhythmic high-voltage delta activity) in stage 4 sleep for seven patients, and decreased total sleep awakenings.

Barabas et al. (1984a) postulate a disorder of arousal associated with a defect in serotonim metabolism for a proposed homogeneous subgroup of Tourette's disorder, based on results in a series of papers and letters. They report 26.6% of 60 Tourette's disorder patients with headaches (defined as "most cases fulfilling the criteria for migraine") (Barabas et al., 1984c); 21.6% of 108 patients with motion sickness (defined as parent report of at least several episodes of car sickness), (Barabas et al., 1984e); 17.5% of 57 patients with somnambulism (not defined) (Barabas et al., 1984a,b); a higher than expected association of somnambulism and migraine (Barabas et al., 1984c); in 15.8% of 57 patients with night terrors (Barabas et al., 1984a), and linkage of a history of migraine in the patient or family and disorders of arousal (defined as sleepwalking, night terrors, and motion sickness) (Barabas and Matthews, 1985), a finding somewhat similar to a report of an association between sleep disturbance and a family history of Tourette's disorder (Nee et al., 1980). A primary disturbance in dopamine metabolism is proposed for patients who do not have migraine or a history of migraine. In contrast to their finding that patients with migraine did not have EEG abnormalities, another study reported that five of six patients with migraine had EEG abnormalities (Verma et al., 1986).

These initial results require replication, especially because of the small sample size, inadequately defined criteria for the symptoms, absence of blind assessment, and evidence of reliability, since they are based on parental reports, and absence of adequate controls and confirmation by other investigators (Krumholz et al., 1983; Erenberg, 1985). We and other investigators have not noted those symptoms to be more frequent in Tourette's disorder. More careful assessment is necessary to evaluate the merits of the hypothesis.

The hypothesis of a generalized arousal disturbance in wakefulness was studied by Bock and Goldberger (1985) who used physiological and neurometric techniques to measure tonic and phasic arousal mechanisms. They reported less change in tonic arousal during habituation paradigms, but failed to find evidence for a global arousal disturbance.

Although the evidence supporting a globally disturbed attention-arousal mechanism is inadequate, some of the previously described preliminary findings warrant further evaluation.

Tics During Sleep

We had previously reported that tics disappeared during sleep (Shapiro et al., 1978). Current evidence indicates that although tics are infrequent, markedly decrease, and are unnoticed by informants, they do occur during sleep. In our sample of 394 informants, tics decreased slightly in 0.8%, decreased markedly in 2%, and disappeared during sleep in 97.2%, a higher percentage than the 86% reported by Erenberg (1986).

It may be difficult to differentiate sleep myoclonus and other adventitious movements from tics. In a sleep study of body movements, not explicitly tics, various measures of body movement increased in Tourette's disorder children compared with controls. Motor and occasional vocal tics (not defined) occurred in all sleep stages in 11 of the 12 children with this disorder but not in the adults. Three patients, treated with tetrabenazine, had a significant decrease in percent of total sleep, number of awakenings, and number of tics during sleep (Glaze et al., 1983). Diverse measures of body movement were reported to increase in another study of children with Tourette's disorder compared to controls (Hashimoto et al., 1981).

Although it appears likely from the few available, primarily clinical reports that tics occur during sleep, additional controlled studies are necessary. This finding that tics do occur during sleep provides further evidence that tics are involuntary, and have a subcortical origin. Identifying the neurochemical or other cause of decreased tics during sleep may have implications for the etiology and treatment of Tourette's disorder (Sandyk, 1985b,c).

CONCLUSION

Although we are committed to a neuropathological hypothesis for the etiology of Tourette's disorder, our review leads us to the conclusion that current neurological data are inadequate to explain its etiology. Shortcomings include methodological problems and speculations based on a series of questionable observations and assumptions. The findings are weakened by inclusion of a high percentage of patients with ADD, hyperactivity, learning and other CNS disorders, often with an unknown number of patients on medication, and the absence of appropriate and adequate controls. Despite these limitations, many clinical observations, preliminary findings, and speculations warrant further study.

We have concluded that EEG abnormalities, nonlocalizing neurological signs, ADD (including hyperactivity and learning disorders), and psychopathology are not intrinsic to Tourette's disorder. Therefore, EEG studies, skull X-rays, CAT, PET, and MRI studies, chemistries, and neuropsychological testing are not necessary for routine evaluation of patients with Tourette's disorder and should only be done if there are other clinical indications for their use or for research purposes.

8

Genetics

This chapter focuses on the history of genetics, and models, theories, and future directions for genetic research in Tourette's disorder. The clustering of Tourette's disorder in families has been observed by investigators since the time it was originally reported by Trousseau and Gilles de la Tourette a century ago. However, systematic efforts to establish and define these familial influences did not begin until the 1970s. At that time, several factors converged to stimulate and guide clinical genetic research on Tourette's disorder.

The sample sizes available for study increased, and old reports of familial patterns began to be reconsidered because tics denied by family members were often observed by experienced clinicians. There was also the recognition of the existence of chronic tics in family members that failed to fulfill criteria for Tourette's disorder, and suggested the possibility that chronic motor tic (CMT) disorder was a form *fruste* or lesser variant of the disorder. Another factor was the well-known fact that Tourette's disorder is characterized by a preponderance of males, which prepared the way for considering a sex effect on the mode of transmission. Other factors were the availability of more sophisticated clinical genetic methods and mathematical models for analysis of data; the return to the concepts of penetrance and expressivity when attempting to interpret familial aggregation data; and the refinement of methods for obtaining data. The latter was the change from the family history method (one or a few family members give the clinical history for all family members) to the family interview method (each family member is directly interviewed). These factors cumulatively ignited a search for the missing pieces that would fill in the genetic puzzle of Tourette's disorder.

The "Genetics" section of Chapter 4 reviews family studies in the literature, sex ratio of relatives, twin research, genetic markers, and describes genetic data on a large sample of patients studied by the Shapiro group. This chapter focuses on recent clinical genetic studies and discusses their hypotheses, methods, and results in relation to potential modes of inheritance.

FAMILIAL AGGREGATION, CLASSIC PEDIGREE METHOD, AND SEGREGATION ANALYSIS

Type of Genetic Disorders

Genetic disorders are conventionally categorized as single gene disorders, chromosome disorders, or multifactorial disorders. Single gene defects are caused by mutant genes whose effects are typically evident on inspection of pedigrees. They are relatively rare, having a frequency of one in 2,000, or less. Chromosome disorders are due to an excess or deficiency of whole chromosomes or chromosome segments. They are common, approximately seven in 1,000 live births, and associated with half of all spontaneous first trimester abortions. Multifactorial disorders are characterized by no single gene error, but, instead, several lesser changes (polygenic) that, together with environmental effects, produce a serious abnormality. They tend to recur in families, but lack the signature of pedigree patterns characteristic of single gene disorders. They are common among developmental disorders (Thompson, 1986).

Difficulties in Interpretation of Pedigree Patterns

Diagnosis and Clinical Criteria

Study of Tourette's disorder, like other potentially genetic disorders, is hampered by the absence of biological markers for the illness. Rigorous segregation analysis is then reliant on clinical phenotypic features as the best available "markers" of a possible genetic defect. This carries significant risk of unreliable observations and misclassification because symptoms are defined arbitrarily, especially for behavioral and cognitive disorders. This may not be a problem if the disorder can be well defined clinically. Nevertheless, the requirement for meticulous assessment and diagnosis is obvious if investigators are to accurately perceive segregation patterns within families. The failure of many clinicians to observe and appreciate CMT in relatives of Tourette's disorder patients is an example of the confusion wrought by such clinical errors.

A similar problem that continues to confound genetic studies of Tourette's disorder is the fact that tics have a high prevalence, estimated from 16 to 25%, in the general population (see Table 3.1). Because in most cases tics are mild and do not come to medical attention, prevalence figures may actually be too low. This is illustrated in a recent study (described previously in Chapter 5) of 159 members of a large Mennonite kindred in which 34 males and 20 females were diagnosed as definite or probable Tourette's disorder or CMT subjects (Kurlan et al., 1986, 1987). Among these 54 subjects, 16 (30%) were unaware of their tics and only two (3.7%) had been given a diagnosis of a tic disorder by local physicians, although not a diagnosis of Tourette's disorder. A small number, ten (18.5%), had turned to a physician for treatment for their tic disorder, and seven (13%) had received medication. These investigators emphasize that most patients had mild Tourette's disorder and CMT that do not require treatment, are not seen in any medical setting, and when they are, the disorder is frequently not diagnosed. Three conclusions can be drawn from this study: the prevalence rates of Tourette's disorder and CMT are probably higher than previously estimated; severity characteristics of tic disorders have profound effects on prevalence rates; and familial aggregation research, even studies using direct interview methods for all family members, are beset by the problem of arbitrary definition for the diagnosis of CMT, particularly in those individuals with relatively mild tics.

Inadequate Clinical Information

The inability to acquire important clinical information on all family members is a common major problem in studies attempting to establish modes of inheritance. Family members may live at a distance, be unlocatable, refuse to cooperate, have incapacitating illnesses, or have died. For these and other reasons, the data are incomplete and can complicate the anticipated segregation analysis.

Variation in the Clinical Expression of the Genotype

Clinicians evaluating a series of patients with a disorder presumed to have a genetic origin are often confronted with highly variable clinical expression of the disorder. The complexities of the clinical diagnosis of Tourette's disorder already described make it imperative that genetic research on this disorder be attentive to the sources of this variability.

Genetic heterogeneity

Different mutations can produce the same phenotype, or one so similar as to be easily confused clinically. This genetic heterogeneity could produce disorders of abnormal involuntary movements that are superficially alike, but have distinct etiologies.

Pleiotropy

A single gene mutation can alter a gene product—an enzyme or structural protein—that will cause multiple phenotypic effects in an individual (pleiotropy). A developmental disorder such as Tourette's disorder is characterized by an abnormality that makes itself evident early in development, and the gene defect can have diverse phenotypic results in fully differentiated structures at a later time. These clinical features may at first appear unrelated;

once they are established as components of the clinical disorder, understanding of the full breadth of its expressivity will enhance the genetic analysis of the disorder (Vogel and Motulsky, 1982; Thompson, 1986).

Concepts of penetrance and expressivity

Variability is common in the expression of a genetic disorder and includes factors such as clinical features, age of onset, the influence of environmental factors, and medications. The mutation of a gene does not necessarily lead to an altered phenotype; when it does, the degree of phenotypic change can be variable. Two concepts designate these effects: penetrance and expressivity.

Penetrance is an all-or-none concept that describes whether the genotype is expressed in individuals. When some individuals carry the gene, but do not express it, it is nonpenetrant in these individuals and there is reduced penetrance in the total group. The mathematical representation of penetrance is the percentage of individuals carrying the gene in whom the clinical phenotype is evident. Expressivity, on the other hand, refers to the variability in form and severity characteristic of the expression of some genes. Individuals in the same family can express a genotype quite differently, due either to the expression of different types of abnormalities or to a range of severity of the abnormalities. Variable expressivity of a genotype is found to be greater across different families than within a family in some disorders; this might reflect either the effects of other modifying genes or an unrecognized genetic heterogeneity. Both variable expression and a failure of penetrance have been observed to be more common in autosomal dominant disorders, causing diagnostic confusion and obscuring the interpretation of pedigrees (Thompson, 1986).

Sex-limited and sex-influenced traits

The sex ratio of affected subjects is not 1:1 in X-linked disorders, as is well known; it is sometimes not appreciated that the sex ratio can be abnormal in autosomal disorders as well. This might reflect the effects of different hormonal environments on the gene defect in the developing individual or other prenatal or perinatal effects. A sex-limited trait is expressed only in a single sex in an autosomal disorder. In contrast, sex-influenced traits are expressed in both sexes, but with markedly different frequencies. Multifactorial traits are often sex-influenced.

Age at onset

Genes are expressed at different times during development, not only during fetal life and at birth. Consequently, genetic disorders have varying ages of onset, extending even into adulthood, that are often characteristic for specific disorders. This must be taken into account in clinical research on the disorder which requires designation of affected or nonaffected status among family members. The simple question concerning whether relatives have reached or not reached the age of expression of a disorder can create formidable problems for the investigator.

Gene interaction and environmental effects

Most discussion of genetic disorders adopts the hypothetical position that a gene acts in isolation while the investigator attempts to define its effects. This pretense is overlooked because of the great complexity introduced when two major sources of influence are considered: gene interaction and environmental effects. Gene interaction refers to modification of the effects of a gene by its own allele or by genes at other loci. Modification of the expression of a gene or the metabolism of its genetic product should always be anticipated; at its most general level this is a reference to the "genetic background." It can contribute to a variable phenotype that may confuse family studies. Similarly, environmental effects on genetic processes and products are pervasive and must be carefully examined if a genetic disorder is to be understood.

Chromosomal Abnormalities

Karyotype analyses of patients with Tourette's disorder generally have not demonstrated chromosomal abnormalities (Shapiro et al., 1978). However, the use of more sophisticated high-resolution banding techniques for karyotype examination might identify occasional individuals who are a Tourette's disorder phenocopy with a chromosomal aberration. For example, a patient was recently described with fragile-X syndrome and clinical diagnoses of Tourette's disorder, autism, and moderate mental retardation (Kerbeshian et al., 1984). Other reports of Tourette's disorder in association with chromosomal abnormalities have included a case with XXX and 9_p mosaicism (Singh et al., 1982) and another with an XYY karyotype (Merskey, 1974). Further investigation along these lines might identify a small subgroup of Tourette's disorder patients with chromosomal aberrations. It would be of interest to assess the association of Tourette's disorder with other genetic disorders; examples are an individual in whom both Tourette's disorder and Duchenne muscular dystrophy were reported (Louis and Bertorini, 1982) and two brothers with Tourette's disorder and tuberous sclerosis (Mathews, 1981).

CLINICAL RESEARCH ON FAMILIAL AGGREGATION IN TOURETTE'S DISORDER

Review of the Literature Up to 1978

The strategy for research on genetic contributions to Tourette's disorder during the early and mid-1970s was to collect cases from genetic research reported in the literature and add families from the authors' patient cohorts as a means of rapidly creating a larger "sample" (Torup, 1962; Corbett et al., 1969; Lucas, 1973; Sanders, 1973; Friel, 1973; Guggenheim, 1979; and Hajal and Leach, 1981). Reports describing a total of 34 families with two or more members with either full or partial syndrome over a 16-year period led to an effort to contact and evaluate new multiplex families (Eldridge et al., 1977). A review of previous genetic research on Tourette's disorder uncovered familial clustering of both motor and vocal tics in 42 families dating from Gilles de la Tourette's original report in 1885. An additional 20 families with Tourette's disorder index case had been reported to have one or more other family members with either motor or phonic tics, but not both; these reports dated from a study by Trousseau in 1873. A new study of 21 multiplex families suggested vertical transmission. However, ascertainment bias, the high prevalence of simple tics in the population, and small sample size left the mode of transmission unclear. An X-linked mechanism was rejected because of several instances of male-to-male transmission. Autosomal dominant, autosomal recessive, and polygenic modes of inheritance were all considered, with no definite conclusion. (Eldridge et al., 1977).

It was appreciated that family studies did not include many individuals with tics that did not fulfill all of the criteria for Tourette's disorder. It was also recognized that tics were common in childhood, making the significance of simple tics unclear, and that base-line prevalence estimates for normative population samples were not available. Estimates at the time suggested a prevalence of tics in childhood ranging from 12 to 23% in various studies (Shapiro et al., 1978). A survey of the literature at that time indicated a prevalence of tics in family members of patients with tics that ranged from 24 to 29%. The prevalence of tics among family members of Tourette's disorder patients was even greater; while the estimates varied widely among studies, one study described a 34.5% prevalence of tics in family members of these patients (Shapiro et al., 1978). When family members were assessed for the full Tourette's disorder, 15 of 392 patients (3.8%) had an additional family member with the disorder. This provided substantial evidence that Tourette's disorder clusters in families, encouraging further research, but a mode of transmission was not clarified. (Shapiro et al., 1978).

The potential significance of sex differences in the rate of positive family histories was also recognized at this time. A review of a series of patients reported that 47% of female patients had a positive family history of tics compared to 28% of male patients. When restricted to only first-degree relatives, 32% of female patients had a family history of tics compared to 24% of male patients (Shapiro et al., 1978).

Another review of genetic research on Tourette's disorder at this time considered the ambiguity of the literature on familial clustering (Wilson et al., 1978). Approximately 30% of patients with Tourette's disorder had a positive family history for tics in the reviewed studies. However, determination of the significance of these findings was dependent on a knowledge of both the prevalence of chronic tics in the population and the number of relatives in each family. The size of the families was usually not reported. The authors estimated the prevalence of chronic tics to be 10%. From this estimate, they suggested that it was fair to conclude that approximately 30% of families would have someone who previously or currently had tics by chance alone. On this basis, they concluded that reports of familial clustering did not support the hypothesis of a significant genetic component for Tourette's disorder. Nevertheless, it was later pointed out that these findings also fail to provide evidence against a genetic hypothesis unless the percentage was quite small. Previous research on Tourette's disorder suggested a high rate of affected family members, so the genetic hypotheses remained tenable (Kidd et al., 1980).

Research Since 1978: Familial Aggregation Studies

Studies using family history methods

Clinical genetic studies of Tourette's disorder by the Yale group (Kidd et al., 1980) provided support for CMTs being a mild manifestation of Tourette's disorder associated with a threshold phenomenon, the familial transmission of Tourette's disorder, the existence of sex difference in the prevalence of this disorder, and the concept that the sex difference is related to a threshold effect in the transmitted susceptibility. The authors confirmed previous reports that the risk to relatives of female probands was greater than the risk to relatives of male probands. A self-report questionnaire was developed and sent to a random sample of patients and families belonging to the Tourette Syndrome Association (TSA). The return rate was disappointing, only 75 questionnaires were completed out of 200 sent, with 66 families providing information about 231 first-degree relatives. The authors considered their study to be pilot, hypothesis-generating research because of the small sample size and the possibility of a self-selection bias. The preliminary findings led to several suggestions about the design of biochemical research on Tourette's disorder. They recommended that data from patients who have relatives with Tourette's disorder or CMT be analyzed separately from those who do not have either Tourette's disorder or CMT because the latter may be sporadic cases with less likelihood of having biochemical abnormalities. They also suggested that an optimal comparison of biochemical indices among subject groups would be within families with more than a single affected individual.

A second systematic genetic study by the Shapiro's group (Baron et al., 1981), provided the first preliminary evidence of single major locus transmission in Tourette's disorder and corroborated the importance of sex effects. It assembled pedigree data with the aim of analyzing it in relation to two genetic hypotheses, single major locus and polygenic-multifactorial modes of inheritance, both incorporating sex effect as a threshold phenomenon. They evaluated 127 consecutive Tourette's disorder patients (93 males and 34 females). Probands had 444 relatives, among whom 11 were determined to have Tourette's disorder and 38 to have CMT. They combined these two groups of relatives into a single "affected" category. The risk for Tourette's and CMT was higher among relatives of female probands than relatives of male probands, consistent with a sex-related threshold phenomenon in which females have a higher genetic loading than males. Using the two-threshold single major locus and polygenic-multifactorial models they found that the polygenic-multifactorial model did not provide a satisfactory fit to the data. The best-fit solution for the single major locus model described a rare allele (0.3%) and there were many nongenetic phenocopies: 79% of affected males and 53% of affected females, leaving many cases of Tourette's disorder and CMT unexplained by this model. The model predicted a population prevalence for Tourette's disorder and CMT, excluding transient tic disorder (TTD), of 0.8% for females and 2.3% for males. This study documented a familial predisposition to Tourette's disorder and CMT whose pattern fit a two-threshold single major locus model of inheritance incorporating sex effect.

The Yale group (Pauls et al., 1981) then attempted to replicate their initial results using a clinic patient sample, and to probe further into severity and risk factors. They utilized the same questionnaire (including a section concerning symptoms of relatives) for the evaluation of 52 consecutive Tourette's disorder patients. In addition, the patient and/or a parent was interviewed and questioned about the presence of Tourette's disorder and CMT in first-degree relatives. Although this family history method was not viewed as optimal, the authors pointed out that it tended to underestimate the actual frequency of a disorder among family members. The data from their initial questionnaire study was reanalyzed among first-degree relatives for the presence of Tourette's disorder and CMT separately. The results of the two studies were then compared in some analyses and combined for others.

They reported that the frequencies of Tourette's disorder and CMT among the 190 first-degree relatives of the 52 probands in the clinic study were similar to the frequencies observed in their questionnaire study. Combining the results for both samples, they concluded that relatives of female probands are at greater risk than relatives of male probands; siblings of probands are at greater risk when at least one parent is affected; brothers of probands are at greater risk than sisters of probands; Tourette's disorder and CMT are etiologically related, CMT appearing to be a mild form of Tourette's; a predisposition to Tourette's disorder and CMT is transmitted from parent to child; there is an actual sex difference for Tourette's disorder and CMT that is not due to ascertainment bias; and the sex difference is related to the transmitted susceptibility as a threshold effect. They emphasized the strength of the evidence for the etiologic relationship between Tourette's disorder and CMT by pointing out that the increased risk for Tourette's in those families with affected parents was observed in the families in which the affected parent had CMT. In addition, the risk for both Tourette's disorder and CMT is increased in relatives of female probands. On the other hand, the fact that the disorder has a higher prevalence among males whereas male probands have fewer affected relatives gives strong support to the concept that the sex effect is a threshold phenomenon related to the transmission of susceptibility for the two traits. Although their results were thought to be similar to another study of aggregation for CMT alone in families, together with a sex difference (Abe and Oda, 1980), they emphasize that no genetic relationship had been demonstrated between those families in which CMT occurs alone, and those in which Tourette's disorder is observed, that CMT is characterized by etiologic heterogeneity, and that further research is required. Also meriting further scrutiny were attentional dysfunction and compulsive phenomena, which according to these investigators are common in Tourette's disorder families; etiologic heterogeneity would again be expected. The authors concluded that a precise mode of inheritance had not yet been adequately demonstrated because none of the genetic models incorporating both sex and severity differences had been excluded by their analyses (Pauls et al., 1981).

Major investigations of the genetic basis of Tourette's disorder were also conducted by the Comings group in the Department of Genetics at the City of Hope Hospital, Duarte, California (Comings et al., 1984). These investigators examined both nuclear families and extended pedigrees. They utilized complex segregation analysis to include the possible influences of both a major gene locus and multifactorial inheritance of the background variation. Their sample included 242 consecutive singly ascertained families of Tourette's disorder patients studied in a clinic (194 male and 48 female probands), comprising 897 first-degree relatives (including 197 brothers and 216 sisters) of probands. Semistructured interviews and review of medical records were used for diagnostic assignment. The probands, parents, siblings, and other relatives, were interviewed. Extended pedigrees (three and four generation) were then separated into nuclear family units for segregation analysis. This was carried out using a mixed model of transmission incorporating possible contributions of a major autosomal locus, as well as a multifactorial variation in the background of each major locus genotype.

The authors reported that 15.5% of first-degree relatives are affected by either Tourette's disorder or CMT, with CMT (11.3%) more common than Tourette's (4.2%). The presence of either Tourette's disorder or CMT in parents increased the recurrence risk of both Tourette's and CMT in siblings. Matings in which both parents have one or the other form of the trait produce more children with the full syndrome than matings in which one parent, but not the other, is affected. Once again, a carefully organized genetic investigation gave evidence for vertical transmission in which a liability for CMT and

Tourette's disorder is transmitted across generations. Segregation analysis of nuclear families and extended pedigrees indicated an incompletely dominant major gene and a multifactorial background variation that is minimally heritable as the favored mode of transmission. Strict multifactorial inheritance with no major locus was rejected in three-generation pedigrees in which the lifetime risk of Tourette's disorder and/or CMT is less than 8/1,000 in the general population. The analyses also rejected a pure recessive major gene effect. Penetrance estimates were reported as 94% for the high-risk homozygote (Ts/Ts), 47% in the Ts/ts heterozygotes, and 0.03 for the low-risk homozygote (ts/ts). Their data indicated that two out of every three cases were heterozygotes, and essentially all other cases would be phenocopies or new mutations. This estimate of the proportion of phenocopies is substantially lower than reported in an earlier study (Baron et al., 1981), and the two studies were not in agreement about the estimate of lifetime risk in the general population.

Their analyses also did not support earlier findings that relatives of female probands have a greater risk for Tourette's disorder or CMT than relatives of male probands (Comings et al., 1984; Shapiro et al., 1978; Kidd et al., 1980). This suggested that the sex-related differences in Tourette's disorder was not related to familial differences, and they judged the familial pattern of Tourette's disorder and CMT to be explained by an autosomal locus with sex-modified penetrances. CMT was viewed as a mild form of the same disorder in Tourette's disorder families. They recommended more intensive study of families with both parents affected, so that children with all three possible allele combinations can be observed. These investigators described the results of these analyses as the first demonstration of a major gene (by segregation analysis) in a human neuropsychiatric disorder with a frequency close to 1%.

Current study

A final study that used the family history method is the current study by the Shapiro group which has not been published previously. The results are comprehensively described in Chapter 4; only the main conclusions are summarized in this section.

The sample size for the Shapiro sample has increased to 641 consecutive clinical patients with Tourette's disorder and 2,630 first-degree relatives. Using a carefully and comprehensively conducted semistructured interview designed to elicit a history of Tourette's disorder or tic disorder (CMT and TTD) in the primary family, a history of Tourette's disorder was obtained in 1.5%, tic disorder in 9.3% and Tourette's or a tic disorder in 10.8% of individuals (Tables 4.9, 4.10). A history of one or more primary family members with Tourette's disorder was reported in 5.5% while 32.3% had a tic disorder and 35.4% had either Tourette's and/or a tic disorder. For all family members, primary and secondary, there is a history in one or more family members of 7.8% for Tourette's disorder, 42.3% for tics, and 46.7% for Tourette's and/or a tic disorder. A history of Tourette's disorder in one or more family members was more frequent in the maternal family (71.4%) than in the paternal family (27.3%); a history of tic disorders was more frequent in the maternal (55.4%) than in paternal (43.9%) members (Table 4.10). Males exceeded females among both primary and secondary affected family members: 70.5% males and 29.5% females with Tourette's disorder among the total group; 59.4% males and 40.6% females for tic disorders; and 60.8% males and 39.2% females for Tourette's and/or tic disorders (Table 4.10). Similarily, more brothers were affected (8.8%) than sisters (4.0%) (Table 4.12) (See Chapter 4 for additional discussion of these relationships and comparisons with other reports in the literature). The results are essentially similar to those reported by Pauls et al. (1981) and Comings et al. (1984). Further support for the heritability of tic disorders is a history of tic disorder in 35% of the primary biological relatives and in 47% of all biological family, compared to relatives' history of a tic disorder in nonbiological relatives for 22 adopted children.

Review of studies in the literature indicates that Tourette's disorder probands with an affected parent are more likely to have siblings with a tic disorder than those without afflicted parents (Table 4.14), monozygotic (MZ) twins are more likely to be concordant for a tic disorder than dizygotic (DZ) twins and siblings (Table 4.15), and that adopted patients with Tourette's disorder have significantly less (none of 22 adopted Tourette's disorder patients) of a family history of tic disorders in their adopted or nonbiological families (Table 4.11). Moreover, many speculative correlates of a history of Tourette's or tic disorder in the family were not confirmed by univariate, correlational, and stepwise regression analyses (SRA Table 4.16). A history of Tourette's disorder and tics was associated with a younger age at onset of Tourette's ($p = 0.05-0.01$), and a family history of Tourette's was associated with less severe Tourette's disorder ($p = 0.01$) and a history of fewer tics of the arm or leg, and less echolalia. Tourette's disorder with attention deficit disorder and with hyperactivity (TS + ADD + H), obsessive compulsive disorder (OCD), obsessive-compulsive symptoms (OCS), and psychopathology were unrelated to a family history of Tourette's disorder or tic disorders. Very few meaningful variables were selected by the SRA indicating essentially that genetic vulnerability is unrelated to the variables, at least those used in this study, or that the variables were not reliably measured. Data were also presented that indicate that the source of samples influence the percent of family members with tic disorders (Table 4.13). The average percent of Tourette's disorder in one or more family members with Tourette's disorder for 12 samples of consecutive, clinical patients is 7.0%. This is 50% lower than the 13.3% in six samples of selected TSA volunteers. A history of one or more family members with either Tourette's or a tic disorder was present in 32.9% of consecutive clinical patients compared to 43.5% (32% higher) for selected referral of volunteer patients. For a family history of tic disorder alone, the percent was about 30% for both sample types (Table

4.13). The difference might be due to selected, volunteer patients having more severe forms of Tourette's disorder and other complications such as TS + ADD, mental deficiency, autism, and other neuropathology or psychopathology. The data suggest reservations about data derived from selected referral of volunteer patients and questionnaire studies.

Direct family interview method

The results from all of these studies were derived from use of the family history method in which information about the family was obtained from only one or two family members. Such studies tend to underestimate the frequency of neuropsychiatric disorders (Andreasen et al., 1977; Orvaschel et al., 1982; Cohen and Cohen, 1984) and are likely to yield less reliable and valid data. These considerations led to a study using direct interviews of all or most family members (Pauls et al., 1984).

Reasoning that the direct family interview method would give substantially more valid and reliable diagnostic assignments, they compared the two methods. Direct interview information was obtained from 86 of 103 first-degree relatives of 27 probands, as well as diagnostic information about all 103 relatives. Comparison of frequencies from this study to those reported in their previous study documented that the direct interview method resulted in an increased number of affected relatives compared to the indirect interview method. Although the two studies are not directly comparable because of different procedures and samples, the frequency of Tourette's disorder among directly interviewed relatives was five times greater than in their indirect family history study (10.7% versus 1.9%). The combined frequencies for Tourette's disorder and CMT using direct interviews was approximately two times higher than for Tourette's disorder and CMT diagnosed through the family history method (29.2% versus 16.2%). In addition, 60% of probands had an affected parent, substantially more than the 26% of probands with an affected parent in the study using the family history method. An interesting result was that affected siblings clustered in the families in which there was an affected parent.

They concluded that further research must utilize the direct family interview method. They also suggest that the risk of Tourette's disorder in families in which Tourette's disorder and CMT clusters is greater than previously recognized, but the small sample size cautioned against generalization of the results. If the results were replicated, several aspects of earlier reports using the family history method would have to be reconsidered. Obviously, parameter estimates used in prior genetic analyses would be too low, and the morbid risk rates derived from earlier research would be revised upwards. New calculations on a sample of sufficient size might lead to a more definitive genetic model for transmission. As might be expected, a large number of the Tourette's disorder cases diagnosed in the families were mild, and many had never sought treatment and few received medication. This reflects diagnostic problems encountered when conducting epidemiologic studies of Tourette's disorder. Those families participating in a clinic, or volunteering in response to requests for participation (TSA) would be likely to have more severe Tourette's disorder and possibly other symptoms in some of their members, leading to an ascertainment bias that would confound genetic analyses. This possibility is supported by the analysis of Table 4.12 which demonstrates that tic disorders in the family are significantly lower ($p = 0.000$) in consecutive clinical patient samples than in selected referral of nonconsecutive, nonclinical volunteer (TSA) samples. All of these considerations, derived from improved clinical assessment methods, promise to generate better understanding of the mode of inheritance of Tourette's disorder and CMT.

The Yale investigators continued their segregation analyses of direct family interview data (Pauls et al., 1984; Pauls and Leckman, 1986). Research from their own and two other sites increased the evidence of a single major gene as the basis for expression of Tourette's disorder and CMT. Yet, each of these reports had failed to establish a mode of inheritance because the observed rates of the disorder in these families were not in agreement with the expected values derived from the segregation analyses. Having documented the fundamental importance of utilizing only direct interview data (Pauls et al., 1984), they postulated that the lack of a satisfactory solution reflected the family history method employed in the initial genetic analyses in these three laboratories. In addition, they reported an association between Tourette's disorder and OCD in both Tourette's disorder patients and their relatives. This led to their examination of the segregation patterns derived when those relatives with only OCD are considered unaffected by Tourette's disorder, as compared to the patterns observed when these relatives are designated as affected.

Their analyses were conducted on the basis of hierarchical application of three diagnostic classification procedures. Initial analyses included only relatives with Tourette's disorder. The second set of analyses was expanded to include relatives with Tourette's disorder or CMT, while the third analyses included relatives with Tourette's disorder, CMT, and OCD. A broad range of population prevalence estimates (and several separate male to female prevalence ratios) were incorporated into their analytic model. Similarly, identification of participating families through the affected members created a bias that was estimated by employment of three different ascertainment probabilities. Multiple genetic models were investigated, arranged hierarchically.

Multiple analyses were performed, but in all cases the mode of transmission was best explained by a model of autosomal dominant transmission with sex-specific, variable penetrance. The procedures used to define "affected" status for the analyses determined the derived penetrance estimates. Analyses using only relatives with Tourette's disorder gave results consistent with autosomal dominant transmission. The penetrance values estimated in these analyses, without including relatives with only CMT, were consistent with autosomal dominant transmission. Frequencies expected according to values estimated from this analysis predicted observed frequencies among relatives according to the goodness-of-fit test. When both subjects with Tourette's disorder or CMT were entered as "affected", the penetrance estimates for males and females were substantially increased (to a level somewhat higher than in previous studies, presumably reflecting the direct interview method). The chi-square goodness-of-fit test in this case indicated a statistically significant difference in the comparison of expected and observed frequencies: The estimated values from segregation analyses suggesting autosomal dominant transmission did not fit the patterns observed among relatives. The number of affected fathers actually observed was much larger than the number predicted; the number of affected mothers observed was much smaller than the number predicted by the model.

The final category of affected subject entered into the analyses included those with Tourette's disorder, CMT, or OCD. The results were consistent with an autosomal dominant model, suggesting that the spectrum for the syndrome includes OCD. Penetrance estimates were 1.00 for males and 0.71 for females. Many more female relatives (17.2%) than male relatives (6.7%) had OCD alone. The goodness-of-fit test indicated that the observed values were in agreement with the expected values for this model. These results provided evidence for a pattern of autosomal dominant transmission in which there are sex-specific differences in the frequency of the disorder and OCD. Their study predicts 10% of patients with the disorder to be phenocopies, as compared to earlier estimates ranging up to 79%.

The failure of their genetic model to predict observed patterns of the disorder when relatives with either Tourette's disorder or CMT are included could result from a deviation in the frequency of CMT in a specific class of relatives. This was supported by the finding that more fathers were affected by CMT than mothers. However, more mothers have OCD, and when they are included among the affected subjects, the observed familial patterns then fit the expected patterns. This is additional evidence favoring the hypothesis that OCD is part of a continuum of behaviors encompassed within the broad syndrome, and that the expression of specific symptoms is characterized by a sex difference. Their results favor the concept that OCD is a subgroup, with other OCD patients having neither a family history of tics nor an etiological relation to Tourette's disorder. Unfortunately, clinical features that can distinguish between the two or more subgroups of OCD are not currently available (Pauls and Leckman, 1986).

The results, however, are not yet definitive (see Chapter 7 for limitations of this study due to the complexity of reliable and valid measurement and differentiation among OCD, OCS, impulsions, complex tics and other Tourette symptoms). Only three factors are cited here: The prevalence of OCS in the population is high and the percentage with OCS may be similar to the percentage in patients with Tourette's disorder (Table 6.7). This problem therefore requires the use of a blindly evaluated and adequate control sample to compare the results of the experimental and control groups. Moreover, it appears that some symptoms that would be classified as tics were classified by the authors as OCD. If they were in error they would have been observing tics but assigning them as OCDs and inflating symptom frequency in the OCD category.

TWIN RESEARCH

Assessment of twin concordance is another method of examining genetic effects in Tourette's disorder. MZ twins are genetically identical and DZ twins have approximately half their genes in common. Establishing reliable zygosity is crucial to twin research. Certainty about the diagnosis of zygosity is based on genetic markers and blood typing, but when not available, is commonly determined by questionnaire (with items inquiring about perceived physical similarity and confusability) (Cohen et al., 1973, 1975; Sarna et al., 1978).

Twin data from the Shapiro group (20 DZ and MZ), and single cases described in the literature (7 MZ and DZ) representing a total of 27 independent twin pairs, are described in Chapter 4 (Table 4.15). Among same sex 16 MZ pairs, 11 are concordant for Tourette's disorder, three for CMT, and two are discordant. In contrast, only one of 4 same sex DZ pairs were concordant for Tourette's disorder, and none of the opposite sex DZ twins were concordant.

A larger sample of 43 same-sex pairs in which at least one co-twin had Tourette's disorder was examined in a more systematic twin study of Tourette's disorder by the Yale group (Price et al., 1984). A questionnaire mailed to over 8,000 members of the TSA led to the identification of 42 pairs, and one pair from their clinic was added. Two of the sets were triplets; an opposite-sex triplet in one set was treated as an ordinary sibling, as was a DZ triplet among a same-sex set. There was some overlap of this sample with previous reports of twin pairs with Tourette's disorder. A follow-up phone call reviewed the questionnaire and inquired about additional information concerning Tourette's disorder and CMT, previous diagnoses, symptoms among first-degree relatives, presence of obsessive-compulsive behavior, and determination of physical similarity and confusability. The investigators estimated that assignment of zygosity on the basis of mailed questionnaires was likely to misclassify only one or two pairs, which would most likely be MZ pairs erroneously designated as DZ pairs (a conservative error) (Cohen et al., 1973, 1975). The analysis was based on 30 pairs classified as probable MZ and 13 pairs as probable DZ, with the excess of MZ pairs presumably reflecting a higher probability of ascertainment of concordant pairs that is common in volunteer twin studies. There were 35 male pairs and eight female pairs, apparently reflecting the lower prevalence of Tourette's disorder among females. Uncertainty concerning possible ascertainment bias led to a decision to not make estimates of specific genetic parameters such as penetrance and heritability.

The overall pairwise twin concordances did not differ in male and female pairs, but there was a marked difference between MZ and DZ pairs: 53% of MZ pairs were concordant for the full Tourette's disorder, while only 8% of DZ pairs were concordant. Concordance for both Tourette's disorder or CMT was 77% for MZ pairs compared to 23% for DZ pairs. Concordance for Tourette's disorder or CMT same-sex twins was not significantly higher for the Shapiro than for the Price sample for MZ pairs (90% versus 77%) and for DZ pairs (33% versus 23%) (Table 4.15). Among 130 first-degree relatives of the 40 nonadopted twin pairs there were two cases of Tourette's disorder (1.5%); 15% of these relatives had Tourette's disorder or tics. These rates are identical to those obtained in the Shapiro sample of 641 Tourette's disorder probands (Table 4.9) and support the assumption that these twin families are not atypical.

Several of an unknown number of retrospective analyses were briefly described: The age at onset of symptoms was significantly associated in concordant MZ twins; the frequency of motor tics was significantly related in fully concordant MZ pairs; and fully discordant pairs had an earlier age at onset (5.9 years) than partially (9.3 years) and fully concordant pairs (8.3 years). They also reported that obsessive-compulsive behavior, briefly assessed but not formally diagnosed, occurred in 83% of Tourette's disorder patients. In twin pairs with at least one with obsessive-compulsive features, concordance was 52% in MZ pairs and 15% in DZ pairs ($p < 0.06$). These results suggested to the authors that there is a continuity among the features of Tourette's disorder and obsessive-compulsive behaviors, and that obsessive compulsive features may be a symptom of Tourette's disorder.

Although ascertainment methods may have contributed to unreliable results, it provided further support for the vertical transmission of Tourette's disorder in families and for CMT being a mild form of Tourette's disorder. Discordant co-twins had tics (not meeting criteria for Tourette's disorder), and partially concordant twin pairs (Tourette's in one, tics in the other) had a similar age at onset, suggesting a common etiology. The lower than anticipated MZ twin concordance (53% full, 77% partial), as well as the smaller than expected difference in MZ and DZ twin concordances, suggest nongenetic factors in the expression of Tourette's disorder, and that the genetic predisposition can be modified by environmental factors, stresses, or developmental changes which determine whether the individual will have no symptoms, Tourette's disorder, CMT, or associated behaviors (Price et al., 1985).

ASSOCIATED PSYCHIATRIC DISORDERS

There has been a recurrent question whether psychiatric or behavioral disorders such as CMT, ADD+H, OCD, and specific learning disorders are components of or an expression of a Tourette's disorder continuum or spectrum. There is now broad agreement that CMT is an intermediate form of the disorder. Systematic study of a possible association of specific learning disabilities and Tourette's disorder has not been done, although the percentage of cases reported in clinical samples of Tourette's disorder patients appear to be higher than expected in the population and may be related to TS + ADD+H.

Possible Genetic Relationship Between Attention Deficit Disorder and Tourette's Disorder

The possibility that ADD+H might be related to Tourette's disorder was suggested by Mahler et al., (1945) who characterized most of their patients as hyperactive, and by Kelman (1965) who noted that 42% of Tourette's disorder patients had ADD. Shapiro et al. cited the presence of ADD in 30 to 62% of Tourette's disorder patients in a series of papers published between 1972 and 1978, and higher than expected percentages in population samples have continued to be reported (Table 4.24, Chapters 4 and 6).

A series of studies at several centers have provided preliminary evidence for the contribution of genetic factors to ADD+H, but without definitive evidence for vertical transmission or the mode of transmission. Observation of symptoms fulfilling criteria for ADD+H in many Tourette's disorder patients prompted many clinicians to wonder about a possible genetic relationship between the two disorders, or subsets of either.

The Yale group conceived of Tourette's disorder as a neuropsychiatric disorder with attentional difficulties, hyperkinesis, impulsivity, and frustration intolerance (i.e., ADD+H) preceding the onset of Tourette's disorder. They suggested these symptoms are intrinsic to Tourette's disorder and that they should be included in the diagnostic criteria (Cohen et al., 1978, 1980, 1982–1983; Leckman et al., 1983, 1985). In other words, Tourette's disorder represented one form of ADD with a common underlying diathesis. This concept was made explicit by Comings et al. (1984) who conceived of both Tourette's disorder and ADD as having the same gene.

At about this time, the Shapiro group began to reconsider their previous conclusions about ADD+H and TS. Subsequently, with a larger sample, and especially with patients with milder forms of Tourette's disorder, the percent of patients with TS + ADD decreased. They began to question whether ascertainment factors were responsible for the high percentages of ADD, and whether, in fact, the percent of ADD among Tourette's disorder patients might not be higher than expectations in the population (Shapiro and Shapiro, 1986) (see Chapters 4 and 6).

Investigators at the City of Hope, Duarte, California studied the possible relationship between Tourette's disorder and ADD+H (Comings and Comings, 1984). A large data set of 250 consecutive clinical Tourette's disorder patients were divided into three grades of Tourette's disorder symptom severity, and the TS + ADD+H patients were allocated into three grades of ADD+H symptom severity. A family history was obtained for all patients, and direct interviews were done as often as possible on an unspecified number of family members. The frequency of ADD+H among Tourette's disorder patients was much higher than in the general population, especially in the 6- to 21-year-age group in which documentation was possible: 62% of males and 42% of females. The grades of severity of Tourette's disorder did not differ between male and female patients. As the grade of severity increased, the severity of ADD+H also increased, particularly in the males. Six pedigrees were presented that mapped the coexistence of Tourette's disorder and ADD+H in the same families. In addition, a MZ twin pair was described in which one had both Tourette's disorder and ADD+H, and the other twin had ADD+H alone. Comparison of Tourette's disorder patients with and without ADD+H suggested that the only differences between the two groups reflected severity, and this was consistent with a formulation that Tourette's disorder with ADD+H is a more severe expression of the TS gene, rather than an indication of two separate types of Tourette's disorder. The authors also emphasized the similarity of many ADD symptoms (even without hyperactivity) to symptoms described in Tourette's disorder patients.

An examination of the question whether stimulants precipitated tics in this sample led to compelling observations that they played no role, or a minor one at most. They estimated that the period of time from onset of hyperactivity to onset of Tourette's disorder symptoms was actually greater in those patients treated with stimulants before tic onset than in the group treated with stimulants after tic onset. Both had a similar family history of Tourette's disorder, approximately three-quarters in each group. They concluded that those individuals developing Tourette's disorder subsequent to stimulant treatment for ADD+H were expressing symptoms of the Tourette's disorder gene that would have appeared regardless of the medication.

Several possibilities for the genetic relationship between Tourette's disorder and ADD+H were proposed: (a) Same gene, same allele: Tourette's disorder and ADD, with or without hyperactivity, express the same mutation of the same gene; (b) same gene, different alleles: Tourette's disorder and a subset of ADD are caused by different mutations of the same gene; (c) different genes, different alleles: A subset of ADD is caused by genes unrelated to Tourette's disorder; and (d) genetic phenocopies: A subset of ADD does not have a genetic etiology. They suggest that although one or more of these four possibilities might occur, the results suggest that within a family the Tourette's disorder gene can be expressed as (a) Tourette's disorder without ADD+H; (b) Tourette's disorder with ADD+H; (c) motor tics with or without ADD+H; (d) vocal tics with or without ADD+H; or (e) ADD + H only. These suppositions are based on six pedigrees and a MZ twin pair whose patterns of symptoms are consistent with other interpretations of genetic relations. For example, it remains a possibility that the MZ twin pair (one with Tourette's disorder and ADD+H, and one with ADD+H alone) reflect the presence of two separate genes responding to similar environmental influences favoring expression of the ADD+H phenotype. Other interpretations are also possible. This report provided a more coherent set of data indicating the necessity of meticulous examination of the possible genetic relationship between Tourette's disorder and ADD+H, but ultimately left the question to be answered by subsequent research.

The Yale group re-evaluated the potential genetic relationship between Tourette's disorder and ADD+H by further analyzing data from their previously described direct family interview study of 27 probands with Tourette's disorder and their 103 first-degree relatives (Pauls et al., 1986a). Their analyses were based on the proposition that a common genetic etiology for Tourette's disorder and ADD+H should manifest itself through fulfillment of three hypotheses: (a) Relatives of Tourette's disorder probands should have higher ADD+H frequency than the population prevalence of ADD+H (3–10%); (b) relatives of probands with Tourette's disorder and ADD+H should have the same risk for ADD+H as relatives of probands with Tourette's disorder without ADD+H; (c) Tourette's disorder plus ADD+H could be a distinct genetic subtype of Tourette's disorder; if so, affected relatives of patients with Tourette's disorder plus ADD+H should demonstrate a higher frequency of Tourette's disorder (or CMT) plus ADD+H than predicted by random assortment of the two disorders. In other words, the two disorders should cosegregate within families.

Their assessments indicated that 11 of 103 (10.7%) first-degree relatives of Tourette's disorder probands met diagnostic criteria for ADD. This frequency was not different from the higher estimate of the population prevalence for ADD. Relatives with only ADD (no Tourette's disorder or CMT) should have an increased frequency among relatives of probands with Tourette's in comparison to the population prevalence for ADD. In fact, only seven (6.8%) of the relatives had ADD in the absence of a tic disorder, indicating no difference from the expected prevalence. Therefore, the first hypothesis, that relatives of Tourette's disorder probands would have a greater frequency of ADD+H than in the general population was not confirmed. The expectation that a high number of Tourette's disorder patients would also have ADD+H was borne out by their finding that 17 of 27 Tourette's probands (63%) met criteria for ADD+H, which is a very high frequency suggesting deviant characteristics for their sample. The second hypothesis (related to the possibility that Tourette's disorder and ADD+H have a common genetic etiology) states that the risk for ADD should be the same for relatives of Tourette's without ADD probands as for relatives of probands with Tourette's disorder and ADD+H. They found that 17.2% of relatives of probands with Tourette's disorder and ADD had ADD themselves, substantially more than the 2.2% of the relatives of probands with Tourette's disorder without ADD.

These findings do not support the existence of a genetic relationship between Tourette's disorder and ADD+H. Nevertheless, Tourette's disorder plus ADD+H could be a subtype of Tourette's disorder with a separate etiology (hypothesis 3). However, the number of relatives with Tourette's disorder and ADD+H or with CMT and ADD+H was not higher than expected by random assortment of the two disorders. There was no evidence of cosegregation of the disorders within the families.

The three hypotheses were not confirmed, and the two disorders do not appear to share common genetic factors. The reason for the high frequency of ADD+H symptoms among some Tourette's disorder samples requires further study, but might be due to the characteristics of selected TSA volunteers. Study of larger samples may, unlike this research, demonstrate a genetic relationship between the two disorders. Other explanations suggested by these investigators include ascertainment bias due to the likelihood that patients with both Tourette's disorder and ADD+H would be more severely impaired and more likely to be evaluated and diagnosed as having Tourette's disorder. Explanations other than this help-seeking bias are not obvious, and the answer will come only through additional research that confirms or denies these findings.

Possible Genetic Relationship Between Obsessive Compulsive Disorder and Tourette's Disorder

The study of OCS and OCD is a hazardous undertaking; the study of the relationship of Tourette's disorder to OCS, OCD, and impulsions is doubly difficult. No study of Tourette's disorder and OCD has been done that adequately fulfills well known basic methodological requirements. The major difficulties, described previously in Chapter 6 and in this chapter, include:

1. There is insufficient agreement about inclusion and exclusion critera, definitions, and reliable and valid measures of OCS, OCD, impulsions, and Tourette's disorder symptoms.
2. Different researchers use different criteria, definitions, and measures.
3. Nonclinical OCSs are frequently interpreted as OCDs.
4. Tourette's disorder symptoms are frequently misclassified as OCS or OCD, which confirms the presence of Tourette's disorder but is erroneously interpreted as OCS or OCD.
5. Inclusion of obsessive-compulsive personality traits, symptoms, or disorder as Tourette's disorder symptoms.
6. Absence of control samples which are essential because of the high percentage of OCS in normal or nonclinical samples.
7. Absence of a matched and appropriate control group rather than healthy volunteers.

8. Absence of blind evaluations to control for bias of observations.
9. Use of questionnaires completed by selected volunteers solicited by members of lay organizations.
10. Absence of power analysis to determine adequate sample size for studies.
11. Use of retrospective analyses, thus capitalizing on chance findings and type I errors.

The use by the Yale group of the direct family interview method was an improvement over previous studies which used the family history method. However, because the study did not include the previously discussed methodological safeguards, the results are controversial, but are useful for the development of hypotheses for future definitive study. With these caveats, the Yale study will be described for heuristic purposes (Pauls et al., 1986b).

The Yale research group examined the relationship between Tourette's disorder and OCD in their direct family interview study. The data were analyzed through procedures that paralleled those for the study on Tourette's disorder and ADD+H. The patients in the study of Tourette's disorder and OCD were 32 probands, five of whom were adopted. There were 103 biologic and 19 adoptive relatives. All probands were randomly ascertained members of the Connecticut Tourette Syndrome Association who volunteered to participate in the study. Diagnoses utilized the "best estimate procedure" in which multiple data sources are examined as the basis for assignment of diagnoses (Leckman et al., 1982). Of 32 probands, 16 (50%) were diagnosed as having OCD. Demographic features were similar in probands with and without OCD in both groups except for an older average age (25.0 years) for probands with Tourette's disorder and OCD compared to those with Tourette's disorder without OCD (16.5 years). Other investigators had previously reported an increase in OCD symptoms among older Tourette's disorder patients (see Chapter 6). The Tourette's disorder probands with OCD were also characterized by lower socioeconomic status than those without OCD. The clinical features of the two Tourette's disorder groups (with or without OCD) were similar in relation to symptom history, symptom severity, and medication history.

Three family groups were formed for comparison: (a) biologic families of Tourette's disorder and OCD probands; (b) biologic families of Tourette's disorder without OCD probands; and (c) adoptive relatives of the five control Tourette's disorder probands. The hypotheses stated that, if Tourette's disorder and OCD had a common genetic etiology, it would be expected that: (a) biologic relatives of Tourette's disorder probands should have a higher frequency of OCD than the relatives in the adoptive families; (b) relatives of Tourette's disorder probands with Tourette's disorder and OCD should have the same risk for OCD as relatives of probands with Tourette's disorder without OCD; and (c) if Tourette's disorder plus OCD is a distinct genetic subtype of Tourette's disorder, then cosegregation of the two disorders within families should be observed.

The interviews with first-degree relatives confirmed a significantly higher frequency of OCD among the 103 biologic relatives of the Tourette's disorder and OCD probands compared to the 19 adoptive relatives. In addition, the rate of OCD among the biologic relatives of the probands with Tourette's disorder without OCD was higher than the rate among the control adoptive relatives. In contrast, there was no difference in the frequency of OCD among biologic relatives of Tourette's disorder plus OCD probands. There was no difference in the risk of these two types of biologic families for Tourette's disorder, CMT, or OCD.

A retrospective breakdown of the frequencies for the various diagnostic categories compared the rates for "pure" OCD (with no tics) in the two family groups. Although the cell sizes are too small for adequate statistical comparisons, the rate of OCD alone (no tics) is increased in the biologic families of Tourette's disorder probands whether they have OCD themselves or do not have OCD. To describe it differently, the frequency of OCD without tics is increased in first-degree relatives of Tourette's disorder probands, even when the proband himself has no symptoms of OCD. In contrast, none of the adoptive relatives had a diagnosis of OCD. The conclusion was that an etiological relationship exists between Tourette's disorder and OCD within biologic families of Tourette's disorder patients, and that OCD is a manifestation of genetic factors contributing to the expression of the full spectrum of Tourette's disorder.

The authors are careful to emphasize the diagnostic problems clouding any research on OCD. Their review of the literature suggests that no satisfactory diagnostic procedure has been determined, and the optimal approach for current use is to apply multiple clinical methods for diagnostic assignment of each subject. Their rate of OCD among the 103 biologic relatives was 12.6%, which is higher than the 2% prevalence rate for nonclinical samples reported in epidemiological studies.

Additional support for a genetic relationship between OCD and Tourette's disorder was derived from the previously described analysis of family data (Pauls et al., 1986b,c). Inclusion of family members with OCD alone strengthened the evidence for autosomal dominant transmission in their segregation analysis, and suggested that the underlying predisposition is characterized by sex-specific differences in the expression of the disorder, which includes Tourette's disorder, CMT, and OCD as manifestations.

These preliminary results provide useful hypotheses for future evaluation, but will require the use of careful and sophisticated methodological procedures. Substantial additional research, with refined diagnostic methods, reliable and valid measurement, and blindly evaluated control samples are necessary to confirm these heuristic hypotheses.

GENES AND ENVIRONMENT

Different sensitivities of Tourette's disorder patients to environmental stimuli implies that environment has an influence on symptom expression in Tourette's disorder. For example, a recent report comments on the 23% discordance among the 30 MZ pairs; six of seven unaffected co-twins had a higher birth weight than the affected twin (Leckman et al., 1987). Improved genetic mathematical models for the interaction of genes and environment may spur research in this area. Currently, however, these models are at an early stage of development, and significant effort will be required to bring this to fruition (Cloninger et al., 1983; Kendler and Eaves, 1986; Roubertoux and Nosten, 1907; Weissman et al., 1986).

CONCLUSION

Several conclusions are suggested by this review of genetic research in Tourette's disorder. There is vertical transmission of Tourette's disorder, with one or more intermediate forms of expression (Table 8.1). Chromosomal aberrations are very rare and insufficient to explain the observed familial clustering of Tourette's disorder. CMT is a lesser variant of Tourette's disorder; some subgroups of CMT may be unrelated to Tourette's disorder. There is initial but controversial evidence that OCD and ADD+H are related to Tourette's disorder. The relationship of TTD and specific learning disorders to Tourette's disorder has not yet been adequately studied. Sex-specific differences in the frequency of Tourette's disorder have been documented, and there are possibly sex-specific differences in the expression of associated disorders and behaviors.

Research on the inheritance of Tourette's disorder has rejected an X-linked mechanism. Polygenic/multifactorial and mixed models have received some support, but a single major locus model best fits the existing data. An autosomal recessive mechanism has been rejected. Preliminary but controversial data suggests that Tourette's disorder and associated disorders may be inherited through an autosomal dominant mode of transmission.

The search for possible genetic markers for Tourette's disorder is at an early stage. Studies utilizing HLA typing have not determined any types to be associated with Tourette's disorder (Arena et al., 1974; Shapiro et al., 1978; Caine et al., 1985; Comings et al., 1982a). Using 21 standard blood marker loci, it was possible to rule out linkage to 16 of the 21 markers. This excluded approximately 15% of the human genome (Pauls and Kurlan, 1986). A neurochemical measure that can act as a marker for Tourette's disorder would be very important, but none are currently available. Linkage analysis may soon lead to localization of the Tourette's disorder gene (Kurlan et al., 1986). However, it has been emphasized that linkage analyses are quite sensitive to

TABLE 8.1. *Genetic models for mode of transmission of Tourette's disorder*

Mode of inheritance	Current status	Study
Vertical transmission	Confirmed	Eldridge et al. (1977)
		Shapiro et al. (1978)
		Kidd et al. (1980)
		Nee et al. (1980)
		Baron et al. (1981)
		Pauls et al. (1981)
		Comings et al. (1984)
		Devor (1984)
		Price et al. (1985)
		Pauls and Leckman (1986)
Chromosomal abnormalities	Very rare	Shapiro et al. (1978)
		Mersky (1974)
		Singh et al. (1982)
		Kerbeshian et al. (1984)
X-linked	Rejected	Eldridge et al. (1977)
		Kidd et al. (1980) and others
Single gene	Confirmed	Baron et al. (1981)
		Comings et al. (1984)
		Devor (1984)
		Pauls and Leckman (1986)
	Probable	Price et al. (1985)
	Possible	Kidd and Pauls (1982)
Autosomal recessive	Rejected	Comings et al. (1984)
		Pauls and Leckman (1986)
Autosomal dominant	Confirmed	Pauls and Leckman (1986)
Polygenic/multifactorial	Rejected	Baron et al. (1981)
		Comings et al. (1984)
		Devor (1984)
	Possible	Kidd and Pauls (1982)
Mixed model	Probable	Comings et al. (1984)
	Possible	Kidd and Pauls (1982)

changes in genetic model factors entered into the analyses; meticulous clinical methods are required to assure that data with the highest possible accuracy are utilized for linkage analyses (Pauls and Leckman, 1986; Chapters 10 and 13). Many technical challenges must be met before the future hope for eventual gene therapy for tic disorders can be realized.

9

Neural Mechanisms

GENERAL ORGANIZATION OF THE MOTOR SYSTEM

Elucidation of underlying neurochemical abnormalities is essential in order to clarify the etiology of Tourette's disorder and guide pharmacological treatment. With increased knowledge of the genetic basis of Tourette's disorder, the objective of neurochemical research is to determine mediators of the genetic defect and the environmental influences on its expression. The question is now rephrased to ask what enzyme(s) or structural protein(s) is (are) impaired through the genetic fault, and how do environmental influences aggravate or mitigate this defect?

Hypotheses about neurochemical abnormalities in Tourette's disorder hinge upon current understanding of the organization of motor function by the brain. Although the symptoms of Tourette's disorder are not limited to the motor sphere, they are most visibly available for investigation and hypothesis formation. Proper function of the motor system is achieved through exquisite control exerted through its hierarchical organization.

1. The spinal cord generates a variety of automatic, stereotyped responses to stimuli known as reflex responses, and acts as the final common pathway for descending influences from the brain.
2. The brainstem integrates descending motor inputs from higher levels and processes information from the spinal cord and the special senses, particularly afferent input related to cranial nerve nuclei and postural adjustments.
3. The motor cortex issues motor commands to the brainstem motor nuclei and the spinal cord through the corticobulbar and corticospinal systems, respectively. It is the point of convergence of cortical influences on motor function.
4. The premotor cortex is closely related to the prefrontal and posterior parietal cortices, and is the highest level of the hierarchy. It acts through the

motor cortex, but has some additional direct influence on brainstem and spinal motor systems (Ghez, 1985).

REGULATORY CONTROL AND COORDINATION OF THE MOTOR SYSTEM

Cerebellum

Two other large divisions of the brain lie outside this formal motor hierarchy, but have a vital influence on the coordination of motor behaviors: the cerebellum and basal ganglia. The cerebellum contains more than half of all the neurons in the brain and is thought to regulate posture and movement by comparing intention (commands for movements) with performance (the actual movements). It receives both movement programming and sensory feedback information and projects to the descending motor systems, where it adjusts their output. The comparative function of the cerebellum consists of an update and control of movement when it deviates from the intended trajectory. The cerebellum is apparently critical to motor learning. Pathology of the cerebellum is evident in particular involuntary movements and disturbances in posture: decreased muscle tone, dyscoordination of limb and eye movements, and impaired balance. Specific clinical phenomena indicative of cerebellar pathology are hypotonia, lack of check, intention (terminal) tremor, titubation, dysmetria, decomposition of movement, dysdiakokinesia, ataxia of gait, scanning speech, and nystagmus (Ghez and Fahn, 1985).

Basal Ganglia

Structural Anatomy

The motor regulatory functions of the basal ganglia are not as well understood as those of the cerebellum. The basal ganglia lack direct afferent or efferent connections with the spinal cord. Afferent input from all areas of the cerebral cortex contribute to efferent influences of the basal ganglia, which are primarily exerted through the thalamus on the premotor and prefrontal cortical areas of the frontal lobes. Basal ganglia pathology is reflected in postural disturbances and abnormal involuntary movements of a different nature than observed in cerebellar disorders. The differences are essential for a clinical appreciation of tics, because they suggest a major role of the basal ganglia in tic disorders (Cote and Crutcher, 1985).

The five anatomical components of the basal ganglia include three major subcortical nuclear structures (caudate, putamen, and globus pallidus) which are functionally interrelated to two other subcortical nuclei (subthalamic nu-

TABLE 9.1. *Anatomical components of the basal ganglia*

Caudate
Putamen
Globus pallidus (or pallidum; consists of internal and external segments)
Subthalamic nucleus (of Luys)
Substantia nigra (consists of pars reticulata and pars compacta)

Alternative terminology
  Neostriatum (or striatum) = caudate + putamen
  Paleostriatum = globus pallidus
  Corpus striatum = neostriatum + paleostriatum
  Archistriatum = amygdaloid nucleus
  Lenticular nucleus = putamen + globus pallidus

cleus and substantia nigra (Table 9.1). The role of the basal ganglia in motor regulation was initially recognized through clinical observations and postmortem examinations of individuals with Parkinson's disease, Huntington's disease, and hemiballismus. Three types of motor abnormalities were recognizable in these disorders: (a) involuntary movements and tremor, (b) slowness and poverty of movement without paralysis, and (c) altered muscle tone and posture. Parkinson's disease was the first brain disorder in which abnormal neurotransmitter metabolism was demonstrated to play a significant role.

Functional Anatomy

Excitatory and inhibitory neuronal circuits

Knowledge of specific components of anatomical circuits of the basal ganglia organizes our understanding of the functional implications of neurochemical research on Tourette's disorder. Afferent projections to the basal ganglia are directed entirely to the striatum. The efferent systems of the basal ganglia are derived from the globus pallidus (internal segment) and the substantia nigra (pars reticulata). The various brain systems whose functions affect motor activity are exquisitely balanced through a series of interacting neuronal circuits capable of fine-tuning each motor act. Excitatory feedback circuits maintain the activity of motor cortex cells whereas inhibitory circuits modulate this activity. Several circuits have been identified and, in most cases, the principal neurotransmitter of each has been specified (Table 9.2).

The functional anatomy of the basal ganglia can be considered as two organizing maps, neuronal feedback circuits, and somatotopic relationships. An overall function of the basal ganglia is regulation of motor activity. The requirement that motor activity be capable of being sustained long enough to execute commands, but also responsive to the modulation that will confer precision in movement, is met by the function of neuronal circuits that pro-

TABLE 9.2. *Maintenance of motor behavior: Cortical and basal ganglia neuronal circuits*

Circuit	Influence	Neurotransmitter	Postulated function of circuit
Excitatory neuronal circuits			
Direct excitation			
1. Collaterals of corticospinal tract to thalamus (ventral anterior and ventral lateral nuclei: VA and VL) Thalamus (VA and VL) to corticospinal tract cells	Excitatory	Glutamate	Positive feedback circuit to sustain activity through corticospinal tract
Excitation by disinhibition			
3. Cortical projections to striatum	Excitatory	Glutamate	Faciliation of cortico-thalamocortical circuits by inhibition of inhibitors (excitation by disinhibition)
Striatum to globus pallidus (internal segment)	Inhibitory	GABA	
Globus pallidus to thalamus (VA and VL) Thalamus to cortex	Inhibitory Excitatory	GABA ??	
Inhibitory neuronal circuits			
2. Globus pallidus (internal segment) and substantia nigra (pars reticulata) output to thalamus (VA and VL) (partial circuit, tonically active)	Inhibitory	GABA	Tonic inhibition of VA/VL cells of thalamus to dampen positive feedback between the cortex and thalamus
4. Striatal output to substantia nigra (pars reticulata) through	Inhibitory	GABA	Negative feedback reducing disinhibition of the thalamus, i.e., facilitating tonic inhibition of the thalamic VA/VL cells
Nigral interneurons to substantia nigra (pars compacta) and	Inhibitory	GABA (or glycine)	
The nigrostriatal projection	Inhibitory	Dopamine	

vide feedback. A positive feedback circuit maintains the activity of two or more cells in a circuit when each cell re-excites the other. The major excitatory circuit for motor function is cortico-thalamocortical. Collaterals of corticospinal tract neurons excite thalamic cells (VA/VL) that project to the premotor and motor cortex, where they, in turn, are excitatory on corticospinal tract cells. This reinforcing circuit sustains motor activity, but can be functional only in a context of intermittent inhibition for regulatory purposes. The major source of this modulation is a projection from the globus pallidus (internal segment) and substantia nigra (pars reticulata) that is inhibitory to thalamic VA/VL cells. The cells of this inhibitory projection are tonically active and appear to dampen the excitatory feedback in the cortico-thalamocortical circuit (Penney and Young, 1983) (Table 9.2).

An override of the tonic activity of this pallidal/nigral-thalamic inhibitory projection might occur through either (a) a pronounced increase in the excitation of the VA/VL cells of the thalamus through other circuits, or (b) an inhibition of the pallidal/nigral-thalamic inhibitory projection. This inhibition of an inhibitory pathway, known as disinhibition, occurs through the activity of striatal cells that project to the pallidal/nigral cells. Each of these inhibitory projections appears to utilize gamma-aminobutyric acid (GABA) as neurotransmitter. Cortical projections to the striatum excite the striatal GABA output cells, and the two sequential inhibitory GABA neurons lead to disinhibition of the cortico-thalamocortical circuit (Penney and Young, 1983) (Table 9.2). This is a significant excitatory circuit essential to the maintenance of ongoing movements.

A fourth neuronal circuit appears to provide modulatory negative feedback to the disinhibitory (striatal-pallidal/nigral-thalamic) circuit. This fourth circuit is composed of striatonigral cells (GABA) projecting to inhibitory nigral interneurons (GABA?) that form synapses on nigrostriatal inhibitory dopamine neurons. The three sequential inhibitory neurons (GABA, GABA, dopamine) constitute an inhibitory feedback loop onto the disinhibitory circuit just described (Penney and Young, 1983) (Table 9.2).

The disinhibitory circuit would favor unmodulated activity, resulting in the maintenance of ongoing activity and difficulty initiating new behaviors. The nigrostriatal dopaminergic projection may regulate the ease of transmission through the disinhibitory circuit, facilitating both maintenance of ongoing activities and the initiation of new activities. This appears to be a tonic modulation of striatal activity by dopamine (Penney and Young, 1983). It may be a significant component of the basal ganglia's role in the stabilization of motor systems (Ito, 1986).

The interposition of a cholinergic excitatory cell in this loop provides a further mechanism for amplification of modulatory capacities in these circuits. The acetylcholine interneuron excites the inhibitory GABA output neuron of the striatum. The cholinergic cell is itself under the influence of (a) excitation by corticostriatal (glutamate) projections, and (b) inhibition by nigrostriatal (dopamine) projections.

Local axon collaterals

Further refinement of the modulated control of motor systems is achieved through the function of local axon collaterals of the GABA striatal output cells that suppress the activity of some output neurons (e.g., some of the pallidal-thalamic inhibitory neurons described above), but not others. This leads to a differentiated disinhibition of some VA/VL thalamocortical projection cells simultaneous with continuing inhibition of others. This represents an important means for striatal control over the selective maintenance (e.g., extension of specific muscles) and suppression (e.g., flexion of the muscles) of cortical motor activities. These operations appear to be significant in striatal influences on other parts of the cortex as well. The patterning of agonistic and antagonistic motor activities by the basal ganglia establish a basis for the "behavioral set" hypothesized as required for a specific movement (Buchwald et al., 1979; Penney and Young, 1983), and for the species-specific behaviors fundamental to orientation to innate set-goals.

Somatotopic organization

Somatotopic organization is the second basis for a functional mapping of the basal ganglia. Frontal lobe cells project largely to the head of the caudate and output cells from more posterior regions of the cortex project prominently to the putamen and the tail of the caudate nucleus (Groves and Young, 1985). Viewed somewhat differently, the sensorimotor cortex projects somatotopically to the putamen, while the association cortex projects to the caudate and the limbic cortex to the nucleus accumbens. These nuclei, in turn, maintain these relations in their efferent output to the globus pallidus and substantia nigra. Pallidal neurons are primarily active in relation to limb movement and nigral neurons with axial and cranial movements. The relationships continue in the remainder of the circuit to the thalamus and returning to the cortex. This enables the maintenance or inhibition of movements of specific, selected parts of the body independent of other parts (Penney and Young, 1983).

These concepts of excitatory and inhibitory circuits, somatotopic organization, and local axon collaterals infer the necessity of considering neural organization at levels beyond the molecular and cellular functions. Methods for examining the functional behavior of populations of multiple interacting neurons are relatively undeveloped in relation to single cell techniques, but this level of conceptualization is essential to clarifying the relation of activities of specific neural assemblies and associated behaviors. Novel electrophysiological and imaging methods (e.g., topographical mapping of event-related potentials and the application of Positron emission tomography (PET scan methods) have begun to chart population responses of very large neural sets in relation to selected functional demands. In addition, the pathophysiology of certain diseases illuminates neural-functional relations; classical examples are the effects of degeneration of the dopaminergic afferents to the neostriatum in Parkinson's disease and degeneration of neurons within the neostriatum in Huntington's disease.

Spiny Neurons and Differential Refinement of Motor Regulation. A single morphologic type of neuron constitutes fully 96% of the neurons in the neostriatum: the spiny neuron, of which there are over 100 million on each side of the human brain. The several other types of nerve cells in the neostriatum are much less plentiful. The dendrites of spiny cells have multiple spines dispersed on each, and the sum of 5,000 to 10,000 spines on each spiny neuron are each the postsynaptic element of an axospinous synapse formed with an afferent fiber. The three major afferent systems to the neostriatum (dopaminergic nigrostriatal projection, thalamic afferents, and corticostriatal fibers) converge onto different spines of the spiny neuron in a topographically organized fashion. Neuroanatomic regions that are functionally related through reciprocal anatomic connections converge onto similar areas of the neostriatum. This allocates an integrative function to the spiny neurons receiving the convergent input of diverse, but anatomically and functionally related, components of the cerebral cortex, thalamus, and substantia nigra (Groves and Young, 1985).

The major afferent projections to the neostriatum form type I synapses, which typically exert excitatory effects on the postsynaptic neuron. Cortical and thalamic inputs to the (postsynaptic) spiny neuron are excitatory. However, there has been controversy about the nature of the action of one class of these inputs, the dopaminergic nigrostriatal projection at the spiny neurons. Both the type I structure and the intracellular response to stimulation of dopaminergic neurons suggests that the snyapse is excitatory, but exogenous application of dopamine or other agonists appears to cause an inhibition at the synapse and a reduced firing rate of spiny cells. The basis for this apparent discrepancy is not clear, but hypotheses have included (a) different receptors on the spiny cell, with excitatory effects at axospinous synapses and slower inhibitory effects at receptors on the initial segment of the spiny neuron; or (b) inhibitory effects of exogenous dopamine on dopamine receptors on the nerve endings of afferents to the neostriatum. This has led to the hypothesis that, in addition to the conventional exitatory effects at axospinous synapses, there may be a "remote," possibly tonic inhibitory influence of the dopaminergic projection on the neostriatal network.

The major axonal branch of the spiny neuron projects outside the neostriatum, while there are also extensive axon collaterals that form inhibitory synapses on neighboring spiny neurons. The neurotransmitter of these inhibitory synapses appears to be GABA. The marked predominance of the spiny neurons among the cells of the neostriatum, together with the extensive collateral network of these spiny cells suggests a fundamental importance of these inhibitory interactions. Such inhibitory networks in the central nervous system apparently enhance the capacity of the network to differentiate among inputs. The convergence of multiple excitatory synapses onto the spiny neuron facilitates a summation of excitation from these afferent systems if they arrive near-simultaneously. Neighboring cells also receive convergent excitatory input from afferent fibers. The collateral network of each spiny cell refines this influence to neighboring spiny cells because the spiny cells receiving the greatest amounts of excitation in turn exert the strongest inhibition on neighboring cells. This heightens the difference between the response of the particular spiny cell and its neighboring nerve cells, through this process enhancing the differentiation of convergent input in a manner that filters and refines the output (Groves and Young, 1985).

Nonprimary Motor Cortex: The Premotor Cortex and the Supplementary Motor Cortex

The frontal lobe of the brain is traditionally divided into three regions: the motor cortex (area 4), the "prefrontal" cortex, and the area lying between, the nonprimary motor cortex (area 6). The functional roles of the nonprimary motor cortex (consisting of the premotor cortex and the supplementary motor cortex) is the subject of current research. These areas appear to be essential to the preparation for movement and the sensory guidance of movement. The preparation for movement involves several component features. Motor programming is conceptualized as the assembly of motor subroutines for later execution, as well as the specification of appropriate force and time specifications for the muscles required for a movement. "Motor set" is a more encompassing concept, involving the state of readiness to perform a specific movement, and includes programming, postural stabilization, and reflex suppression. Arousal, goal selection, selective attention, and strategy formulation are other behavioral components contributing to the planning and execution of movements, and are related to the general function of planning for future action that is characteristic of many frontal lobe functions (Wise and Strick, 1984; Wise, 1985).

Novel anatomical research has illuminated the function of these regions by demonstrating patterns of connectivity. It appears that feedback loops to the cortex are organized as parallel channels in which the deep nuclei of the cerebellum, the globus pallidus, and the substantia nigra have separate thalamic targets, with this separation preserved in their destinations in the motor (from the cerebellum), premotor (from the globus pallidus), and prefrontal (from the substantia nigra) cortices. The coordination of these independent circuits may be accomplished by local cortical fibers that connect various subdivisions within the frontal lobe (e.g., topographical connections between the motor and premotor cortices, or multisynaptic prefrontal-premotor pathways to the motor cortex. The premotor and prefrontal regions have rich cortico-cortical processing networks that communicate with sensory and motor cortices; they are characterized by columnar interdigitation of ipsilateral and contralateral cortico-cortical connectivity (Goldman-Rakic, 1984).

Prefrontal Cortex

The prefrontal cortex has been of special interest to investigators because of its contribution to abstract thought, synthetic reasoning, and the organization of individual behaviors sequentially in time and space. However, extensive research has not been done because of methodological problems associated with the complexity of these functions.

Research indicates that the prefrontal cortex has an important role in verbal fluency, the organization and monitoring of material to be remembered and responded to, and the use of environmental stimuli to regulate behavior (e.g., the ability to overcome previously established response tendencies according to new external cues) (Milner and Petrides, 1984). Many of its functions appear to be related to the general capacity to form elaborate and temporally extended behavioral sequences, i.e., the organization of goal-directed actions in the time domain. Two activities in which the prefrontal area participates are short-term memory and anticipatory set (Fuster, 1984). The integration of sensory data and motor activity is reflected in two types of cells discharging in the prefrontal cortex, one related to environmental stimuli associated with short-term memory, the other related to response, and preparation for response (Fuster, 1984). Thus, neuronal activity is synchronous with this cue, delay, and response sequence of a delayed-response trial. Connections have been demonstrated among prefrontal cortex and other regions involved in short-term memory (Goldman-Rakic, 1984).

Alterations in neuronal discharge in the striatum, globus pallidus, and substantia nigra pars reticulata precede specified movements in certain situations: some neurons in relation to a remembered target but not to a target currently present, others in response to a behaviorally significant stimulus but not an insignificant one. This suggests that a system including the basal ganglia may be uniquely involved in the internal initiation of movement in the absence of sensory guidance. The intimate anatomical connections between the basal ganglia and the frontal cortex suggests that the latter may be a component of this system (Evarts et al., 1984). The prefrontal and premotor cortices have intense and diffuse projections throughout the caudate nucleus. Deficits on delayed response tasks can be produced by caudate lesions, and these deficits are as severe as those spawned by prefontal lesions. This connectivity between neostriatum and prefrontal cortex appears to be essential to the regulation of voluntary motor behavior (Goldman-Rakic, 1984).

NEURONAL LOCALIZATION OF NEUROTRANSMITTERS: PERSPECTIVES ON PATHOPHYSIOLOGY AND NEUROPHARMACOLOGY

Dopaminergic Neuronal Systems

Anatomy and Function

The discussion of the intrinsic and extrinsic neuronal systems of various components of the basal ganglia identified an individual neurotransmitter associated with each system; there is actually greater complexity because multiple neurotransmitters in single neuronal systems in the basal ganglia have been demonstrated. However, the dopamine-containing neuronal systems have been examined in more detail than others and have been more directly implicated in both the pathophysiology of Tourette's disorder and its amelioration by pharmacological agents.

Dopaminergic activity is known to have important effects on motor regulation, cognition, arousal, and other essential phenomena. Its discrete anatomical organization has been mapped.

Distribution of the terminal fields of the dopaminergic neuronal systems has led to a general classification of four relatively discrete subsystems: the nigrostriatal, mesolimbic, mesocortical, and tuberoinfundibular dopaminergic systems. Determination of the intrinsic properties of these subsystems, as well as of the related dopamine receptors, have clarified many aspects of both pathophysiology and pharmacological actions of related drugs.

Dopamine Receptors

Receptor binding studies

The direct investigation of postsynaptic effects of dopamine has been made possible by the development of radioligand binding techniques. The utilization of classical functional assays of receptor activation (e.g., adenylate cyclase activity, muscle contraction, etc.) in association with radioligand binding data identifying putative dopamine receptors has provided substantial information about dopamine receptors and their subtypes. These advances developed against a background that included two major areas of research that fundamentally altered our understanding of dopaminergic function and the dopamine receptor in human disorders. The first was the identification of a dopamine-sensitive adenylate cyclase in both the peripheral and central nervous systems. The enzyme is distributed in brain areas rich in dopaminergic innervation, suggesting an association with dopaminergic transmission. The second research area demonstrated parallel effects between binding characteristics of phenothiazines and other neuroleptics at dopamine binding sites and their clinical potencies in relation to specific symptom dimensions. The phenothiazines have been shown to be competitive inhibitors of dopamine stimulation of adenylate cyclase, and the range of this inhibitory capacity parallels the antipsychotic potencies of the drugs. However, the correlation of inhibitory capacity and antipsychotic potency does not extend to the butyrophenones, such as haloperidol and spiroperidol. Their inhibition of dopamine-stimulated cyclic adenosine monophosphate (AMP) production is quite weak in relation to their antipsychotic potency. Eventually, several explanations for this discrepancy were considered, including one which hypothesized that butyrophenones did not block dopamine receptors, but reduced dopaminergic activity indirectly. Another theory postulated the existence of more than one kind of dopamine receptor. Further research has supported the view that there are at least two subtypes of dopamine receptors, D1 and D2. Activation of D1 receptors is accompanied by stimulation of dopamine-sensitive adenylate cyclase activity, while agonist occupation of the D2 receptor elicits either no effect or a decrease in adenylate cyclase activity. More complex categorization of dopamine receptors has included description of D3 and D4 receptors, but, in some studies, they appear to be different states of the first two receptors. Many investigators find that the D1, D2, and D3 categorization fits the cumulative data on dopamine receptor research best at the moment. Antipsychotic agents appear to exert their beneficial effects through blocking D2 receptors (Creese et al., 1983; Jenner and Marsden, 1983; Bunney, 1984).

Autoreceptors

At an early stage of the investigation of dopamine receptors evidence accumulated that suggested the presence of dopamine-sensitive presynaptic receptors on the axons of central dopamine neurons projecting to the striatum. Subsequently, receptors on neurotransmitter-specific neurons that respond to the neuron's own transmitter have been designated as "autoreceptors"; this terminology applies regardless of the location of the autoreceptors relative to a specific synapse. Dopamine autoreceptors occur on the soma and dendrites of midbrain dopamine neurons, as well as the nerve terminals of nigrostriatal and mesolimbic neurons.

Autoreceptors on dopamine neurons modulate the rate of dopamine biosynthesis and impulse-induced release of dopamine through a negative feedback mechanism. Stimulation of these autoreceptors reduces the physiological activity of the dopamine neurons, while blockade of the autoreceptors augments dopaminergic effects on postsynaptic cells (Bunney and Aghajanian, 1978). Autoreceptors are not present on all four dopamine systems in the brain, possibly accounting for significant clinical phenomena theoretically related to these differences. Tuberoinfundibular and some mesocortical (mesoprefrontal and mesocingulate) dopamine neurons appear to lack autoreceptors, and this is hypothesized to be the basis for the relative failure of mesocortical dopamine neurons to develop tolerance during prolonged neuroleptic treatment (Cooper et al., 1986; Roth, 1984).

The most interesting feature of autoreceptors is their greater sensitivity to agonists when compared to postsynaptic receptors. The dopamine agonist apomorphine is 10 to 20 times more potent at dopamine autoreceptors than dopamine postsynaptic receptors (Skirboll et al., 1979). Pharmacological exploitation of this differential sensitivity is essential to treatment strategies attempting to diminish dopaminergic activity through low doses of agonist to activate dopamine autoreceptors without effects at postsynaptic sites (Cooper et al., 1986; Roth, 1984). New drugs tailored to increased specificity of action at autoreceptors and postsynaptic receptors may have useful clinical applications in the treatment of Tourette's disorder.

Noradrenergic Neuronal Systems

Anatomy and Function

Noradrenergic fibers from the locus coeruleus (LC) are diffusely distributed to essentially all parts of the brain and spinal cord. This widespread terminal field of the LC is paralleled by the broad effects of the noradrenergic system on behavior, including arousal, selective attention, mood, sleep, learning and memory, behavioral reinforcement, anxiety, and other dimensions. Although noradrenergic neurons are not an intrinsic component of the basal gangila or cerebellum, their broad activity is the basis for the attention given them in research on Tourette's disorder.

The LC has two major subdivisions, the ventral and dorsal bundles, and projects to all major areas of the neuraxis. More recent research has designated five tracts emanating from the LC, three ascending to midbrain and forebrain structures, one to the cerebellum, and one descending to the spinal cord. Many other noradrenergic neurons, separate from the LC, are found scattered in the lateral ventral tegmental fields and generate fibers that intermingle with those from the LC (Aston-Jones et al., 1984; Cooper et al., 1986). The afferent projections to the LC are quite limited, arising largely from two nuclei (the paragigantocellularis and the prepositus hypoglossi) with possible minor inputs from two other nuclei. Structures previously thought to project to the LC now appear to innervate neighboring areas instead. Afferents to the LC appear to utilize multiple neurotransmitter systems (Aston-Jones et al., 1986).

Systematic research on the LC-norepinephrine (NE) system in many laboratories has suggested that stimulation of the LC causes inhibition of most target cells, depressing their spontaneous activity. The underlying mechanism of this inhibition includes hyperpolarization of the target cell with an increase in membrane resistance (a decrease in passive ionic conductance across the membrane). This is in contrast to the hyperpolarization with decreased membrane resistance commonly observed with such classical inhibitory transmitters as GABA. These effects of LC-NE activity appear to lead to a reduction in endogenous or "background" spike activity, at the same time enhancing evoked activity to afferents. This has suggested that LC activity may augment the signal-to-noise ratio of the target cells. Other characteristics of its physiological effects are in agreement with this type of conceptual description of LC-NE functions. They emphasize the integrative function of the diffusely distributed LC-NE system on cellular systems in the brain. (Aston-Jones et al., 1984). This is in harmony with the restricted afferent input to the LC, providing highly preprocessed signals to the LC. Rather than processing complex signals from diverse sources, the LC would appear to respond to influences from two sources and project a uniform, synchronous message through its broad efferent network (Aston-Jones et al., 1986).

These coordinating activities may primarily be directed to contrasting states of tonic vegetative behavior and phasic intense excitation driven behavior. Strong tonic afferent inhibition of the LC-NE system may underly vegetative function and the global orientation of brain programs to visceral processes. Interruption by intense phasic afferent excitation may facilitate response to the external world, particularly unexpected stimuli and events. This capacity of the LC-NE system to respond to internal and external stimuli by favoring a global orientation of behavior either to the external or internal environment fits well with previous observataions of its domains of behavioral influence, such as vigilance and arousal (Aston-Jones et al., 1984; Robbins, 1984).

Noradrenergic Receptors

Each of the two major classes of noradrenergic receptors, alpha and beta, includes two subtypes (alpha$_1$, and alpha$_2$; and beta$_1$ and beta$_2$). All but alpha$_1$ receptors are linked to the adenylate cyclase system as biochemical effector in signal transduction in the membrane. A large number of beta-receptors have been demonstrated in the cerebral cortex and the cerebellar cortex. (Lefkowitz et al., 1984; Aston-Jones et al., 1984).

Autoreceptors on central noradrenergic neurons modulate impulse-induced transmitter release, but have not yet been demonstrated to regulate biosynthesis of norepinephrine. Low doses of drugs blocking adrenergic receptors (e.g., yohimbine) act selectively to block autoreceptors (alpha$_2$ receptors), while increase of dosage interferes with this specificity and effects at alpha$_1$ receptors are observable.

Serotonergic Neuronal Systems

Serotonin-containing neurons are located near the midline of the pons and upper brainstem, particularly in the raphe nuclei. Caudal cell groups project to the medulla and spinal cord, while rostral nuclei generate diffuse innervation of the diencephalon and telencephalon. The distinct pattern of noradrenergic innervation of the cerebral cortex is not characteristic of the more heterogenous terminal fields of serotonin neurons in the cerebral cortex. The predominant effect of serotonin on target cells is to decrease their discharge rate, although serotonin is known to cause activation in specific regions. It is not yet clear whether serotonin has effects on target cells that modulate the response of these cells to other afferent input.

Multiple receptors for serotonin have been identified. While serotonin receptor classification systems are the subject of active research, a conservative approach would specify 5-HT_{1A}, 5-HT_{1B}, and 5-HT_2 subtypes. Serotonin does not activate adenylate cyclase in mammalian brain, although it is known to do so in other specific tissues. Serotonergic activity appears to influence a wide range of behavioral dimensions, although distinguishing them from effects mediated by other neuronal systems has often posed a problem (Cooper et al., 1986; Aghajanian, 1981).

Cholinergic Neuronal Systems

Determination of the anatomy of cholinergic tracts in the brain has been impeded by technical difficulties until the past few years. Recent methods have identified ascending cholinergic pathways from several pontine and forebrain nuclei, as well as interneurons in areas such as the striatum and cerebral cortex. The cellular effects of acetylcholine suggest that it may be a hormone as well as a neurotransmitter. Muscarinic cholinergic receptors have been classified as M_1 and M_2 types. The nicotinic cholinergic receptor has been isolated and characterized in great detail.

Amino Acid Neurotransmitters

The amino acid transmitters are the major transmitters in the mammalian CNS from a quantitative viewpoint; the monoamines, in contrast, act as transmitters at a small percentage of synapses. The excitatory amino acids depolarize neurons in the mammalian CNS, and include glutamic acid, aspartic acid, cysteic acid, and homocysteic acid. The inhibitory amino acids hyperpolarize mammalian neurons, and include GABA, glycine, taurine, and beta-alanine.

GABA is present in high concentrations in the brain and spinal cord (measured in micromoles per gram, rather than nanomoles), and is a transmitter at approximately 30% of brain synapses. The greatest concentrations in the human brain are found in the substantia nigra, globus pallidus, and hypothalamus, but GABA is present in widespread regions of the brain. In most brain areas, GABA is associated with local inhibitory neurons; it is located in longer projections in only two regions. There are large numbers of GABA receptors in the brain. Because GABA binds to a great number of sites in the brain, it is difficult to distinguish which should properly be designated as GABA receptors. Antianxiety drugs, such as the benzodiazepines, alter the function of GABA receptors to facilitate GABAergic transmission. (Tallman and Gallager, 1985; Cooper et al., 1986).

The involvement of glutamate in intermediary metabolism (e.g., one of its functions is as precursor for GABA) has made it difficult to conclusively demonstrate its role as an excitatory transmitter in mammalian brain. However, these technical problems are now being overcome and it is clear that glutamate is present in high concentrations in brain and has powerful stimulatory effects on neuronal activity. The excitatory amino acids are widespread throughout the neuraxis. Three excitatory amino acid receptor subtypes have been designated as N-methyl-D-aspartate (NMDA), quisqualate, and kainate (Cooper et al., 1986).

CLINICAL NEUROCHEMICAL RESEARCH

Neuropharmacological and Neurochemical Methods

Dopaminergic Function

The consistent response to drugs affecting dopamine release and receptors is the most compelling evidence for dopaminergic involvement in Tourette's disorder. Haloperidol, a dopamine-receptor blocking agent, is the principal medication used in the treatment of Tourette's disorder. Approximately 80% of Tourette's disorder patients have a good response to haloperidol, suggesting that an excess of dopaminergic activity contributes to symptom formation. Other neuroleptics that block dopamine receptors have a similar effect (e.g., pimozide, fluphenazine, penfluridol). Congruent with this theory, although controversial (see Chapter 11), are reports that stimulant medications, which release dopamine, can trigger or exacerbate tics. Stimulant medications can also induce complex stereotypies in animals which may be amplified by stress, adding further credence to this model (Knott and Hutson, 1982). Tics occasionally have been reported to appear during neuroleptic therapy or neuroleptic withdrawal, providing additional support for dopaminergic mechanisms (hypothesized as supersensitivity of postsynaptic receptors) in the genesis of tics (Klawans et al., 1978, 1982; Gualtieri and Patterson, 1986).

Studies measuring homovanillic acid (HVA), the principal dopamine metabolite, in the cerebrospinal fluid (CSF) are inconsistent. Post-probenicid

HVA levels were reported as high in two studies of five and 12 Tourette's disorder patients (Van Woert et al., 1976; Han-bai and Han-quin, 1983), as normal in seven patients before and after probenicid (Shapiro et al., 1978), and other studies of one, nine, and ten Tourette's disorder patients reported lower levels (Johansson and Roos, 1974; Buter et al., 1979; Cohen et al., 1979a; Singer et al., 1982b). Singer et al. (1982b) reported a significant increase in CSF HVA following treatment with haloperidol compared to baseline values. They were unable to confirm a previous report (Cohen et al., 1978) of low 5-hydroxyindoleacetic acid (5-HIAA) levels relative to probenicid and severity of symptomatology.

The inconsistency in the data on HVA levels may be largely the result of procedural differences. Obviously, there is a need for a uniform method to measure HVA. Interpretation of the data would also be enhanced if controls were matched for age, sex, and other variables. Nevertheless, despite the small sample size used in these studies, the majority report that HVA levels are decreased in Tourette's disorder patients, suggesting that the increased dopaminergic activity may be due to supersensitivity of postsynaptic dopamine receptors with a subsequent reduction in presynaptic dopamine release.

Friedhoff (1982) has attempted to test the hypothesis of an overactive dopaminergic system in the pathogenesis of Tourette's disorder. Using a technique of pharmacological intervention in fetal rats, Friedhoff produced a state of enduring hyperdopaminergia secondary to an increase in the number of dopamine receptors. L-DOPA was administered to Tourette's disorder patients to produce an increase in central dopamine and a decreased number of postsynaptic dopamine receptors. The termination of L-DOPA resulted in temporary improvement in six patients with Tourette's disorder although other clinicians report having treated patients in whom this technique has been unsuccessful.

Karson et al. (1985) studied blink rate, a putative correlate of central dopamine activity in 19 Tourette patients and 49 controls. Blink rate was not elevated compared to controls and was not reduced by treatment with pimozide, but did correlate with the number and severity of tics. The results are not consistent with elevated brain dopamine activity.

Individual differences among patients are suggested by a study using challenge doses of a drug and simultaneous behavioral observations. The mean results for a group of six Tourette's disorder patients indicated predictable behavioral responses to stimulants and haloperidol. Examination of the behaviors of individual patients showed a surprising diversity of responses. Patients did not always improve with haloperidol or worsen with stimulants. The etiological heterogeneity of disorders, and individual differences among patients, make predictions concerning single patients hazardous (Caine et al., 1984).

Clinicians have come to this conclusion through a number of observations. Not all patients respond to haloperidol and there is a wide therapeutic dose range among those who do. Some clinicians have observed beneficial effects of stimulants in Tourette's disorder patients, possibly by reducing hyperactivity or improving attentional function. A transient beneficial effect has been reported for apomorphine, a potent dopamine agonist; this has been interpreted as a presynaptic inhibitory influence on dopaminergic turnover through preferential stimulation of dopamine autoreceptors (Feinberg and Carroll, 1979).

Serotonergic Function

There is less direct evidence supporting a serotonergic contribution to Tourette's disorder symptoms. CSF levels of 5-HIAA, the major serotonin metabolite, have been reported as normal in several studies (Cohen et al., 1974, 1979a; Van Woert et al., 1976; Shapiro et al., 1978; Butler et al., 1979). Lower 5-HIAA levels were reported in one study without probenicid administration (Butler et al., 1979), and in two studies following probenicid administration (Cohen et al., 1978; Han-bai and Han-quin, 1983).

Several investigators suggested that serotonergic activity may have a balancing modulatory relationship to dopaminergic influences on motor function (Cohen et al., 1978; Butler et al., 1979; Singer et al., 1982b; Koslow and Cross, 1982; Jacobs et al., 1982). Reduced CSF-5-HIAA in Tourette's disorder has been hypothesized to reflect inadequate modulation of dopaminergic activity by serotonergic neurons. This might reflect such problems as a dysfunction or reduction in the number of serotonergic neurons, or augmented feedback inhibition. The response of CSF 5-HIAA to *d*-amphetamine in an individual Tourette's disorder patient was in agreement with this hypothesis, as it increased after the stimulant induced activation of dopaminergic receptors. When group means were examined the CSF 5-HIAA/HVA ratio was correlated with the degree of clinical impairment in the patients; inadequate serotonergic compensatory balance is postulated to contribute to the dysregulation of motor and impulse control (Cohen et al., 1978). Other strategies for studying the effect of serotonin on the pathophysiology of Tourette's disorder have left the picture clouded. Peripheral serotonin measures in Tourette's disorder (i.e., plasma tryptophan and blood serotonin) have not been useful (Leckman et al., 1984). Several drugs affecting serotonergic activity, including a precursor of serotonin (5-hydroxytryptophan), a serotonin receptor blocker (methysergide), and a serotonin reuptake blocker (chlorimipramine) all failed to demonstrate reliably useful effects (Sweet et al., 1976; Van Woert et al., 1977b, 1982; Crosley, 1979; Yariyura-Tobias, 1979).

Noradrenergic Function

Attempts to demonstrate noradrenergic abnormalities in Tourette's disorder have been unsuccessful. Urinary 3-methoxy-4-hydroxyphenethyleneglycol (MHPG) was normal in one patient, but levels were reduced in 24-hr urine excretion during exacerbation of symptoms (Sweeney et al., 1978). Low levels of urinary MHPG were reported in 21 medication-free Tourette's disorder outpatients compared to controls (Ang et al., 1982), but elevated values have been reported in occasional patients (Cohen et al., 1979a; Yeragani et al., 1983). Normal MHPG concentrations in CSF were reported in five Tourette's disorder patients (Singer et al., 1982b) and elevated levels in two patients (Cohen et al., 1980).

Normal values have been reported for vanillylmandelic acid in CSF and urine (Shapiro et al., 1978; Han-bai and Han-quin, 1983), dopamine-beta-hydroxylase (Lake et al., 1977; Eldridge et al., 1977; Shapiro et al., 1978, 1984; Cohen et al., 1979a), plasma norepinephrine (Lake et al., 1977; Eldridge et al., 1977), plasma amine oxidase activity, platelet monoamine oxidase (MAO) activity (Lake et al., 1977; Cohen et al., 1979a; Shapiro et al., 1984), and erythrocyte catechol-O-methyltransferase (COMT) (Lake et al., 1977; Cohen et al., 1979a). However, in a carefully controlled study of potential genetic markers in Tourette's disorder, platelet MAO was significantly ($p < 0.001$) higher in 24 untreated Tourette's disorder patients compared to a matched control group (Shapiro et al., 1983c). The evidence from clinical pharmacotherapy does not suggest abnormalities for NE, 5-hydroxytriptamine, and acetylcholine (Shapiro et al., 1981).

Clonidine, an imidazoline derivative used widely as an antihypertensive agent, stimulates alpha$_2$-presynaptic adrenergic inhibitory receptors, reducing spontaneous firing in the LC, although effects at alpha$_1$-adrenergic receptors must also be considered (Bunney and De Riemer, 1982; Kehne et al., 1985). These observations led to the clinical use of clonidine for the treatment of Tourette's disorder and several biochemical studies. Although initial reports of 80% effectiveness in Tourette's disorder (Cohen et al., 1979b, 1980; Bruun, 1982; Leckman et al., 1982b), have not been confirmed by subsequent studies (see Chapter 11), a subset of patients, not clinically identifiable other than by medication trial, may respond to treatment with clonidine.

Acute clonidine challenge reduces urinary total MHPG; plasma MHPG levels are normal at baseline and are not reduced following clonidine challenge (Young et al., 1981a,b). However, challenge with clonidine after a 12-week course of clonidine treatment does elicit a significant reduction in plasma MHPG. This research has also suggested that the therapeutic effects of clonidine might, in part, be exerted through indirect effects on dopaminergic function. Following a 12-week course of clonidine, base-line plasma HVA levels are increased (Leckman et al., 1983). This finding is similar to the rise in plasma HVA which occurs after chronic administration of haloperidol. Elucidation of the neurochemical basis of clonidine's therapeutic effects may require determination of noradrenergic-dopaminergic interactions (Bunney and De Remier, 1982).

Plasma NE levels were measured in five boys with Tourette's disorder who were treated successfully with clonidine. Base-line levels were similar to controls, but decreased 11 to 89% in four of the five boys (one showed a 23%

increase) after 2 weeks of clonidine treatment. The reduction below base line continued during 3 months of clonidine therapy, but by 6 months plasma NE had increased to levels somewhat above baseline. Platelet alpha$_2$-adrenergic receptor number and affinity were measured at the same time points in these boys, as discussed below (Silverstein et al., 1985).

Cholinergic Function

Attempts to specify the role of the cholinergic system in Tourette's disorder have produced contradictory results. Elevated levels of red blood cell choline have been reported in Tourette's disorder patients and their relatives, but no clear relation to brain cholinergic function has been established (Hanin et al., 1979; Comings et al., 1982b). Responses to physostigmine (an acetylcholinesterase inhibitor which increases cholinergic activity) are inconsistent. Physostigmine, given subcutaneously, was largely without effect in one study (Shapiro et al., 1978), decreased tics when given intravenously in a second study (Stahl and Berger, 1980, 1981), and increased tics in a third study (Tanner et al., 1982). The parasympatholytic agent scopolamine reduced tics in one study (Tanner et al., 1982). The use of choline and lecithin to enhance cholinergic activity has been unsuccessful (Shapiro et al., 1978; Barbeau, 1979; Polinsky et al., 1980; Moldofsky and Sandor, 1983). Blockage of cholinergic receptors led to mixed responses, leaving the overall status of the cholinergic system in Tourette's disorder unclear (Stahl and Berger, 1980, 1981, 1982a,b).

Opioid Peptidergic Function

Individual patients have treated themselves with opiates and noted improvement in their symptoms. Enkephalin-containing neurons have been identified in the basal ganglia, establishing a neuronatomical basis for further study of opioid peptide systems in Tourette's disorder (Buck and Yamamura, 1982). The effect of naloxone, which prevents and reverses the effects of opioids, may have implications for clarifying the role of the opioid system in Tourette's disorder. Clonidine is an effective agent for treating withdrawal symptoms after narcotic abuse, presumably through its inhibition of the adrenergic overactivity characteristic of the withdrawal state; this is further encouragement for careful study of opioid peptide neuronal systems in Tourette's disorder. However, clinical results on a small number of patients given naloxone or morphine are inconsistent (see Chapter 11).

Response to Clonidine Challenge

There are direct noradrenergic projections from the LC to the striatum, and raphe serotonergic systems connect the LC and dopaminergic areas in the substantia nigra and striatum. Previous research and a review of the literature by the Yale group suggested that the effect of clonidine might not be restricted to the noradrenergic system, but might include interaction with the dopaminergic and serotonergic systems. Support for the concept included (a) a positive therapeutic response to haloperidol predicted a beneficial response to clonidine in one double-blind cross-over study; (b) increased plasma HVA levels following 12 weeks of clonidine treatment of Tourette's disorder patients; (c) increased CSF HVA levels after long-term clonidine treatment of alcohol amnestic syndrome (Martin et al., 1984); and (d) beneficial effects on the symptoms of tardive dyskinesia.

These concepts were evaluated in a study (Leckman et al., 1986) of seven children with Tourette's disorder (ages 9–13 years) who were treated in an open 12-week trial with clonidine and then abruptly withdrawn from clonidine. Tics were markedly aggravated in five patients following withdrawal, and motor restlessness, blood pressure, and pulse rate increased. Return to prewithdrawal level of tic symptom severity required 2 weeks to 4 months of treatment with clonidine. Plasma-free MHPG levels were not altered during the 12 weeks of clonidine treatment, but abrupt clonidine withdrawal precipitated a 61% increase. Unlike their previous results, there was a 28% decrease in plasma HVA levels by the end of 12 weeks of clonidine treatment, and an increase in plasma HVA levels to pretreatment levels after abrupt withdrawal of clonidine. Urinary MHPG, NE, epinephrine, and dopamine were not significantly altered during clonidine treatment, but abrupt withdrawal caused an increase in urinary MHPG (28%), NE (59%), and epinephrine (72%). Urinary dopamine levels were unchanged during clonidine withdrawal. While blood serotonin and tryptophan levels were unchanged during clonidine therapy, they increased (but not significantly) after withdrawal of clonidine.

Active compensatory mechanisms are suggested by the failure of clonidine to suppress adrenal medullary, central noradrenergic, and sympathetic nervous system neurochemical measures during the treatment period. Findings during the withdrawal phase, however, were in agreement with theoretical expectations: the hypothesis that withdrawal symptoms reflect a rebound increase in central noradrenergic, sympathetic, and adrenal medullary activity, was supported by increased plasma-free MHPG and urinary MHPG, NE, and epinephrine. These findings parallel those reported for adult hypertensive patients.

Altered plasma HVA levels, particularly after withdrawal of clonidine, suggest modulatory effects of central noradrenergic neurons on dopaminergic systems, although the use of plasma HVA as a measure of central dopaminergic activity is controversial, and plasma HVA is not significantly related to tics or motor restlessness. In addition, these investigators have evidence of variability in morning plasma HVA levels and there is marked individual variation in the response of plasma HVA to long-term clonidine administration (Leckman et al., 1986). In sum, there is preliminary clinical neurochemical evidence of interactions among the noradrenergic, dopaminergic, and serotonergic systems, but current indices and methods to clarify the interactions are unsatisfactory. Obviously, the presence of cotransmitters in neurons, other neurotransmitter neuronal systems, and receptor changes are potential sources of compensatory activities that are difficult to monitor simultaneously with these indices.

Enzyme Activities

Familial aggregation of tics and Tourette's disorder encouraged a search for abnormal gene products, including several studies of enzyme activities in Tourette's disorder patients. This has been conceptualized as a possible method to utilize a biological marker to identify subgroups of Tourette's disorder.

Monoamine Enzymes

Synthetic Enzymes. Enzymes function as membrane components or within the cell, so that their activities are not easily accessible for measurement. One method for circumventing this is to culture specific cell lines. For example, fibroblasts, obtained by punch biopsy of the skin, can be cultured. An additional advantage of cell cultures is that they are not subject to acute influences such as stress or medications, so that measures of enzyme activities and other indices may be more accurate (Giller et al., 1980; Comings et al., 1981; Goetz et al., 1981). However, procedures associated with maintaining cell cultures are difficult and expensive.

An exception to the problem of inaccessibility of intracellular enzymes is dopamine-beta-hydroxlase (DBH), the catalyst for the conversion of dopamine to NE. This essential enzyme for the synthesis of NE is in vesicles within sympathetic nerve endings which are released into the blood. While it was thought to be released in amounts proportional to NE, other data have not supported this idea and serum DBH is no longer used as an index of acute sympathetic activity. However, it may be related to long-term sympathetic activity, and research on CSF DBH suggests that it may have clinical utility.

Early studies reported normal serum DBH activity in Tourette's disorder patients (Lake ete al., 1977; Eldridge et al., 1977; Shapiro et al., 1978; Young et al., 1980a). A subsequent investigation of several enzymes in Tourette's disorder was more carefully controlled and included an age-and sex-matched control group. The plasma DBH activity of the Tourette's disorder group was no different than the control group. However, a small group of seven patients with both Tourette's disorder and attention deficit disorder had significantly higher DBH activity (Shapiro et al., 1984).

Catabolic Enzymes

Preliminary research on erythrocyte COMT activity indicated that it was within the normal range in Tourette's disorder patients (Lake et al., 1977; Eldridge et al., 1977; Giller et al., 1980). In more carefully controlled subsequent research, there was no difference in COMT activity between Tourette's disorder patients and age- and sex-matched control subjects. A small group of seven patients with both Tourette's disorder and ADD had significantly reduced red blood cell COMT activity (Shapiro et al., 1984).

Similarly, early studies indicated normal activities of platelet MAO (Lake et al., 1977; Giller et al., 1980) and plasma amine oxidase (Lake et al., 1977). In a better controlled study, platelet MAO activity and plasma amine oxidase activity were higher than those of age- and sex-matched controls. The small group of seven patients with both Tourette's disorder and ADD also had greater activity for each of these enzymes than the control subjects (Shapiro et al., 1984).

These studies on enzyme activities have not indicated an association among any of the enzyme activities and symptom severity, age of onset, family history of tics and Tourette's disorder, or ethnic-religious background (Shapiro et al., 1984).

Other Enzymes

An early study of hypoxanthineguanine phosphoribosyltransferase (HGPRT) suggested an abnormality in enzyme function (decreased stability and an abnormal pattern on isoelectric focusing, Van Woert et al., 1977b), but another laboratory failed to replicate these findings with HGPRT (Johnson et al., 1977).

Receptor Binding Research

While it is not possible to directly measure receptor function in brain tissue of patients, indirect measures of receptor characteristics in other tissues such as blood cell receptors have been widely utilized as models for neuronal receptors. Although extrapolation from blood cell to neuron is laden with potential misinterpretations, they can be a useful guide because of shared functional, regulatory, and binding characteristics. For example, exposure of platelet membranes to clonidine causes a decrease in the number of binding sites for an alpha$_2$-adrenergic receptor antagonist, ^{3}H-yohimbine, both *in vitro* and *in vivo* (Brodde et al., 1982). Another study demonstrated clonidine-induced reduction in the number of binding sites for ^{3}H-yohimbine during treatment of hypertensive adults (Schneider et al., 1984).

The effect of clonidine on platelet alpha$_2$-adrenergic receptor number and affinity was measured in five boys with Tourette's disorder, age 8–11 years. All five were described as having a good clinical response to clonidine (Silverstein et al., 1985). Both clonidine (agonist) and yohimbine (antagonist) were employed as radioligands in the pretreatment, base-line assessment. The number of binding sites (B MAX) and affinity (KD, dissociation constant) for both ^{3}H-clonidine and ^{3}H-yohimbine were similar to those of normal young adult controls and a contrast group of children. This suggests that alpha$_2$-adrenergic receptors are neither subsensitive nor supersensitive in Tourette's disorder patients. Yohimbine binding was then assessed after 2 weeks, 3 months, and 6 months of treatment with clonidine. Receptor affinity did not change in any systematic way during treatment. The number of yohimbine binding sites decreased significantly (a range of 10% to 35% in the five patients) after 2 weeks of treatment. The receptor number changes were more variable after 3 and 6 months of treatment; the mean reduction of 19% of the group (compared to pretreatment levels) was less than the reduction at 2 weeks. The initial reduction in the number of alpha$_2$-binding sites (downregulation) after 2 weeks of clonidine therapy, followed by a gradual return to pretreatment number of binding sites at 3 and 6 months was paralleled by an initial reduction of plasma NE at 2 weeks and at 3 months and return to pretreatment plasma NE levels at 6 months.

Neuroendocrine Indices and Dynamic Drug Challenge Procedures

Another method for assessing receptor function is indirect measurement through drug challenge of neuroendocrine indices. For example, the secretion of human growth hormone (HGH) is regulated through central adrenergic mechanisms, and clonidine has become a useful probe for HGH function in patients with endocrinopathies. The HGH response to clonidine is robust and lacks the potentially severe problems that characterize insulin hypoglycemia. Initial studies indicated its utility in the assessment of Tourette's disorder patients (Young et al., 1981b; Leckman et al., 1983). Clonidine appears to elicit HGH release through activation of alpha$_2$-adrenergic receptors, although there has been controversy concerning whether this involves a presynaptic or postsynaptic hypothalamic site of action.

The Yale group explored this approach to receptor function in Tourette's disorder through a clonidine challenge of HGH in 18 medication-free (at least 2 months) Tourette's disorder patients (mean age of 12.3 years). These results were contrasted to those with 26 medication-free children (mean age of 11.0 years) with short stature (SS) and normal hypothalamic-anterior pituitary function. HGH response to clonidine was evaluated before treatment and following either 3 weeks or 12 weeks of clonidine therapy in the Tourette's disorder patients. The single-dose challenge procedure included two base-line measures (−30 and −10 min) and eight post-clonidine measures (30, 60, 90, 120, 150, 180, 210, and 240 min).

The Tourette's disorder group had a mean peak HGH response to clonidine that was 28% lower than that of the SS group (20.1 ng/ml versus 27.7 ng/ml) and was delayed compared to the SS group (86.5 min. versus 71.5 min). Age and dosage of clonidine did not alter these results and clonidine blood levels did not differ in the two groups. The apparent blunted HGH response to clonidine in Tourette's disorder subjects could reflect either subsensitive postsynaptic receptors or supersensitive presynaptic receptors (Leckman et al., 1984c). The results for HGH response in SS subjects are similar to another clonidine challenge study in SS children (Laron et al., 1982). In addition, children with attention deficit disorder with hyperactivity (ADD+H), who were given a clonidine challenge of HGH response using an identical procedure, had a similar response pattern to the SS group (Hunt et al., 1984; 1985). The Tourette's disorder group included 12 patients with a concurrent diagnosis of ADHD, and provides further support for the hypothesis that the HGH response to clonidine is blunted in Tourette's disorder patients.

The mean peak HGH response to treatment of Tourette's disorder subjects with clonidine at 3 and 12 weeks was higher than in the pretreatment condition, but not significantly higher when controlled for age and dosage of clonidine. Although it is unclear whether there is up-regulation of postsynaptic receptors and an enhanced HGH response during clonidine treatment, there is clearly no evidence for blunted HGH response (Leckman et al., 1984b).

This research suggests new perspectives for the neurobiological assessment of Tourette's disorder patients, although it did not illuminate underlying pathophysiological mechanisms. There was no relation between Tourette's disorder symptoms and the magnitude or timing of the HGH response. In addition, the pretreatment HGH response to clonidine challenge failed to predict either long- or short-term therapeutic response. Once again, meticulous surveys of multiple indirect neurochemical indices appear to be the optimal strategy for clarifying brain function in Tourette's disorder rather than reliance upon a single measure (Leckman et al., 1984c).

Associated Behavioral Symptoms and Disorders

Associated behavioral disorders may be a basis for subgrouping Tourette's disorder patients. It is possible that attention, hyperactivity, learning, compulsive, and other behavioral disorders have different neurochemical correlates in Tourette's disorder patients compared to those without such psychopathology. Study of parallel neurochemical and behavioral changes in these groups would be of interest, especially because these associated disorders occasionally are associated with particularly severe forms of Tourette's disorder, and the associated neurochemical alterations may be of greater magnitude.

NEURAL FUNCTION AND DYSFUNCTION IN TOURETTE'S DISORDER: HYPOTHESES FOR RESEARCH

Neurotransmitter Function

Intensive research on dopaminergic activity in Tourette's disorder, spurred by the beneficial clinical effects of neuroleptics, is often mistaken to imply that dopaminergic neurons are a site of primary pathology in Tourette's disorder. Contributing to this concept is the documented loss of dopaminergic neurons in Parkinson's disease, which encourages a search for structural pathology in Tourette's disorder. At the current time, however, no comparable evidence of dopaminergic pathology in Tourette's disorder exists. On the other hand, the function of dopaminergic neurons in the regulation of movement makes it clear that they are a potential site for altering impaired regulation of motor activity by drugs. If dopaminergic inhibition of the effects of the disinhibitory circuit on the cortico-thalamocortical circuit is increased, then modulation of ongoing motor activity will occur. The reverse occurs when drugs reduce dopaminergic effects and there is an augmentation of sustained motor activity and a reduction in the variety of new movements. This implies that the blockade of dopaminergic activity would promote a reduction of normal or abnormal new movements; abnormal involuntary movements, including tics, would generally decline in frequency regardless of their pathophysiological origin.

Similar reasoning applies to possible roles for noradrenergic functions. The use of clonidine was initially suggested by preliminary data indicating noradrenergic dysfunction, but subsequent research failed to confirm the noradrenergic system as a site of primary pathology in Tourette's disorder. Review of physiological and behavioral effects of activation of the LC-NE system indicates that it does not function as a specific component of the motor divisions of the brain. Instead, it appears to have an integrative function, affecting the signal-to-noise characteristics of target cells which are spread diffusely throughout the brain. Clonidine might be theorized as a nonspecific means of diminishing the response of brain neuronal systems to stimuli. This would be an especially apt and practical therapeutic effect in Tourette's disorder, in which the general impairments may fit the concept of disinhibition and unmodulated response to external and internal stimuli. Therefore, although primary pathology in some aspect of noradrenergic function remains a possibility, it is not necessary to postulate such a primary pathology to explain how clonidine exerts its clinical effects.

Although there is a neuroanatomic basis for serotonergic influences on motor regulation, more systematic research is required to utilize the potential usefulness of this knowledge in pharmacotherapy. The results of limited trials of serotonergic agents for the treatment of Tourette's disorder were disappointing, and their potential usefulness has not been fully evaluated. The conceptual basis for considering more thorough trials of serotonergic agents is based on preclinical research demonstrating the capacity of serotonergic neuronal systems to reduce the discharge rate of multiple neuronal systems, and clinical research demonstrating reciprocal, balancing interactions (neurochemical and clinical) between dopaminergic and serotonergic systems in several severe neuropsychiatric disorders, including Tourette's disorder.

Drugs affecting opioid peptide neuronal systems had mixed results in Tourette's disorder patients, but they have not been systematically studied. Naltrexone, a potent, oral long-acting narcotic antagonist, has had beneficial effects in a small number of autistic and retarded individuals. Its capacity to reduce repetitive self-injurious behaviors, stereotypies, impulsivity, and hyperactivity (Campbell et al., 1985) suggests that naltrexone and other drugs affecting the opioid system merit evaluation in Tourette's disorder patients.

Other specific neurotransmitter systems have received less attention in neuropharmacological research on Tourette's disorder. The cholinergic neurons appear to facilitate the disinhibitory circuit and might be a target for therapeutic efforts in Tourette's disorder. However, as indicated previously, the treatment results with various agents affecting cholinergic activity have been mixed.

Drugs altering GABAergic activity are sedative or increase wakefulness, anxiolytic or stimulate anxiety, and anticonvulsant or facilitate seizures. Several structurally unrelated compounds act on the complex of proteins associated with postsynaptic GABA responses to produce this spectrum of clinical actions. Interacting binding sites for GABA, benzodiazepines (BDZ), and chloride channel blockers (picrotoxin, TBPS) mediate these pharmacological effects. Benzodiazepines act at their binding site to enhance the inhibitory actions of GABA at the GABA/benzodiazepine complex (Tallman and Gallager, 1985). The prominent role of GABA neurons in basal ganglia components of motor regulatory circuits suggests their potential as a target for drug treatment of Tourette's disorder. Little systematic research of the effects of GABAergic drugs in Tourette's disorder has been undertaken, and may be a fruitful area for future investigation.

The symptoms of myoclonus suggest a close relationship to tics: "myoclonus, one type of involuntary movement, is a quick muscle jerk arising from dysfunction of the CNS" (Hallett, 1987). Although there are many types of myoclonus and multiple physiological etiologies, there is some evidence that hyperexcitability of neuronal systems essential to motor function characterize many types of myoclonus. The potential parallel role of excitatory neuronal systems in myoclonus and tics warrants further study. For example, glutamate is an excitatory neurotransmitter that is utilized in a large percentage of brain synapses. It plays a prominent role in excitatory circuits of the basal ganglia regulating movement and contributes to memory formation and learning. Considering the apparent hyperexcitability of specific neuronal circuits in Tourette's disorder, a possible glutamatergic role should be pursued as appropriate technical methods become available (Lynch and Baudry, 1984; Maragos et al., 1987).

Although other neurotransmitters might play a role in Tourette's disorder, development of clinical methods for identifying molecular function and dysfunction is the essential challenge. The most informative clinical research methods have been pharmacological challenge procedures and assessment of CSF metabolites. Receptor binding techniques utilizing blood cells also may be useful but little work has been done in Tourette's disorder.

Single-dose pharmacological challenge in Tourette's disorder patients has several advantages: (a) It provides information about the integrity of neuronal systems regardless of the actual primary locus of pathology; (b) it illuminates dynamic, functional characteristics of neuronal systems, possibly identifying abnormalities not identifiable through stable base-line measures; (c) indices for functional responses of several neuronal systems can be obtained, and comparative response profiles for different probe medications can be generated; it may be possible to identify identical patterns in response to different drug probes; (d) repeated single-dose challenge at baseline, during treatment, and following withdrawal can clarify the associated acute and chronic behavioral and neurochemical effects of a medication.

Assessment of neurotransmitter and metabolite levels in the CSF has the obvious advantage of measuring predominantly central neuronal function rather than the peripheral contribution in blood and urinary measures. This can generate more accurate information to guide our understanding of the plasma and urinary indices. The optimal procedure for accomplishing this is to obtain near-simultaneous CSF, plasma, and urinary measures under challenge conditions. As new methods for clinical assessment of neuronal function emerge, such as the use of salivary fluid indices (Selinger et al., 1984; Cohen et al., 1987), they can be more sensibly interpreted. It is essential to develop efficient, practical, nonintrusive means for neurochemical research with children. The requirement for CSF measures deserves emphasis as controversies concerning the meaning of various plasma and urinary measures continue.

Currently there is preliminary agreement between clinical and animal research for CSF HVA and 5-HIAA. Plasma and urinary measures of dopaminergic and serotonergic function are not adequate substitutes for the CSF indices. The behavioral-neurochemical correlations are not specific to Tourette's disorder but have been observed in several other disorders. A positive correlation between CSF HVA and both motor activity level and abnormal involuntary movements has been demonstrated but requires more refined study. Serotonergic activity appears to affect the expression of a disorder rather than determine the specific components of a disorder. A reduction in CSF 5-HIAA levels is associated with impulsivity and a failure of regulatory or control mechanisms in several disorders (autism, violent suicide, antisocial disorder, aggression, possibly Tourette's disorder), especially in relation to a reciprocal balance of dopaminergic effects. There is now sufficient understanding of these effects to guide future research.

Neuroanatomical Perspectives

Neuropathologic studies of brains of Tourette's disorder patients have been reviewed in Chapter 7. Intensive efforts to apply current neuropathologic techniques to autopsy specimens are among the highest priorities in current research on Tourette's disorder.

Research on proposed neuroanatomical sites for pathology in Tourette's disorder has centered on the basal ganglia and midbrain, and theories have implicated the dopaminergic, noradrenergic, and other midbrain neuronal systems. A more extensive effort to localize possible brain abnormalities through the application of findings from several disease models exemplifies the nature of these hypotheses concerning the midbrain.

One hypothesis about possible abnormal loci in Tourette's disorder is based on the pathology in encephalitis lethargica and the anatomy of vocalization. Encephalitis lethargica commonly leads to sequelae including a parkinsonian syndrome, obsessive-compulsive behaviors, motor and vocal tics, and respiratory and oculogyric crises (OGC). Emotional factors often precipitate OGC, appear to be associated with parkinsonian symptoms of rigidity and bradykinesia, and may represent the ocular form of these symptoms. They may have a similar origin in unopposed disinhibition of excitatory motor regulatory circuits, causing maintenance of ongoing activity while dopaminergic mechanisms facilitating initiation of new activities are lacking. It has been hypothesized that dopaminergic systems play a significant role in OGC because L-DOPA relieved the symptoms of OGC in these patients with postencephalitic parkinsonism. If OGC result from diminished dopamine release (due to destruction of dopamine neurons), then the postulated hypersensitivity of the postsynaptic dopamine receptors could cause a heightened response to L-DOPA or other dopaminergic agents in the follower cells; in fact, tic-like symptoms have been observed during L-DOPA therapy. In agreement with this line of reasoning is the observation that OGC and other dystonias are commonly observed shortly after the administration of neuroleptics. In addition, OGC and other dystonic phenomena are thought to indicate decreased dopaminergic activity and reduced effects on follower cells, while tics are thought to be due to dopaminergic overactivity (whether through supersensitivity of dopamine receptors or other mechanisms) (Devinsky, 1983). This is supported by the pharmacological and neurochemical studies described earlier in the chapter, and by the occasional appearance of tics during neuroleptic treatment, tardive dyskinesia, and withdrawal dyskinesia (Klawans et al., 1978; Gualtieri and Patterson, 1985).

The origin of dopaminergic projections in midbrain cell systems within the substantia nigra (SN) and ventral tegmental area (VTA) suggests further consideration of neuroanatomical approaches to Tourette's disorder. Similar midbrain pathways are involved in the genesis of OGC and accompanying emotional phenomena. In addition, the periaqueductal gray (PAG) and midbrain tegmentum are major loci of pathology in encephalitis lethargica; the SN and lenticular nuclei are also involved, although less frequently. The anatomy of vocalization suggests participation of a similar set of structures, including the cingulate gyrus, mesencephalic central gray, PAG, and midbrain tegmentum. (Devinsky, 1983). Devinsky concludes that the mesencephalic central gray (or periaqueductal gray), midbrain tegmentum, and certain limbic structures are involved in the generation of tics, obsessive-compulsive behaviors, OCG, and emotional vocalization. He proposes that research on the neuroanatomical locus of pathology in Tourette's disorder focus on these sites.

A broad array of data implicates midbrain structures in the genesis of Tourette's disorder. Further research is certainly warranted. However, expanding knowledge about the functional anatomy of motor regulation, and extended and interacting neuronal circuits, requires novel approaches to the neuroanatomy of dysregulation in Tourette's disorder. This is especially evident when considering the contributions of the frontal lobes. Interaction of the frontal lobes with the basal ganglia in behaviors such as motor programming, motor set, initiation of movement, temporal elaboration of behavioral sequences, nonmotor functions, etc., indicates that the premotor and prefrontal cortices may be involved in the pathogenesis of Tourette's disorder. Demonstration of dopaminergic axon terminals in the frontal lobes supports this view.

These considerations indicate that any neuroanatomically based hypothesis about the etiology of Tourette's disorder can be heuristcally useful for selecting pathways for future research, but that all theories and studies will be subject to considerable revision with advances in technical methods.

Several strategies are likely candidates to increase our understanding of neuroanatomic areas affected in Tourette's disorder. First, further neuropathological examination of autopsy brain specimens with novel technical methods must be given the highest priority. Second, it would be highly desirable to develop animal models for Tourette's disorder. Improved methods, such as the use of voltammetry *in vivo* and push-pull perfusion in conscious, freely-moving animals, will yield more precise data about the association between behavior and neurotransmitter release (Myers and Knott, 1986). Third, imaging methods such as the PET scan and magnetic resonance imaging will provide functional neuroanatomical information that may identify metabolic abnormalities in Tourette's disorder in the absence of structural damage. These methods may contribute important clues to the etiology of Tourette's disorder.

10

Proposed Nosology, Criteria, and Differential Diagnosis

In this chapter we propose a revised nosology for tic disorders, and more precise definitions and criteria for simple and complex motor, vocal, sensory, coprophilic, echophilic, and other tics, signs and symptoms associated with tic disorders. Although the nosology and criteria in DSM-III (American Psychiatric Association, 1980) and the criteria in DSM-III-R (American Psychiatric Association, 1987) are useful guides for the clinical diagnosis of tic disorders, they are inadequate for research. More precise description of and criteria for the signs, symptoms, and classification of tic disorders are necessary to develop reliable and valid measures, to improve the comparability among studies, to increase the generalization of results in order to reduce heterogeneity in studies and to provide more meaningful hypotheses about the neuropathological loci for tic disorders.

HISTORY

Tourette's disorder (TS) has had a checkered course historically. Although Itard (1825) described the first patient with Tourette's disorder in 1825, Gilles de la Tourette (1885) provided the first useful description and criteria for the syndrome in 1885 based on the records of three patients who were evaluated by other physicians and on observation of six patients. He characterized the syndrome as a chronic, progressive, fluctuating, hereditary, nervous affliction, with onset in childhood of generalized motor incoordinations, noises, and echolalia, often with coprolalia. The description and criteria were essentially correct except for errors, largely corrected in 1899, describing the movements as motor incoordinations rather than tics, specifying that the inarticulate sound occurred at the culmination of a movement, incorrectly characterizing the progression of symptoms, overemphasizing the frequency of echolalia, and including the startle conditions, jumping Frenchmen, latah, and myriachit, in the syndrome. Criteria for the diagnosis of Tourette's disorder since that time variously included childhood onset, motor, vocal, echophilic, coprophilic, obsessive-compulsive symptoms, and dementia. The etiology was attributed to demonic possession, neuropathic antecedents, unconscious oral, anal, narcissistic, aggressive, and obsessive-compulsive neurotic or psychotic conflicts (Shapiro et al., 1978). Tic was cited as a supplementary term in DSM-I (American Psychiatric Association, 1952) and as a special symptom in DSM-II (American Psychiatric Association, 1965). Neither manual defined a tic or mentioned Tourette's disorder.

By 1976 we had intensively evaluated and studied 145 patients and reviewed published reports on 76 other patients (Tourette, 1885; Shapiro et al., 1978; Eisenberg et al., 1959; Feild et al., 1966; Challas et al., 1967; Lucas et al., 1967; Morphew and Sim, 1969; Abuzzahab and Anderson, 1973). Our book was reviewed by a member of the DSM-III Task Force and criteria were derived for tic disorders in DSM-III (American Psychiatric Association, 1980). The resulting criteria were somewhat arbitrary and inadequate, ignored important data, and were seriously limited by clinical pragmatism, requirements of the nomenclature and various logistic and philosophic constraints. These criteria, nonetheless, were a major improvement over previous criteria, and clarified many previously confusing concepts about Tourette's disorder. The criteria in DSM-III, their subsequent inclusion in many texts and use in studies, focused attention on Tourette' disorder and contributed to the increase in the number of evaluated and diagnosed patients. Tic disorders in DSM-III were classified as stereotyped movement disorders, with four disorders: transient tic disorder, chronic motor tic disorder, Tourette's disorder, and atypical tic disorder.

The following proposed changes rely heavily on our extensive data base and give more emphasis to controlled studies and reports in the literature of a large number of patients than to single case reports and clinical speculation. The discussion focuses on the concepts and content in DSM-III and in DSM-III-R. Although the procedure for deriving criteria in DSM-III and DSM-III-R compared to DSM-I and II has been immeasurably improved by including data-oriented researchers on the Task Force Panel, many serious limitations remain. Criteria in DSM-III and DSM-III-R are derived only partially from carefully controlled studies. Equally important is the clinical background, biases, and theoretical orientation of participating individuals, the limited time for discussion, the pressure to arrive at closure, often premature, despite many differences of opinion and somewhat arbitrary final decisions by officials of the Task Force. Moreover, methodological procedures for evaluating the evidence from studies are not used and references supporting decisions about the criteria are not included in DSM-III or III-R.

In our opinion, DSM-III and III-R are useful, but limited, guides for clinical diagnosis but not for studies of tic disorders. Since the pathophysiology of tic disorders is unknown, unreliable diagnosis can contribute to problems of heterogeneity, irresolvable problems in research, clinical misdiagnosis, and inadequate treatment of patients. To aid clinicians and improve studies, it is important, therefore, to develop more precise criteria. By so doing, we hope to reduce the uncertainty that often plagues the clinician and researcher when making a diagnosis (Shapiro and Shapiro, 1986, 1987).

CHANGE OF DIAGNOSTIC CLASSIFICATION FROM STEREOTYPED MOVEMENT DISORDERS TO TIC DISORDERS

The diagnostic classification in DSM-III-R has been changed from stereotypic movement disorder to tic disorders based on the following considerations. The term "stereotype" is ambiguous and has a pejorative connotation. Stereotype is defined as "an unvarying form or pattern, fixed or conventional expression, notion, character, or mental pattern" (*Webster's Dictionary*, 1966), "constant or abnormal repetition of an action . . . or phrase" (*Psychiatric Dictionary*, 1960; *Webster's Dictionary*, 1966), "meaningless gestures or movements" (*Stedman's Medical Dictionary*, 1966), and "observed in catatonic schizophrenia . . . or dementia praecox" (*Psychiatric Dictionary*, 1960; *Webster's Dictionary*, 1966). The term stereotypy should be reserved for abnormal symptoms observed in schizophrenia, autism, mental deficiency, and some patients with attention-deficit hyperactivity disorder (World Health Organization, 1977).

This change also brings the diagnostic classification closer to the designation of tics (307.2) in the WHO Glossary (1977), and the designation of TICS (307.2), tic disorder, unspecified (307.20), transient tic disorder of childhood (307.21), chronic motor tic disorder (307.23), and Gilles de la Tourette's disorder, motor-verbal tic disorder (307.23) in ICD-9 (World Health Organization, 1978). In addition, the appelation, stereotyped movement disorders, may be confused with stereotypic symptoms which are described as stereotyped repetitive movements (307.3) in WHO, as atypical stereotyped movement disorder (307.30) in DSM-III, and has been differentiated and excluded from tic categories in WHO, ICD-9, and DSM-III-R.

Tic disorders are separated from stereotypic movements which are now designated as stereotypy/habit disorder in DSM-III-R. The essential features of this disorder are intentional and repetitive behaviors that serve no purpose, such as body-rocking, head-banging, hitting or biting parts of one's body, etc.

CRITERIA FOR TICS

We propose a general definition and criteria for all tics associated with tic disorders. Because the pathophysiology for tics is unknown the criteria are derived primarily from clinical observations. Although the criteria may not encompass all of the observed phenomena, as with all signs and symptoms for

TABLE 10.1. *Definition of tics*

Criteria
1. Involuntary movement, vocalization or sensation, which is
2. Rapid, brief, quick, sudden, ejaculatory,
3. Recurrent, repetitive, stereotypic,
4. Nonrhythmic, occuring at irregular intervals,
5. Purposeless, inappropriate, an end in itself, and
6. Experienced as irresistible but can be suppressed for varying periods of time.

Characteristics
1. Tics may be single or multiple.
2. Motor and vocal tics can be simple or complex.
3. The number, frequency, type, location, or severity of tics change over time.
4. The clinical course is variable, characterized by chronic life-long course, periodic remissions, or complete remission.
5. Stimuli can increase, decrease, or have no effect on tics.
6. Tic disorders are classified as Tourette's disorder, sensory tic subtype of Tourette's disorder, chronic motor or vocal tic disorder, transient tic disorder, tic disorder not otherwise specified, and movement disorder not otherwise specified.

syndromes without established etiology, they provide state of the art operational definitions which are believed to be more precise and useful than previous descriptions.

The cardinal features for the definition of tics include the criteria and characteristics listed in Table 10.1.

Involuntary Movement, Vocalization, or Sensation

An essential feature for all tics, in our opinion, is that they are involuntary, unintended, have no psychodynamic purpose, and are an end in themselves. The involuntary nature of tics is similar to other physiological processes such as eye-blinking, breathing, and excretion; and neuropathology such as convulsions in epilepsy, catalepsy in narcolepsy, tonic movements in blepharospasm, spastic torticollis and torsion dystonia, tetanic contractions, fibrillations, fasciculations, myokymia, and other neuronal damage (see Table 7.4). Some of the volitional or intentional aspects associated with tics, such as their inhibition for varying periods of time, or allowing or even facilitating an incipient or subliminally beginning tic to occur, have contributed to the erroneous concept that tics are intentional, voluntary, or psychodynamically determined. However, the ability to inhibit a tic may not be preceded by perception of its imminence. For example, although a normal eye-blink which is involuntary and is not preceded by a sensation, can be intentionally inhibited for brief periods by a general counter-contraction of ocular muscles, in Tourette's disorder, symptoms are often inhibited in the same way, using general muscular vigilance to inhibit the tic.

Concepts about whether tics are intentional, voluntary, or involuntary may involve several factors: the Freudian view of unconscious motivation, the current counter-reaction to the brain-mind dualism of Aristotle and Descartes, and semantic or epistemological issues.

Freudian Unconscious Motivation

The Freudian view tends to conceive of behavior as unconsciously motivated and that tics are caused by unconscious conflicts. The unconscious determinants of behavior, however, are by definition unknowable except to well trained and thoroughly analyzed psychoanalysts. For example, the interpretation by the psychoanalyst that the patient unconsciously wishes to kill his father and sleep with his mother is not consciously experienced by the patient, but may finally be accepted intellectually by the patient as a plausible and logical explanation of unconscious behavior. However, since the reliability and validity of the Freudian concept of the unconscious has not been substantiated, it is irrelevant to the question of whether tics are voluntary or involuntary.

Brain-Mind Dualism

We have the impression that current neurobehavioral concepts, in part a reaction to the unfashionable dualism of Aristotle and Descartes, have contributed to blurring the distinction between psychological and physiological events and differences between intended or voluntary and involuntary tics. It is apparent that some organic or physiological events are quite distinct and separate from motivational, cognitive, and psychological factors. Events in the brain, such as astrocytoma, initially may have no effect, and slowly or suddenly cause primary neurological or anatomically induced psychological symptoms, as well as psychological symptoms secondary to the perception of or reaction to the symptoms or the diagnosis. A progressive atherosclerotic carotid artery can cause scotoma, dizziness, and sudden strokes, without psychological interactions. Similar differentiation of symptoms apply to many medical illnesses: diabetes, myxedema, pernicious anemia, ruptured lumbar disc, encephalitis lethargica, neurofibromatosis, infections, collagen diseases, and so on. In this sense, a tic is defined as a primary involuntary symptom that may or may not have psychological interactions.

Semantic Factors

DSM-III-R has adopted the distinctions for voluntary, intended, and involuntary actions described by Culver and Gert (1982). Based on semantic derivatives and concepts, "A voluntary action is one that is willed by someone with the volitional ability to will to do that action," and "An intended action is one that is willed." Actions are further categorized as "intentional voluntary actions" illustrated by malingering; "intentional unvoluntary actions" illustrated by some phobias, factitious disorder, obesity, alcoholism, kleptomania, and several types of ego-dystonic behavior; "nonintentional actions" illustrated by accident proneness and slips of the tongue; and "nonactions" illustrated by epilepsy, eye-blinking, neurological reflexes, and the motor and vocal tics of Tourette's disorder. An epileptic movement is a "nonaction" because it is "independent of the will" of a patient "who is unconscious, and has physical rather than mental causes," and "Tourette's disorder is a similar condition occurring in patients who are not unconscious." Thus, compulsions are described as "intentional" in DSM-III-R rather than "voluntary" as in DSM-III. The term "involuntary," in the sense of nonintentional, involuntary nonactions, is retained in DSM-III-R, and used in our discussion and criteria to describe the symptoms of Tourette's disorder.

Involuntary Sensation

The definition of tics is expanded to include sensory tics which are described more fully later in this chapter.

Rapid, Brief, Quick, Sudden, Ejaculatory

Most involuntary tics are rapid, brief, quick, sudden, and ejaculatory. Some, however, have the appearance of being slower, more prolonged, and less ejaculatory. Possible explanations include the possibility that some tics originate or are associated with other neuronal pathways, involve a mechanism similar to that observed in sensory tics, or the tic is intentionally prolonged to reduce discomfort.

Recurrent, Repetitive, Stereotypic

These characteristics have obvious face validity.

Nonrhythmic, Occurring at Irregular Intervals

Involuntary tics are nonrhythmic and occur irregularly as in normal eye-blinking. These characteristics help differentiate tics from tremors, convulsive movements, myokamia, and other symptoms, and movement disorders of unknown etiology which superficially resemble tic disorders. Bearing these and other differential features in mind is desirable because of the potential problems of heterogeneity among tic disorders.

Purposeless, Inappropriate, An End in Itself

These characteristics differentiate tics from compulsions and intended or psychologically motivated behavior. The symptom resembles a sneeze, which is purposeful and an end in itself.

Irresistible but Can Be Suppressed for Varying Periods of Time

These criteria are supported by clinical observations, reports by patients, and the change in severity of symptoms associated with stimuli (Table 5.22).

Characteristics of Tics

Characteristics 1 to 5 listed for tics in Table 10.1 are supported by clinical observations and the data described in Chapter 5. The diagnostic classification listed in characteristic 6 follows the proposed nomenclature in DSM-III-R, except for our addition of the category "movement disorder not otherwise specified." This category is needed to classify patients who have a movement disorder, but whose symptoms do not fulfill the criteria for a tic (Table 10.1).

Waxing, Waning, and Fluctuation

The number, frequency, type, location, or severity of tics vary over time (waxing, waning, and fluctuation of symptoms). For 666 of our patients, 97% had waxing and waning, and 96% had fluctuation of symptoms (Table 5.17), all having one or the other. The degree of these changes vary widely among patients. Some patients report no waxing, waning, or fluctuation of symptoms, but detailed inquiry and information from informants usually elicits minimal changes (see Chapter 5).

Stimuli-Induced Changes in Tics

As with many other movement disorders, stimuli can increase, decrease, or have no effect on tics. The type of stimuli and the effect of stimuli vary among patients. Tics markedly decrease or disappear during sleep, usually decrease with nonanxious absorption in a task and in the presence of strangers, and increase with anxiety, pleasurable anticipation, fatigue, and in the presence of family or close friends (see Chapters 5, 7, and Table 5.22).

MOTOR TICS

Motor tics, which are involuntary contractions of both agonist and antagonist muscles in one or more parts of the body, fulfill the six criteria for tics and

TABLE 10.2. *Definition of motor tics*

Criteria
    Fulfill criteria 1–6 (Table 10.1) for tics.
Characteristics
    Motor tics are involuntary contractions of agonist and antagonist muscle groups.
    Motor tics are classified as simple or complex. Although the boundaries are not well defined, classification is easier at the extremes, e.g., clonic contractionn of one muscle group such as eye-blinking compared to echopraxia, copropraxia, or twirling while walking.
Simple motor tics
    Electromyograms for simple motor tics consist of short muscular bursts usually lasting up to 100 msec and occasionally up to 200 msec.[a]
    Simple motor tics resemble normal physiological eye-blinking.
    The most frequent simple motor tics are eye-blinking (80%), horizontal or vertical head-shaking (69%), shoulder-shrugs (55%), facial grimace (36%), mouth-twitching (34%), hand tics (34%), and others totaling at least 26 different tics.[b]
Complex motor tics
    Electromyograms for complex tics consist of many different patterns over a short period of time, variable duration of both short and long EMG bursts, irregular frequency, cocontraction, reciprocal or nonreciprocal activation of antagonist muscles and the independent or simultaneous presence of simple and complex tics.[a]
    Complex motor tics involve a number of coordinated muscle groups and appear more elaborate than simple motor tics.
    The most frequent complex motor tics are hitting self (22%), jumping (20%), copropraxia (15%), touching self (13%) and others (11%), smelling hands (12%) and objects (11%), echopraxia (8%) and others totaling at least 54 different tics.[b]

[a]Obeso et al (1981).
[b]Order and frequency of tics based on 666 patients from current study.

have the characteristics outlined in Table 10.2. One tic or multiple tics may be present at any one time. Motor tics are classified arbitrarily as simple or complex.

Simple Motor Tics

The first physiological evidence supporting the concept that simple motor tics are involuntary was provided by Obeso et al. (1981) who demonstrated the absence of a premovement potential that is always present with voluntary or intended movements. These electromyograph (EMG) studies were consistent with the clinical observation that tics are of short duration usually lasting less than 100 msec and occasionally up to 200 msec. The authors suggest "a subcortical origin for tics in Tourette's syndrome since most patients did not have cortical activity preceding and time-locked to the spontaneous jerks," and "show that the simple muscle jerks of Gilles de la Tourette's syndrome are physiologically distinct from normal self-paced willed movements," and should "be classified as true abnormal automatic movements, which reinforces the idea of a neurological basis for Gilles de la Tourette's syndrome."

From our data base of 666 patients, the most frequent simple tics are eye 80%, head 69%, shoulders 55%, facial grimace 36%, mouth 34%, hands 34%, and others totaling at least 26 different tics.

Complex Motor Tics

Complex tic replaces the term complicated tic in DSM-III-R. Whereas the term complicated tic implies volition and psychological motivation, the term complex tic is more neutral. EMG activity, more complex for complex than for simple tics, is described by Marsden et al. (1983) as consisting of

> many different EMG patterns. Burst length may be considerably prolonged and cocontraction may be present. Normal reciprocal activation of antagonist muscles may also be seen during some fast complex tics, which give the appearance of a normal ballistic movement. The frequency of tics recorded electromyographically is quite irregular, and any one individual may exhibit a number of different combinations over a short period of time. Indeed, simple and complex tics can occur simultaneously or independently of each other.

Studies of premovement potentials to evaluate whether these movements are involuntary have not been done for complex tics.

Because physiological evidence for differentiating simple and complex tics is not available, and it may not be feasible to conduct EMG studies in clinical patients, we rely on clinical phenomenology in our discussion.

Complex tics, as described previously (see Chapter 5), are briefly mentioned in "Associated Features" for Tourette's disorder in DSM-III. They are described as "compulsive impulses to touch things or perform complicated movements, such as squatting, deep knee-bends, retracing steps, and twirling when walking." This description is imprecise, the symptoms are miscategorized, and the use of the phrase "compulsive impulses" has caused considerable confusion in the literature. Fortunately the term "compulsive impulses" has been deleted in DSM-III-R and symptoms formerly described as "compulsive impulses" are now classified as complex tics.

Complex tics are frequent in patients with Tourette's disorder. In fact, they occur more frequently than many simple motor tics. For example, 7.1% of 666 patients had complex tics as their initial symptom, and cumulative lifetime complex tics were present in 68.6% of patients, a higher percentage than the 40.7% with simple tics of the lower limbs, and 46.5% with tics of the torso. Fifty-four movements were classified as complex tics in our sample. Of these, most frequent were hit self 21.6%, jumping 19.8%, copropraxia 15% (involuntary obscene gestures), touch self 13.2%, smell hands 11.8%, touch others 11.4%, smell objects 10.9%, and echopraxia 8% (involuntary imitation of the movement of another) (Table 5.9). Complex tics listed in "Associated Features" in DSM-III occurred less frequently: squatting 7.2%, retracing steps 5.1%, twirling 4.8%, and deep knee bends 4.4%. Complex tics are characterized by patients as involuntary and are similar in all respects to simple tics except that they appear more complicated.

A major problem, however, is establishing clinical criteria for classifying a tic as simple or complex because the boundaries are not well defined. Classification is easier at the extremes, for example, a simple contraction of a single or limited number of synergistic muscle groups, such as eye-blinking, lip-twitch, shoulder-shrug, head-nod, or flicking of the hands, or a more complex movement that includes a coordinated contraction of several muscle groups, such as sudden deep knee bends, or twirling while walking. A reasonable proposal, if the extremes are used, is that a simple tic be defined as a contraction of one muscle group, and that a complex tic be defined as the contraction of more than one muscle group (Comings and Comings, 1984). The classification of other symptoms which blend into each other is difficult, however. A sudden contraction of the arm, leg, or torso has the appearance of a simple tic but may include contraction of muscle groups in the shoulder, elbow, or hands, hip, knee, or foot, and the whole body for a torso tic. Equally imprecise are terms such as more purposeful or deliberate appearance. The difficulty of reliably classifying complex tics is illustrated by the range of symptoms classified as complex by different authors (Shapiro et al., 1978; American Psychiatric Association, DSM-III, 1980; Fahn, 1982b; Jagger et al., 1982; Comings and Comings, 1984).

Another basis for classifying complex tics implies and interprets tics as intended or voluntary compulsive impulses that seemingly have a psychodynamic purpose, such as a patient touching sexual or nonsexual parts of another person or of themselves. However, there is no support for the concept that these symptoms have psychodynamic determinants (Shapiro et al., 1978); they do not fulfill the criteria for intended compulsive symptoms and patients describe the symptoms as similar to simple tics.

Since there does not appear to be a reliable anatomic or physiological basis for the classification, and the pathogenesis for simple and complex tics is unknown, for heuristic purposes, complex tics are included in the category of involuntary motor tics and subcategorized as simple and complex tics, but they should be specifically cited and described. These problems could be minimized if a panel of experts were to classify and define the range of symptoms that may be present in tic disorders for use by clinicians and researchers.

VOCAL TICS

Vocal tics, similar in character to motor tics, fulfill the same criteria as motor tics except that the symptom is expressed as an inarticulate sound or articulate word, phrase, or sentence (Table 10.3). Vocal tics, usually but not always, occur between important phrases, concepts, or sentences, possibly because vocal tics, like motor tics, can be inhibited somewhat. They usually appear as interjections without interfering with normal speech, rhythm, and resemble the ejaculatory sounds or words that occur in aphasics searching for a word. These clinical observations were confirmed by Ludlow et al. (1982) in a well-controlled linguistic study comparing 54 Tourette's disorder patients with a matched control sample. Vocal tics occurred mainly in "phase junctions in speech, the same points where interjections, starters and hesitations occur in normal speech." These findings are similar to other reports (Martindale, 1976; Frank, 1978). The authors cite the interesting observation that normal subjects during pauses in speech frequently have "extraneous movements of the larynx, lips, and tongue," (two of the normal controls had verbal tics), which may indicate that "vocal tics in TS have their origin in normal behavior," the main difference being the "increase in the force and frequency" of the vocal tics in Tourette's disorder. The authors point out that since vocal tics occur "in synchrony with the overall speech rhythm . . . and . . . do not occur randomly . . . their origin must be related to speech planning" in the cortex with coordination in the cerebellum and basal ganglia. They also report impairment in language expression and in written and oral reading scores for Tourette's disorder subjects, but without separating those with ADHD or other CNS impairment, and comprehensively review the physiology of language as it relates to Tourette's disorder. Vocal tics can be simple or complex.

Simple Vocal Tics

Simple vocal tics include inarticulate noises and sounds such as throat clearing 57%, grunts 46%, sniffs 33%, high-pitched noises 33%, coughs 25%, screams 21%, snorts 20%, shouts 20%, barks 19%, humming 18%, spitting

TABLE 10.3. *Definition of vocal tics*

Criteria
  Fulfill criteria 1–6 (Table 10.1) for tics.
Characteristics
  Vocal tics are involuntary sounds, words, phrases, or sentences.
  Vocal tics are classified as inarticulate sounds (simple vocal tic) or articulated words, phrases, or sentences (complex vocal tic).
  The most frequent vocal tics are throat clearing (57%), grunting (46%), sniffing (33%), high-pitched noises (33%), coughing (25%), screaming (21%), snorting (20%), shouting (20%), barking (19%), word accentuation (10%), humming (18%), spitting (18%), clicking noises (14%), stuttering or stammering (13%), and others totaling at least 77 different tics.[a]
  The most frequent complex vocal tics are articulate words, phrases, or sentences such as coprolalia (32%), echolalia (18%), palilalia (17%), and occasionally nonspecific exclamatory phrases such as "oh, right, right-on, say it again," mental echophilia, mental echo tics, and others totaling at least 157 tics.[a]

[a]Order and frequency of tics based on 666 patients from current study study.

18%, hissing 15%, clicking 14%, stuttering or stammering 13%, and word accentuation 10%. Some symptoms such as word accentuation, stuttering and stammering noises, unlike most vocalization, can occur at the beginning or within words and seriously impair speech.

Complex Vocal Tics

Complex vocal tics include articulate words, phrases, or sentences such as echophilia, coprophilia, and occasionally nonspecific exclamatory phrases such as "oh; right"; "right on"; "say it again"; and more than 157 other symptoms.

ECHOPHILIA

Echophilia, which occurs in 33% of patients with Tourette's disorder, is defined as involuntary repetition of sounds, words, phrases, sentences, or movements. Although echophilia is classified as a complex tic, it is unclear whether echolalia and palilalia should be classified as a complex articulated vocal tic and echopraxia as a complex motor tic, or whether echophilic tics should be classified separately. Criteria for echophilic tics are described in Table 10.4.

Echophilic Complex Vocal Tics

Echophilic symptoms can be classified as articulated complex vocal tics such as echolalia (involuntary repetition of the last sound, word, phrase, or sen-

TABLE 10.4. *Definition for echophilia (echo tics)*

Criteria (1 and either 2, 3, 4, or 5)
  1. Fulfill criteria 1–6 (Table 10.1) for tics.
  2. Echopraxia (involuntary imitation of the movements of another).
  3. Echolalia (repetition of the last sound, word, phrase, or sentence of another).
  4. Palilalia (repeating one's own last sound, word, phrase, or sentence).
  5. Mental echophilia (mental repetition of one's own or another's sound, word, phrase, or sentence).

Characteristics
  Echopraxia is classified as a complex motor tic.
  Echolalia and palilalia are classified as articulated complex vocal tics.
  An estimated frequency for echophilia is echolalia (18%), palilalia (17%), echokinesis (8%), and mental echoing (5%).[a]

[a]Order and frequency of tics based on 666 patients from current study.

tence of another person), occurring in 18% of patients, palalalia (involuntary repetition of one's own last sound, word, phrase, or sentence), occurring in 17% of patients, and mental echophilia (mental repetition of one's own or another's sound, word, phrase, or sentence), occurring in less than 1% of patients (Tables 5.13, 10.4).

Echophilic Complex Motor Tics

Echopraxia, also referred to as echokinesis, which occurs in 8% of patients, is defined as involuntary imitation of the movement of another person (Tables 5.11, 10.4).

COPROPHILIA

Coprophilia, which occurs in 37.4% of patients, can take the form of an articulated complex vocal tic such as coprolalia and mental coprolalia, or as a complex motor tic such as copropraxia. As with echophilia, coprophilia is classified as a complex vocal or motor tic. Criteria are listed in Table 10.5.

Coprophilic Complex Vocal Tics

Coprophilic complex vocal tics include coprophilia (involuntary socially unacceptable or obscene words, phrases, or sentences) occurring in 18% of patients, and mental coprolalia (involuntary sudden thoughts of socially unacceptable or obscene sounds, words, phrases, or sentences) occurring in 4% of patients (Tables 5.12, 10.5).

TABLE 10.5. *Definition of coprophilia*

Criteria (1 and either 2, 3 or 4)
  1. Fulfill criteria 1–6 (Table 10.1) for tics.
  2. Coprolalia (involuntary socially unacceptable or obscene sounds, words, phrases, or sentences).
  3. Copropraxia (involuntary obscene gestures, such as an obscene finger or elbow gesture, and touching or pointing at genital areas).
  4. Mental coprolalia (sudden thoughts of socially unacceptable or obscene sounds, words, phrases, or sentences).
Characteristics
  Copropraxia is classified as a complex motor tic.
  Coprolalia and mental coprolalia are classified as articulated complex vocal tics.
  An estimated frequency for coprophilia is coprolalia (32%), copropraxia (13%), and mental coprolalia (4%)[a]

[a]Order and frequency of tics based on 666 patients from current study.

Copropraxic Complex Motor Tics

Copropraxic complex vocal tics (involuntary obscene gestures, such as giving someone "the finger" or touching genitals) occurs in 13% of patients (Tables 5.13, 10.5).

Echophilia and coprophilia should be removed from citation in "Associated Features" and included in the general description of tics. Whereas echophilia and coprophilia could be classified in a separate symptom category, they are classified for heuristic purposes as complex motor and vocal tics. Whether they should be included in one or another category requires empirical study. Of course, determination of the neuropathology will resolve the question.

SENSORY TICS

We refer to a pattern of recurrent, involuntary, somatic sensations in joints, bones, muscles, or other parts of the body as sensory tics. The sensation is described by patients as feelings of heaviness, lightness, emptiness, tickle, cold, hot, weird, or other sensations in skin, bones, muscles, and joints. The sensations evoke a dysphoric feeling to which the patient responds by executing an intentional (or voluntary) movement to relieve the disturbing internal sensation. The movements, which utilize voluntary muscles in any part of the body, are intentional, usually tonic squeezes, stretches, tightening of muscles, or other movements often lasting 1 sec or more. Relief is temporary, however, and the movements recur persistently. Occasional patients do not have a preliminary sensation, but have a need to feel or squeeze the muscle sometimes to the point of pain. A small number of patients exhibit intentional vocalizations which are different from the usual involuntary sudden and brief vocalizations common in tic disorders. They are intentional responses to a sensory stimuli in the larynx or throat, frequently in the form of more prolonged and lower humming, gurgling, or "mm" sounds.

Although the tonic symptoms are less noticeable than tics because they are more easily inhibited, patients experience them as very troublesome since they cause constant tension. Only 51 (4.1%) of 1,237 with tic disorders had sensory tics. Another 4.4% had both: predominantly fast and involuntary tics characteristic of classical Tourette's disorder and sensory tics (Table 2.1). The actual precentages are much higher, however, because we were less sensitive to the existence of these symptoms when evaluating our early patients.

As early as 1972, we characterized these symptoms as dystonic (Shapiro et al., 1978), later as segmental dystonia (Shapiro and Shapiro, 1982) according to the classification of Marsden (1976), more recently as sensory dystonia because the involuntary sensory stimuli were experienced as dysphoric by patients and caused a voluntary or intended, tonic movement (Shapiro and Shapiro, 1982a). We currently refer to these symptoms as sensory tics (Shapiro and Shapiro, 1986), a name which reflects both the involuntary character of the sensation and a similar hypothesized pathophysiology for both motor or vocal tics and sensory symptoms.

Because the sensory stimuli are involuntary, the symptoms are much less obvious than in Tourette's disorder because the motor component is under greater intentional control and patients inhibit the motor movements in the presence of observers. Despite the benign appearance of the manifest symptoms, most patients experience them as very disturbing, due to the need to constantly squeeze, squirm, and move. Since the symptoms were minimally noticeable and often not noticeable at all, we frequently discouraged treatment with neuroleptics. However, most patients request treatment because of the unremitting nature of the symptoms. Patients with sensory symptoms alone, as well as those with both sensory symptoms and classical Tourette's symptoms, respond equally well to neuroleptics. Based on these observations we conclude provisionally that the neuropathology of these symptoms is the same as Tourette's disorder, and we heuristically classify these patients as having a sensory subtype of Tourette's disorder.

The severity of symptoms, similar to Tourette's disorder, varies from very mild to severe. Most patients are classified as having mild severity. A case vignette of a 36-year-old married, successful businessman illustrates severe symptoms. The patient is the second child of four children in an Ashkenazi family. A younger brother has severe Tourette's disorder and his father and sister have a mild chronic motor tic disorder. The family and patient's medical history are otherwise noncontributory. The symptoms began at age 8 with a nonspecific and vague dysphoric feeling that was temporarily relieved by a slow, 1- to 2-sec long, tonic-like contraction of abdominal muscles. Many other dysphoric sensations developed over the years and resulted in intentional squeezing, rolling, and undulating movements of the trapezius muscles to the point of pain, movements of the calf muscles, extension and flexion of the toes, inward and outward movement of the ankles, squeezing of the thigh muscles, manneristic movement of the wrists, stretching arm and shoulder muscles, flexing lumbar muscles, slow movements of the nose, eyebrow, jaw, and mouth, contraction of the buttocks, and many other movements. The only vocal symptom was an intended throat-clearing, lower in volume and more prolonged than the usual throat-clearing symptom in Tourette's disorder. Only two involuntary typical tics were present: a rapid side-to-side head movement followed by slow stretching, and typical eye tics which were followed by slow furrowing of the eyebrows. The abdominal symptoms were severe before the age of 13, all symptoms were less distressing in college, and have become more severe since age 21. Although waxing, waning, and fluctuation of symptoms were apparent, these changes were not as marked as in Tourette's disorder. Despite the presence of many symptoms, only slow, squeezing, and undulating movements of the abdomen, shoulder, and neck, and an occasional eye tic were observed during the consultation. The symptoms decreased markedly when he was under direct observation and increased considerably when he was observed indirectly on a video screen.

Sensory symptoms appear similar to those identified by Fahn (1982b), who described "tonic-sustained (dystonic) motor tics" which "may be preceded by irresistible urge, followed by relief," and to symptoms described in two clinical reports.

Bliss et al. (1980) provides a very detailed description of "sensory experiences of Gilles de la Tourette syndrome" experienced over 62 years. Although he erroneously generalizes to all Tourette's disorder patients, the observations about sensory tics are relevant. Bliss describes slowly becoming aware of "faint signals that preceded a movement," which then were experienced as "vague, unfulfilled feelings" and finally as "discrete sensations." The initial sensation is described as beginning on the surface of the skin, which "generally transfer rapidly and imperceptibly to deeper muscle tissues." All of the movements are "preceded by certain preliminary sensory signals . . . and . . . is the result of a voluntary capitulation to a demanding and relentless urge . . . As soon as the senses become aware of any site . . . a very rapidly escalating desire to satisfy the sensation with movements intended to free oneself from the insistent feeling ensues." The sensation is "perceived as an unsatisfied or unfulfilled sensation that immediately translates into a craving for relief. Relief of the impulse seemingly can be achieved only by movement . . . Yet no single muscular movement ever completely satisfies the urge." The "movements are intentional bodily movements. The intention is to relieve a sensation, as surely as the movement to scratch an itch is to relieve the itch."

The sensory tic is actually described as an itch in a paper by Bullen and Hemsley (1983), *"Sensory Experience as a Trigger in Gilles de la Tourette's Syndrome."* The authors describe a 19-year-old girl with "fairly continuous, fidgety movements with various sudden, intense movements," involving the "head, neck, left shoulder, left arm . . . occasionally her torso and legs . . . eye twitching, sniffing, etc." The patient "described a 'horrible' sensation in her upper back which she could only 'get rid of by moving.' The closest analogy we could agree on was to compare the sensation to an 'itch.'. . . such sensations also appearing, although more rarely, in other parts of her body." Her movements "never occurred without being preceded by the itch and that the itch was always followed by movement . . . giving her a feeling of relief."

The effect of treatment and attempts to control the patient's symptoms are consistent with our formulation about sensory tics. Behavioral techniques such as "habit reversal" and relaxation were unsuccessful, and "exposure and response reversal" (breaking the association between the itch and the movement) was only partially successful, and, similar to the results of behavioral treatment of Tourette's disorder, did not generalize to periods outside the therapy sessions. Similarly, Bliss, who was more successful at controlling his secondary movements, could never extinguish the sensory stimuli. He states that his methods of control "are merely useful methods of control and are not to be viewed as satisfactory treatment . . . symptoms will constantly recur and need to be confronted and extinguished endlessly—the only time relief comes is in moments when no urge at all is perceived."

These observations suggest to us that both the classical tics of Tourette's disorder and the sensations that give rise to sensory tics, are involuntary, physiological, and have a similar pathophysiology. The conclusion by Bullen and Hemsley (1983) that these sensory experiences are not epiphenomena is similar to ours. Two factors which provide further support for this conclusion are the dual presence of both involuntary motor or vocal tics and involuntary sensations in many patients, and the effectiveness of treatment with neuroleptics for both types of symptoms. This formulation does not fully account for involuntary motor or vocal tics alone, involuntary sensations alone, simultaneous involuntary motor or vocal tics and sensations, prodromal feelings that a tic is imminent, various urges, impulses, fixations, preoccupations, echoing, blocking, and other polymorphous (sometimes perverse) symptoms. We characterize these symptoms as epiphenomena, reflecting secondary neuropathological and psychological interactions with the basic or primary neuropathology manifested principally by motor, vocal, or sensory tics. Criteria for sensory tics are outlined in Table 10.6.

Comparison of Sensory Tic with Tourette Samples

Our clinical hypothesis is that sensory tics should be included within the rubric of tic disorders because of the concurrent presence of both clonic motor tics and sensory tics in 45 patients, and because both types of tics respond to treatment with neuroleptics. Preliminary support for the hy-

TABLE 10.6. *Definition of sensory tics*

Criteria
- Fulfill criteria 1–5 (Table 10.1) for tics.
- Involuntary sensations in joints, bones, muscles, or other parts of the body.
- The sensations are experienced as dysphoric and include feelings of heaviness, lightness, emptiness, tickling, cold, hot, or other sensations, and occasionally as a need to squeeze or feel the muscle.
- To relieve the dysphoric sensation an intended or voluntary movement is executed such as squeezing, stretching, tightening, or other tonic movement of the head, neck, torso, limbs, or other parts of the body. Less frequent movements include snapping of the fingers, wrist, or other joints, or quick movements of the shoulders, head, or other body areas. Sensory tics that effect the larynx or throat may result in inarticulate sounds, such as humming, throat clearing, and other sounds that are lower and longer-lasting than typical vocal tics.
- The primary sensation or sensory stimulus cannot be suppressed, but the secondary or resulting movement can be suppressed for varying periods of time.

pothesis is available from analysis (ANOVA, chi-Square) of data for patients with sensory tics (ST) ($N = 15$), Tourette's disorder and sensory tics (TS+ST) ($N = 33$) and Tourette's disorder alone (TS-alone) ($N = 633$). As expected, the sex ratio, range for age at onset, and family history of Tourette's disorder or tics were similar for the three groups. The only significant variables (Table A.1) are more complex tics, total number of cumulative tics, fluctuation of tics, and attention deficit disorder (ADD) in the Tourette's disorder group. The most frequent tics are facial, head, and upper limb for the ST group (79%–93%), and limbs, torso, and complex tics (55%–73%) for the TS+ST group.

If these preliminary results are confirmed on a larger sample, concepts about the pathophysiology of Tourette's disorder warrant revision. It is possible that the etiology of Tourette's disorder involves a basic neurophysiological focus (in the basal ganglia, for example) but symptoms can be expressed differently based on the anatomic location or neurophysiological pathway: involuntary tics if the pathophysiology is limited to motor areas, STs if the pathophysiology is limited to sensory areas, and concurrent involuntary and STs if both areas are involved. This formulation also may account for the incredible variety of symptoms, such as over 300 different simple and complex motor and vocal tics, and other less frequent symptoms such as impulsions and obsessive-compulsive-like symptoms, the prodromal sensation that a tic is imminent, and the almost simultaneous appearance of an involuntary tic.

Conclusion

Our proposal to include sensory tic subtype of Tourette's disorder was presented to the DSM-III-R Task Force. However, other clinicians did not agree with us and the proposal was rejected. Thus, according to the criteria for tic disorders in DSM-III-R, patients with ST would not fulfill criteria for a tic disorder because the movements are intended rather than involuntary. The diagnosis would have to be tic disorder not otherwise specified, but only if the clinician is aware of the sensory symptoms. This may result in missed diagnoses for a sizeable number of patients with these symptoms. Similar to our early experience with Tourette's disorder, many patients with STs have been told by clinicians that their symptoms did not fulfill the criteria for a tic disorder, that the symptoms were psychologically induced and should be treated with psychotherapy. Because of our increased sensitivity to ST symptoms, we have the impression that there are more patients than previously estimated by us who have only STs, and many more who have a combination of both Tourette's disorder and STs. Since the ST symptoms can be treated successfully with neuroleptics, as well as for theoretical reasons, future study of these symptoms has high priority.

OBSESSIVE COMPULSIVE DISORDER, OBSESSIVE-COMPULSIVE SYMPTOMS, AND IMPULSIONS

The rationale for differentiating obsessive compulsive disorder, obsessive-compulsive symptoms, and impulsions is discussed in Chapter 6. Differences among the three symptom types are of course somewhat arbitrary and they may in fact have the same pathophysiology, differing only in degree, severity, or secondary characteristics. However, because they may have a different pathophysiology, we feel it is important to keep our options open by studying the similarities and differences among the three symptom types. It is recognized that any set of criteria will not completely separate the three groups, that some patients may fall into more than one category and others may not fit perfectly into any of the categories. Sophisticated psychometric scales will have to be developed. However, for heuristic purposes, we propose the following criteria which probably will separate most patients into relevant groups.

Obsessive Compulsive Disorder

Criteria for obsessive compulsive disorder are listed in Table 6.7. All criteria should be fulfilled.

Associated features for Tourette's disorder in DSM-III-R states that "in clinical samples, other mental disorders are frequently associated, particularly . . . . obsessive compulsive disorder. It is not clear if this comorbidity also exists in representative community samples." For reasons comprehensively described in Chapter 6, we prefer the statement "The relationship of behavioral problems and psychopathology to Tourette's disorder is controversial. It has not been demonstrated in adequately controlled studies that obsessive compulsive disorder or symptoms are more frequent in Tourette patients than in the population."

We also disagree with the statement in the section concerning familial pattern that "In addition, there is some evidence that obsessive compulsive disorder is more common in first-degree biological relatives of people with Tourette's disorder than in the general population and is another expression of the same underlying disorder." Since the statement is based on only one unreplicated and methodologically flawed study (Pauls et al., 1986b) (Chapter 6). We prefer the statement "There is controversy as to whether or not obsessive compulsive disorder is more common in family members than in the general population." A surprising last minute addition to the differential diagnosis of obsessive compulsive disorder in DSM-III-R is the statement: "In some individuals with Tourette's disorder an associated diagnosis is obsessive compulsive disorder." This statement was included without consultation with the four subcommittee members (A.K.S., E.S., Drs. Rachman, and Insel).

Obsessive-Compulsive Symptoms

The criteria for obsessive-compulsive symptoms are the same as for the disorder except that the symptoms do not cause marked distress, are not time-consuming (take less than an hour a day), and do not interfere with occupational functioning, or with usual social activities or relationships with others.

Impulsions

Criteria for impulsions are differentiated from obsessive-compulsive symptoms because the behavior is an end in itself, is performed without discernable purpose, lacks intellectual content, is not designed to neutralize or prevent a dreaded event or situation, but is connected in a realistic way with what it is designed to prevent (e.g., appropriately neutralize an impulsion), and is not associated with clinically significant guilt, anxiety, resistance, and interference with psychosocial functioning. For a small number of patients who fulfill these criteria, but in whom the behavior is excessive and interferes with functioning, the diagnosis should be impulsive disorder (Table 10.7). (See Chapter 6 for comprehensive discussion of impulsions.)

ORGANIC FACTORS

"Associated Features" in DSM-III states that "Nonspecific EEG abnormalities, soft neurological signs, central nervous system psychological test abnormalities, hyperactivity or perceptual problems during infancy and childhood, or organic stigmata occur in about half the individuals with the disorder." The estimate of 50% of patients with such abnormalities was derived primarily from our sample of 114 patients who were evaluated between 1965 and 1974

TABLE 10.7. *Criteria for impulsions*

Criteria
- Repetitive, purposeful, and intended behavior that is performed according to certain rules, or in a stereotyped fashion.
- The behavior is an end itself, either performed automatically without discernible purpose or designed to neutralize discomfort, but not to neutralize or prevent a dreaded event or situation. The activity may or may not be connected in a realistic way with what is designed to neutralize or prevent, but it is excessive.
- The individual recognizes that the behavior serves no useful purpose.
- The impulsions do not cause marked distress, are not time-consuming (take less than an hour a day), and do not interfere with occupational functioning or with usual social activities or relationships with others.
- If the impulsions cause marked distress, are time-consuming (take more than an hour a day), or interfere with occupational functioning or with usual social activities and relationships with others, the diagnosis should be impulsion disorder.

(Shapiro et al., 1978). However, as documented in Chapters 4, 5, 6, and 7, this sample included more severely afflicted patients with Tourette's disorder who had significantly more organic CNS stigmata than does our current sample. Our present analyses indicate that most organic stigmata can be accounted for by the diagnosis of attention deficit disorder (ADD), and the frequency of organic stigmata in patients with Tourette's disorder without ADD does not differ from population estimates.

Although the above statement was not retained in DSM-III-R, there is considerable confusion about the relationship of organic findings in Tourette's disorder and we recommend the following statement:

> Attention-deficit hyperactivity disorder, specific developmental disorder, non-localizing neurological signs, nonspecific EEG abnormalities, ambidexterity or left-handedness and central nervous system neuropsychological test abnormalities have been reported in a range of from 17% to 60% of patients in various samples. These abnormalities may be largely associated with the diagnosis of attention-deficit hyperactivity disorder and other coexisting disorders such as mental retardation, autism and Down's syndrome.

BEHAVIORAL SYMPTOMS AND PSYCHOPATHOLOGY

Reports in the literature citing an association of behavioral problems and psychopathology with Tourette's disorder are based on retrospective clinical impressions, use of unreliable measures, small nonrandom samples, absence of or inadequate comparison with control groups, and a failure to separately study Tourette's disorder patients with and *without* ADD (see Chapters 4, 5). As previously discussed, our clinical impression and studies indicate that patients with both Tourette's disorder and ADD+H have significantly more behavioral problems and psychopathology (often associated with ADD+H), compared to Tourette's disorder patients without ADD+H, who for the most part do not differ from a normal control sample. In other words, observed psychopathology in patients with Tourette's disorder is an artifact of having ADD+H, and not intrinsically associated with Tourette's disorder.

However, although our recommendation to the DSM-III-R task force was not accepted, the controversial nature of the issue is implicit in the statement which will appear in Associated Features:

> In clinical samples, other mental disorders are frequently associated with Tourette's disorder, particularly attention-deficit hyperactivity disorder and obsessive compulsive disorder. It is not clear if this co-morbidity also exists in representative community samples.

We recommend the following:

> The relationship of behavioral symptoms or psychopathology to Tourette's disorder is controversial. They may be more frequent in patients with an associated diagnosis of attention-deficit hyperactivity disorder than in patients with uncom-

plicated Tourette's disorder. An association between psychopathology and uncomplicated Tourette's disorder has not been demonstrated in controlled studies.

DIAGNOSTIC CRITERIA FOR TIC DISORDERS

The limitations of the DSM-III-R revision procedure for arriving at criteria, the necessity of compromise among participants, space limitations, the primary usefulness of DSM-III-R for clinical diagnosis, but not for research, have been cited previously. Our proposal for tic disorders gives greater weight to data and controlled studies. Where the data leave off, we rely on clinical experience and reasonable conjecture. We believe that this approach will result in criteria that are more useful for clinical diagnosis, management, and treatment of patients, and enhance meaningful research. Obviously, others may develop different criteria, highlighting one aspect or another, but agreement should increase as the data from studies accumulate.

The criteria in DSM-III-R incorporate many of our proposals, but not all of them. The revised DSM-III-R criteria, including some of our proposals, are outlined in Table 10.8. We propose that the six criteria for tics (Table 10.1) be included as a criteria for Tourette's disorder (TS), chronic motor or vocal tic disorder (CMT or CVT) and transient tic disorder (TTD). Other proposed changes are described in the sections discussing each of the tic disorders.

Tourette's Disorder

Criteria in DSM-III-R specify the age at onset as before 21 years of age, the number of vocal tics necessary for diagnosis as one or more, and that the anatomic location, number, and complexity of tics change over time; in other words, there is fluctuation of symptoms. DSM-III-R criteria (A to E) for Tourette's disorder are listed in Table 10.8.

We propose that category C describing waxing, waning, and fluctuation be modified to include the possibility for change of tics within anatomic locations, such as eye-blinking, eyeball-rolling, or tics and eyebrow tics, or mouth-opening, puckering, and lip tics. The addition of the word "type" to the criteria would account for this variability. We also question the use of the word "and" in category C since all characteristics (location, number, frequency, complexity, and severity) are required if this criteria is to be fulfilled. However, empirical data indicates that not all of these characteristics are present (see later section), although one or more of the characteristics is always present. We therefore have added the word "type" and changed the word "and" to "or" in the criteria listed in Tables 10.8, 10.11 and 10.13.

Symptoms cited in Associated Features in DSM-III as "compulsive impulses to touch things or to perform complicated movements, such as squatting, deep knee bends, retracing steps, and twirling while walking" have been deleted in DSM-III-R; these symptoms are now classified as complex tics. Symptoms previously referred to as "complicated movements" are now referred to as complex tics. Both motor and vocal tics are classified as simple and complex; echopraxia is classified as a complex motor tic; coprolalia, echolalia, and palilalia are classified as a complex vocal tic. Based on semantic concepts, DSM-III-R uses the word intended instead of voluntary actions (Culver and Gert, 1982).

As previously described we propose that sensory tics be included in criteria A for all tic disorders. For continued study of possible heterogeneity among tic disorders, minor deviations from the criteria should be specified as indicated in Table 10.11. If there are major deviations from criteria for Tourette's disorder, the diagnosis should be tic disorder not otherwise specified or movement disorder not otherwise specified.

Chronic Motor or Vocal Tic Disorder

Although only 74 or 5% of 1,467 patients with tic disorders fulfilled criteria for either chronic motor tic disorder using DSM-III criteria or chronic motor tic disorder using the revised DSM-III-R (Table 2.1), the prevalence is believed to be much higher than for Tourette's disorder. For example, 32.3% of 641 patients reported a family history of tic disorder in one or more primary family members, 5.9 times more frequently than for Tourette's disorder and 4.3 times more tics than Tourette's disorder in other family members (Table 4.10). For the number of individuals, the ratio of tic disorder to Tourette's disorder is 6.3:1 for primary family and 8.6:1 for other family members (Table 4.10). An indirect estimate of the prevalence for both Tourette's disorder and CMT derived from a subsample of our patients is 1.55% of the population (Baron et al., 1981). It is likely that the prevalence for Tourette's disorder and CMT is much higher in the population than the frequency estimated from clinical samples. Mildly afflicted patients may never seek treatment and be unaware that they have tics. It is not uncommon for a parent during intake to deny that anyone in the family has tics, at the same time displaying mild and occasionally moderate tics which are obvious to other family members. A more direct assessment of the discrepancy is reported by Kurlan et al. (1987) who interviewed 159 Mennonite kindred, of which 54 were diagnosed as having Tourette's disorder or CMT. Sixteen or 29.6% were unaware of tics, 28 or 51.9% were aware of tics but never sought help, and only 10 or 18.5% sought treatment. The ratio of untreated patients with tics to treated patients with tics is 4.4:1. Similar results are reported in many family genetic studies which consistently cite many more relatives with CMT than Tourette's disorder (Chapter 4). Despite the large number of potential patients, there are no studies in the literature of patients with non-Tourette's disorder tic disorders.

TABLE 10.8. *Diagnostic criteria for Tourette's disorder (307.23)*

Criteria in DSM-III-R with proposed changes by the authors
  307.23 Tourette's disorder
   A. Fulfill the six criteria for tics in Table 10.1.[a]
   B. Both multiple motor and one or more vocal tics have been present at some time during the illness, although not necessarily concurrently.
   C. The tics occur many times a day (usually in bouts), nearly every day or intermittently throughout a period of more than 1 year.
   D. The anatomic location, number, frequency, complexity, type[b], or[c] severity of the tics change over time.
   E. Onset before age 21.
  Proposed comments[a]
   Age at onset: The mean age at onset is 7 years but the disorder may appear as early as 1 year, and almost always before 20 years of age. Onset occurs before the age of 11 years in 90% and before the age of 14 years in 99% of patients.
   Sex: The disorder is approximately three times more common in boys than girls.
   Familial pattern: Tic disorders are more common among family members than in the general population. Tourette's disorder has been reported in 8% of families, other tic disorders in 42%, and a tic or Tourette's disorder in 47%. Monozygotic twins are 75 to 85% concordant for tic disorders. Adequately controlled studies have not demonstrated that obsessive compulsive disorder or symptoms are more frequent in families or individuals with Tourette's disorder than in normal control samples.
   Echophilia: Occurs in approximately 33% of patients and includes echokinesis (8%), echolalia (18%), and palilalia (17%).[d]
   Coprophilia: Occurs in approximately 37% patients and includes coprolalia (32%), copropraxia (18%), and mental coprolalia (4%).[d]
   Impulsions: An impulsion is defined as an impulse to perform a repetitive act, that is an end in itself, and not designed to prevent a dreaded event or situation. Inhibition of the act causes discomfort. The frequency is estimated to occur in 9% to 22% of patients with Tourette's disorder.[d]
   Organic central nervous system stigmata: Nonlocalizing neurological signs, nonspecific EEG abnormalities, ambidexterity or left-handedness, central nervous system neuropsychological test abnormalities, and attentional, learning and perceptual problems have been reported in 17% to 60% of patients. These abnormalities may be largely associated with coexisting disorders such as attention-deficit hyperactivity disorder, specific developmental disorder, mental retardation, autism, Down's syndrome, and other disorders with known central nervous system pathology. The reports of a higher than expected frequency of attention-deficit hyperactivity disorder is probably due to ascertainment bias.
   Behavioral problems and psychopathology: The relationship of behavioral problems and psychopathology to Tourette's disorder is controversial. They may be more frequent in patients with an associated diagnosis of attention-deficit hyperactivity disorder than in patients with uncomplicated Tourette's disorder. An association between psychopathology and obsessive compulsive disorder or symptoms in uncomplicated Tourette's disorder has not been demonstrated in adequately controlled studies.
   Stimuli-induced change in symptoms: As with many other movement disorders, tics markedly decrease or disappear during sleep, usually decrease with nonanxious absorption and in the presence of strangers, and increase with anxiety, pleasurable anticipation, fatigue, and with close friends and family.
   Predisposing factors: There are no known predisposing, precipitating, or psychodynamic factors. A controversy exists about whether exposure to neuroleptics, head trauma, or the use of central nervous system stimulants can precipitate tic disorders. The severity of symptoms can be exacerbated temporarily by central nervous system stimulants in approximately one-third of patients, possibly a dose-related phenomenon, may decrease in one-third, or remain unchanged in one-third of patients.

TABLE 10.8 *(Continued)*

Clinical course: Symptoms typically vary in number, frequency, type, location, or severity over months. They may decrease during adolescence in approximately 30% of patients and after adulthood in most patients. The symptoms of the disorder may disappear entirely in approximately 8% of patients in childhood or adolescence. Periods of spontaneous remission from 1 week to 7 years occur in approximately 27% of patients.
Complications: Possible complications include rare orthopedic disorders, blindness, excoriation or brusies of the skin, self-injury from complex motor tics such as biting or hitting self, and suicide. Withdrawal, interference with psychosocial and vocational functioning, and depression may occur in predisposed individuals, especially those with severe forms of the disorder.
Prevalence: The prevalence is unknown but has been estimated to be at least 0.05%

---

[a]Proposed by authors but not included in DSM-III-R.
[b]We propose inclusion of the word "type" of tic which is not included in DSM-III-R to account for changes within anatomic locations such as eye-blinking, eyeball-rolling, and eyebrow tics, or mouth-puckering, opening, and lip tics.
[c]DSM-III-R uses the word "and"; whereas we propose use of the word "or." The use of the word "and" implies that all characteristics (location, number, frequency, complexity, type, and severity) must be present to fulfill the criteria. However, empirical data analysis indicates that all of these characteristics frequently are not present, although one or more of the characteristics are always present.
[d]Order and frequency of tics based on 666 patients from current study.

Chronic Motor Tic Disorder

DSM-III criteria for CMT include (a) no more than three motor tics at one time, (b) unvarying intensity of the tics over weeks or months, (c) can be suppressed, and (d) duration of at least 1 year.

There were a number of problems with this diagnostic entity. In our clinical sample of patients with CMT who were diagnosed using DSM-III criteria, the muscular contractions appeared to be stronger or more vigorous than in Tourette's disorder. Vocal symptoms were absent or were loud, vocal, expiratory, grunt-like noises secondary to a vigorous contraction of diaphragmatic, abdominal, or torso muscles. Patients reported much less waxing, waning, and fluctuation of symptoms and fewer tics. Only five patients in our total sample of 742 patients with tic disorders met these criteria. Moreover, neuroleptics were less effective in these patients than in those with other tic disorders. Many more of our patients, however, had tic symptoms similar in all respects to those of patients with Tourette's disorder, but they only had motor symptoms. DSM-III-R has revised the criteria and renamed the category chronic motor or vocal tic disorder.

Clinically, the symptoms and criteria of CMT are indistinguishable from Tourette's disorder in most patients except for the absence of vocal symptoms (Tables 10.1, 10.2). Most patients have only multiple motor tics. A smaller number have only a chronic single motor tic, but subsequently may develop other motor tics or vocal tics. If both motor and vocal tics develop subsequently the diagnosis of Tourette's disorder should be made. Although considerable indirect evidence has accumulated from genetic studies reporting family clustering of both Tourette's disorder and CMT (Eldridge et al., 1977; Golden, 1978; Shapiro et al., 1978; Baron et al., 1981; Nee et al., 1980; Kidd et al., 1980; Pauls et al., 1981, 1984), studies directly comparing patients with CMT and Tourette's disorder have not been done because of the small number of patients with CMT who seek treatment and are available for study. For these reasons, although the sample size is small, we describe preliminary results comparing patients with complete data who met DSM-III criteria for CMT disorder ($N = 3$), and those who met DSM-III-R criteria for CMT disorder ($N = 24$), the total sample subsequently referred to as CMT disorder ($N = 27$), with the sample of 666 patients with Tourette's disorder.

Preliminary study of chronic motor tic and Tourette's disorder

Our clinical hypothesis is that CMT should be included within the rubric of tic disorders because family clustering, symptoms, clinical course, and response to treatment for CMT is similar to Tourette's disorder. Additional support for the hypothesis is available from analysis of the 54 variables described in Table A.1 for 27 patients with CMT compared with 666 with Tourette's disorder. Statistical tests included 2-tailed *t*-tests and chi-Squares; only selected and significant variables are presented in the table; variables not included in the table are not significant (Table 10.9). Our expectations were that the null hypothesis would hold for sex ratio, family history of Tourette's or tic disorders, age at onset of Tourette's disorder, and other relevant characteristics.

Although the results only partially confirmed our expectation, significant differences were interpreted as primarily associated with secondary factors. The sex ratio and a family history of Tourette's disorder are similar for both CMT and Tourette's disorder. The significantly fewer family members with a history of tics reported by patients with CMT is probably artifactual. The symptoms of CMT are frequently less severe and patients often are unaware of having them. Moreover, patients with Tourette's disorder may be more likely to inquire about a history of the disorder in other family members, thus more readily identifying those with Tourette's disorder than with tics. Although the average age at onset of symptoms was 9.1 for CMT and 6.6 for Tourette's disorder ($p < 0.0001$), the range was similar, 4 to 14 for all CMT patients except for one patient whose symptoms began at age 21. Patients with CMT also had less previous diagnoses and consultations ($p < 0.01$), less ADD ($p < 0.01$), and lower hyperactivity factor score (FS) scorers ($p < 0.05$). Other differences are largely related to less severe symptoms ($p < 0.05$), reflected by fewer symptoms in most categories and more or longer periods of remissions. Vocal, coprophilic, and echophilic symptoms were excluded by diagnosis. Less frequent fluctuation of symptoms may be related to having fewer symptoms, and less frequent waxing and waning may be due to having less concern

TABLE 10.9. *Comparison of variables for patients with chronic motor tic disorder and Tourette's disorder*[a]

Variables	Chronic motor tic disorder ($\bar{X}$ or %)	Tourette's Disorder ($\bar{X}$ or %)	t or χ^2 $p<$
Demography			
Year of evaluation	1978	1976	0.001
Age	22.4	19.8	—
Sex (% males)	77.9%	76.3%	—
Genetics (family history of:)			
Tourette's disorder	7.4%	7.8%	—
Tics	19.2%	42.0%	0.05
TS or tics	26.9%	46.7%	0.10
Other movement disorders	7.1%	13.3%	—
Medical history			
Parents age at birth FS	31.4	29.0	0.05
Neurological			
Attention-deficit hyperactivity disorder	7.4%	25.1%	0.10
Behavior			
Hyperactivity FS	0.8	1.2	0.05
Illness variables			
Duration of illness FS	16.0	13.7	—
Previous diagnosis-consultation FS	2.9	3.3	0.01
Age at onset	9.1	6.6	0.0001
Symptoms (history of tics:)			
Face	85.2%	93.1%	—
Head	81.5%	91.1%	0.10
Upper limb	22.2%	68.6%	0.0001
Lower limb	14.8%	40.7%	0.01
Torso	22.2%	46.6%	0.01
Complex	11.1%	68.5%	0.0001
Inarticulate sounds	0.0%	98.5%	—
Coprolalia	0.0%	32.0%	—
Copropraxia	0.0%	12.8%	—
Mental coprolalia	0.0%	3.9%	—
Echophilia	0.0%	32.7%	—
Total current tics	3.2	6.9	0.0001
Total cumulative tics	4.7	15.7	0.0001
Waxing and waning	77.8%	97.2	0.0001
Fluctuation	33.3	96.0	0.0001
Severity of tics	2.2	2.7	0.05
Remission of symptoms FS	1.4	0.9	0.01
Stimuli-induced change			
Interpersonal FS	3.8	3.3	0.01
Non-anxious absorption FS	3.4	3.0	0.10
Seasonal stimuli FS	3.8	3.9	0.10

[a]Only significant and selected variables included in the table; all other variables in the Variable List (Table A.1) were not significant. Chronic motor tic disorder, $N = 27$; Tourette's disorder (TS), $N = 666$.

[b]Three patients had very low intensity sounds that lasted less than 1 year.

about and awareness of mild changes. The latter is supported by less decrease of symptoms with interpersonal stimuli FS ($p < 0.01$), and nonanxious absorption stimuli FS ($p < 0.10$). The most frequent tics involve the face and head.

Variables identified by the stepwise regression analysis (Table 10.10) tend to be epiphenomena. These preliminary results support the concept of a continuum of types and severity of symptoms and similar etiology for CMT and Tourette's disorder. Confirmation requires study of a larger sample and clinical course over many years.

Chronic Vocal Tic Disorder

The diagnosis of CVT is reserved for the small number of patients who have only one or several involuntary vocal tics. Patients who develop motor tics

TABLE 10.10. *Chronic motor tic vs. Tourette's disorder: Stepwise regression analysis*

Variables	Simple r	Multiple R^2	Parameter estimate
Demography			
Year evaluated	0.12[b]	0.02	0.01[c]
Genetics			
Family history of tics	−0.09[d]	0.01	−0.03[d]
Medical history			
Parents' age at birth FS	0.09[d]	0.01	0.00[d]
Neurological			
Attention deficit disorder	−0.11[b]	0.01	−0.04[d]
Behavior			
Hyperactivity FS	−0.12[d]	0.02	−0.03[b]
Illness Variables			
Previous diagnosis-consultation FS	−0.10[d]	0.01	−0.03[b]
Symptoms			
Fluctuation	−0.26[e]	0.24	−0.34[e]
Complex tics	−0.44[e]	0.26	−0.04[b]
Remission of symptoms FS	0.12[c]	0.26	0.01[b]
Age at onset	0.17[e]	0.27	0.01[b]
Upper limb tics	−0.19[e]	0.28	−0.03[d]
Summary SRA[a]			
Fluctuation	0.26[e]	0.23	0.33[e]
Complex tics	−0.44[e]	0.24	−0.04[b]
Family history of tics	−0.09[d]	0.25	−0.03[b]
Upper limb tics	−0.19[e]	0.26	−0.04[b]
Parents' age at birth FS	0.09[d]	0.27	0.00[b]
Remission of symptoms FS	0.12[c]	0.28	0.01[b]
Age at onset	−0.17[e]	0.28	−0.01[b]
Adjusted R^2	—	0.27	—

[a]Hyperactivity FS, EEG, and neurological variables were omitted from the summary SRA because of missing data.
[b]$p < 0.01$.
[c]$p < 0.001$.
[d]$p < 0.05$.
[e]$p < 0.0001$.

subsequently are diagnosed as having Tourette's disorder. We have seen only seven such patients who were followed into middle age. However, the vocal symptoms were very different from those of patients with Tourette's disorder and would not fulfill the criteria for a vocal tic. One patient, with a past history of severe alcoholism, chronic pancreatitis, and diffuse psychopathology had prolonged, singsong, or undulating noises, and shrieks only when alone in the evening. A middle-aged woman, with diffuse nonpsychotic psychopathology, had similar symptoms throughout the day which were completely inhibited when in the presence of others. Two elderly patients had an organic mental syndrome, one was addicted to benzodiazapines, and two had a habit of sporadically filling sentences with "mm" or "tsk" sounds. A possible clinical indication that the etiology is different from Tourette's disorder is that none of the patients responded adequately to treatment with haloperidol.

The differential diagnosis includes diverse vocal symptoms unsystematically associated with various organic disorders (pervasive developmental disorder, mental deficiency, schizophrenia, senility, strokes, addiction), habits or mannerisms, and chronic cough of adolescence.

Chronic Cough of Adolescence

Chronic cough of adolescence is a rare disorder of unknown etiology, which usually occurs during puberty or adolescence without discernable psychopathology, respiratory, medical, or other organic pathology or symptoms (Bernstein, 1963; Minnegerode and Polyzaidis, 1981), and should be differentiated from CVT Disorder. In response to a feeling of irritation in the throat the patient inspires deeply and emits one or more loud and harsh coughs which resembles the cough of pertussis. The symptoms are not responsive to treatment with psychotherapy, benzodiazepines, neuroleptics, or other drugs. We have evaluated four males and one female with this disorder.

Our suggested criteria for chronic motor or vocal tic disorder in DSM-III-R are outlined in Table 10.11.

Transient Tic Disorder

Although TTD is the most common tic disorder, with a life-time prevalence estimated between 4% and 25% (Table 3.1), we have diagnosed only 28 (2.6%) patients with this disorder between 1965 and 1985, and there is little available information about TTD in the literature. Three studies that included a large number of patients with transient tics were conducted before DSM-III criteria were established, and it is not possible to separate the TTD group from other tic disorders (Zausmer, 1954; Torup, 1962; Corbett et al., 1969; Corbett, 1976). Because of the dearth of data in the literature, and although the sample size is small, a preliminary and retrospective study was designed (in collaboration with A. Shenker, M.D., Ph.D.) to retrospectively provide

TABLE 10.11. *Diagnostic criteria for chronic motor or vocal tic disorder (307.22)*

DSM-III-R Criteria with Proposed Changes by the Authors
Fulfill the six criteria for tics in Table 10.1.[a]
Either motor or vocal tics, but not both, have been present at some time during the illness.
The tics occur many times a day, nearly every day, or intermittently throughout a period of more than 1 year.
The anatomic location, number, frequency, complexity, type,[b] or[c] severity of the tics change over time.
Onset before age 21.

Proposed comments[a]
This diagnosis is reserved for patients who have either motor or vocal tics, but not both. The diagnosis should be changed to Tourette's disorder if motor and vocal tics develop subsequently.
Chronic motor tic disorder is much more common than chronic vocal tic which is infrequent.
Genetic and other studies indicate that this disorder is similar to Tourette's disorder.
The associated features of this disorder are less well known but believed to be similar to Tourette's disorder.
The prevalence is estimated to be 2–10 times as frequent as Tourette's disorder. The prevalence of both disorders is estimated as 1.6%.

[a]Proposed by authors but not included in DSM-III-R.
[b]We propose inclusion of the word "type" of tic which is not included in DSM-III-R, to account for changes within anatomic locations such as eye-blinking, eyeball-rolling, and eyebrow tics, or mouth-puckering, opening and lip tics.
[c]DSM-III-R uses the word "and"; whereas we propose use of the word "or." The use of the word "and" implies that all characteristics (location, number, frequency, complexity, type and severity) must be present to fulfill the criteria. However, empirical data analysis indicates that all of these characteristics are frequently not present, although one or more of the characteristics are always present.

information about three issues: (a) description of demographic and clinical characteristics of a sample of children with TTD; (b) comparison of these characteristics with a sample of children initially diagnosed as having TTD who subsequently developed Tourette's disorder; and (c) determine if there are specific features that can differentiate children with TTD from children with early Tourette's disorder. Accordingly, the clinical course for 29 patients was evaluated one to 11 years after an initial diagnosis of TTD. The sample included nine children in whom all symptoms disappeared within 1 year, with a final diagnosis of TTD, and 17 children whose symptoms did not remit and subsequently fulfilled criteria for Tourette's disorder. Three patients were excluded from the analysis: one had a diagnosis of CMT, and two patients could not be located. The clinical status of patients was evaluated by telephone using a structured interview conducted by Dr. Shenker. The data were reviewed by E.S. who confirmed diagnoses using DSM-III criteria. Nonparametric tests were used to compare the two groups (Mann-Whitney rank sum test and two-tailed Fisher exact test) (Table 10.12). Power analysis to determine adequate sample size was not done.

TABLE 10.12. Comparison[a] of selected variables for children initially diagnosed as transient tic disorder and subsequently diagnosed as transient tic disorder or Tourette's disorder[b]

Variables	Transient tic disorder[c] ($\bar{X}$ or %)	Tourette's disorder[d] ($\bar{X}$ or %)
Sex (% males)	78%	69%
Race (% white)	89%	100%
Family history of TS or tics	50%	44%
Attention-deficit hyperactivity disorder	24%	11%
Behavior problem	18%	22%
Age at onset of tics		
Mean	7.2	6.4
Range	3–10	4–12
Duration of illness (months)		
Mean	4.8	5.5
Range	>1–10	>1–12
Length of follow-up (years)		
Mean	3.8	3.8
Range	>1–10	>1–11
Initial tics[e]		
Eyes	62%	41%
Face	25%	25%
Head, neck	13%	44%
Shoulders	0%	19%
Upper limb	0%	19%
Lower limb	0%	13%
Torso	0%	13%
Complex	0%	18%
Sounds	25%	41%
Coprolalia	0%	0%
Total number of motor tics		
Mean	3.8	4.0
Range	1–8	1–8
Total number of vocal tics		
Mean	1.4	2.1
Range	0–2	0–8
Cumulative symptoms		
Eyes	89%	59%
Face	44%	56%
Head, neck	67%	81%
Shoulders	22%	50%
Upper limb	22%	41%
Lower limb	0%	25%
Torso	33%	25%
Sounds	78%	94%
(three or more vocal tics)[f]	0%	47%
Coprolalia	22%	13%

[a]Mann-Whitney rank sum test or 2-tailed Fisher exact test.
[b]One patient could not be located; one patient subsequently diagnosed chronic motor tic disorder omitted from analysis. Initially diagnosed as transient tic disorder, $N = 26$; subsequently diagnosed as transient tic disorder, $N = 9$ or Tourette's disorder, $N = 17$.
[c]$N = 9$.
[d]$N = 17$.
[e]$N = 8$.
[f]Fisher exact test, $p = 0.023$.

Based on our concept that TTD, CMT, and Tourette's disorder have a similar etiology that is symptomatically expressed on a continuum of duration of illness, type of symptoms and severity, our expectation was confirmed that prediction of the clinical course and the final diagnosis could not be made from background and symptom variables during the first year of the illness.

Only one of 32 variables, within chance expectations, was significantly different. Children were more likely to develop Tourette's disorder if they had three or more vocal symptoms during the first year (8 or 17 children); all of the children with less than three vocal symptoms had a final diagnosis of TDD ($p = 0.02$). Several nonsignificant retrospective trends warrant mention. The cephalic concentration of initial tics (including vocal tics) in both groups resembles the distribution of initial tics in our total Tourette's disorder sample and for patients with diverse tic disorders (Corbett et al., 1969). None of the children with a final diagnosis of TTD had initial tics originating below the head or neck, and none had leg tics during the first year. The better prognosis for children without leg tics confirms the observation by Corbett et al. (1969). The occurrence of coprolalia in two patients eventually diagnosed as TTD tends to confirm the concept of similar etiology for both Tourette's disorder and TTD, and indicates that coprolalia during the first year does not

TABLE 10.13. *Diagnostic criteria for transient tic disorder (307.21)*

DSM-III-R criteria with proposed changes by authors
Fulfill the six criteria for tics in Table 10.1.[a]
Single or multiple motor and or vocal tics.
The tics occur many times a day, nearly every day for at least 2 weeks but not for longer than 12 consecutive months.
The anatomic location, number, frequency, complexity, type[b], or[c] severity of the tics change over time.
Onset before age 21.
No history of Tourette's or chronic motor or vocal tic disorder.
Specify: single episode or recurrent.

Proposed Comments[a]
The only differentiating feature between transient tic disorder and other tic disorders is that the tics in transient tic disorder completely and permanently disappear within 1 year.
The associated features for this disorder are less well known but believed to be similar to other tic disorders.
The prevalence is estimated as 4% to 25% of the population.

[a]Proposed by authors but not included in DSM-III-R.
[b]We propose inclusion of the word "type" of tic which is not included in DSM-III-R, to account for changes within anatomic locations such as eye-blinking, eyeball-rolling, and eyebrow tics, or mouth puckering, opening and lip tics.
[c]DSM-III-R uses the word "and"; whereas we propose use of the word "or." The use of the word "and" implies that all characteristics (location, number, frequency, complexity, type and severity) must be present to fulfill the criteria. However, empirical data analysis indicates that all of these characteristics are frequently not present, although one or more of the characteristics are always present.

warrant a diagnosis of Tourette's disorder or a poor prognosis. These preliminary results are limited by the small sample and do not reflect characteristics of nonclinical patients with tics in the general population. They are congruent, however, with the clinical impression that the age of onset, sex ratio, signs, symptoms, and etiology of TTD are similar to CMT and Tourette's disorder. Our suggested criteria for TTD are outlined in Table 10.13.

Tic Disorder Not Otherwise Specified

DSM-III-R defines "tic disorder not otherwise specified" as "tics that do not meet the criteria for a specific tic disorder." We suggest the addition of: This category is for a disorder that includes tics or symptoms that resemble tics and that fulfill some but not all the criteria for a specific tic disorder. Examples are a tic disorder with onset in adulthood, without waxing, waning, or fluctuation of symptoms, with tonic rather than clonic movements, with symptoms that cannot be inhibited even for short periods of time, and which occur rhythmically or regularly rather than arhythmically and irregularly, etc. Criteria that are or are not fulfilled should be specified (Table 10.14).

Movement Disorder Not Otherwise Specified

Our experience with this category reminds us of the story about an 85-year-old lighthouse keeper. Every morning the tides came in at 6 a.m. and without fail for the past 65 years set off the fog horn. One morning something went wrong and the fog horn did not sound. The lighthouse keeper awoke from a sound sleep, exclaiming "What's that!"

We had a similar experience with 37 (2.5%) of our patients over the past 22 years. Although the symptoms usually include various movements and often sounds, some partially resembling tics, and usually diagnosed by others as Tourette's disorder or CMT, the symptoms and clinical course, in our opinion, did not fulfill criteria for a tic or other known movement disorder. The most frequent characteristics of this group are movements that do not resemble or

TABLE 10.14. *Criteria for tic-disorder-not-otherwise-specified (307.20)*

Tics that do not meet the criteria for a specific tic disorder.
This category is for a disorder that includes or resembles tics and that fulfills some but not all criteria for a specific tic disorder. Examples are a tic disorder with onset in adulthood, that does not have waxing, waning, or fluctuation of symptoms, that has tonic rather than clonic movements, that cannot be inhibited even for short periods of time, that occur rhythmically and regularly rather than arrhythmically and irregularly, etc.[a]
Specify: criteria that are not fulfilled.[a]

---

[a]Proposed by authors but not included in DSM-III-R.

fulfill the criteria for tics, and an inability to suppress the movements. They also have little or no response to treatment with haloperidol and other dopamine-blocking drugs. Frequently absent are waxing, waning, and fluctuation of symptoms and little or no response to stimuli that usually affect tic symptoms. Because the specific etiology for tic disorders is unknown, and the diagnosis is based on syndromal characteristics, the possibility of heterogenous etiologies is a major problem. For heuristic purposes and to keep clinical, research, and treatment options open, patients who do not fulfill criteria for tic disorders should be classified as movement disorder not otherwise specified.

To discern patterns among these 29 atypical patients, we periodically review our records and obtain information about the clinical course subsequent to our evaluation. Although the signs, symptoms, and other characteristics are extremely varied, three syndromal patterns are suggested in a small number of patients.

Paroxysmal Myoclonic Dystonia with Vocalization

Six patients were identified with a pattern of similar symptoms which we refer to as paroxysmal myoclonic dystonia with vocalization (PMD). The predominant feature is the sudden appearance of paroxysmal bursts of involuntary, regular, repetitive, rhythmic, bilateral, coordinated, simultaneous, stereotypic, myoclonus, with less apparent background dystonia, lasting 2 sec to 20 min. This pattern is clinically quite different from the symptoms of Tourette's disorder which are discrete muscular contractions that occur intermittently and randomly in a pattern like normal eye-blinking. They are never repetitively and regularly rhythmic. For example, a 21-year-old male subject, suddenly, without apparent stimuli, developed mild opisthotonic arching of the back with the arms held in front bent at the elbows and the onset of vigorous, bilateral, alternate flexion and extension of the forearms at the elbow. The very regular and rhythmic pattern resembles an exaggerated stereotypic playing of drums, and the periodicity, regularity, and rhythmicity is similar to the tremor observed in parkinsonism, senile and essential tremor, but much more vigorous and extending over a large amplitude of 90 degrees in the arms and through 30 to 40 degrees in the head. Proximal and distal muscle groups are involved in all movements, with proximal groups demonstrating more tonic and distal groups more myoclonic movements. Myoclonic movements involve a muscle group and its synergists, whereas tonic movements simultaneously involve agonists and antagonists. Occasional myoclonic jerks occurred in isolation or were superimposed on spasm of the same muscles. Guttural grunts and nasal exhalations often occurred synchronously in a nearly one-to-one relationship. Moreover, unlike Tourette's disorder, the movements continued in this stereotypic fashion for as long as 20 min, could not be intentionally or voluntarily stopped, prevented other intended or voluntary activity, and were minimally or not influenced by stimuli. Five other patients, described in greater detail by Feinberg et al. (1986), had similar symptoms, although the individual pattern for each patient was different. All of these patients also had ADD, and none responded to many different treatments including dopamine-blocking drugs. PMD may represent a hitherto unknown disease entity or a variant or combination of myoclonic, dystonic, or tic syndromes. Comparison of PMD movements with other movement disorders is outlined in Table 7.4.

Other Movement Disorders

Among the remaining 23 atypical patients, two groups, all previously diagnosed as Tourette's disorder or CMT, were classified by us as having a movement disorder of unknown etiology rather than a tic disorder.

The first group comprised five patients, three males and two females, with a pattern of symptoms characterized largely by fascicular, fibrillar, choreiform, and athetoid movements. Symptoms were confined to facial muscles in four patients and to the back in a female patient; vocal symptoms were not present. The muscular movements were not discrete as in Tourette's disorder. The overall pattern appears stereotypic, but closer examination reveals a continually changing pattern of undulating muscular movements. The predominant muscle contractions involve a part of a muscle in waves seemingly running over a portion of a muscle, or undulation over groups of muscles, in a continuous arrhythmic pattern, with both slow, sometimes worm-like, and fast features, and occasionally involve a whole muscle group. The symptoms occur unilaterally or bilaterally and are synchronous or asynchronous. The shifting pattern resembles the movements occasionally present in hemifacial spasm, Huntington's chorea, Sydenham's chorea, and tardive dyskinesia. The symptoms are involuntary, but unlike Tourette's disorder, can rarely be inhibited, are not usually affected by stimuli, have little waxing, waning, and fluctuation, and do not respond adequately to many different psychological and drug treatments, including dopamine-blocking drugs. Treatment with clonidine reduced symptoms markedly in one patient, minimally in another, and was ineffective in a third patient. The occasional contraction of a whole muscle group which resembles a tic probably contributed to the initial diagnosis of a tic disorder. Because the total pattern is so different, these patients were classified as atypical movement disorder, but would now be classified as movement disorder not otherwise specified.

The second group consisted of three patients with involuntary truncal dystonia which could not be inhibited. Symptoms were mild in one patient, moderate in another, and extremely severe in a third. The symptom in the severely afflicted patient began with a slight opisthotonic movement of truncal muscles which rapidly escalated to a rigid backward, slightly tilted to the left, contraction accompanied by an increasingly loud moan-like sound which paralleled the severity of the muscular contraction. Haloperidol, up to 500 mg daily, had no effect on these symptoms. Lower dosages of haloperidol had no therapeutic effect on two other patients.

The remaining 15 patients had some symptoms that would fulfill the criteria for motor or vocal tics, but also had atypical symptoms such as choreiform, athetoid, ballismic, and dystonic movements, spasms, tremors, incoordination, or other neurological stigmata. Not included in this group are 47 patients diagnosed as having another movement disorder (Table 2.1), many who had been previously diagnosed as having a tic disorder, and approximately a dozen patients who were secretly addicted to various drugs.

The reader may have noticed our frequent reference to a positive response to treatment with haloperidol or other dopamine-blocking drugs. It is perhaps clinically significant that none of the 29 patients diagnosed as atypical tic or movement disorder or the 47 patients diagnosed as other movement disorder (Table 2.1) who were treated by us responded adequately to haloperidol, even at high dosages. Comparatively low dosages of haloperidol usually have a dramatic effect on tic disorders. Higher dosages, although causing adverse effects, always reduce tic symptoms, but have no effect on patients in the atypical category. These clinical observations, which of course, require confirmation, have implications for both the etiology and heterogeneity in tic disorders. The effectiveness or ineffectiveness of haloperidol for tic disorders has the same implication as treatment with low dosages of thyroid for myxedema, antibiotics for bacterial infections, insulin for diabetes, and so on. The effectiveness of dopamine-blocking drugs, especially at low dosages, and their ineffectiveness, even at high dosages for other disorders, may be considered presumptive clinical evidence (albeit backward) that we are treating or dealing with a homogeneous syndrome or disorder.

It is important therefore to use the new DSM-III-R classification tic disorder not otherwise specified for patients who fulfill some but not all of the criteria for other tic disorders. Not included in both DSM-III or DSM III-R, however, is the classification movement disorder not otherwise specified. Since not every movement or noise signifies a tic disorder, we feel the inclusion of this diagnosis is important.

Criteria for movement disorder not otherwise specified are outlined in Table 10.15. For heuristic purposes, we also propose that unusual features be specified as outlined in Table 10.16.

TIC DISORDERS AS A CONTINUUM OR SPECTRUM

Many clinicians hypothesize that Tourette's disorder, TTD, and CMT represent an underlying disease with the same etiology. The continuum hypothesis is supported by the similarity of initial symptoms, age at onset, sex ratio,

TABLE 10.15. *Diagnostic criteria for movement disorder not otherwise specified*[a]

This is a residual category for movement disorders that does not meet the criteria for a tic disorder or other known CNS movement disorder.
This category includes a movement disorder characterized predominantly by non-tic-like movements, such as choreiform, athetotic, dystonic, ballismic, or myoclonic symptoms, that may be rhythmic, regularly repetitive, and occur in prolonged paroxysms. Less prominent tic-like movements may be present.
Vocalization may occur but tends to be prolonged rather than brief sounds.
Variation in number, frequency, type, location, or severity of symptoms may occur over time.
Inhibition of symptoms is usually less than for tic disorders.
Age at onset in childhood, adolescence or adulthood.
Associated features are unknown for this disorder, but frequently are associated with signs and symptoms of other CNS disorders.
Specify: the signs and symptoms of the movement disorder.

[a]Proposed by authors but not included in DSM-III-R.

Table 10.16. *Specification of Unusual Features for Tic Disorders*[a]

Specify if age at onset is older than 13 years.
Specify if symptoms include predominant involuntary tics and the presence of less frequent sensory tics, or only sensory tics.
Specify or describe the presence and type of induced voluntary movement.
Specify if vocal sounds are secondary to a sensory tic or to a vigorous diaphragmatic, abdominal, or torso contraction.
Specify if only one or two vocal symptoms are present.
Describe vocal symptoms if not tic-like.
Describe movements if they are not tic-like, such as choreiform, athetotic, dystonic, rhythmic, regularly repetitive, paroxysmal lasting one or more seconds, etc.
Specify if symptoms cannot be suppressed.
Specify if spontaneous waxing, waning, or fluctuation of symptoms are absent.
Specify associated symptoms and diagnoses if present, such as attention-deficit hyperactive disorder, specific developmental disorder, perceptual problems, behavior symptoms, psychopathology, or other associated diagnoses.
Specify other differentiating features not specified above.

[a]Proposed by authors but not included in DSM-III-R.

signs, symptoms, clinical course (except for the type of symptom and duration of illness), and the response to treatment with haloperidol and other neuroleptics. It is not possible to predict whether new symptoms will develop subsequently, fulfilling the criteria for one or another tic disorder. Patients with early symptoms of CMT frequently develop other symptoms years later which then fulfill the criteria for Tourette's disorder. Vocal symptoms in a patient with Tourette's disorder may disappear and the residual motor symptoms may then fulfill the criteria for CMT. A family history of Tourette's disorder or tics is more common in all tic disorders than is expected in the population. One type of tic disorder, for example CMT, may be present in a family member or in one monozygotic twin, whereas Tourette's disorder may be present in a second family member or in the co-twin. Family genetic studies suggest that Tourette's disorder and CMT are similar disorders.

Factors supporting the spectrum hypothesis include the discordance of tic disorder in 13 to 23% monozygotic twins and the ineffectiveness of treatment with neuroleptics, even at high dosages, in some patients. These speculations require carefully controlled studies of larger samples with TTD, CMT, Tourette's disorder, tic disorder not otherwise specified and movement disorder not otherwise specified. Better yet, would be identification of the neurophysiology of tic disorders.

However, although studies of Tourette's disorder have increased, the etiology still eludes us. The development of precise definitions and criteria for tic disorders has high priority. Reliable and valid criteria will reduce the heterogeneity of samples and improve generalization of results. Reliable and valid data about the signs, symptoms, and other variables are also important to provide hypotheses about the neuropathological loci for tic disorders. Carefully controlled and replicated studies are necessary to accomplish these goals.

11

Studies of Treatment

The treatment of Tourette's disorder is reviewed in this chapter. Each medication is classified according to its effect on neurotransmitters and pharmacological systems. This approach may provide insight into the neuropathology and site of the disturbance in Tourette's disorder and identify possible directions for future research. The psychological treatment of tic disorders and the results for a miscellaneous group of therapies are also described. Treatment recommendations and the recognition and management of adverse effects are discussed in Chapter 12.

EARLY HISTORY OF TREATMENT

The early history of treatment of Tourette's disorder was characterized by valiant although impotent attempts to treat the condition. Trousseau (1873) recommended an early form of behavior therapy consisting of gymnastic exercise of the involved muscles to the rhythmic accompaniment of a metronome. However, he insightfully observed that the arrest of a tic in one part of the body would be replaced by the development of a tic in another part. He and others, such as Pryol, Duchenne of Boulogne, Axenfeld, Troisier, Meige and Feindel (1907) and Gilles de la Tourette (1884, 1885), were pessimistic about treatment. Tourette felt that isolation, hydrotherapy, electricity, and constitutional treatment had minimal effects and that effective treatment was unavailable. By turn of the century many treatments had been tried and were being recommended. Tourette (1899), in his last statement about Tourette's disorder unenthusiastically recommended isolation and quiet rest in the country. Other unenthusiastic recommendations included hydrotherapy and gymnastics (Charcot, 1888, 1889) and hydrotherapeutics combined with isolation (Guinon, 1887). Meige and Feindel (1907), in their comprehensive work on tics, were equally pessimistic about the treatment of Tourette's disorder and described the illness as of a graver nature . . . peculiarly resistant to treatment. Patients suffering from these forms of tic present in the most advanced degree physical instability and volitional fickleness and betray an irresistible tendency to impulsion and obsession, calculated to render the institution of any methodological treatment futile . . . . patience and perseveration may be rewarded, but they never consent to undergo for a sufficiently long period the discipline indispensible for their cure.

Meige and Feindel, despite their pessimism about severe forms of Tourette's disorder, comprehensively reviewed the literature on the treatment of tics and other movement disorders, some of which would now be classified as Tourette's disorder. They concluded that "all the ordinary medicinal agents in vogue in nervous and mental diseases have at one time or another been applied to the cure of tics; all have proved equally inefficacious." The drugs used at one time or another included conium, bromides, chloral hydrate, opium, morphine, laudanum, the basic extract, atropine, curare, chloroform, ether, zinc valerianate, valerian, gelsemium, quinine, cannabis indica, arsenic, strong mustard plasters, cautery to the vertebral column, cold, hot and tepid douches, warm fomentations, cocaine, kola, coca, antipyrine, sulfonal, and lecithin.

Surgical treatment included tonsillectomy, elongation, section or ligature of the spinal accessory nerve, and resection of the trigeminal and spinofacial anastamoses. Other treatment included rhythmic traction of the tongue, thoracic compression, phrenic electrization, static sparks, diet, nutrition, general hygiene, hydrotherapy, tepid douche preferable to cold, morning and evening bath followed by energetic friction of the skin, massage, electricity, and waking and hypnotic suggestion.

Meige and Feindel had more faith in an appeal to the intelligence, good sense and will of the patient, and many procedures which are similar to those currently used by behavior therapists, such as systematized mental discipline, forced immobility (Brissaud, 1899), motor discipline, training antagonists, respiratory drill, or gymnastics (Cruchet, 1901), systematized exercises, mirror drill, systematic discipline, isolation, and bed rest. Psychotherapy was considered of "capital importance" and included encouragement, explanation, kindly counsel, unlearning, education, and discipline.

Meige and Feindel insightfully observed that many of these therapies, particularly respiratory drill, were effective because of

the bestowal of the attention on the allotted task. Whatever be the movements, they demand of the patient a momentary halt, a momentary interruption of those ill-timed motor reactions that make concerted action impossible. Observations show that the degree of successful control is in proportion to the degree of concentration of the attention. The novelty of the exercise in itself acts as a stimulus, but when this novelty wears off, faults are prone to reappear. Hence the necessity of varying the procedures and of rendering them always interesting; in the end the habit of supervision is contracted, and the patient feels increasing satisfaction in watching his physical infirmities daily diminish and the resources of his will daily widen.

Change the words around slightly and you have a procedure and explanation that would justify a behavioral analysis and treatment. What Meige and Feindel, as many therapists, hypnotists, behavioral therapists, and psychotherapists of today, did not appreciate is that nonanxious absorption in a task always decreases symptoms. This phenomenon is characteristic of the illness. It has been a "red herring" or "blind alley" for many therapies since the phenomenon is valid, but decrease in symptoms unfortunately does not generalize to other situations and activities.

After Meige and Feindel's book in 1907, few papers on tics appeared in the literature. The paper by Ferenczi (1921), discussed previously, and other analytical papers contributed little to an understanding of and much to the confusion about tics and Tourette's disorder. An influential paper by a prominent neurologist, Wilson (1927), the translator of Meige and Feindel's book, unfortunately contained several erroneous observations and conclusions which influenced many future authors. Wilson, in 1927 and subsequently (Wilson, 1940), characterized the tic as an act initially caused by an external act or idea, which with repetition became habitual and involuntary. Such patients show mental and volitional instability, degeneration, mental infantilism, idiocy, imbecility, paranoia, schizophrenia, and, in psychoanalytic parlance, a narcissistic fixation leading to degeneration and insanity. Tics were confused with tonic movements characteristic of the dystonias and torticollis, and many absurdities were intermixed with occasional appropriate observations. Treatment did not progress very much subsequent to Meige and Feindel, and included hygienic measures, sedative drugs, bromides, isolation, seclusion, re-education through Brissaud's muscular drill, Cruchet's respiratory exercises, Meige and Feindel's mirror drill, hypnotic or suggestive treatment, and psychoanalysis. Brain's (1928) paper is not very different and emphasizes treatment with psychotherapy and exercises involving muscular relaxation, immobility, and orderly movement of the affected muscles, along with a common-sense, early type of conditioning.

As indicated in many histories of psychiatry, psychological treatment was part of the zeitgeist during the 19th century (Janet, 1924, 1925; Bromberg, 1954). It included embryonic forms of behavior therapy. Hypnosis (Bernheim, 1889) preceded the psychotherapies, which became more prominent after the turn of the century (Parker, 1908, 1909); Tourette's disorder was treated with persuasion, re-education, autogenic training, psychoanalysis (Mahler et al., 1945, 1946); group therapy, family therapy, hundreds of other types of psychotherapy, and, more recently, behavior therapy, biofeedback, and transcendental meditation. The turning point in the history of treatment of Tourette's disorder occurred in the 1950s with the advent of neuroleptic treatment. Early papers describe the use of phenothiazines in the treatment of Tourette's disorder, and the success with haloperidol heralded a new and effective treatment method and eventually led to important new insights into the etiology and management of this disorder.

PHARMACOTHERAPY

The number of published studies of treatment with drugs and other modalities has increased dramatically during the past 25 years, stimulated in part by the need to find more effective medications with minimal adverse effects, and to gain insight into neurochemical systems underlying the disorder and its pathophysiology.

Dopamine Antagonists

Butyrophenones and Diphenylbutylpiperidines

Haloperidol

Haloperidol, a butyrophenone, is an antagonist at dopaminergic receptor sites. Its greater effectiveness compared to the phenthiazines is probably related to the fact that it binds more specifically to D_2 than to D_1 receptors. It also has some effect on norepinephrine which may account for some of the adverse effects reported with haloperidol.

The first successful use of haloperidol in a patient with Tourette's disorder was reported by Seignot (1961) in France and by Caprini and Melotti (1961). Challas, a fourth-year medical student at the University of Iowa, reported the successful use of haloperidol in two patients (Challas and Brauer, 1963). A year later, Chapel et al. (1964) reported similar success in two additional patients. Challas et al. (1967) confirmed initial favorable results in a second report.

Abuzzahab and Anderson (1973) conducted an exhaustive search of the world's literature and described the results for approximately 600 treatments of various types received by 430 patients. The percent improvement, without regard to length of treatment, was 89% for haloperidol, 48% for other neuroleptics, 20% for other chemotherapy, 22% for various somatotherapies, and 35% for assorted psychological treatment.

In 1973 we conducted a retrospective study of the treatment of 34 consecutive patients (Shapiro et al., 1973a) which we extended to the first 80 consecutive patients treated for 7 months to 8.5 years from 1965 to 1974 (Bruun et al., 1976; Shapiro et al., 1978). Patients treated with an average dosage of 5.0 mg/day haloperidol had an average of 80% (median 90%) decrease of symptoms compared with 24% (median 0%) in the non-haloperidol-treated group ($p < 0.001$). Improvement of at least 50% was reported in 97% of patients treated with haloperidol and in 40% of the non-haloperidol-treated group ($p < 0.005$). The amount of improvement variance accounted for by haloperidol was 44%. This study, thoroughly described in the first edition of our book, will not be repeated. We also reviewed the results of treatment with haloperidol for 144 patients reported in 41 publications between 1961 and 1975. The results suggested that treatment with haloperidol improved 78–91% of patients; only 8 to 22% failed to improve.

Other uncontrolled studies report improvement in 62 to 84% (Nee et al., 1980), 73% (Wassman et al., 1978), 70% (Nomura and Segawa, 1982), and 90% (Golden, 1978a). However, some clinicians report less favorable results (Ford and Gottlieb, 1969; Cohen et al., 1980; Tibbetts, 1981; van Woert et al., 1982; Leckman et al, 1985). Borison et al. (1982) reported haloperidol to be significantly better than placebo and equally efficacious to fluphenazine and trifluoperazine in ten patients with Tourette's disorder. Nevertheless, because of the largely favorable clinical reports, haloperidol has become the drug of choice for the treatment of Tourette's disorder.

Our conclusion, based on a review of the literature and clinical experience, is that haloperidol is an effective treatment for the symptoms of Tourette's disorder. Our results indicate that 25% of patients have at least 70% reduction of symptoms at a low dosage without significant adverse effects. Another 50% of patients develop adverse effects when treated with therapeutic dosages of haloperidol, but these can be successfully managed over time. The remaining 25% are treatment failures because adverse effects nullify therapeutic benefit. The limiting factor in the use of haloperidol are adverse effects which tend to correlate with dosage. Adverse effects and their management are discussed in Chapter 12.

However, despite reports of clinical effectiveness, there are no carefully controlled, randomized, double-blind studies in a large sample of patients supporting the effectiveness or superiority of haloperidol over placebo or other medications. We are currently comparing the clinical response to haloperidol, pimozide, and placebo using a double-blind cross-over design in 60 patients with Tourette's disorder. The results are now being analyzed.

Pimozide

Pimozide is reported to selectively block central dopamine receptors but has no effect on norepinephrine receptors (Anden et al., 1970; Nyback et al., 1970; Matthysse, 1973; Seeman and Lee, 1975; Nose and Takemoto, 1975). It preferentially binds to dopamine (D_2) receptors (Casamenti et al. 1980; Goldberg, 1985). The absence of norepinephrine antagonism and more specific dopamine antagonism may result in more improvement and fewer and less severe sedative, depressive, dysphoric, motivational, and cognitive adverse effects. Peak plasma concentrations occur in a range of 4 to 12 hr, and the elimination half-life averages 55 hr (McNeil Pharmaceutical, 1985).

The clinical literature provides some evidence that pimozide may be more effective and have a lower potential for adverse effects than haloperidol. Messerschmitt (1972) treated 186 children with various behavior problems, including tics, with pimozide. Pimozide was reported to have the same range of effectiveness and duration of action as haloperidol, and to have less sedative and extrapyramidal adverse effects. In a clinical study of the treatment with pimozide of 33 children with various types of tics, Debray et al. (1972) reported that 22 (67%) recovered, four (12%) improved, and seven (21%) were failures. In an acute double-blind cross-over study by Ross and Moldofsky (1977, 1978) of nine patients with Tourette's disorder, both haloperidol and pimozide equally reduced tics, but pimozide had significantly fewer sedative effects than haloperidol. Nomura and Segawa (1979) reported that seven (87.5%) of eight patients on pimozide showed more than moderate improvement. Pimozide compared to haloperidol was better in two patients, equal in three patients, worse in one patient, and one patient responded to neither drug. We have treated over 200 Tourette's disorder patients with pimozide since 1977. An initial report appeared in 1982 (Shapiro and Shapiro, 1982a), and we subsequently reported the results of an open clinical trial of 31 patients who were treated initially with haloperidol and subsequently with pimozide (Shapiro et al., 1983b). Pimozide yielded significantly more improvement of symptoms and had less akinesic adverse effects than haloperidol. This open trial was succeeded by a randomized, double-blind, cross-over, prospective study comparing pimozide with placebo in 20 patients (Shapiro and Shapiro, 1984). Multiple dependent variables of improvement were all highly significant (mainly $p < 0.0001$), favoring pimozide over placebo. Of 16 patients who had been treated previously with haloperidol, 13 reported that pimozide was better than haloperidol, two rated both drugs as equivalent, and one rated haloperidol as better than pimozide.

In a recent study by Reguer et al. (1986), pimozide was used alone in 69 patients with Tourette's disorder, in combination with tetrabenazine in five and with clonidine in four patients. Forty-three percent of patients on pimozide alone experienced good clinical response. If the patients treated with combination therapy are included, the percent improvement increases to 81% of patients. Daily dosages of pimozide varied from 0.5 to 8 mg. Dosage of tetrabenazine varied between 25 and 50 mg, and clonidine between 100 and 225 mg. Eleven patients developed moderate to marked side effects; four patients had intolerable sedation, four had weight gain, one restless legs, and two became depressed. The authors concluded that pimozide is superior to haloperidol causing less adverse effects.

Pimozide appears to be an effective alternative treatment for Tourette's disorder, possibly yielding greater improvement with fewer adverse effects than haloperidol. However, its superiority over haloperidol has yet to be demonstrated. We are conducting a study comparing the clinical response of 60 patients to pimozide, haloperidol, and placebo, using a double-blind cross-over design. The results are being analyzed.

Penfluridol

Penfluridol, a long-lasting diphenylbutylpiperidine, is thought to be a specific blocker of dopamine without significant norepinephrine or 5-hydroxytryptamine blocking effects (Seeman and Lee, 1975; Nose and Takemoto, 1975). This mode of action may result in more improvement than with haloperidol and fewer and less severe sedative, depressive, dysphoric, motivational, and cognitive adverse effects.

These speculations are supported by an open clinical study of seven patients in which six reported more improvement and fewer adverse effects compared to previous treatment with haloperidol (Holomboe, 1977). Almost complete remission has been reported in a single Indian patient at a weekly dosage of 160 mg (Parikh et al., 1979).

We have treated 15 Tourette's syndrome patients with penfluridol between 1979 and 1985. All patients had been treated previously with one or more of the following medications: haloperidol, pimozide, clonidine, chlorpromazane, trifluoperazine, clonazapan, amitriptyline, fluphenazine, thiothixine, metoclopramide, and physostigmine. Penfluridol yielded significantly more improvement than haloperidol, and there was a similar trend to greater improvement than with pimozide. Initial reports on eight patients treated were published in 1982 and 1983 (Shapiro and Shapiro, 1982a; Shapiro et al., 1983b). Since that time we have treated more patients. The results for the total sample of 15 patients, excluding three patients who were resisters to all treatment, are that penfluridol was better than haloperidol in nine (75%), equal in one (8%), and less effective than haloperidol in two (17%). For nine patients who were treated with penfluridol and pimozide, penfluridol was superior to pimozide in six (67%), equal in two (22%) and less effective in one (11%). The results of these open and uncontrolled clinical studies suggest that penfluridol is a worthwhile and alternative drug for the treatment of Tourette's disorder, yielding more improvement and less akinesic adverse effects than haloperidol. An additional advantage of penfluridol is weekly or biweekly administration. However, pancreatic and mammary tumors have been reported in studies of rats given high oral dosages of penfluridol. Although the significance of these findings for humans is unknown and there have been no published reports of carcinogenesis in the literature for any class of neuroleptics, the Food and Drug Administration and McNeil Pharmaceuticals have discontinued investigatory use of penfluridol in the United States, although it is available in many other countries.

Phenothiazines

Fluphenazine

The adenylate cyclase-linked D_1 receptors have a higher affinity for certain phenothiazines than do the butyrophenenome compounds which are more potent as antagonists at the D_2 receptor. In a double-blind, placebo-controlled study comparing haloperidol, fluphenazine, and trifluoperazine in ten patients, the three active drugs were significantly better than placebo, but no one drug was significantly better than the other. However, sedative and extrapyramidal adverse effects were reported to be significantly higher for haloperidol than for the other drugs (Borison et al., 1982). The dosages ranged from 5 to 20 mg for haloperidol, 8 to 24 mg for fluphenazine, and 10 to 25 mg for trifluoperazine. The failure to demonstrate differences in efficacy among the three drugs may be related to small sample sizes. Power analysis indicates that at least 52 subjects are necessary to demonstrate differences among neuroleptics in a cross-over design. Other limitations of this study were the failure to report previous treatment, whether the patients were haloperidol resisters, the length of the therapeutic trial, and whether medication was used to control adverse effects. Another study of 21 patients, who had been treated with an average dosage of 6.75 mg/day haloperidol (range 1–20 mg) for an average of 2.7 years (range 3 months to 8 years), and were considered to be resistant to haloperidol, reported a 35% decrease of tics without significant adverse effects (Goetz et al., 1984). No other medications were used for the control of adverse effects. They were subsequently treated with fluphenazine in an open study for an average of 2.3 years (range 10 months to 4.5 years) at an average dosage of 7 mg/day (range 2–15 mg). Improved efficacy and fewer adverse effects were reported in 11 (52%), similar efficacy and fewer adverse effects in 5 (24%), similar efficacy and adverse effects in 2 (10%), similar efficacy and more adverse effects in 1 (5%), and less efficacy and more adverse effects in 2 (10%). These studies suggest that fluphenazine, and possibly trifluoperazine, cause fewer adverse effects than haloperidol. Large-scale double-blind studies, selecting patients who have not been previously treated, and excluding resisters to haloperidol treatment, are warranted. Although we have not conducted a study comparing these drugs with haloperidol, our clinical experience with these drugs indicates that they do not have advantages over haloperidol.

Other phenothiazines

Favorable clinical response to other phenothiazines such as chlorpromazine and thiopropazate has been reported in occasional patients with Tourette's disorder. Clinical experience suggests that phenothiazines are less effective overall compared to haloperidol and pimozide. This impression should be verified in a carefully controlled clinical trial. The major limitations to the use of phenothiazines are the adverse effects of increased sedation, photosensitivity, seizures, dermatitis, and blood and liver dyscrasias for the aliphatic group, such as chlorpromazine; significantly more extrapyramidal symptoms such as akathesia, akinesia, dyskinesia, and parkinsonism for the piperazine subgroup, such as trifluoperazine, perphenazine, and prochlorperazine; and in the piperidyl group, increased sedative and sexual adverse effects, and limitation of dosage to 800 mg for thioridazine. The pattern of adverse effects for the butyrophenones and diphenylbutyliperidines are similar to the piperazine subgroup of phenothiazines.

Miscellaneous Dopamine Antagonists

Tetrabenazine

Tetrabenazine is a benzoquinolizine derivative that depletes brain storage of catecholamines. Fourteen patients were treated by us in an open study with oral dosages up to 300 mg/day (Shapiro et al., 1978). Initial improvement in 12 patients, associated with sedation and akinesia, was not sustained after 2 months. One patient reported improvement on 25 to 75 mg/day for 5 years, but there was no difference when reserpine and placebo were substituted. It was our impression that sedation accounted for the initial improvement which was not sustained as adverse effects remitted (Sweet et al., 1976; Shapiro et al., 1978). However, a more positive result was reported by Jankovic et al. (1984) in nine patients who had not responded adequately to previous treatment. In an open clinical trial patients were treated an average of 9.4 months (1–20 months) with dosages that ranged from 25 to 100 mg/day. Marked improvement was described for four (44%), mild transient improvement in three (33%), and minimal or no response in two (22%). Patients who improved in this study were younger than those in our study while two patients who failed to improve were over 48 years old. Additional controlled studies are necessary to resolve these reported differences in efficacy.

Metoclopramide

Metoclopramide is a selective D_2 receptor antagonist. We treated four patients with metoclopramide at a maximum dosage of 240 mg/day, but only one had an excellent response of 95% decrease of tics. A favorable result was reported in a single patient treated at a dosage of 240 mg/day for 12 weeks with complete remission of clinical symptoms (Desai et al., 1983). Dosage reduction to 120 mg/day resulted in a return of symptoms. The potential efficacy of metoclopramide has important theoretical implications because of its exclusive D_2 blocking properties and should be further evaluated using higher dosages. Although adverse effects were minimal in our patients, parkinsonism, tardive dyskinesia, and acute dystonic reactions have been reported (Grimes et al., 1982; Patel, 1986; Bateman et al., 1983; Pollera et al., 1984; Leopold, 1984; Jankovic and Glass, 1985).

Tiapride

This medication, not available in the United States, is reported to have dopaminergic blocking action, mainly on D_2 receptors. It is related to both sulpiride and metoclopramide of which it is a derivative. There have been several reports of its use in children with tics and Tourette's disorder. Nonhospitalized patients (15 with tics, one with tics and psychoses, one with tics and mental retardation, two with stammers, three with chronic chorea, and two with abnormal movements) were treated with tiapride, 100 mg/t.i.d. (Pasquier and Pouplard, 1977). Excellent results were reported in six, moderate in five, and poor in one of the 15 patients with tics. Seven patients relapsed as medication was either reduced or stopped prematurely, and one patient had a severe relapse while still on therapeutic dosages. The other groups obtained no benefit from tiapride. Although it is the authors' impression that the therapeutic effect is no greater than with haloperidol, adverse effects were clearly less severe. Tiapride was administered in an open placebo study at a daily dosage of 5 mg/kg to ten children with tics and Tourette's disorder for 7 days and then again for 6 months after 7 days on placebo (Eggers et al., 1983). Tics were rated three times a day for 15-min intervals during meals and during video-taped play and testing after each treatment segment. No significant difference was found when active drug was compared to the initial 7 days of placebo, although there was a decline in tic frequency. Adverse effects were minimal. A more favorable response was reported in a 17-year-old female patient with disabling Tourette's disorder who was treated initially with 300 mg tiapride intramuscularly, and subsequently with 900 mg/day orally (Lipcsey, 1983). Hyperkinesis and vocal tics were sharply reduced.

Clozapine

Clozapine, an antipsychotic, which blocks dopamine receptors and has few extrapyramidal effects, was ineffective in seven patients. A double-blind cross-over study over 4 to 7 weeks using dosages varying between 8 and 10 mg/kg/day found clozapine without therapeutic benefit (Caine et al., 1979b). These negative results are inconsistent with the dopamine hypothesis for Tourette's disorder, and it is significant that six of the seven patients had a previous good response to haloperidol. Adverse effects included drowsiness, marked somnolescence, salivation, and leukopenia.

Alpha-methylparatyrosine

Alpha-methylparatyrosine, which inhibits tyrosine hydroxylase, the rate-limiting enzyme in catecholamine synthesis, was administered to six Tourette patients at a maximum dosage of 3,000 mg/day (Shapiro et al., 1978). Tics improved in three patients, especially dystonic neck and trunk movements in two of the patients. There was no improvement in three patients. The major limitation of this medication are urinary effects, consisting of microscopic, needle-like crystals which appeared in the urine of four patients, and crystalluria associated with decreased creatine clearance (50–60 ml/min) in two patients. In addition, akinesia, akathesia, lethargy, and enuresis were sufficiently pronounced to nullify therapeutic effects. We also used a combination of alpha-methylparatyrosine in combination with resperine in one patient without effect.

Disulfiram

Disulfiram inhibits the enzyme dopamine-beta-hydroxylase (DBH) which catalyzes the conversion of dopamine to norepinephrine. Based on the theory that inhibiting DBH should decrease the concentration of norepinepherine and enhance the accumulation of dopamine, two Tourette patients were given 1.5 mg/day disulfiram. Both patients reported an increase in tics while on the medication. However, the increase in tics persisted and was not reversed when one patient stopped the medication. The second patient remained on the medication for only 4 days without increased tics (Shapiro et al., 1978).

Piquindone

Piquindone, a D_2 receptor antagonist, was reported to be effective in three patients with Tourette's disorder in an open clinical trial and in a subsequent 1-month double-blind cross-over study which included three patients who participated in the initial open trial (Uhr et al., 1984, 1986). Dosage varied from 20 to 50 mg/day. There was a marked to moderate reduction in motor tics and mild reduction of vocal tics. The only adverse effect was mild sedation. The authors relate the efficacy of the drug to its specific D_2 blockade. Unfortunately, clinical trials by the drug company have been terminated because of long-term toxic effects in animals.

Dopamine Agonists

Apomorphine

Two clinical studies report a transient but theoretically interesting decrease of Tourette's disorder symptoms with subcutaneous apomorphine (Shapiro et al., 1978; Feinberg and Carroll, 1979). The results suggest the possibility of an inhibitory effect on presynaptic dopamine receptors. The effect is brief and therefore not clinically useful.

Piribedil

Piribedil is a putative stimulator of dopamine receptors. We gave 3 mg piribedil intravenously to two patients. This dosage resulted in drowsiness and a slight decrease in tics in one patient. An oral dosage of up to 160 mg/day resulted in nausea but no effect on tics. Feinberg and Carroll (1979) used piribedil in doses from 40 to 240 mg/day in two patients without effect.

Levodopa

Levodopa (L-DOPA), a precursor of dopamine and norepinephrine which increases brain dopamine concentration, should result in increased tic activity. We gave three Tourette patients L-DOPA in increasing doses to a maximum of 3,000 mg/day (Shapiro et al., 1978). At the maximum dosage of 3,000 mg/day, tics in a 26-year-old man increased forcefully up to twice their original frequency. The movements, however, were choreoathetoid and dystonic and clearly different from tics. Tics in a second patient on 1,000 to 1,500 mg/day did not increase. A patient on 1,500 mg/day discontinued the medicine because of irritability and nausea, and the effect on his tics could not be evaluated. L-DOPA was also given to a 38-year-old man in doses up to 6 mg/day without increase in tics, although the effect of L-DOPA might have been mitigated by the concomitant use of 900 mg/day chlorpromaxine (DiGiacomo et al., 1971). A single report of L-DOPA inducing a syndrome similar to both klazomania and Tourette's disorder in a brain-injured patient was reported by Klempel (1974).

Friedhoff et al. (1982) developed a receptor sensitivity modification approach to the treatment of Tourette's disorder based on the theory that if the disorder is caused by a hyperdopaminergic state, L-DOPA should increase dopamine initially but later result in a compensatory decreased sensitivity of dopamine systems. L-DOPA is given in gradually increasing doses over a period of 4 to 6 weeks, beginning with 500 mg/day and increasing to a final dosage of 3 to 6 g/day. After 2 weeks, medication is withdrawn. Significant improvement is described in a brief note (no details given) for six patients who improved for 4 months to several years, a few successfully being retreated. Several treated patients seen by us subsequently, however, reported the method to be of little benefit. Confirmation of these initial results requires more detailed description of the results and replication.

Serotonin Agonists

L-5-Hydroxytryptophan

Although the serotonin agonist, L-5-hydroxytryptophan (5-HTP), in combination with carbidopa, was reported to ameliorate tics and self-mutilation (tongue- and lip-biting) in one patient, it was ineffective in nine others (Van Woert et al., 1977b, 1982). Dosage was 400 to 1,900 mg/day L-5HTP and 200 mg/day carbidopa. In addition to worsening hyperactivity, in patients with attention deficit disorder and hyperactivity (ADD+H), irritability, akathesia, anxiety, and agitation were reported.

L-Tryptophan

We treated two patients with L-tryptophan (LTP), an amino acid precursor of serotonin (Shapiro et al., 1978). Nausea was reported by a 46-year-old patient on 6.5 g/day but disappeared when the dosage was decreased to 5.5 g/day. The second patient, an 18-year-old boy, was evaluated in a double-blind procedure alternating placebo and LTP, and as well as MK 486 and 100 mg/day of pyridoxine. LTP had no significant effect on tics in both patients.

Tricyclic antidepressants

Tricyclic antidepressants, which block the reuptake of serotonin in presynaptics neurons, are discussed in the section entitled *Antidepressants*.

Methysergide

Methysergide in doses to 10 mg/day for 2 weeks was given to two of our patients. An initial reduction in tics was not sustained.

Cholinergic Agonists

Physostigmine

Physostigmine, an inhibitor of cholinesterase, was given subcutaneously to five patients at a dosage of 1 mg together with 1 mg of methylscopolamine. There was no effect on tics in three patients although two others had transient improvement (Shapiro et al., 1978). Physostigmine was administered intravenously to six Tourette's disorder patients in a double-blind, placebo-controlled study (Stahl and Berger, 1981, 1982a). Motor and vocal tics significantly decreased in all patients. These results prompted us to use oral physostigmine which has been reported to be slightly effective in the treatment of Alzheimer patients. Oral physostigmine was titrated to a maximum dosage of 15 mg/day (the maximum dosage permitted by the FDA) in two adult Tourette's disorder patients. There were no beneficial or adverse effects. Further testing with higher dosages are required to determine efficacy. Blood levels are suggested to titrate appropriate dosages.

Deanol

Deanol, a possible generator of acetylcholine in the CNS, was given to two Tourette patients at a maximum dosage of 2 g/day without altering the frequency of tics from base-line levels (Shapiro et al., 1978). Adverse effects included lightheadedness and nervousness. The addition of deanol (1,200 mg/day) to perphenazine (36 mg/day) in a 31-year-old male patient did not result in improvement of tics (Pinta, 1977).

Choline

Three patients were treated with choline by us. A 20-year-old male was given 40 g/day of choline as an outpatient. Tic frequency was decreased approximately 40% without adverse effects, but the patient discontinued using choline because of the offensive fish odor that invariably occurs. A 16-year-old male was given 1.2 g/day choline as an inpatient but the medication induced nausea and emesis and was discontinued before an adequate clinical trial could be conducted. Choline at a dosage of 20 g/day was also ineffective in a 26-year-old patient.

Lecithin

Two patients were treated with lecithin without benefit (Barbeau, 1979). In a more recent study, lecithin was administered in higher concentrations to five patients without benefit on tics (Moldofsky and Sandor, 1983). These patients had been either refractory to previous treatment with haloperidol and pimozide or had stopped the medications because of adverse effects. Lecithin was administered at bedtime and dosage was increased every 4 days to a maximum dosage of 35 g/day. Length of treatment varied from 19 to 35 days. Serum prolactin and serum growth hormone levels did not change suggesting that lecithin has no direct effect on the CFS neurotransmitters that influence their secretion. A double-blind cross-over study of lecithin in six Tourette's disorder patients was also negative (Polinsky et al., 1980). Our experience parallels these reports. Lecithin used by several of our patients was ineffective. The role of cholinergic mechanism in Tourette's disorder is currently indeterminate.

Cholinergic Antagonists

Benztropine mesylate

Benztropine mesylate, 2 mg subcutaneously, was associated with brief but marked increase of tics in one of our patients, brief increase in two, and no effect in a fourth patient (Sweet et al., 1976; Shapiro et al., 1978). Clinically, we have noted no effect on tics with the oral use of many different anticholinergic medications.

Stimulants

The effects of stimulants are discussed in another part of this chapter.

Antidepressants

The effect of antidepressants on Tourette's disorder is unclear. A literature review reported worsening of Tourette's disorder symptoms in 13 of 17 patients (Abuzzahab and Anderson, 1973), but the medications were not separated into categories according to their neuropharmacologic properties.

Imipramine

Imipramine has both norepinephrine and 5-HT reuptake blocking properties. One report described improvement in a 44-year-old patient on varying dosages of haloperidol (1–30 mg/day together and alternating with 75 mg/day of imipramine and placebo) (Messiha and Knopp, 1976). In contrast two other reports describe an exacerbation of Tourette's disorder with imipramine (Fras and Karlavage, 1977; Fras, 1978). The first patient was treated with 25 mg/day imipramine, the second with a combination of haloperidol and 25 mg t.i.d. The addition of the tricyclic antidepressant caused an increase in tics in two patients. With discontinuation, patients returned to their previous level of tic symptomatology. However, another report indicated that imipramine at a dosage of 50 mg/day did not worsen tics in a 12-year-old male patient with a history of ADD and Tourette's disorder. There was a substantial improvement in the ADD but no improvement or worsening of tics (Dillon et al., 1985).

Amitriptyline

Amitriptyline has predominant 5-HT reuptake blocking properties. A negative effect on treatment was reported in a 38-year-old male with Tourette's disorder who was treated initially with 4 mg/day haloperidol and 40 to 60 mg/day amitriptyline (Fras and Karlavage, 1977). Although tics exacerbated when dosage was raised to 75 mg/day, it is difficult to ascribe the increase of tics to medication alone because of general clinical worsening.

Chlorimipramine

This non-FDA approved medication, frequently used to treat obsessive compulsive disorder, has 5-HT receptor blocking properties. Clinicians in one study but not patients reported 80 to 90% improvement of tics (Yaryura-Tobias, 1975; Yaryura-Tobias & Neziroglu, 1974, 1977). Six patients in another study were treated with 105 mg/day of chlorimipramine or desimipramine and placebo, in a double-blind cross-over study (Caine et al., 1979a). Neither of the active medications were effective and one patient had a marked worsening of tics with chlorimipramine. This otherwise well-designed study may have had too few patients to adequately test the hypothesis about the effectiveness of chlorimipramine. Our experience with chlorimipramine in eight patients used in dosages up to 300 mg/day indicated no benefit or worsening of tics.

Desimipramine

This tricyclic has predominant norepinephrine reuptake blocking properties in the CNS. As noted above, desimipramine was reported to be ineffective in reducing tics in a double-blind cross-over study. Treatment of a 10-year-old male with Tourette's disorder and ADD+H, who had previously failed on imipramine, was reported to benefit from 4 mg/kg of desimipramine, the plasma level reported as 30 mg/ml (Hoge and Biederman, 1986). Its possible effect in the 10-year-old with TS+ADD+H may be a compensatory effect of reduced hyperactivity, since other reports indicate that it is ineffective for tic symptoms. Desimipramine has been reported as improving the symptoms of ADD in adolescents (Gastfriend et al., 1984).

Monoamine oxidase inhibitors

These agents increase brain levels of norepinephrine, dopamine, and 5-HT. Positive or adverse effects when used below the toxic level have not been reported.

Lithium

The reports on the effectiveness of lithium in Tourette's disorder have been both positive and negative. Two patients experienced benefit at blood levels of lithium between 0.8 and 1.0 mEq/liter, which was maintained for 3.5 months (Erickson et al., 1976). Lithium was used in combination with haloperidol (blood levels between 0.8 and 1.5 mEq/liter) by us in six patients with no therapeutic benefit or worsening of tic symptoms. However, four patients in a single-blind placebo-controlled study of ten patients had a worsening of symptoms on lithium (Borison et al., 1982). Patients were treated in increments of 300 mg/weekly to blood levels of 0.8 to 1.0 mEq/liter. Improvement was reported in only one subject. Hamra et al. (1983) reported a positive effect of lithium up to 1,500 mg/day (plasma level 0.63 mEq/liter) in a patient with multiple tics and cyclothymic disorder. The tics gradually resolved and completely disappeared after 2 months. These clinical reports suggest that lithium is generally ineffective but controlled clinical trials are recommended.

Anticonvulsants

Carbamazepine

Following a preliminary report from Poland of a positive response to carbamazepine in five male patients (Zawadski, 1972), we used carbamazepine initially in combination with alpha-methylparatyrosine. Two patients with a history of a seizure disorder and Tourette's disorder, were given carbamazepine added to other anticonvulsants but the combination was ineffective. Subsequently, we used this medication in a range of 1,000 to 1,800 mg/day in

11 Tourette patients. Adverse effects were frequent and there was no improvement of tics.

The possible triggering of the onset of Tourette's disorder with carbamazepine has been reported (Neglia et al., 1984). The authors used carbamazepine for seizure control in three patients. Two had an exacerbation of previously noted infrequent tics and one, a female patient who was previously tic-free, developed tics. Discontinuation of the medication did not resolve the tics. We treated 14 patients with carbamazepine and none experienced a worsening of their tic symptoms. Several reports have implicated carbamazepine in the onset of orofacial dyskinesias, dystonia, and myoclonus.

Other anticonvulsants

Our clinical experience suggests that other anticonvulsants, such as phenytoin, ethoxucimide, primidone, and valproic acid, are ineffective for the treatment of tic disorders. Burd et al. (1986a), however, reported that anticonvulsants either caused or exacerbated existing tic disorders in five patients, and that tics decreased but did not remit when medication was discontinued.

Antianxiety-Sedative-Hypnotics

All drugs with sedative properties decrease tics linearly with the degree of sedation. These drugs include antihistaminics, barbiturates, benzodiazepines, meprobamate, piperidenediones, tertiary alcohols, carbamates, chloral derivatives, paraldehyde, bromides, methaqualone, and so on. However, the therapeutic benefit is offset by sedation, development of tolerance, potential addiction, and other adverse effects. Clonazepam is the only one of many benzodiazepine derivative that is currently recommended by some physicians (Gonce and Barbeau, 1977; Kaim, 1983; Voulters et al., 1985).

Clonazepam

An open clinical trial of clonazepam in seven patients with Tourette's disorder reported potential benefit on vocalizations in three patients and some reduction of tics in two others (Gonce and Barbeau, 1977). Clonazepam, at 2 mg/day, but not at 1.5 mg/day, was reported to be effective in reducing tics in a 16-year-old male who had been treated initially with phenobarbitol (Kaim, 1983).

A brief note described positive results in 17 of 25 patients treated with clonazepam in an open clinical trial (Voulters et al., 1985). Significant improvement was rated as reducing tics at least 50% for 3 months. Average dosage was 2.5 mg/day and patients were evaluated from 3 months to over 4 years. Adverse effects included drowsiness and behavioral changes which were moderate to severe in seven patients (28%). However, four of the 17 patients with good response had to discontinue the drug. Insufficient details about length of follow-up were given, thus making it difficult to evaluate whether improvement was sustained. The findings are provocative, but confirmation using a double-blind methodology is necessary to fully evaluate the effectiveness of clonazepan. A single-blind study of 20 Tourette's disorder patients reported that patients with low red blood cell to plasma choline ratios responded better to clonazepam than to haloperidol (Merikangas et al., 1985).

We have used clonazepam in many patients but only in those who did not respond to haloperidol and other neuroleptics primarily because of adverse effects. Clonazepam was generally ineffective except in an occasional patient with tics or other clinical characteristics that retrospectively were somewhat different from patients with classical tics. These clinical reports, which require confirmation, suggest that clonazepam may be effective in some patients.

Other benzodiazepines

Other benzodiazepines such as diazepam, chlordiazepoxide, flurazepam, chlorazepate, and so on, have been used in many patients without evidence of clinical effectiveness.

Other Medications

Clonidine

Clonidine, an alpha$_2$-adrenergic agonist, which inhibits presynaptic norepinephrine release, has been used to treat Tourette's disorder and many other neurological and psychiatric disorders. The data about effectiveness of clonidine for tics is contradictory. Our review identified five favorable (Cohen et al, 1980; Dorsey, 1981; McKeith et al., 1981; Bruun, 1982; Borison et al, 1982) and four unfavorable reports (Dysken et al., 1980; Abuzzahab, 1981; Shapiro et al., 1983c; Gilles and Forsythe, 1984). In an open clinical trial, we compared the percent improvement of tics for clonidine compared to neuroleptics such as haloperidol, pimozide, penfluridol, and fluphenazine in 68 patients who were divided into two groups (Shapiro et al., 1983c). The first group was treated initially with haloperidol and subsequently with clonidine; the second group of previously untreated patients began treatment with clonidine and then went on to treatment with a neuroleptic. The results for the two samples were similar. Patients treated with neuroleptic medications improved significantly more ($p < 0.0001$), an average of 68.8%, compared to 13.5% with clonidine. Fifty of the 68 patients treated had no response at all to treatment with clonidine. It has been postulated that clonidine has its greatest effect on behavioral or attentional symptoms. However, this was not confirmed in our study. In addition, significantly ($p < 0.0001$) more patients rated the neuroleptic medication as better than clonidine. A small subgroup of patients may have benefited from treatment with clonidine but the claims about its overall effectiveness have not been confirmed. Our experience with over 200 patients is that only occasionally is clonidine associated with improvement of tics. Clonidine has been reported to be effective for ADD+H. If this report is confirmed, reducing hyperactivity, which is correlated with Tourette's disorder severity (see Chapter 4), may secondarily reduce the severity of tics (Hunt et al., 1985). Carefully controlled, randomized, and double-blind studies are necessary to resolve the divergent views about clonidine.

Propranolol

Propranolol is a beta-adrenergic blocking agent that has antagonistic effects on both the noradrenergic and serotonergic systems. We used propanolol in seven patients in an open clinical trial in dosages which varied from 100 to 1,000 mg/day. Propranolol at a dosage of 400 mg/day had a beneficial effect of 60 to 80% in one patient with a chronic motor tic which lasted for 8 months. A second patient had 40% decrease in symptoms on 100 mg/day. Another patient had no therapeutic effect on dosages up to 1,000 mg/day. Four others either had no beneficial effect or adverse effects which necessitated stopping the medication. We concluded propranolol was not useful for the treatment of Tourette's disorder.

Two additional negative reports of the effectiveness of propranolol have been published (Sverd et al., 1983; Sverd and Kupietz, 1984). In the initial report, none of the five patients with Tourette's disorder had a positive response to treatment with low dosages (120 mg/day) of propranolol. In a subsequent study using higher dosages (540 mg/day), the therapeutic effect was minimal in one, and two patients experienced no change in tics.

Naloxone

Naloxone, which prevents and reverses the effects of opioids, may have implications for the treatment of Tourette's disorder (Berecz et al., 1979; Sanydk, 1985a,b,c; Sanydk, 1986; Gillman and Sandyk, 1985, 1986; Sandyk et al., 1986). A marked increase in tics in a 15-year-old boy with Tourette's disorder caused by nitrous oxide used at analgesic concentrations was reversed following administration of an intravenous bolus (0.8 mg) of naloxone. A single-blind administration of 1.2 mg naloxone intramuscularly on two other occasions resulted in a decrease of tics in 10 min with symptom return in 45 min. In another double-blind trial of both naloxone, same dosage, or placebo, naloxone but not placebo had a beneficial effect on tics within 10 to 15 min. A single-blind trial of naloxone and saline repeated three times on separate occasions was conducted in two male patients. In one, tics and aggressive behavior were exacerbated within 10 min of administration. The effect lasted 35 to 40 min. The second patient, an 11-year-old child, experienced an amelioration of echolalia and motor tics with the administration of naloxone. The contradictory findings are said to implicate both an under- and overactivity of the opioid system in Tourette's disorder perhaps related to different phases of the illness or subgroups of the disease. These findings are provocative but their limited nature indicates that further work is necessary to clarify the role of the opioid system in Tourette's disorder.

Corticosteroids

Prednisone has been reported to be effective in four patients (Popielarska et al., 1972) and in an 11-year-old by who developed tics after an acute infection (Kondo and Kabasawa, 1978). He was treated with 30 mg/day prednisone for 2 weeks and 15 mg/day for 3 months. Symptoms disappeared after 3 days and did not recur after prednisone was discontinued after 30 months. The patient has been asymptomatic for 4 years. A history of arthritis suggests a residual encephalitis which provoked the tic symptoms. Interpretation of the effects of treatment and its etiological implications are difficult. Tics could have been the result of a transient tic disorder, provoked by the residual encephalitis, or caused by the streptococcal infection which resulted in rheumatic fever and the symptoms of Sydenham's chorea. Improvement in the symptoms could have been spontaneous or possibly from the use of corticosteroids. The long-term adverse effects of corticosteroids, however, limit their possible use for Tourette's disorder.

Baclofen

This drug, an analog of the putative neurotransmitter inhibitor gamma-aminobutyric acid (GABA), was ineffective in seven of our patients.

Calcium channel blockers

Calcium antagonists have been reported as effective in preliminary open clinical trials. Walsh et al. (1986) reported the successful use of verapamil at a dosage of 20 mg t.i.d. in an 11-year-old male with Tourette's disorder. The motor and vocal tics improved, and irritability and compulsive symptoms decreased. A second patient, a 19-year-old female with chronic motor tic, experienced a decrease in her involuntary movements with nifedipine (10 mg t.i.d.) but the medication caused chronic flushing and tachycardia. Her symptoms did not respond to diltiazem (180 mg/day). Two other Tourette's disorder patients were treated successfully with nifedipine; a young male patient experienced improvement of tic symptoms, as did a 22-year-old male on a dosage of 10 mg in the morning and 5 mg t.i.d. thereafter (Goldstein, 1984; Berg, 1985). We have used verapamil up to 80 mg t.i.d. in four patients without therapeutic benefit.

Allergic desensitization

Lanier (1985) discussed the relationship between allergy and Tourette's disorder. He noted that although standard allergic testing may be positive in Tourette's disorder, it reflects the widespread incidence of allergy in the general population. Additionally, to indicate a valid relationship, studies should demonstrate the antigen, a causal relationship between the antigen and the disease and the mechanism underlying the immunological response. The evidence supporting a relationship between allergy and Tourette's disorder is lacking at present, and allergic desensitization or other allergic treatment is not recommended without further evidence of such a relationship (Lanier, 1985; Finegold, 1985).

Diet and nutrition

Studies of the effect of withdrawing or limiting common foods, flavorings, and colorings for the treatment of children with hyperkinesis or ADD have produced equivocal results. There are at present only anecdotal reports of success with special diets in Tourette's disorder patients. Unless scientific, well-controlled studies attest to the relationship between a specific diet and amelioration of the symptoms of Tourette's disorder, our opinion is that the imposition of such a diet can be potentially stressful for the child already burdened with a chronic illness.

Megavitamins

Although individual, anecdotal reports attest to the efficacy of megavitamins in other disorders, there are no data supporting their effectiveness in Tourette's disorder.

Orthomolecular mineral therapy

Several of our patients had an expensive analysis of their mineral status and hair. None of them reported improvement in Tourette's disorder following mineral therapy. Controlled studies supporting an abnormality in trace elements or the use of mineral supplements in diet is not available.

Miscellaneous treatment

Miscellaneous therapies such as electroconvulsive shock, insulin coma therapy, fever therapy, arsenic therapy, and hydrotherapy are ineffective.

Surgical Procedures

Surgical ablation procedures of localized areas of the extrapyramidal system have included bilateral coagulation of the rostral intralaminar and medial nuclei of the thalamus (Hassler and Dieckmann, 1970), bilateral cryothalomectomy (Cooper, 1969; Shapiro et al., 1978), bilateral coagulation of the cerebellar dentate nuclei (Nadvornik et al., 1972), and bifrontal surgical lesions (Baker, 1962). Two patients underwent stereotactic surgery in puberty with transient relief of symptoms but both experienced postoperative neurological defects (Asam and Karrass, 1981). Neurosurgical procedures are not recommended because of the equivocal, limited, and unsustained therapeutic benefit and the possibility of irremediable central nervous system damage. Precisely identifying the cause of Tourette's disorder might lead to the development of more specific and useful surgical procedures.

CONTROVERSY ABOUT STIMULANTS AND TIC DISORDERS

This section focuses on the controversy about stimulants. The issues have important implications for the treatment of patients with ADD+H and tic disorders and for the etiology of both conditions.

Stimulants were used to treat Tourette's disorder in the past. Kelman (1965), in a review of 44 patients in the literature between 1906 and 1964, noted that of six patients treated with amphetamines, tics increased in two, decreased in one, and were unchanged in three. Abuzzahab and Anderson (1973), in a review of the world's literature, cited decreased tics in 3 of 17 patients. Our review of the literature after 1960 is summarized in Table 11.1.

Increased tics following the use of stimulants were noted in single patients by Singer (1963) and by Meyerhoff and Snyder (1973), who postulated mediating effects of norepinephrine in Tourette's disorder and dopamine in ADD+H based on the differential effects of d-amphetamine and l-amphetamine (results which have not been confirmed) (Caine et al., 1984). The possibility that stimulants could cause Tourette's disorder in vulnerable individuals was first proposed by Golden in 1974 based on description of a 9-year-old hyperactive child who had marked behavioral benefit from treatment with methylphenidate, 10 mg b.i.d., but who developed Tourette's disorder 8 weeks later, which persisted after discontinuation of the stimulant. Similar cases were described by Golden (and others throughout the years; see Table 11.1), culminating in his report of a larger number of patients in 1977 (Golden, 1977b). A questionnaire about the use of stimulant drugs prior to the onset of Tourette's disorder was sent to an unspecified number of members of the Tourette Syndrome Association (TSA). The sample included three private patients and 85 who responded to the questionnaire survey. Seven (8.0%) had been treated with stimulants prior to the onset of Tourette's disorder. Exacerbation of preexisting tics occurred in approximately 52.8% (or approximately 13) of patients who used stimulants after the onset of Tourette's disorder. Golden favored the interpretation that although it "cannot be absolutely proved," stimulants "triggered the onset of the syndrome in susceptible patients." Other case histories and reports followed eventually causing alarm about using stimulants in patients with ADD+H, patients with tics, Tourette's disorder and a family history of this disorder or to counteract adverse effects of neuroleptic treatment of Tourette's disorder. These reports stressed the possibility that stimulants would permanently exacerbate Tourette's disorder by altering norepinephrine and dopamine receptors and warned about the imprudent use of stimulants (Lowe et al., 1982). Finally the FDA, uncritically, based entirely on *post hoc* or retrospective reports, issued alarming directives about the dangers of using stimulants, and a citation in the adverse reactions section of the *Physicians' Desk Reference* (1985) that "There have been rare reports of Tourette's syndrome." There has also been an increase in malpractice suits (one for 140 million dollars against a pediatrician and Ciba Pharmaceutical Company, recently lost by the plaintiff) and innumerable inquiries to us at the Tourette and Tic Laboratory and Clinic from physicians all over the country about this issue.

Is the alarm and concern warranted or has it been premature, causing confusion among physicians and contributing to inadequate treatment of patients? To answer the question about whether stimulants trigger, provoke, cause, or permanently exacerbate tics and Tourette's disorder, the evidence must be carefully evaluated.

Do Stimulants Cause Tourette's or Tic Disorders?

Stimulants Preceding the Onset of Tourette's Disorder Cited in Questionnaire Surveys

Much of the data about the use of stimulants and the onset of Tourette's disorder was reported by investigators using questionnaire surveys of TSA membership. The use of stimulants preceding the onset of Tourette's disorder averaged 14.5% (range 7.6% to 18.5%) in three surveys (Table 11.1). Several factors (see Chapters 3, 4, 5, 6) suggest that the percentages reported in surveys of volunteer TSA patients are higher than expected in the population.

Not all Tourette's disorder patients contacted responded to the questionnaire. It is common experience that only 10% to 30% of questionnaires sent to Tourette's disorder patients are returned. The response rate was 18% to 25% in one study (Price et al., 1985) and is unknown in another study (Golden, 1977b). Since some patients respond and others do not, ascertainment bias might be responsible for the reported increased percent of patients thought to have stimuli-induced Tourette's disorder.

Information about the possible relationship between stimulants and Tourette's disorder was available to patients through lay sources since 1974, and most patients believe that stimulants cause Tourette's disorder. Imagine patients or parents of children with ADD+H who were treated with stimulants prior to the onset of Tourette's disorder receiving a questionnaire about whether stimulants caused Tourette's disorder. It is reasonable to assume that they would be more likely to complete the questionnaire than those without a similar history. Moreover, as described in Chapter 4, responders compared to nonresponders are more severely afflicted with Tourette's disorder, have more symptoms in all categories, more organic stigmata, more ADD+H, less abilities and assets, and are in a lower social class. These factors may contribute to a higher percent of stimulant use prior to the onset of Tourette's disorder reported in questionnaires compared to other sources, and lead to the erroneous impression of a strong relationship between the use of stimulants and Tourette's disorder.

This possibility is supported by the data for consecutive clinical patients.

Stimulants Preceding the Onset of Tourette's Disorder Cited for Consecutive Clinical Patients

Our expectation is supported by the significantly lower percentage of 5.3% (range 1.3–15.0%) of consecutive clinical patients reported in the literature with a history of stimulant use prior to the onset of Tourette's disorder compared to the percentage of 14.5% (range 7.6% to 18.5%) for patients in questionnaire surveys ($\chi^a = 35.5$, df = 1, $p = 0.000$) (Table 11.1). Even this percent may be too high. Since most patients with ADD+H are treated with stimulants, the percent of Tourette's disorder patients with a history of stimulant use would be related to the percent who have ADD+H. This relationship is borne out by the higher percentages for stimulant use in samples that include a high percentage of patients with Tourette's disorder and ADD+H. The percentage of Tourette's disorder patients with ADD+H is 54% in the Comings and Comings study (1984), 35% in the Erenberg et al. study (1985), 26.4% in the Shapiro and Shapiro study (1981b), and unreported in the two other studies (Bachman, 1981; Lowe et al., 1982). The correlation for the three studies is 0.9988, $p = 0.03$. Thus, because stimulant use is strongly associated with the percent of ADD in samples, reports of Tourette's disorder following use of stimulants are artifactually elevated.

However, we still do not know whether the lower percent of 1.3% to 1.6% (Shapiro and Shapiro, 1981b; Bachman, 1981) of patients with a prior history of stimulant use is significantly higher than expected in the population. Determination of the frequency of stimulant-induced Tourette's disorder in the population requires a large sample of children who were treated with stimulants for ADD+H. Fortunately, such data are available in the important study by Denckla et al. (1976).

Study of Children with Attention Deficit Disorder and Hyperactivity Who Develop Tourette's Disorder or Tics After Treatment with Stimulants

The most persuasive data counter to the hypothesis of stimulant-induced Tourette's disorder is the extensive clinical experience of Denckla et al.

(1976) with more than 5,000 cases of ADD+H (formerly minimal brain dysfunction). The results and clinical observations for a subset of 1,520 children who were treated with methylphenidate for ADD+H have important implications for the controversy about stimulant-induced Tourette's disorder. None developed the disorder, although one child had pre-existing Tourette's disorder. Only 14 or 0.9% developed tics. It is noteworthy that this percentage is much lower than the range of 4% to 25% reported in epidemiological studies (Table 3.1). No particular pattern was apparent for duration of treatment (tics occurring in a range of 1 day to after 1 year of treatment) or dosage range (10 mg to 60 mg/day). Moreover, tics subsided in 13 of the 14 patients, and persisted in only one patient after discontinuing methylphenidate. Tics appeared with increased dosage and subsided with reduced dosage in three patients. They did not recur in four patients who had substantial benefit for the symptoms of ADD+H when subsequently retreated with the same dosage of methylphenidate. In two patients, tics recurred spontaneously while not receiving medication (after a 2-year drug-free period in one patient). None of the children required treatment with haloperidol, "as the symptoms did not seem to warrant it, and the tics were ameliorated following discontinuation of methylphenidate treatment." Moreover, of clinical significance for the management of children with ADD+H, "Seventeen, or 85% of the 20 children with tics, benefited from methylphenidate therapy (improved attention, control, and organization)." We concur with the conclusions of Denckla et al. (1976) that "Tics related to methylphenidate administration appear to be rare," and "While there does appear to be a relationship between tics and methylphenidate treatment in rare instances, the nature of this relationship remains obscure."

This clinical study is a more direct evaluation of the hypothesis about stimulant-induced Tourette's disorder and in our opinion does not support the conclusions in the previously reviewed retrospective reports. This opinion is also supported by two recently published stories.

Study of the Length of Time to Develop Tourette's Disorder After the Use or Nonuse of Stimulants to Treat Children with Attention Deficit Disorder with Hyperactivity

Comings and Comings (1984) reasoned that if stimulants were associated with the development of Tourette's disorder, children treated with stimulants for ADD+H should develop the disorder sooner than children with ADD+H not treated with stimulants. Using a dependent measure of years to develop Tourette's disorder after the onset of hyperactivity, they found, however, that children treated with stimulants developed the disorder after 5.3 years compared with 3.3 years for children not treated with stimulants ($t = 4.3$, $df = 56$, $p < 0.001$). Despite the limitations of the study (the difficulty of establishing the onset of hyperactivity, possible differences between treated and untreated patients) the results do not support the general hypothesis that stimulants cause Tourette's disorder, or the hypothesis that stimulants trigger Tourette's disorder in susceptible children. In fact, the results could be interpreted as possibly indicating that the use of stimulants in ADD+H delays the onset of Tourette's disorder. This possibility is also suggested by the results of the Denkla et al. study (1976) in which only 0.9% of ADD+H children treated with stimulants developed tics. This percentage is much lower than the percentage of 4% to 25% reported in surveys (Table 3.1). The authors conclude that, "The combined data suggest that patients with hyperactivity who develop tics after treament with stimulants had ADD due to a Tourette's disorder gene and probably would have developed tics without stimulant treatment." They strongly differ with the suggestion "that there be an absolute restriction on the administration of stimulants to patients with Tourette's disorder (Golden, 1982; Lowe et al., 1982). Our feeling is that the hyperactivity in these children is often such a severe problem that it desperately needs attention; we have a number of individuals whom we first treated with haloperidol and then with stimulants to help control the hyperactivity. In these, the use of both medications offered significantly more in the total management of the patient than use of haloperidol alone."

Study of Identical Twins with Tourette's Disorder Discordant for Use of Stimulants

It is reasonable to assume that the hypothesis of stimulants causing Tourette's disorder would not be supported if identical twins both developed this disorder whether or not they were pretreated with stimulants. In a national study of twins, Price et al. (1986) described six identical twins with ADD+H, in which one twin but not the other twin was treated with stimulants. Both twins, whether or not treated with stimulants, developed Tourette's disorder (defined as the presence of motor and vocal tics). Although the onset of Tourette's disorder was slightly later for the untreated twin, the difference was not significant. However, the twin samples were not identical because four of the stimulant-treated twins had a previous history of motor and vocal tics, and two had motor tics at the time stimulants were used. It is also of interest that only one (16.7%) of the six twins had an exacerbation of their tics. The authors conclude that "There are few cases in which stimulants can be associated unequivocally with the induction or precipitation of Tourette's disorder." and "The full concordance for Tourette's disorder in all six twin pairs discordant for stimulant treatment in our study and one other case (Waserman et al., 1983) suggests that stimulant treatment may not substantially increase the risk for developing or permanently exacerbating tics in many individuals, because the tics also appear in untreated co-twins." They also add, somewhat inexplicably to us, "On the other hand, the close temporal association of treatment and exacerbation of symptoms in a few cases and the clear evidence from animal studies" (we are not aware of any studies demonstrating tics in animals, or relevant evidence from animal studies) "imply real danger of exacerbation of tics in some cases." Their speculation that "genetic vulnerability and duration and timing of treatment may mediate response," requires confirmation.

Do Stimulants Increase or Permanently Exacerbate Tics?

Review of the literature does not support the widespread clinical impression that stimulants are dangerous, contraindicated, likely to increase tics, or permanently exacerbate them. Although conclusions about these controversial issues are not possible from the reviewed reports because of methodological limitations, such as retrospective clinical reports of small samples, different or unspecified dosages, length of treatment, or drug-free periods before the onset or increase of tics, absence of placebo controls, and so on, they do provide clinical indications that the alarm about the use of stimulants is exaggerated and unfounded.

Children with Attention Deficit Disorder, Hyperactivity, and Pre-existing Tics Who Are Treated with Stimulants

Only the Denckla et al. (1976) study provided meaningful data about the effect of stimulants on children with ADD+H and pre-existing tics. Of 45 children who were treated with methylphenidate, tics increased in only six (13.3%) and decreased to pretreatment levels after discontinuing medication. Four of these children were treated subsequently with methylphenidate, two at lower and two at the same dosage, without tics recurring, and with substantial improvement of ADD+H symptoms which could not otherwise be controlled. However, one child developed tics which persisted, and one had a return of tics 2 years after discontinuing the stimulant.

Patients with Tourette's Disorder Treated with Stimulants

For 111 Tourette's disorder patients treated with stimulants described in six papers (which reported more than one patient), the percent of increased tics averages 34.2%, consistently ranging from 21.4% to 33.33%, except for 100% reported in one study (Lowe et al., 1985) (Table 11.1). A higher percentage of increased tics is reported in 75% of 16 retrospective single case histories. All of the studies, except one, report no change in tics for 60% to 70% of patients, and decreased tics for 6.3% (range 0% to 9.3%).

We treated 43 children who required treatment with haloperidol for TS and stimulants for ADD+H (Shapiro and Shapiro, 1981b, 1985c). Dosages of haloperidol varied from 2 to 10 mg/day; the dosage of methylphenidate varied

TABLE 11.1 Studies citing use of stimulants preceding and following the onset of tics and Tourette's disorder

Studies	Total sample N	Use of stimulants preceding TS or tics				Effect of stimulants on TS or tics						
		Preceding TS		Preceding tics		Total sample N	Increased tics		No change		Decreased tics	
		N	%	N	%		N	%	N	%	N	%
Questionnaire surveys of patients with TS[a]												
Golden (1974, 1977b)[b]	88	8	8.0%	—	—	25	13	52.0%	—	—	—	—
Stefl (1983)[c]	425	79	18.5%	—	—	—	—	—	—	—	—	—
Price et al. (1986)[d]	170	13	7.6%	—	—	21	8	38.1%	—	—	—	—
Total	683	99	14.5%	—	—	46	21	45.7%	—	—	—	—
Consecutive Clinical Patients with ADD+H												
Denckla et al. (1976)	1,520	0	0.0%	14	0.9%	45	6	13.3%	—	—	—	—
Consecutive clinical patients with TS[ae]												
Shapiro and Shapiro (1981a)[f]	134	2	1.3%	—	—	43	13	30.2%	26	60.5%	4	9.3%
Bachman (1981)	64	1	1.6%	—	—	14	3	21.4%	10	71.4%	1	7.1%

Study	N	n	%			n	n	%	n	%	n	%
Rapoport et al (1982)	40	6	15.0%	—	—	6	2	33.3%	4	66.7%	0	0.0%
Lowe et al. (1982)	100	6	6.0%	—	—	9	9	100.0%	0	0.0%	0	0.0%
Comings and Comings (1984)	250	18	7.2%	—	—	?	?	some	?	some	?	some
Erenberg et al. (1985)	200	9	4.5%	—	—	39	11	28.2%	26	66.7%	2	5.1%
Total	788	42	5.3%	—	—	111	38	34.2%	66	59.5%	7	6.3%
Case reports of patients with TS[a,g]												
—	7[g]	—	—	—	—	16	12	75.0%	4	25.0%	0	0.0%
Literature reviews of patients with TS												
Kelman (1965)	—	—	—	—	—	6	2	33.3%	3	50.0%	1	17.0%
Abuzzahab and Anderson (1973)	—	—	—	—	—	17	—	—	—	—	3	19.0%
Total	—	—	—	—	—	23	2	33.3%	3	50.0%	3	17.4%

[a] An unknown number of patients reported in more than one study.
[b] Sample included unknown number of private patients and respondents to a TSA questionnaire survey (number of questionnaires sent and returned not specified).
[c] Ohio TSA questionnaire survey (response 78%).
[d] Sample included 8 patients responding to a Canadian TSA questionnaire survey (18–25% response) and 90 responses to a US TSA twin questionnaire survey (32 monozygotic. 15 dizygotic twin pairs).
[e] Includes reports of at least 10 consecutive clinical patients.
[f] Consecutive patients in 1 year from 1979 to 1980, which included 21 patients with a history of stimulant use before our evaluation and 22 patients who were treated with stimulants for haloperidol-induced adverse effects.
[g] Singer, 1963; Meyerhoff and Snyder, 1973; Fras and Karlavage, 1977; Pollack et al., 1977; Feinberg and Carroll, 1979; Bremness and Sverd, 1979; Mitchell and Matthews, 1980; Sleator, 1980; Bachman, 1980; Rapoport et al., 1982; Caine et al., 1982; Lowe et al., 1982; Volkmar et al., 1985; Dillon et al., 1985.

from 10 to 60 mg/day; both drugs were titrated separately and slowly to final dosages that resulted in control of both tics and hyperactivity without adverse effects (see Chapter 12 for details of our treatment). Tics decreased in 9%, were unchanged in 60.5%, and increased, usually only slightly, in 30.2%, and always returned to pretreatment tic levels on lowering the dosage. We also have successfully treated over 100 patients with stimulants who had recalcitrant adverse effects such as akinesia, sedation, lethargy, depression, amotivation, cognitive dulling, and weight gain (see Chapter 12 for method of treatment).

Conclusion

Our conclusion, similar to others (Comings and Comings, 1984; Butler, 1985; Licamele and O'Leary, 1986), is that the available evidence does not support the concept that stimulants cause Tourette's disorder. Clinical observations, however, suggest the possibility that stimulants can prematurely trigger Tourette's disorder in a small number of vulnerable individuals who would have developed Tourette's disorder in the future (Erenberg et al., 1985). Clinical observations and data from the literature indicate that tics can be increased at dosages that vary for each individual, but that the effect is temporary and tics return to previous levels within 1 day with decrease of dosage. These clinical hypotheses, which are based entirely on uncontrolled retrospective clinical observations, require confirmation from carefully controlled studies. Before postulated variables such as genetic vulnerability and timing of treatment can be considered, more mundane variables would have to be controlled and standardized: variables such as the daily dosage of methylphenidate which now varies from 5 to 60 mg, duration of treatment which varies in reports from a few days to many years, onset of Tourette's disorder concurrent with stimulant treatment or onset years after stimulant treatment is discontinued, the age and sex of patients, diagnosis of ADD+H, and more reliable data about the population prevalence of tics and Tourette's disorder. Such studies are difficult to conduct, however, because of the very few patients who develop Tourette's disorder after the use of stimulants. Their rarity raises the important question of why more patients or even all patients do not develop stimulant-induced Tourette's disorder. The answer may be simple: The hypothesis that stimulants cause Tourette's disorder is incorrect, the frequency is more apparent than real and may be due to the absence of adequate controls and poor methodology.

Premature Acceptance of Concept that Stimulants Cause and Permanently Exacerbate Tics and Tourette's Disorder

If we are correct that clinical data, observations, and studies do not support the conclusion that stimulants cause or permanently exacerbate tics and Tourette's disorder, what accounts for the uncritical acceptance of the concept?

Post Hoc, Ergo Propter Hoc Logical Fallacy

Part of the answer is due to the *post hoc, ergo propter hoc* logical fallacy, or the almost universal psychological inclination of physicians to uncritically interpret retrospective observations as indicating a causal relationship, a common problem in the history of medicine (Shapiro, 1960, 1964, 1971a, 1974, 1984; Shapiro and Morris, 1977a,b, 1978). Appreciation of this problem in the 1950s, now universally accepted, led to the specification that an adequate study employ random allocation, control groups, double-blind procedures, reliable and valid measures, sophisticated statistics, and other methodological safeguards. These methodological safeguards are totally absent in reports of stimulant-induced tics and Tourette's disorder. They ignore other factors, such as the high percentages of patients with spontaneous waxing, waning, and fluctuation of symptoms, the high percentages with diurnal, seasonal, and stimuli-induced changes, the significant percentage with temporary remission of symptoms and the high increase of symptoms (15% to 55%, averaging 36%) when patients are treated with placebos (Table 11.2). It is possible, likely in our opinion, that these factors alone account for more of the reported increase in tics than stimulants.

In our opinion, given the major limitations of the studies and data, it is remarkable that the hypothesis that stimulants cause and permanently exacerbate tics and Tourette's disorder has been so uncritically accepted by investigators and clinicians.

Neuropathology of Stimuli-Induced Tics or Tourette's Disorder

Another factor is the conceptually appealing but superficial concept that because Tourette's disorder is caused by sensitivity to catecholamines, and stimulants increase catecholamines, therefore stimulants increase tics, cause Tourette's disorder, and permanently exacerbate tic disorders. All of these assumptions, however, are hypothetical constructs which have not been proven. In fact, the evidence is inferential and inadequate to support the concept that Tourette's disorder is caused by excessive amounts of, or sensitivity of, postsynaptic receptors to catecholamines. Stimulants do not always increase tics and sometimes tics decrease with their use. Stimulants cannot be a major factor causing Tourette's disorder because so few patients develop the disorder or tics after their use, and the reported prevalence may be artifactually inflated because of sampling problems. The data for stimulant-treated children with ADD+H does not support the concept that stimulants permanently exacerbate tics, and tics are not increased in 67% of Tourette's disorder patients (Table 11.1).

Moreover, the effects of stimulants (amphetamines, methylphenidate, pemoline, etc.) on neuronal systems are complicated and not fully understood.

They can both increase or decrease catecholamines, can inhibit or activate norepinephrine, D_1 and D_2 presynaptic or postsynaptic receptors in mesocortical, mesolimbic, and nigrostriatal brain areas, can depress at low dosages and stimulate at high dosages, and can induce multiple perturbations of neurochemical systems. Stimulants have multiple, sometimes contradictory effects, such as elevated mood; increased attention, vigilance, and learning; depressed appetite, and decreased hyperactivity in patients with ADD+H (Goff, 1986). Although papers frequently cite tics or stereotypy in animals treated with stimulants as evidence for the catecholamine hypothesis for Tourette's disorder and tics, no study has ever demonstrated the existence of tics in animals, and in fact the resulting stereotype and hyperactivity do not resemble tics.

In addition, although stimulants and neuroleptics have many antagonistic effects, many of their effects are not antagonistic and may even be synergistic. For example, neuroleptics do not antagonize and may, in fact, improve the beneficial effects of stimulants on the symptoms of ADD+H. Moreover, carefully titrated dosages of stimulants can ameliorate or control neuroleptic-induced adverse effects such, as akinesia, sedation, lethargy, depression, amotivation, cognitive dulling, and increased appetite, without increasing tics.

Furthermore, it is not known whether stimulant-induced tics are directly caused by increased norepinephrine or dopamine, or whether they are an indirect effect of neuronal pathways mediating general arousal or anxiety. This possibility is suggested by the effect of anxiety alone, without the use of stimulants, which significantly increases tics (92%) in patients (Table 5.17) compared to the 34% increase in tics following the use of stimulants (Table 11.1) ($\chi^2 = 177$, df $= 1, p < 0.0001$).

These factors suggest considerable inadequacy about concepts of simple and direct relationships between stimulants and tics, the norepinephrine or dopamine hypothesis about the etiology of Tourette's disorder or tics and that stimulants cause the disorder or permanently exacerbate tics.

Conclusion

We conclude that the alarm about the dangers of using stimulants is unwarranted and the beneficial effects of stimulants for the treatment of ADD+H and the management of neuroleptic-induced adverse effects outweigh their possible disadvantages. We are not alone in this view. Others have opined that the evidence does not support the concept of stimulant-caused Tourette's disorder (Butler, 1985; Erenberg et al., 1985, Licamele and O'Leary, 1986; Comings and Comings, 1984), that stimulants are not contraindicated in children with ADD+H (Butler, 1985; El-Defraw and Greenhill, 1984; Erenberg, 1982; Comings and Comings, 1984; Lees, 1985), or for children with symptoms of ADD+H that may be more disabling than the tic or Tourette's disorder symptoms (Erenberg, 1982; 1985; Comings and Comings, 1984, Golden, 1984). Moreover, the current revision of DSM-III-R acknowledges that "A controversy exists as to whether or not the onset of some cases of tic disorders are precipitated by exposure to . . . the administration of central nervous system stimulants. In many cases the severity of the tics may be exacerbated by administration of CNS stimulants, which may be a dose related phenomenon."

PSYCHOTHERAPY

In Chapter 1 we reviewed the psychological and psychoanalytic papers on tics and Tourette's disorder from the 1920s to the 1970s. Some authors postulated a direct correlation between symptoms and inhibition of aggression, displacement of sexual impulses, underlying psychosis, and so on. The belief in a psychological etiology for tics and Tourette's disorder was accompanied by the recommendation for psychotherapeutic intervention.

Mahler and her co-workers (1946) described the outcome for 18 patients treated with psychotherapy as generally poor and unrelated to the method, thoroughness, or length of psychotherapy. Various shortcomings are apparent in the outcome study. No information was provided about whether drugs or other treatments were used during psychotherapy given in the hospital. Only sketchy information was provided about the therapy, the psychotherapists, and the intensity of the therapy. It is difficult to evaluate the effect of treatment on the primary tic symptoms for which the child had been hospitalized because patients were evaluated at discharge only as improved or unimproved, but not whether the improvement referred to psychopathology or tics. The presence or absence of tics was mentioned in the case descriptions, but the observations were made some time after discharge. No information was provided about which tics disappeared, or when. Patients' age at follow-up ranged from 12 to 23.5 years, and they were evaluated 1.5 to approximately 11 years after discharge. The possibility of spontaneous improvement was not considered.

The authors' clinical impression was that outcome was not related to the method, thoroughness, or length of psychotherapy, and whether or not the symptoms were of short duration and treatment begun at an early age. These poor results were theoretically expected because, according to Freud, organ-neurotic symptoms are "not directly accessible to psychoanalysis."

Based on two patients whose tics completely disappeared, but who had the worst outcome otherwise, tics were explained as a morbid release or discharge of dammed-up instinctual impulses. In other words, patients whose tics are cured will become psychotic or deteriorate psychologically since they are defenseless against their instinctual impulses. However, there is no evidence that Tourette patients deteriorate psychologically with successful treatment. In fact, the reverse is more often observed: Patients function more adequately in all ways and their general adjustment improves after disappearance of their tics.

For patients without personality deterioration, the crucial variable was believed to be adequate postdischarge management concentrated on organized physical activity and performance. The authors therefore recommended sustained muscular activity to discharge motor impulses. The authors discouraged the use of deep psychotherapy with children because intensive therapy weakened the controlling powers of the child ticqueur and was especially contraindicated during adolescence. If treatment began early enough, the outcome was fairly favorable. If untreated there would be no resolution in self-restitution of the personality. If the condition remits during adolescence, a severe personality maladjustment will occur. These clinical observations and the effectiveness of these therapeutic procedures are not supported by clinical data.

Nevertheless, despite the poor outcome data and the inability to specify the factors responsible for both cure and noncure, the authors inexplicably maintain that psychotherapy with organized activity is helpful to relieve if not cure the tic syndrome.

Reports about the efficacy of psychotherapy for tics or Tourette's disorder are limited by failure to provide adequate follow-up data (Latimer, 1945; Menaker, 1945; Asher, 1948; Aarons, 1958; Gerard, 1946; Rosenheim, 1948). A recent report by Negishi (1983) described 29 children who were treated with psychotherapy for various tic disorders. Children were followed up for more than 5 years. Prognosis was best for children who had a neurotic personality and were treated with intensive psychotherapy. Other modalities included activity and milieu therapy. The study was flawed by the lack of clear diagnostic criteria for both tics and Tourette's disorder and the personality groups and the use of multiple therapeutic methods in the same patient.

Asam (1982) described four patients who were treated with analytically oriented psychotherapy. Three were able to develop self-control to overcome their symptoms, although no patient undergoing any form of psychotherapy was able to obtain complete relief of symptoms. She concluded that definitive evidence for the efficacy of this approach was lacking.

Psychological treatment was not limited to individual psychotherapy. Family dynamics were stressed by some (Latimer, 1945; Dunlap, 1960; Downing et al., 1964; Kurland, 1965; Robinson, 1966; Bradnan, 1972; Tiller, 1978) and group treatment by others (Faux, 1966). Most of the published reports were clinical case studies of one patient or family and the therapeutic results were mixed.

Following the advent of drug treatment, many physicians used a combination of drugs and psychotherapy. Treatment reports were open studies of very few patients making it difficult to ascertain whether the therapeutic effects were due to psychotherapy, drugs, or spontaneous factors. The papers were of interest, however, because they indicated that psychotherapy alone was an ineffective treatment for tics.

The outcome data as a whole fail to support the effectiveness of psychotherapy as a primary treatment for tics or Tourette's disorder. Although individual patients have been reported to benefit from psychotherapy, most patients' report little therapeutic benefit on tics. The remarkable overall improvement afforded by medication, especially haloperidol (Shapiro et al., 1978), underscores the inefficiency of psychotherapeutic treatment as a primary treatment for tics and Tourette's disorder. In patients with behavioral or academic problems, counseling or remediation, of course, may be indicated.

Hypnosis

Many patients have been treated with hypnosis although few reports have appeared in the literature, probably because of poor results. Schneck (1960) attributed a failure of hypnosis to a defense against explosive hostility and psychosis. The successful use of hypnosis was reported in two patients described as having, but clearly not fulfilling, the criteria for the diagnosis of Tourette's disorder (Erickson, 1964). Hypnosis and a combination of CO_2 treatment was unsuccessful in a 15½-year-old male. Treatment was effective during the hypnotic sessions, but after discharge symptoms continued and coprolalia increased (Politis et al., 1965). In another report hypnotherapy was used to treat a 19-year-old patient, but was discontinued prematurely by the parents (Lindner and Stevens, 1967). Follow-up after 9 years was inadequate to evaluate therapeutic response. Clements (1972) described the course of a patient with Tourette's disorder over a 13-year period from age 4 to 17. Treatment was complicated and included a combination of intensive psychotherapy, hypnosis, and haloperidol. Symptoms were in remission at age 17, but the length of follow-up was not specified. Approximately 20% of our total sample have been treated unsuccessfully with hypnosis. It is our impression based on present evidence that hypnosis is an ineffective treatment for tics and Tourette's disorder.

Behavior therapy

The literature of behavior treatment for tics and Tourette's disorder through 1976 was extensively reviewed and critiqued in our previous book (Shapiro et al., 1978), and only the post-1976 literature is evaluated in this section.

Massed practice to eradicate coprolalia in an 18-year-old female increased the behavior and the clarity of the uttered coprolalic word, which had initially sounded like a bark (Hollandsworth and Bausinger, 1978). According to the authors, some of the factors contributing to the poor response included the patient's resistance, family lack of support, and the negative effect of practice on the behavior.

Habit reversal versus negative practice was compared in the treatment of diverse groups of patients with tics (Azrin et al., 1980). The authors classified tics as nonmedical or "nervous" tics, and did not use standard diagnostic criteria. They report excellent therapeutic benefit using the habit reversal technique which consists of two steps: immediate control of the tic and then exerting isometric pressure on the muscles opposed to the tic. Follow-up was done by telephone and no objective measures were used to verify tic counts making it extremely difficult to evaluate therapeutic response. While the results are interesting, replication using a standard diagnostic criteria, reliable and valid outcome measures, controls, and double-blind methodology is necessary.

Massed and enhanced massed practice of a single obscenity and right-sided facial tic and relaxation through decrease of muscular tension and mental imagery were used to treat a patient with Tourette's disorder (Canavan and Powell, 1981). The authors report an increase in tic frequency with both massed practice techniques and no generalization with relaxation. Oral feedback consisted of saying "no" each time a tic appeared with and without time out. There was no long-term therapeutic effect with both feedback methods.

Self-control techniques were used in one 11-year-old female (Friedman, 1980). She was taught to substitute nonobscene phrases whenever she felt an urge to vocalize an obscenity and to control body tics. This procedure was effective for only short periods. Relaxation techniques were also used but despite therapeutic benefit, the patient had to be eventually treated with medication. Another negative report by Turpin and Powell (1984) used massed practice and cue-controlled relaxation in three single case studies.

A habit-reversal paradign was utilized in patients with muscle tics (Miltenberger et al, 1985). Patients were volunteers, without a formal diagnosis except for an observable, high rate of muscle tics, the majority did not have Tourette's disorder and several were taking medication. It is difficult to generalize the results to specific tic disorders or to evaluate the specific therapy in a mixed group of patients without specific diagnoses, and some not medication-free.

Massed negative practice was used to treat three patients with Tourette's disorder (Storms, 1985). Some benefit was noted in the first patient, although it was the therapist's impression that improvement was incomplete and may have been due to fluctuations expected in the course of this disease. The second patient did not benefit from massed negative practice, and was treated with haloperidol subsequently. After some time haloperidol was withdrawn, and massed practice resumed. Patient's tics were virtually absent after 5.5 months of treatment. However, improvement was not sustained and the patient was treated subsequently with individual psychotherapy. Mansdorf (1986) described the successful use of assertiveness training in a child with tics who was also unassertive.

The studies of behavior therapy, similar to the conclusion in our previous review (Shapiro, 1976a; Shapiro et al., 1978), continue to be methodologically inadequate. Control groups, specific diagnostic criteria, standardized outcome measures and double-blind procedures were not used. While the individual case reports using habit reversal are interesting, they require confirmation using more rigorous methodology.

TREATMENT HISTORY OF PATIENTS IN CURRENT STUDY

The extensiveness of the treatment history for Tourette's disorder patients is documented in Tables 11.2, 11.3. Most patients (87.5%) had a previous consultation or treatment for Tourette's disorder; over 50% had their first consultation before 8 years of age; and approximately 49% had consulted at least three physicians. The many therapies tried by most patients are listed in Table 11.3. Many treatments were not remembered, especially by older patients. The extensiveness of the treatments indicates the desperation of patients seeking help for their symptoms and the ineffectiveness of many of these methods.

SPONTANEOUS, NONSPECIFIC, AND PLACEBO EFFECTS

The difficulty of evaluating the effectiveness of treatment for tics and Tourette's disorder is complicated by spontaneous changes and nonspecific or placebo effects.

TABLE 11.2. *Treatment history of Tourette's disorder sample*

Treatment history	N	%	Cumulative %
Previous consultation or treatment for tics[a]	583	87.5	—
Age at first consultation (years)[b]			
2–6	142	24.7	24.7
7–8	186	32.3	56.9
9–12	113	19.6	76.6
12–49	135	23.4	100.0
Number of physicians consulted[c]			
7–10	35	5.3	5.3
6	42	6.3	11.6
5	52	7.8	19.4
4	82	12.3	31.7
3	112	16.8	48.5
2	129	19.4	67.9
1	135	20.3	88.1
None	79	11.9	100.0

[a]$N = 666$.
[b]$N = 576$.
[c]$N = 666$.

TABLE 11.3. *History of drug and non-drug treatment of Tourette's disorder*[a]

Treatment	N	%
Neuroleptics		
Haloperidol	203	48.2
Chlorpromazine	33	7.8
Thioridazine	20	4.8
Trifluoperazine	8	1.9
Fluperazine	3	0.7
Prochlorpromazine	2	0.5
Perphenazine	1	0.2
Pimozide	1	0.2
Reserpine	1	0.2
Total	270	64.1
Benzodiazepines		
Diazepam	55	13.1
Chlordiazepoxide	10	2.4
Other	10	2.4
Total	11	2.6
Other Drugs		
Meprobamate	2	0.5
Antihistamine	6	1.4
Hydroxazine	13	3.1
Anticonvulsants	13	3.1
Stimulants	23	5.5
Steroids	3	0.7
Imipramine	1	0.0
Psychological Therapies		
Supportive psychotherapy	270	78.7
Intensive psychotherapy	11	3.2
Psychoanalysis	15	4.4
Group psychotherapy	31	9.0
Family psychotherapy	41	12.0
Play therapy	4	1.2
Hypnosis	42	12.2
Behavior therapy	42	12.2
Biofeedback	8	2.3
Relaxation	12	3.5
Meditation	11	3.2
Yoga	2	0.6
Physical Therapies		
Electroconvulsive therapy	9	2.6
Insulin coma therapy	4	1.2
Fever therapy	2	0.6
Arsenic therapy	2	0.6
Ultraviolet therapy	1	0.3
Hydrotherapy	2	0.6
Cold and hot showers	1	0.3
Habitual showers	1	0.3
Surgical Therapies		
Cryothalamectomy	2	0.6
Chemothalamectomy	1	0.3
Hospitalization		
General treatment	37	10.8

TABLE 11.3. (Continued)

Treatment	N	%
Other		
Chiropractic therapy	13	3.8
Vitamin therapy	4	0.3
Dietary therapy	2	0.6
Exorcism	3	0.9
Herbal medicines	1	0.3

^aDrug treatment, N = 421; nondrug treatment, N = 343.

Spontaneous changes are reported in a high percentage of the 666 Tourette's disorder patients in our sample. These changes include 97% with spontaneous change in the severity of symptoms (waxing and waning of symptoms), 96% with spontaneous change in the type of symptoms (fluctuation of symptoms), and 27% with spontaneous remissions lasting from 1 month to 7 years (Table 5.17). Other factors contributing to changes in the severity of symptoms are diurnal variation, seasonal factors, situational stimuli, diagnosis of TS+ADD+H (Table 5.22, 5.23) and other possible nonspecific or placebo effects. In fact, the magnitude of these spontaneous changes often exceeds the percent of improvement reported in many uncontrolled clinical studies. Moreover, waxing, waning, and fluctuation and remission of symptoms are criteria for all tic disorders and are described as characteristic of the clinical course in DSM-III-R.

This problem can be illustrated by a retrospective analysis of the effect of placebo in a recent carefully designed double-blind cross-over comparison of pimozide and placebo (see Chapter 13 for details) (Shapiro and Shapiro, 1984). Twenty patients were treated with placebo for 6 weeks. The percent of change for seven dependent variables at endpoint compared to base line is summarized in Table 11.4. Each dependent variable was trichotomized into percent patients improved, unchanged or worse.

The percent change for the seven dependent variables averaged 36% (10–55%) improved, 31% (0–60%) unchanged, and 43% (0–80%) worse after 6 weeks of treatment with placebo. Thus, if the results are taken as a whole, tics increased, decreased, or were unchanged in approximately one-third of patients, respectively. These results suggest that nonplacebo effects should exceed improvement in more than one-third of treated Tourette's disorder patients. However, the range for improvement varies from 10 to 55% with different dependent variables (Table 11.4). Since controlled and uncontrolled studies in the literature largely report results for only one dependent variable, improvement reported in such studies may be related more to the type of dependent variable used in the study than to the effect of the treatment. In

TABLE 11.4. *Percent of patients improved, unchanged, or worse after treatment With placebo for 6 Weeks*[a]

Dependent variables	Improved %	Unchanged %	Worse %
Judges' ratings			
Total motor and vocal tic counts	35	0	65
TS severity scale	55	15	30
Clinician Ratings			
TS severity scale	50	40	10
Clinical global improvement	35	45	20
Physician global evaluation scale	25	50	25
Patient ratings			
Percent change of tics	40	60	0
Patient global evaluation scale	10	10	80
Average of all ratings	36	31	43

[a]$N = 20$.

addition, it is important to note that although a report of improvement in 50% to 55% of patients would be quite impressive, none of the percentages for the seven dependent variables are significant (see Table 13.5). Even worse is the tendency to retrospectively select a dependent improvement variable, usually based on which variable shows the most improvement.

These factors underscore the necessity of conducting carefully designed studies which include multiple dependent improvement measures to evaluate the efficacy of treatment in Tourette's disorder. Also contributing to spontaneous and placebo effects are the patients' expectations that the new medication will result in symptomatic improvement. In fact, patients generally change to a new medication when they are at their worst and the likelihood of spontaneous improvement is maximized. Thus, symptomatic change may be fortuitous due to a natural, spontaneous waning of symptomatology or exaggerated because there are decreased adverse effects after the first the medication is discontinued and the change is misinterpreted as improvement. These methodological problems underscore the need for well controlled double-blind studies of both drug and psychological treatment of tic disorders (Levine et al., 1971, Levine, 1979).

CONCLUSION

This review of studies and clinical experience reported in the literature strongly indicates that the most effective drugs for the treatment of tics and Tourette's disorder are neuroleptics, such as haloperidol, pimozide, fluphenazine, penfluridol, probably sulpiride, and, possibly, metoclopramide. Although clonidine, clonazepam, and tetrabenazine are largely ineffective, their possible benefit for a small subcategory of patients, whose clinical characteristics have not been identified, should be evaluated further. The effects reported for apomorphine, oral physostigmine, naloxone, and calcium channel antagonists require replication. The effectiveness of dopamine-blocking neuroleptics, particularly those with predominant D_2 blocking effects, is the major empirical finding implicating dopamine in the etiology of Tourette's disorder. Spontaneous waxing and waning of the severity of symptoms in 97%, spontaneous fluctuation of symptoms in 96%, spontaneous remissions lasting from 1 month to 7 years in 27% of patients, and possible spontaneous or positive placebo effects (averaging 36%) and spontaneous or negative placebo effects (averaging 31%) underscore the limitations of uncontrolled studies and the necessity of conducting carefully controlled studies to evaluate the effectiveness of treatment for tics and Tourette's disorder.

12

Treatment of Tic Disorders

In this chapter we discuss indications for treatment, general principles of treatment with specific drugs, the recognition and management of adverse effects, and the role and use of psychotherapy.

INDICATIONS FOR TREATMENT

Based on our extensive clinical and research experience and the evaluation of published studies, we have concluded that the only effective treatment for tics is pharmacological, and that the treatment of Tourette's disorder should be directed primarily at reducing tic symptoms. Other problems such as psychopathology, learning and attentional problems may require other types of remediation. These may include neuropsychological and intellectual assessment to identify and remediate learning and school problems; psychotherapeutic treatment for problems of low self-esteem, depression, or anxiety secondary to having the disorder; and family counseling for problems that may arise with siblings, discipline, etc.

Pharmacological treatment, however, is indicated only if the symptoms impair psychosocial, educational, or occupational functioning. Since treatment is palliative, it is not recommended if the symptoms are mild, do not elicit comments and the curiosity of others, or interfere with psychosocial functioning. Treatment of patients with mild to moderate symptoms is elective and should be determined by the patient and family based on the degree of distress caused by the tics.

GENERAL PRINCIPLES OF TREATMENT

Dosage of all neuroleptics requires individual titration to achieve maximum effectiveness with minimal adverse effects (Campbell, 1985). Endpoint dosage is arrived at by pragmatic trial and error. There is no standard dosage for everyone as there is for aspirin or penicillin. This clinical observation is supported by recent findings that enzymes governing the metabolism of these drugs are genetically determined.

Haloperidol, for example, is used at considerably higher dosages in psychotic patients in contrast to a dosage range of 2 to 10 mg/day for Tourette patients. Nevertheless, Tourette patients report frequent, bothersome adverse effects even at these low dosages.

Other pharmacodynamics contribute to variable dosage, clinical response, and elimination of medication from the body. Blood levels of haloperidol may plateau for as long as 72 hr and tend to accumulate in the body, so that the same dosage over time results in higher cumulative blood levels. A steady blood level state is reached in approximately 4 days. Thus, the clinical effect should be evaluated on the fourth day during initial titration, and dosage changed appropriately on the fifth day. Although the elimination half-life in acute single-dose studies varies from 12 to 38 hr (mean 24 hr) and from 13.4 hr to 21.2 days (Rubin et al., 1980; Campbell and Balderessini, 1985; Hubbard et al., 1987), in clinical treatment elimination of the drug appears to take approximately 4 days during initial acute treatment, but with chronic treatment, elimination increases to approximately 14 days or a range of 4 to 30 days. With acute withdrawal, adverse effects tend to decrease and disappear before tics return to their pre-existing level. Because neuroleptics have a long half-life, the total dosage can be administered at bedtime for most patients. Akinesic or sedative effects may increase after intake and are often better tolerated by patients during sleep. Once-a-day, night-time administration contributes to ease of administration and improves compliance. Occasional patients have a better response and fewer adverse effects if medication is administered at intervals throughout the day.

Dosage is increased until the patient reports at least 70% control of symptoms. Titration of dosage should be directed primarily, at least during initial treatment, at symptomatic reduction outside the home, in school, or at work, to minimize social and psychological difficulties.

Occasionally, during treatment, symptoms exacerbate, either spontaneously or in reaction to stressful external events, such as returning to school in September. If the exacerbation persists beyond 2 weeks, dosage of medication should be increased temporarily. Approximately 6 months after the therapeutic effect is stable, the dosage should be reduced every 2 to 4 weeks to achieve the lowest possible dosage to effect symptom control.

Children and adolescents should be informed completely about the illness and participate in their treatment as appropriate for their age. Not infrequently adolescents may act out their conflict with parents by resisting treatment. They may forget to take their medication which precipitates squabbles, or often refuse to take medication because they feel they do not need it. The adolescent's desire for a trial off medication should be supported. If severe symptoms return, they become highly motivated to resume treatment and cease to act out over this issue. Adults, too, are often curious about whether they need medication and should be supported if they desire to stop treatment. Patients question how they will know if their symptoms have disappeared or have decreased spontaneously while on medication. This issue is easily resolved if dosage is constantly titrated up or down according to the severity of symptoms. When medication is discontinued, symptoms may increase the very next day, more usually by the fourth day, and almost always in 2 weeks. There are no major contraindications to suddenly discontinuing medication. However, because some patients experience withdrawal effects, such as withdrawal dyskinetic symptoms, insomnia, jitteriness, and gastrointestinal symptoms, slow withdrawal is desirable. If symptoms are minimal after withdrawal or do not return, a spontaneous remission can be considered and medication is no longer required. If symptoms return, treatment can be resumed, with the same therapeutic benefit achieved previously.

Some patients report fewer symptoms after discontinuing medication (than while on it), but their symptoms usually return to pretreatment levels after 2 to 3 weeks. Adverse effects usually attenuate and disappear before tic symptoms recur, approximately 4 days after discontinuation of the drug, but they may last for as long as 3 weeks.

HALOPERIDOL

Haloperidol, a butyrophenone type neuroleptic, was approved for use in the United States for adults in 1969 and for children in 1978. Haloperidol is a potent antagonist of dopamine receptor sites. It is the drug of choice for most physicians because of its remarkable effectiveness (see Chapter 11).

Treatment Regimen

Almost all patients are treated as out-patients. Occasional patients with a significant number of associated problems such as self-destructive or suicidal behavior, or those for whom the dosage cannot be stabilized, may require inpatient treatment.

The usual starting dose is 0.25 mg/day haloperidol at bedtime. We administer 0.5 mg/day of benztropine mesylate prophylactically with haloperidol to prevent acute dystonia which occurs in approximately 5 to 9% of patients usually within 72 hr, and akinesia which occurs in 25% of patients usually within the first 2 weeks of treatment.

The initial dose of 0.25 mg haloperidol is taken before retiring every night for 4 to 7 days. The dose is increased 0.25 mg on the fifth to eighth day if there is inadequate therapeutic effect and an absence of adverse effects. The dose should be increased 0.25 mg until one of three possibilities occur: the symptoms decrease 70 to 90% without adverse effects; adverse effects occur without symptomatic benefit; or symptoms decrease and adverse effects occur at the same time. The usual response is the third possibility; symptoms begin to decrease with the onset of adverse effects. Approximately 25% of patients achieve 70 to 90% decrease in symptoms with minimal, nonsignificant, or no adverse effects. The dose for individual patients may vary from 2 to 10 mg/day, probably because of unknown factors about the illness and genetic differences in metabolizing drugs. If there is no therapeutic benefit or adverse effects, it is likely that the dosage is inadequate. In this event, the dosage should be increased until adverse effects appear, indicating that the dosage is adequate.

A slow increase in dosage has many advantages. The onset of adverse effects will be subtle, mild, and well tolerated by patients. If adverse effects are troublesome, the dosage can be increased more slowly, e.g., every 10 to 30 days. Slow increase allows adequate time for the disappearance or development of tolerance to many adverse effects, and patients do not become prematurely discouraged because of temporary adverse effects. In addition, patients learn by experience how to change the dosage, and to recognize and manage adverse effects.

The dosage can be increased more rapidly, 0.25 mg every 1 to 4 days, depending on indications and factors already discussed. The only caution is the recognition that, because of the long half-life of haloperidol, the final dosage will probably overshoot an appropriate endpoint. Dosage should then be reduced 0.25 mg every 4 days until appropriate equilibration between improvement and adverse effects occur.

Patients are encouraged to increase the dosage slowly until slight, but tolerable adverse effects occur. If the increase results in adverse effects on the first day, they may disappear by the fourth day and dosage may again be increased on the fifth day. If adverse effects persist and are uncomfortable, the dosage should be reduced 0.25 mg and they will usually disappear by the fourth day. If they do not, dosage can be lowered by the same amount again. As patients experience the effects of changing dosage, they become more confident and comfortable about titrating the dosage.

Blood Levels to Monitor Treatment

The optimal dosage is determined clinically based on therapeutic effect and/or the appearance of adverse effects. Blood levels are not useful to determine dosage because they are largely unassociated with age, weight, sex, severity, therapeutic response, or adverse effects.

We used a specific radioimmunoassay (Shostak and Perel, 1976) to measure blood levels of haloperidol in 14 Tourette's disorder patients between the ages of 9 to 28 years. These patients had been treated with haloperidol for up to 4 years at dosages ranging from 0.5 to 71 mg/day. The average daily dosage of haloperidol was 2.96 mg (SD 2.04; range 0.5–7.0) and the average blood level was 3.8 ng/ml haloperidol (SD 2.85; range 1.0–10.5). The correlation coefficient between mg/kg haloperidol and blood level was 0.81 ($p < 0.001$). However, the blood level was unrelated to therapeutic response, or adverse effects, sex, age, weight, chronicity of illness, and length of treatment. The minimum effective blood level of haloperidol is approximately 2.0 ng/ml. (Shapiro et al., 1981; Shapiro and Shapiro, 1981a, 1982f). Haloperidol plasma levels and therapeutic response have been reported to be uncorrelated in other pediatric disorders (Morselli et al., 1979) and in schizophrenic patients (Rubin et al., 1980).

Similar findings of a lack of convergence between blood levels and therapeutic response was noted by Singer et al. (1981). They measured serum haloperidol levels in eight patients with Tourette's disorder using a radioreceptor assay. All patients were on a therapeutically effective dosage of medication for an average of 17 months. Dosage ranged from 1.5 to 10 mg/day, average 3.8 ± 1.0 mg/day. Serum levels of haloperidol were also quite low, three of the patients had levels below the limit sensitivity of the assay. Thus, Tourette patients demonstrated symptomatic improvement with dosage values that were significantly lower than those used to control psychotic symptoms, and serum levels tenfold lower than that measured in schizophrenic patients.

A correlation between plasma level and dosage of haloperidol has been demonstrated by radioimmunoassay but with large interindividual variation in children and adults (Goyot et al, 1985).

The relationship of serum prolactin levels to therapeutic efficacy has not been studied with haloperidol. Moldofsky and Brown (1982), however, studied ten Tourette's disorder patients with normal prolactin levels treated with pimozide. They found no significant relationships among magnitude of serum prolactin increase, drug dosage, and decrease in tics. They did find that an optimal clinical response with pimozide occurred when serum prolactin attained a maximum or peak response, which they feel may be a satisfactory objective indicator of therapeutic responsiveness to pimozide.

Rapid Increase of Dosage

Rapid treatment generally requires hospitalization. Occasionally, hospitalization can be avoided if the patient and family are stoic and do not overreact to adverse effects, if a responsible family member can attend the patient, if the patient can visit the doctor frequently, and if the physician is readily available for management. Rapid treatment and hospitalization may be indicated for patients with severe symptoms, which preclude functioning outside the home, or those for whom it is difficult to make out-patient visits to the physician's office, and occasional patients with orthopedic or medical complications that are exacerbated by the tics. Some patients are hypochondriacal and markedly exaggerate the significance of physical changes from medicine or spontaneous body changes, and frequently confuse the origins of these stimuli. Such patients are always difficult to treat. Reassurance, explanations, and competent staff and management in a hospital may be necessary for their treatment.

Parenteral administration is the most rapid method of treatment. The usual base-line laboratory studies (complete blood count (CBC), white blood count (WBC), and differential count) and vital signs (pulse, supine, sitting, and standing blood pressure; temperature) should be recorded before treatment. Neurological, electroencephalogram (EEG), radiological, psychological, and other examinations and tests are optional as discussed previously; their use is dependent on clinical indications. An antiparkinsonian drug, (such as benztropine mesylate), 1 mg orally, should be given 1 hr before initial use of haloperidol to prevent acute dystonia and akinesia, as well as to anticipate its subsequent use for other inevitable extrapyamidal symptoms. The initial dosage of haloperidol is 1 mg i.m. (an injectable form is available at a concentration of 2 mg/cc) at 8 a.m., for example. The dosage is doubled to 2 mg 4 hr later at 12 noon, doubled again to 4 mg 4 hr later at 4 p.m., and 5 mg is given at 8 p.m. If marked benefit or adverse effects (primarily akinesia) do not occur that evening or the next morning, titration of dosage should be continued. After 1 mg oral benztropine mesylate, which is continued thereafter each morning, 5 mg haloperidol i.m. is given at 8 a.m., and doubled at each subsequent 4-hr period until the desired effect is achieved. The patient should be observed clinically and vital signs obtained before each dosage. Marked decrease of symptoms usually occurs in association with akinesia manifested as sedation, sluggishness, tiredness, and lethargy at a dosage ranging from 10 mg to 100 mg or higher if necessary. If the effect persists for 4 hr, the next dosage should be given orally at one-fourth the dosage given in the previous 24 hr. For example, on the first day, the dosages for each 4-hr period, given intramuscularly, would be 1, 2, 4, and 5 mg; on the next day 5 mg at 8 a.m. and 10 mg at 12 noon. If a marked improvement occurs after this dosage and persists for 4 hr, one-fourth of the previous 24-hr dosage (totaling 24 mg) would be 6 mg haloperidol is then given orally at a dosage of 6 mg q.i.d. If improvement persists for 4 days, it is likely that no further increase in dosage will be necessary. If symptoms recur within 4 days, the dosage should be increased 5 mg/day until a therapeutic plateau is reached . After a therapeutic plateau has been maintained for 4 days, the same dosage is continued for another 6 days (total 10 days). During this period, the dosage of benztropine mesylate can be changed each 24 hr, usually increased 0.5 to 2.0 mg/day, as clinically indicated, and the effects observed in the subsequent 24 hr. If the previously described clinical schedule had been followed for our hypothetical patient, 12 days would have elapsed after the beginning of treatment. If adverse effects are not severe, many patients can leave the hospital and be treated as an outpatient. The dosage should be reduced every 5 days as follows: 1 mg between 10 and 15 mg, 0.5 mg between 5 and 10 mg, and 0.25 mg subsequently. Adverse effects will decrease with reduced dosage of haloperidol and the dosage of benztropine mesylate can be varied accordingly at a dosage change of 0.25 mg each day. If acute dystonia occurs (during the first 2 days usually), it can be controlled rapidly by intravenous injection of 60 to 90 mg barbiturate or 1 mg benztropine mesylate. It can also be controlled by giving 1 mg benztropine mesylate orally, but it may take 30 to 45 min. If this fails to control the acute dystonia, which is unusual, another 1 mg orally should be given in 1 hr. The total dosage given to control the dystonia should then be given daily for 2 weeks, after which other clinical signs should determine the dosage of benztropine mesylate.

Treatment can be even more intensive and rapid by beginning with a 5-mg intramuscular injection and repeating it every 4 hr during the first day, and doubling the dosage every 4 hr on subsequent days. This is rarely necessary because it usually takes very few days to get to an endpoint using the lower initial dosage. An advantage of the lower initial dosage is the additional time available for the patient to adjust to the hospital, the procedure, and initial injections.

Giving the medication orally at initial treatment is also feasible and usually does not take much longer than intramuscular treatment, although the starting dosage should be higher. An oral dosage schedule might be 5 mg q.i.d. on the first day, 10 mg q.i.d. on the second day, and so on until the clinical endpoint described previously is reached.

The adverse effects of hospitalization on patients contributed to our treating patients on an outpatient basis with slow increments of medication. Patients were hospitalized in a psychiatric hospital because only there is skillful management of patients treated with high dosages of psychotropics possible. Although some patients with inadequate defenses became upset, much of their upset was iatrogenically induced. Psychiatric staff, overly specialized in psychiatric treatment, would treat Tourette patients, despite the best intentions, as if they were disturbed psychiatric patients. Instead of responding to the patient's questions in a simple matter-of-fact way, the usual psychiatric response was "Why do you ask?" or "What do you think?" or a dynamic interpretation was given. This can be unnecessarily upsetting to a patient with Tourette's disorder, who is undergoing the stressful experience of a new treatment in a strange atmosphere. The exquisitely sensitive, specialized, and prolonged training of psychiatrists often results in loss of clinical judgment in the treatment of nonpsychiatric patients. A less stressful hospital environment would be a neurological or medical ward but, unfortunately, the staff of such a ward may not have extensive experience using psychotropic medication.

Recognition and Management of Adverse Effects

The discussion of adverse effects focuses on those associated with drugs usually prescribed to treat patients with Tourette's disorder.

Acute Dystonia

Acute dystonia occurs in 5 to 10% of Tourette patients treated with haloperidol and in up to 50.4% of psychiatric patients treated with high potency neuroleptics (Winslow et al., 1986; Sramek et al., 1986; Boyer et al., 1987), usually within 48 to 72 hr, occasionally up to 4.5 days (Ayd, 1961) after initial treatment and is unrelated to dosage. Acute dystonia is more frequent in children, teenagers, brain-damaged, and older patients (Winslow et al., 1986; Sramek et al., 1986; Boyer et al., 1987). The symptoms are involuntary, intermittent, or sustained contractions of unilateral or bilateral muscles usually of the upper body, particularly the head, neck, shoulder, and back, resulting in mandibular and oculogyric spasms, speech and swallowing difficulties, torticollis, hyperextension of the neck and trunk, and torsion spasm. To avoid the occurrence of acute dystonia, which can be life-threatening especially if laryngeal-pharyngeal dystonia occurs (Flaherty and Lahmeyer, 1978; Menuck, 1981; McDanal, 1981; Modestin et al., 1981; Winslow et al., 1986), we administer benztropine mesylate, 0.5 mg/day, concomitant with haloperidol or other neuroleptics. An adolescent male we treated with haloperidol developed a thick, swollen tongue which interfered with speech, eating, swallowing, and breathing. Intravenous anti-Parkinson drugs alleviated the symptoms. Acute dystonia can be immediately and completely controlled by intravenous anti-Parkinson drugs, such as benztropine mesylate, followed by oral administration without discontinuing medication. Acute dystonia can also be controlled within an hour with oral benztropine mesylate at a dosage of 1 to 2 mg. Further episodes almost never occur even after the discontinuation of anticholinergic medication. Other medications include antihistaminics and benzodiazepines (Director and Muniz, 1982).

Akinesia

Akinesia is characterized by muscular weakness, general tiredness, aches, pains in muscles or joints when mild; and by apathy, depression, loss of motivation, regression, and dependence when severe. This adverse effect may not be experienced as a loss of alertness but as an inability to perform repetitive muscular acts such as walking or working. Children may become irritable, fearful, disinterested in school, cling to their mother, and develop school avoidance (Mikkelsen et al., 1981; Linet, 1985).

Akinesia can occur acutely during the first 2 weeks of treatment in approximately 25% of patients and is unrelated to dosage. With subsequent chronic treatment akinesic effects are associated with higher dosages and are usually responsive to dosage reduction or the use of anticholinergic drugs. Anticholinergic medication usually can be discontinued within 3 to 8 months of treatment. Persistent akinesic effects may require the use of stimulants.

Akathisia

Akathisia is characterized by motor restlessness, which can range from uncomfortable muscle and skin sensations, to mild jitteriness to severe pacing, as well as an inability to sit quietly, concentrate for longer than moments, and possibly insomnia. It can mimic anxiety, but the restlessness or jitteriness is experienced primarily in the body rather than in the mind. Approximately 25% of patients experience akathesia frequently during the first weeks of therapy. If often lasts for hours, and, usually but not always, disappears within 3 months. Akathisia can be quite severe and is not entirely related to dosage. If severe, the dosage of benztropine mesylate is increased 0.5 mg/day to a dosage ranging from 1 to 6 mg/day. Other alternatives include propranolol, 30 to 80 mg/day (Lipinski et al., 1984) and the temporary use of benzodiazepines, 5 to 15 mg/day (Director and Muniz, 1982; Jeste et al., 1986; Kutcher et al., 1987).

Tardive Akinesia, Dystonia, or Tourette's Disorder

These tardive syndromes are reported infrequently and may essentially reflect atypical symptoms of tardive dyskinesia (TD) that have been misinterpreted. Jeste et al. (1986), in a review of these conditions concluded that "there is satisfactory evidence implicating neuroleptics in the etiology of these so called tardive syndromes." We have never encountered tardive Tourette's disorder and cases referred to us by colleagues were diagnosed by us as TD.

Extrapyramidal Parkinsonian Adverse Effects

Extrapyramidal parkinsonian adverse effects (EPS) are frequent, temporary, reversible, and related to dosage. Akinesia, the most subtle EPS adverse effect, results in an earlier bedtime than usual or difficulty on awakening. Other symptoms may appear as dosage is increased such as blank facial expression, depressive appearance, open mouth, drooling, tremors, rigidity, shuffling gait, loss of associated movements, cogwheeling, and akinesia experienced as daytime sedation. Patients report taking naps during the day, and interference with academic and occupational functioning. One method to detect the onset of these adverse effects is by observing the patient's handwriting which becomes constricted and jerky. Effective management includes reduction of dosage or the use of anti-Parkinson agents. Most adverse effects disappear after 3 to 4 months of treatment.

Extrapyramidal Parkinsonian Hand-Finger Mannerism

We refer to a rare adverse effect that has been observed in approximately 30 of our patients treated with neuroleptics, but not reported in the literature, as EPS hand-finger mannerism. In the past, patients who developed this adverse effect were referred to psychiatrists knowledgeable about neuroleptic EPS. However, none had ever observed the symptom. Several physicians who were consulted recently observed this adverse effect in occasional schizophrenic patients treated with neuroleptics. We stress the rarity of this symptom because when we referred to this adverse effect in several of our papers, its legitimacy was challenged by reviewers who were unaware of its existence.

The cardinal feature is a manneristic positioning of the hands or fingers. It may take the form of slight flexion of one or all of the metaphalangeal joints, sometimes including the wrist; stiff extension of the second or second and third fingers with flexion of the fourth and fifth fingers; stiff extension of the first three digits separated from a similar extension of the fourth and fifth fingers; flexion of the wrist alone; and occasionally slight flexion at the elbow. The symptoms are always bilateral, can readily be stopped voluntarily when attention is directed to the hand position, but always returns when attention is diverted. It is dosage-related, but can occur at low dosages, without other EPSs, and tends not to decrease over time or respond to treatment with anti-Parkinson drugs. This symptom has persisted in some patients for as long as 10 years. There are no other obvious correlates. The symptom always decreases with reduced dosage and completely disappears after discontinuation of the neuroleptic. The cause and significance are unknown.

Cognitive Impairment

Cognitive impairment, reported as impaired attention, motivation, memory and response time, is a subtle and major limitation of the use of haloperidol (see Chapter 13). It occurs at dosages of haloperidol that vary from 2 to 10 mg/day. School grades fall, work performance decreases, and motivation is impaired in both children and adults. Management requires constant titration to the minimal dosage required for maximum improvement outside the home, and possibly the prudent use of anticholinergic or stimulant drugs.

Tardive Dyskinesia

Symptoms of TD include involuntary, rapid, rhythmic, choreiform, occasionally athetoid and dystonic movements of the tongue, neck, face, mouth, jaw (such as grimacing, masticatory, or chewing movements), tongue protrusion, puffing of cheeks, mouth-puckering, and sometimes generalized jerky and writhing movements of other parts of the body. Fine vermicular movements of the tongue is an unreliable early sign of TD since many individuals not on drugs have such movements and neuroleptics almost always increase them. Severe writhing movements of the tongue, usually with perioral spread, however, are frequently observed in TD. TD occurs spontaneously in individuals not treated with neuroleptics and is more likely to occur in older patients and in patients treated with high dosages for a prolonged period of time. These movements may be very mild or severe, and are difficult to differentiate from tics except by physicians experienced with both movement disorders. TD appears or breaks through while the patient is on medication, such as haloperidol, and lasts longer than 3 months. But very few patients develop irreversible or severely incapacitating TD (Baldessarini and Cohen, 1987); it frequently disappears after discontinuation of the neuroleptic, may slowly disappear over years, or be permanent (Baldessarini, 1985). In surveys of schizophrenic patients of all ages, sexes, and neuroleptic dosages (which are much higher than those used in the treatment of Tourette's disorder), the prevalence corrected for spontaneous dyskinesia has been estimated to be 15 to 28%; the incidence is estimated as 2 to 5% per year, and appears to be higher between 6 to 24 months after beginning neuroleptic treatment (Baldessarini, 1985). The symptoms are often indistinguishable from covert dyskinesia (CD) except for their duration. CD appears only after reduction of dosage, is usually suppressed after reinstitution of the neuroleptic, and the clinical course is otherwise similar to TD. Withdrawal dyskinesia (WD), frequently including ataxia of the extremities and trunk, appears only after rapid dosage reduction or sudden discontinuation of medication, and the symptoms usually are transient and always disappear within 3 months. It is not known whether WD, which is more common in younger patients, is pathologically the same as TD or an early development of TD (Baldessarini, 1985).

Although the possibility of TD causes justifiable concern among patients, parents, and physicians, none of the patients with tic disorders treated by us with haloperidol has developed TD, probably because low dosages of medication were used (Shapiro and Shapiro, 1982a). However, nine cases of haloperidol-induced TD in Tourette patients have been reported in the literature (Caine and Polinsky, 1981; Caine et al., 1978; Mizrahi et al., 1980; Golden, 1985; Riddle et al., 1987). Our review of these cases suggests that possibly only four had incipient but not confirmed TD (Shapiro et al., 1982). In all four incipient cases the symptoms suggesting TD were detected soon after their development and disappeared within 3 months after dosage reduction or discontinuation of medication. However, usually TD symptoms increase after lowering the neuroleptic dosage. In two of the cases symptoms appeared following withdrawal of medication and are more consistent with withdrawal emergent symptoms (Caine and Polinsky, 1981). Only one patient, an elderly, depressed man who had been treated with multiple medications, clearly had TD. Differentiating the symptoms of TD from the return of old symptoms or the development of new symptoms can be difficult. For example, a patient who developed lip-puckering was referred to us for evaluation of TD. However, review of our records indicated that lip-puckering was one of his symptoms when evaluated initially.

The difficulties of diagnosing TD are illustrated in a recent report (Riddle et al., 1987). Ten days after discontinuing haloperidol, 7 mg/day, symptoms of Tourette's disorder exacerbated and the patient developed symptoms "suggestive of tardive dyskinesia, including tongue thrusting, lip movements and mouth stretching." The history suggests a diagnosis of CD rather than TD. Moreover, the symptoms "suggesting" TD would be very difficult to differentiate from tics, since they are very common Tourette symptoms, and could have been new symptoms or have been present previously in the history. Haloperidol reinstituted at 2.5 mg/day reduced both tics and TD symptoms, which is consistent with the symptoms being either Tourette's disorder or TD. A further differentiation could have been made by using haloperidol at the previous dosage of 7 mg/day; this dosage should have reduced the tics and completely controlled the "suggestive" TD symptoms. If an anticholinergic drug was used, TD symptoms should increase, but have no effect on tics (Klawans et al., 1980; Gardos et al., 1984).

Six patients chronically treated by us with neuroleptics developed WD when dosage was reduced rapidly. Withdrawal dyskinetic symptoms include unsteady walking or dystonic movements of the limbs and body, facial grimace, closing and rolling back of the eyes, and stentorian breathing. Several had insomnia, hyperactivity, borborygmus, and loose bowels. Three patients had movements resembling those of bobbing rag dolls. The symptoms in all patients disappeared within 3 months.

One of our patients, withdrawn from 2 mg/day haloperidol very slowly over several months, had a marked exacerbation of symptoms after being off medication for 8 days, including marked violence, abrupt mood swings, paranoid thinking, self-abuse, marked irritability, and the onset of impulsions which had been absent formerly. Resumption of treatment controlled these behaviors.

Our experience is that while it is often easy to make a diagnosis of TD in adult psychiatric patients treated with high dosages of neuroleptics over a prolonged period, it is very difficult to differentiate minor symptoms of TD from tics. It requires careful review of the past history and a long period of inquiry and observation of patients in different situations (while distracted, performing neurological tests, etc.), provocative increase, decrease, or discontinuation of medication, and use of anticholinergic drugs which may increase TD symptoms but not tics.

However, because of the possible development of TD, patients treated with neuroleptics should be evaluated periodically, optimally every 3 months, and the benefits and risks including the possible development of TD should be discussed with the patient and family, and their informed consent to treatment documented.

Anticholinergic Adverse Effects

Anticholinergic adverse effects include xerostomia, mydriasis, impaired accommodation for near objects, and constipation. They are related to dosage, associated with both haloperidol and anticholinergic drugs, as well as most antidepressant drugs, and their effects are additive. They are usually not troublesome and can be managed by reduction of dosage, change to another drug, or the use of various corrective measures. Constipation is readily controlled by the use of docusate sodium, 300 mg/hs, for 1 week. Light-sensitivity from mydriasis can be managed by the use of sunglasses. Impaired vision for close objects, sometimes lasting for as long as a year, can be successfully managed by the use of temporary reading glasses. Occasionally, instances of urinary retention may occur, more frequently in males, and nonspecific, aseptic trigonitis in females. Rare instances of toxic confusional states, with visual hallucinations, are associated with higher dosages and older age in predisposed individuals.

Endocrinological Adverse Effects

Endocrinological adverse effects are related to dosage and usually are associated with elevated prolactin levels. Prolactin levels initially rise at the beginning of treatment, but tend to decrease during the first 3 months of treatment and remain constant thereafter (Brown and Laughren, 1981). Galactorrhea, breast engorgement, menstrual irregularities, gynecomastia, and impaired libido improve over time with dosage reduction (Ghadirian, 1982). Hyperglycemic glucose tolerance curves may occur but do not require corrective measures. A major difficulty is increased appetite, which results in a slow, persistent and sometimes alarming increase of weight. General weight reduction regimens including reduction of caloric intake, use of low caloric foods, and exercise should be used initially. They are often ineffective and stimulants may be required to control the drug-induced increased weight.

Decreased libido in adults can be a major difficulty. This adverse effect is dosage-related and is manifested by decreased sexual interest, fantasies, motivation, arousal, activity, and performance (Shapiro and Shapiro, 1975). Dosage reduction may bring sexual functioning back to normal levels.

In adolescence, normal vigorous sexual drive may be muted and may be interpreted as a sign of being "unmanly" or "queer". Adolescents should be informed that sex drive may be blunted so that they are not upset should this adverse effect occur. In some patients there may be rebound or marked surge in libido when medication is decreased or stopped suddenly.

Bromocriptine was ineffective in counteracting either decreased libido or impotency in several of our patients, but has been reported to effectively suppress galactorrhea and amenorrhea (Chang et al., 1982). Brom-ergocryptine has been reported to decrease but not completely control phenothiazine-induced galactorrhea in nine hospitalized psychiatric female patients (Beumont, 1975).

Depressive, Dysphoric, and Phobic Adverse Effects

Depressive, dysphoric, and phobic adverse effects are related to dosage, but may occur at very low dosages in susceptible individuals. Patients frequently complain of sadness, crying spells, and occasional suicidal thoughts (Caine and Polinsky 1979; Bruun, 1982). We have been unable to identify the premorbid characteristics that predispose patients to the development of depression. Symptoms of separation anxiety, school phobias, and other phobias, may occur in children on low dosages (Shapiro and Shapiro, 1980, 1981e, 1982b; Mikkelsen et al., 1981; Linet, 1985). Anticholinergics are usually ineffective to control these adverse effects. If they are ineffective, the dosage of neuroleptics is halved or stimulants or tricyclic antidepressants, such as desipramine, are used. (See section on management of adverse effects.)

Potentiation of Other Drugs

Neuroleptics can potentiate barbiturates, narcotics, anesthestics, antihistaminics, and alcohol. The effects of these substances may be potentiated 25 to 50% with initial use of haloperidol, but there is usually little or no potentiation with chronic use.

Addiction and Withdrawal

Haloperidol is not an addictive drug. The development of tolerance is minimal and withdrawal effects are attenuated. Minor adverse effects such as headaches, perspiration, insomnia, restlessness, anxiety, diarrhea, nausea, and vomiting can occur after haloperidol is stopped suddenly, but can be completely avoided by slow decrease of dosage (Lacoursiere et al., 1976; Gardos et al., 1978).

Fog States

"Fog states," more fully characterized by feelings of depersonalization, paranoia, and slowed mentation, lasting from a few seconds to several hours, has been experienced by several of our patients when on haloperidol or phenothiazines. If these symptoms occur, especially in the presence of a subtle, organic mental syndrome, high dosages of haloperidol should be considered as a possible cause. The dosage should be reduced or trials on and off medication should be used to evaluate whether medication is the cause of the "fog state." The existence of a "fog state" should be further documented and studied. Two of our patients had "fog states" when on more than 15 mg/day haloperidol. One patient, a 16-year-old boy, had a left Babinski sign and mild clumsiness on the left. Some of his tics were atypical because of a dystonic component, although profuse coprolalia was documented. He developed episodes of "rushing thoughts," paranoia, adversive head movements to either side, and frequent tics after 3 years of haloperidol therapy. During several observed episodes, the patient was lethargic and slightly disoriented. His vital signs, postural responses, and blood sugar were normal. Such episodes usually lasted hours, although a short aura of "far-away feeling" sometimes occurred without the episode itself. Skull X-rays and brain scan were normal. The EEG between episodes showed bilateral frontotemporal sharp waves. A pneumoencephalogram was normal, although the cerebrospinal fluid (CSF) protein was 67 mg%. The patient also reported many episodes of having his thoughts fixate on a part of his body, an object, or a word. At these times, despite continuing the conversation and exerting great effort to control this behavior, his thoughts would constantly return to, for example, his knee, which may have been casually mentioned. These incidents would occur sporadically, without warning, last for variable periods of time, disappear spontaneously, and did not appear to be related to psychological stress or conflict. They were more frequent when the patient was on phenothiazine-type medication, particularly haloperidol, and slowly decreased after medication was withdrawn. A second patient, a 17-year-old boy, also described "fog states" and a more elaborate fixating tendency. He would "get stuck" on what appeared to be psychopathological fantasies or thoughts. These included Oedipal thoughts, obsessive thoughts of female feces, repeated sexual arousal following masturbation as if not surfeited, stabbing himself in the abdomen while masturbating, and many others. These episodes would last for a period of weeks or months, disappear, reappear, and continually change. A psychological cause for these fantasies was not obvious. Their presence would ordinarily indicate severe psychopathology, but there were no other indications that this boy was psychotic or obsessive-compulsive. The "fog states" were more frequent on higher doses of medication and disappeared after withdrawal of the medication. The exact extent and relationship of these "fog states" and "fixated ideas" to neuroleptics and Tourette's disorder is unclear.

Paranoid States

Approximately five patients, all intact psychosocially, had "paranoid states" while on low dosages of both haloperidol and pimozide. A 30-year-old accountant described sporadic episodes of paranoid feelings which occurred every 1 to

3 months and did not have obvious precipitants. He felt that strangers or his employer were looking at him, frequently accompanied by a foreboding of danger. He would try consciously to rid himself of these thoughts because he knew they were unreal. He could rid himself of the thoughts only by going to sleep for several hours, or by using diazepam, 5 to 10 mg, to help him sleep. On awakening the paranoid feelings were gone. Both haloperidol and pimozide, at dosages from 3 to 6 mg/day, caused these episodes and they never occurred when not on medication. Gradual titration of clonazepam to 4 mg/day controlled tics adequately and did not result in these paranoid feelings.

Four other patients had similar histories. We have no explanation for these symptoms which occur very infrequently. The characteristics, which we have not observed in other patients treated with neuroleptics, usually for schizophrenia, appear to be different clinically from paranoid symptoms in general psychiatric patients.

The possible existence of neuroleptic-induced fog or paranoid states should be documented and studied in a larger number of patients. They are described to alert clinicians to their existence.

Teratogenicity

Most studies of the teratogenic potential of neuroleptics in humans report few if any birth defects associated with antipsychotic drug use during pregnancy. However, reanalysis of a large epidemiological study by Edlund and Craig (1984) reported a possible increase in birth defects among children whose mothers first took phenothiazenes during the sixth to ninth gestation week. Since the patient population was psychotic women, the dosage level necessary to control the psychosis may have been higher than commonly used in Tourette's disorder and thus may have increased the risk of birth defects. The authors recommend that neuroleptics be avoided during the fourth to tenth week after fertilization.

A general recommendation is to avoid the use of neuroleptics prior to fertilization and throughout pregnancy, if possible. Until sound data are available this appears to be a prudent decision. We have had experience with six women who discontinued haloperidol during their pregnancy. The symptoms decreased markedly in three, moderately in two, and increased in an unmarried woman who had many other anxieties. If treatment cannot be avoided during the total time of the pregnancy, neuroleptics should be avoided between the fourth to tenth week.

Miscellaneous

Possible complications for some of the antipsychotic drugs, but unlikely or not reported for haloperidol, include hypothermia and unexpected deaths from asphyxia during a seizure, ventricular fibrillation, or respiratory or vascular collapse (Risch et al., 1981; Fayer, 1986), jaundice or blood dyscrasias (Cunningham et al., 1968; Winsberg and Yepes, 1978).

Laboratory Testing

Jaundice and agranulocytosis occur infrequently, especially with the use of haloperidol. For phenothiazine drugs, jaundice usually occurs in the first 5 weeks of treatment and agranulocytosis in the fourth to tenth week of treatment. Agranulocytosis cannot be anticipated by serial blood counts and is usually diagnosed by the sudden appearance of a high fever and an overwhelming, usually oral or pharyngeal, infection caused by a precipitous drop in the WBC. It is important to stop medication immediately because the mortality increases to 40% with continued use. The jaundice is usually benign, and patients recover whether or not the medication is continued. Most experienced clinicians do not recommend weekly or routine blood determinations, but use them only with the appearance of the clinical symptoms suggesting or associated with these adverse effects. If agranulocytosis is suspected, a WBC and differential count should be obtained. Prodromal symptoms for hepatitis include malaise, fever, and flu-like symptoms, which may develop into a yellow color of the sclera and skin. Laboratory tests for hepatitis might include bilirubin, serum glutamate pyruvate transaminase (SGPT), serum glutamate oxalocetate transaminase (SGOT), and alkaline phosphatase.

Use of Anticholinergic Medication for Adverse Effects

Anticholinergic medication such as benztropine mesylate are useful for EPS adverse effects. Clinical experience and evidence indicate that initial prophylaxis with anticholinergics prevents acute dystonia, acute akinesia, and significantly reduces the occurrence of other EPSs (Keepers et al., 1983). Anticholinergics generally have a long half-life, are usually excreted after 24 hr and can be administered once a day at bedtime. The effective dosage for mild EPS ranges from 1 to 3 mg/day, but the dose can be increased to 6 mg/day until EPSs are controlled, or anticholinergic adverse effects occur, such as xerostomia, mydriasis, blurred vision, or constipation, without benefit on EPS symptoms. The dosage should be decreased 0.5 to 1 mg/day to the minimal effective dosage if anticholinergic adverse effects occur, or omitted entirely if there is no beneficial effect. Anticholinergics are usually more effective early in treatment, and usually can be discontinued after 3 to 8 months of chronic treatment.

Although we routinely use benztropine mesylate to control anticholinergic adverse effects, other antiparkinsonian agents are probably equally effective. We found amantadine to be ineffective in many of our patients, although it has been reported to be more effective for haloperidol-induced adverse effects than benztropine mesylate in a single-blind cross-over study (Borison et al., 1983).

Control of Adverse Effects by Reducing Dosage

The dosage of haloperidol should be reduced by 0.25 mg every 5 to 7 days until adverse effects decrease or disappear if the patient experiences mild interference with academic, occupational, or psychosocial functioning. If adverse effects become severe, the dosage is halved immediately, i.e., a dosage of 6 mg/day is lowered to 3 mg/day or even less. After adverse effects disappear, usually after 7 days (range 4 to 14 days), dosage can be increased slowly, 1 mg/day every 1 to 4 weeks, until adequate symptomatic control is achieved.

Stimulants to Control Adverse Effects

The rationale for our use of stimulants to treat patients who have both Tourette's disorder and attention deficit disorder with hyperactivity (ADD+H) and to counteract the adverse effects of neuroleptic-induced adverse effects is discussed in Chapter 11. In this section we describe the use of stimulants to treat TS+ADD+H and to manage stimulant-induced adverse effects.

Stimulants have been used successfully by us to counteract the akinesic adverse effects of neuroleptics such as lethargy, dysphoria, depression, impaired cognition, and motivation. The occasional use of small dosages of stimulant drugs is illustrated in the treatment of one of our patients. A 6-foot, husky, male stockbroker achieved 90% decrease of symptoms at a dosage of 2 mg/day of haloperidol, but did not feel inclined to and often did not answer his phone, which was an integral part of his job. Libido was also decreased. An antiparkinsonian drug helped, but not enough. The dosage of haloperidol was lowered to 1.75 mg, to which 5 mg/day of methylphenidate was added, with 75% decrease in symptoms and return to normal functioning. Normal functioning was sustained with an increase in dosage of haloperidol to 1.85 mg and continuation of methylphenidate, with a decrease in symptoms of 80%. After 1 year the dosage of haloperidol was increased to 2 mg/day and methylphenidate was increased to 7.5 mg/day, with 95% decrease of symptoms. One year later methylphenidate was discontinued. Improvement has been maintained at 95%, without adverse effects, for the last 5 years. This case illustrates a major principle of treatment, that is, constant, sensitive, and subtle titration of the dosage so that maximum relief of symptoms can be achieved with minimal discomfort from adverse effects. Similar beneficial effects of stimulants have been reported for schizophrenic patients who were impaired psychosocially by the akinesic effects of neuroleptics (Ayd, 1964).

In our experience stimulants may increase, have no effect on, or decrease tics in approximately one-third of patients, respectively. Similar observations have been made by others (Comings and Comings, 1984; Erenberg et al., 1985; Butler, 1985). Although tics may increase in susceptible patients, especially if higher dosages are used, the increase is short-lived and the potential benefits of stimulants often outweigh their disadvantages. We have successfully treated many patients with a combination of haloperidol and stimulants, and consider them to be necessary agents for the treatment and management of children with Tourette's disorder and clinically significant hyperactivity. Some of these conclusions are supported by a statement in the proposed revision of the American Psychiatric Association Diagnostic and Statistical Manual of Mental Disorders: "In many cases the severity of Tourette's disorder may be exacerbated by administration of CNS stimulants, which may be a dose-related phenomenon" (DSM-III-R, 1987).

Methylphenidate is given at an initial dosage of 2.5 mg on awakening and subsequently titrated in daily increments of 2.5 mg/day, in divided dosages, to a dosage that varies between 5 to 40 mg/day. The results are often dramatic. If tics increase, they readily subside within 8 hr after reduction of dosage. An added benefit is decreased appetite and loss of weight. Other stimulants, such as dextroamphetamine or pemoline, can also be used. Pemoline, a long-lasting stimulant, can be administered once daily, and titrated up or down at weekly intervals, the dosage varying between 18.75 to 150 mg/day.

PIMOZIDE

Pimozide, a diphenylbutylpiperidine, was approved by the Food and Drug Administration (FDA) for use in the treatment of Tourette's disorder in 1984. Clinical data reviewed in Chapter 11 suggest that it is a potentially useful medication for Tourette's disorder.

The FDA cautions that pimozide should not be the first drug used to treat Tourette patients and its use should be limited to severely afflicted patients who fail to respond to standard medication. Dosage should not exceed 20 mg/day or 0.3 mg/kg and patients are required to have initial and periodic electrocardiograms during dosage titration. The dosage ratio is estimated as 2 to 4 mg of pimozide to 1 mg of haloperidol.

For most children and adults the starting dosage is 1 mg pimozide at bedtime. Dosage is increased 1 mg every 5 to 7 days until improvement is optimum with minimal adverse effects. We use benztropine mesylate 0.5 mg/day prophlyactically during initial treatment. Our average dosage was 7.0 mg/day (range 2–12 mg) in patients treated for 6 weeks. For patients treated for 1 year or more, dosage averaged 13 mg/day, although the most frequent dosage was 8 mg/day.

Adverse effects are similar to those reported for haloperidol. They include, in order of frequency: sedation, impaired motivation, interference with cognition, work or school performance, dysphoria or irritability, phobia, weight gain, dilated pupils or blurred near vision, slurred speech, dry mouth or salivation, gynecomastia or lactation, akathesia, and decreased libido. The first five adverse effects were reported to be less severe in patients treated with pimozide compared with haloperidol in our uncontrolled study (Shapiro et al., 1984).

Pimozide may have an adverse effect on the cardiovascular status of patients treated with this agent. Two sudden deaths possibly due to cardiac arrest were reported in a national collaborative acute study of pimozide in schizophrenic patients whose dosage was increased to 80 mg in 2 weeks. These deaths probably prompted the FDA to restrict dosage, limit its use to patients who failed on other medications, and to recommend initial and periodic ECGs. However, only one patient in over 200 treated by us with pimozide had a clinically significant cardiovascular change or abnormal electrocardiogram (ECG). A 12-year-old boy developed nonspecific T-wave changes on a daily dosage of 14 mg, and U waves, and diphasic and inverted T waves when rechallenged at a dosage of 8 mg. The ECG in both instances reverted to normal within a week after medication was discontinued. Prolongation of the Q-T_c interval and other ECG changes cited in the *Physician's Desk Reference* (PDR) for pimozide are similar to reports for other neuroleptics (PDR, 1986). In our double-blind study, currently in progress, we reviewed the ECGs for the first 42 patients at baseline, midpoint, and endpoint while on placebo, haloperidol, and pimozide. There were no clinicallly significant ECG changes, although the Q-T_c interval was significantly prolonged by pimozide, but not by haloperidol or placebo. The differential effect on the Q-T_c interval may be related to the fact that pimozide and other diphenylbutylpiperidines have calcium channel blocking properties but butyrophenones do not. Impeding the influx of calcium delays cardiac repolarization, thereby increasing the Q-T_c interval. The increase in the Q-T_c interval was always within 25% of base-line values and occurred within 3 weeks of starting treatment. These preliminary results indicate that periodic ECG monitoring may be unnecessary for Tourette's disorder patients without histories of cardiac disease or prolonged Q-T_c intervals, and if the dose is titrated gradually to a maximum of 20 mg/day or 0.3 mg/kg/day. However, further study of all neuroleptics is warranted, using 24 hr ECG monitoring and especially after glucose loads, which are associated with T-wave changes during neuroleptic treatment (Chouinard and Annable, 1977). Since an ECG at baseline and unspecified subsequent ECGs are recommended in the PDR, some clinicians may opt to monitor treatment with ECGs. The following conservative guidelines are suggested: Patients with Q-T_c intervals above 0.44 sec should not be treated except after approval by a cardiac consultant. If a T-wave alteration (except T-wave inversion) occurs, the dose should not be increased; ECGs should be repeated and the patient should be closely observed. If during treatment the Q-T_c interval exceeds 25% of base line or 0.47 sec in children and

0.52 seconds in adults, or if other T-wave alterations occur, the dose should be reduced until repeated ECGs are normal. If U-wave or T-wave inversion is observed, or cardiac arrhythmia develops, pimozide should be discontinued and ECGs should be repeated until normal. If bradycardia (less than 50 beats/min) occurs, the dose should be reduced until the pulse is normal.

The recommendations for the management of adverse effects are similar to those outlined for haloperidol.

OTHER DRUGS

Penfluridol

Penfluridol is no longer available for use in the United States but is available in Europe. The indications for treatment and management of adverse effects are similar to haloperidol. Penfluridol has a longer half-life than haloperidol and differs in dosage ratio and frequency of administration.

Penfluridol is administered daily or once every 3 to 7 days, at an initial dose of 10 mg. Dosage is increased usually in 10-mg increments every 3 to 7 days to the point of maximum benefit and minimal adverse effects. At that point the total dosage for the preceding week can be given weekly or in divided doses during the week. After chronic use, dosage can administered at intervals of 2 to 4 weeks. The median weekly dosage is approximately 40 mg with a range of 20 to 140 mg. Adverse effects disappear and clinical symptoms return 1 to 6 weeks after penfluridol is withdrawn because of its long half-life. Adverse effects are similar to those experienced with haloperidol except for less severe akinesic type effects. Management of adverse effects should follow those outlined for haloperidol.

Fluphenazine

The starting dose for fluphenazine is 0.25 to 0.5 mg/day. Dosage is titrated every 5 days to maximum benefit and minimum adverse effects. The usual endpoint dose is 7 mg/day with a range of 2 to 15 mg/day. Management of adverse effects are similar to those proposed for haloperidol.

Clonidine

The dosage of clonidine should be increased slowly to avoid sedative and hypotensive adverse effects. The beginning dose is 0.05 mg/day for 1 week and increased by the same amount until optimum response is achieved. The drug is eliminated in approximately 4 hrs, thus divided doses b.i.d. or q.i.d.

are necessary during waking hours. Endpoint dosage is usually achieved in 6 weeks and a beneficial effect should occur by 3 months.

The usual average total daily dose is 0.25 mg, with a range of 0.1 to 0.4 mg (Cohen et al., 1980; Shapiro et al., 1983c). Adverse effects are infrequent and are linearly associated with dosage. They can easily be managed by dosage reduction and usually disappear in 3 to 4 hr. Sedation, one of the most frequent adverse effects, usually abates after several weeks.

The adverse effects include, in order of frequency: sedation, light-headedness, dizziness or lowered blood pressure, impaired cognition, xerostomia, dry mouth, irritability, excitement, and, less frequently, loss of facial expression, disturbed sleep, weight gain, anorexia, headache, and sensation of body coldness.

Clonazepan

The initial dose for clonazepan is 0.5 mg/day and increased by the same amount every 2 to 5 days. Clonazepan is administered in divided dosages b.i.d or t.i.d. or at bedtime. The average endpoint dose is 5.0 mg/day with a range of 2 to 15 mg/day. To minimize adverse effects, which are similar to those of other antianxiety-sedative-hypnotic drugs, bedtime administration may be helpful. The major limitation to the use of this class of drugs is sedation and the development of tolerance and addiction.

Table 12.1 summarizes the doses for frequently used medications.

Conclusion

Clinical studies and experience indicate that neuroleptics such as haloperidol, pimozide, penfluridol, and fluphenazine are the most effective drugs for the treatment of tics and Tourette's disorder. Each of these drugs has helped

TABLE 12.1. *Dosages for drugs frequently used in the treatment of Tourette's disorder*

Drug	Usual administration	Initial dosage	Usual total daily dosage	Usual dosage range
Haloperidol[a]	h.s.	0.25	5.0	1.5–10.0
Pimozide[a]	h.s.	0.5–1.0	7.5	1.5–30.0
Penfluridol[a,b]	h.s.[b]	10.0	40.0	20–40
Fluphenazine[a]	h.s.	0.25–0.5	7.0	2–15
Clonidine	b.i.d.-q.i.d.	0.05	0.25	0.1–0.4
Clonazepam	t.i.d.-h.s.	0.5	5.0	2–15

[a]Benztropine mesylate, 0.5 mg/day HS, used initially and usually for 3 to 8 months.
[b]Administered daily or every 3 to 7 days.

some patients who fail on other drugs. The effect of clonidine and clonazepam is less predictable. The use of metoclopromide, oral physostigmine, and, possibly, tetrabenazine warrant further evaluation. Although there are several drugs, in contrast to the past, that can help patients with tic disorders, more effective medications, with fewer adverse effects and greater ease of use by nonspecialists are necessary.

PSYCHOTHERAPY OR COUNSELING FOR ASSOCIATED BEHAVIORAL PROBLEMS

Despite our conclusion that psychiatric and psychopathological factors are not intrinsic or etiological to tics or Tourette's disorder, some patients with Tourette's disorder have coexisting behavioral difficulties that require psychotherapeutic, counseling, academic, or vocational interventions (Shapiro et al., 1978; Shapiro et al., 1984; Cohen et al., 1982, 1983; Montgomery et al., 1982; Nee et al., 1982; Wilson et al., 1982; Comings and Comings, 1984; Young et al., 1985).

The behavioral difficulties may arise from several different sources. Epidemiological data (Weissman et al., 1978) indicates that a certain percentage of the population will have a mental disorder including patients with Tourette's disorder (Shapiro and Shapiro, 1981a). Thus, some patients with Tourette's disorder may have two disorders, i.e., Tourette's disorder with schizophrenia, manic-depressive illness, etc. At present there are no data indicating that the percentage of Tourette patients with another mental disorder exceeds population expectations. In fact our data indicates very low prevalence rates for other mental disorders in Tourette's disorder patients (see Chapter 6). If a mental disorder is diagnosed, treatment for the disorder should be integrated with treatment for Tourette's disorder. Remediation for behavior, vocational, and academic problems should be independent of the drug treatment.

A percentage of Tourette's disorder patients varying from 14% to 60% have an associated ADD, characterized by low frustration tolerance, attentional problems, hyperactivity, mood swings, impulsivity, and, in some patients, aggression and destructiveness (see Chapter 4). These behavioral problems should be treated vigorously for they often result in academic failure, poor peer and family relations, low self-esteem, and despair. Management requires careful evaluation with neuropsychological or academic testing, possibly behavioral treatment, counseling, and drugs (Shapiro et al., 1978, Shapiro and Shapiro, 1986; Cohen et al., 1983; Young et al., 1985). Other difficulties may arise from the inherent nature of having a neurological illness. Our studies have demonstrated that patients with Tourette's disorder and ADD+H have higher than expected indices of organic impairment (Shapiro et al., 1973, 1974, 1978; Sweet et al., 1973; Wayne et al., 1972). In addition, learning disabilities and specific neuropsychological deficits have been identified in some patients with Tourette's disorder (Shapiro and Shapiro, 1985b). They include speech and language problems (O'Quinn and Thompson, 1980; Ludlow et al., 1982); difficulty in mathematics, poor perceptual motor skills (Shapiro et al., 1978; Incagnoli and Kane, 1983; Joscho and Rourke, 1982); difficulty taking timed tests (Hagins et al., 1982); and poor handwriting. These deficits, however, may be related to the presence of ADD+H in the patient population (see Chapters 6 and 7).

When a child or adult is seen in initial consultation, the parents are asked to supply us with neurological, EEG, school records, psychological tests, and past treatment evaluations. These data are added to the information supplied by the parent or patient on our Movement Disorder Questionnaire and from the initial interview. If our evaluation indicates the existence of an associated problem, such as ADD+H or learning disabilities, we recommend specialized academic, educational, and vocational testing. If emotional problems are identified, psychiatric evaluation or counseling is suggested.

Academic and educational difficulties can be treated by tutoring and school placement. Suggestions for specific educational approaches include improving students' visual-manual skills, using the typewriter rather than pen for students with poor handwriting or the tape recorder instead of oral presentation, working in smaller groups, examining test performance to detect deficits and strengths, increasing time to take tests, helping the child by avoiding stressful experiences, and assessing the possible need for special school placement or services (Shapiro et al., 1978; Bauer and Shea, 1984, Hagens et al., 1982; Parker, 1985; Stefl and Rubin, 1985).

However, some of the problems faced by patients growing up with a chronic illness fall into the category of "coping" rather than psychopathology (Shapiro and Shapiro 1981c, 1983). Denial or acceptance of the symptoms is rooted in many factors. Frequently, children get upset and feel disparaged and scapegoated when parents describe their behavior during intake. Other patients enter into an intelligent discussion of their symptoms including possible precipitating factors, methods of control they have used successfully, problems that arise because of the symptoms when they are with others, etc. These coping methods appear to be rooted in the personality of the child, as well as in the way parents respond to the symptoms, either by acceptance or by shaming the child, or by being unable to protect the child from others. Certainly a thorough discussion of the symptomatology, causes of exacerbation, the involuntary nature of many of the symptoms, and the need for acceptance often helps the parents understand the nature of the illness and steadies the dynamics within the family. Children, too, need the opportunity to explore the range of their symptoms and to identify the factors that may contribute to their exacerbation and decrease. "Rap sessions" or group therapy may provide clues to management and avenues of acceptance (Shapiro et al., 1978; Parker, 1985).

Although our primary modality is drug treatment for the tic symptoms, and our primary emphasis during treatment sessions is dosage titration and management of adverse effects, we also discuss, family, behavioral, and academic problems. While this may not be considered "formal" psychotherapy, we attempt to help the patient develop coping mechanisms and alternative behaviors.

Recommendations to Parents

Although Tourette's disorder imposes similar problems on all patients, patients react to their illness according to their personalities, background, intelligence, assets, adaptability, and the degree of support and acceptance provided by the family. Problems common to parents of children with Tourette's disorder merit discussion.

An invariable question after the diagnosis of Tourette's disorder is made is: How much control does the child actually have over his symptoms? Although all patients can diminish or control their symptoms, the ability varies and is related to the social situation and the severity of symptoms. A dramatic decrease of symptoms often occurs in the doctor's office. A child who is ordinarily in almost constant motion, making movements and noises, sits perfectly quietly so that the doctor cannot see the symptoms. Parents who would like the doctor to know what they are going through at home will plead with the child to "behave normally" or even imitate the symptoms, but the child may minimize the gravity of his symptoms, sometimes even flatly denying that they exist. The discussion of control usually brings up several related questions: Why are the symptoms so much more pronounced when the patient is at home with the parents than in other environments? If the child can control the symptoms, how can this be truly a neurological condition? And should the parents punish the child to help control the symptoms? Although Tourette's disorder patients have considerable ability to lessen, disguise, or control the symptoms in public, eventually there must be a release of the tension in manifest symptoms. Quite naturally, this occurs at home when the child is most relaxed. Punishment will accomplish nothing except to make the child miserable and the parents guilty. Patients try valiantly to control the symptoms especially if they elicit negative psychosocial comments.

At one time or another most parents have punished or scolded their children for symptoms that could not be helped. After Tourette's disorder is diagnosed and the parents realize that this is a "real illness," they feel guilty and try to make up for their behavior by becoming too lenient and permissive. They may then become confused about what part of the child's behavior is or is not related to Tourette's disorder. If the child is nasty, throws tantrums, shouts profanities, and behaves inappropriately, they are not sure if this is Tourette behavior and may excuse it if they think it is part of the disorder. The child, ready to take advantage of the situation, as all children are, will start "getting away with murder" at home. The parents are soon faced with a spoiled and tyrannical child who secretly despises the parents for tolerating the behavior. Parents, on the other hand, begin to hate their child, who is now ruining their family life; a vicious circle of anger, guilt, and manipulation is set up, which may take years to untangle. A consequence may be that the child is shielded from contact with people outside of the home who may ridicule or mistreat him. He is allowed to make excuses not to go to school or do his homework, and so on. Expectations are generally lowered and less effort is made to encourage the child to live an ordinary life. To shield the child from further stress, the parents may become overprotective and indulgent, creating an atmosphere that encourages regression and isolation. This problem, of varying gravity, is occasionally encountered in the treatment of Tourette patients and their families.

To minimize these secondary effects, parents should be helped to realize that this is an illness, like any other illness, and is not something to be ashamed of. They should resolve their ambivalence about the disorder. A child will be unable to accept his illness realistically until his family is able to do so. The clearest guide for behavioral management is to remember that the specific symptoms of Tourette's disorder are involuntary movements, noises, and words. The behavior as a whole must then be evaluated, putting these symptoms aside. Parents should be instructed that children who are disagreeable, rude, uncooperative, and lazy should be dealt with like any other child showing these traits, and no special excuses for this behavior should be made. Also, parents should expect children to do as well in school as their intelligence and capabilities permit, and they should not be allowed to stop trying because of Tourette's disorder. Of course, a child who is not well controlled on medicine or with persistent tics is functioning with a handicap. To the extent that a child can learn to deal with the symptoms and not be ashamed of or overly preoccupied with them, he can work and socialize effectively. Samuel Johnson (McHenry, 1967), is the most notable example of a successful adaptation to life despite the liability of Tourette's disorder. It is striking how well many patients, even with obvious and severe symptoms, can adjust successfully. It is therefore essential not to allow the child to become emotionally crippled and to "cop out on life."

We strongly recommend that children be informed about Tourette's disorder to the extent that is possible to do so, based on their age. Response to treatment and the possible occurrence of adverse effects should be solicited and heeded. As they grow older, children should take increased responsibility for monitoring the dosage of medication. The previously described adverse effects, especially cognitive impairment, should be carefully and continuously evaluated. Unless marked control of symptoms can be achieved readily at a low dosage, it is essential that initial treatment be managed by a physician, with special competence in psychochemotherapy and, preferably, experience with Tourette's disorder. The subsequent course of treatment, optimally every 3 to 6 months, should be reviewed to insure proper management and maximum effectiveness of treatment.

CONCLUSION

The recommendations in this chapter about the treatment and management of patients with tic or Tourette's disorder disorders are based on 31 years of experience teaching psychopharmacology and treating general psychiatric patients in private practice, 22 years of experience treating tic and Tourette's disorder disorders, and thorough knowledge of published research. These recommendations represent the current "state of the art" treatment of Tourette's disorder. They are not cast in stone and obviously will be modified with additional experience based on the results of controlled studies. During the past 22 years, a major hazard has been the continued publication of very preliminary case studies, or worse yet, poorly or pseudo-controlled studies, leading to the premature use of ineffective medications and recommendations about management and treatment, some of which may be harmful to patients. The most notable examples, in our opinion, include the alarm about the use of stimulants, the extensive use of many ineffective drugs that have not been adequately tested with double-blind methodology, and the premature labeling of Tourette's disorder patients as having behavior problems, obsessive compulsive disorder, and ADD. These dangers can be minimized by the reliance on controlled studies that utilize methodological safeguards (Shapiro, 1971, 1976b, 1978).

13

Measurement in Tic Disorders

The rapid, almost epidemic increase in the number of diagnosed patients and published studies has made the need for reliable and valid measurements, scales, and rating systems a major priority (consensus meeting of the Tourette Syndrome Association (TSA). They are necessary to minimize errors of measurement, ensure comparability of results, and solve differences of opinions about the interpretation of results.

In this chapter we review the literature on measurement in Tourette's disorder and describe our studies of the measurement of its severity, response to treatment, and cognitive impairment associated with neuroleptic treatment.

RELIABILITY AND VALIDITY OF MEASUREMENT IN TOURETTE'S DISORDER

The difficulties of developing reliable and valid measures of the signs, symptoms, clinical course, and response to treatment in tic disorders is reflected in the absence of definitive studies in the literature. We were aware of this problem when we conducted a preliminary study in 1972 of ten Tourette's disorder patients who were hospitalized for at least 30 days in the Clinical Research Center of Cornell University Medical Center in New York City. Patients were evaluated twice daily by nurses and once daily by a psychiatrist, neurologist, and psychologist. Ratings included the number of motor and vocal tics for 5 min, a linear global severity scale, and the Peg Board Test. We could not demonstrate adequate reliability or validity for any of the measures. Although we developed a severity of symptoms scale for Tourette's disorder, we did not empirically evaluate its usefulness (Shapiro et al., 1978).

Subsequently, we reported the results of a retrospective study of the clinical course and response to treatment of 80 consecutive patients who were treated between 1965 and 1973 for 0.5 to 8.5 years after their initial evaluation (Shapiro et al., 1978). Two measures of improvement were used, each completed by both patient and physician. The percent change of symptoms was a rating of the percent decrease (or increase or no change) of current symptoms compared to pretreatment base-line severity. The Severity Scale, a four-point scale which varied from mild to severe, incorporated various components of Tourette's disorder severity. The correlation coefficient between ratings of the percent change of symptoms and severity scale was 0.44 (df = 72), $p < 0.001$ for patients and 0.76 (df = 40), $p < 0.001$ for the physician. Of greater importance was the high level of agreement between the patient and physician, $r = 0.82$ (df = 42), $p < 0.001$ for the Severity Scale, and 0.94 (df = 40), $p < 0.001$ for the percent change of symptoms. A serious limitation of this study was the absence of blind independent ratings and the possible influence of patient ratings on physician ratings.

Other clinical investigators utilized global scales and counts per minute of motor and vocal tics (Ross and Moldofsky, 1978; Feinberg and Carroll, 1979; Cohen et al., 1980; Wilson et al., 1982; Tanner et al., 1982). Limitations of these reports include small samples, inadequately described procedures, incomplete statistical analyses, unstandardized conditions, and inadequate empirical data to support the reliability and validity of the measures.

Recently, investigators at Yale developed the Tourette's Syndrome Global Scale (TSGS), a global scale for measurement of tic and behavioral symptoms associated with Tourette's disorder (Harcherik et al., 1984). An advantage of the TSGS was the attempt to define measures and ratings. The major limitations included use of a global scale based on the total score for disparate domains, not empirically derived, that included four types of tic groups, five categories for frequency of tics, five categories for disruptiveness of tics, and single items measuring behavior, motor restlessness, school and learning problems, and work and occupational functioning. Moreover, the reliability and validity analysis utilized unconventional procedures and was limited essentially to the data for six patients. Further development of the TSGS is in progress.

Our earlier studies identified some of the factors that contributed to the difficulty of developing rating scales for tics. The first factor is the difficulty of rating Tourette's disorder symptomatology because of the number of different symptoms affecting all parts of the body. In Chapter 5 we noted that there were 26 different simple and 54 complex motor tics, 77 sounds, 118 coprophilic symptoms, and nine echophilic symptoms. Seventy-seven percent of patients report from 11 to 60 different symptoms during the course of their illness. The second factor is that 97% of patients report spontaneous variation in symptom severity, 96% report spontaneous change in type of symptoms, and 27% report a total remission varying from 1 month to over 7 years. Diurnal and seasonal variables are a third factor. Symptoms decrease during the morning hours for 40% of patients, and in the summer for 19%. Lastly, situational variables can affect severity. Symptoms decrease with strangers or with the physician in 63% of patients, and in school or at work in 46%, but increase in 54% of patients when with the family, and in 92% when anxious. In addition, many patients have the capacity to substitute inconspicuous symptoms for conspicuous ones. These data suggested to us that situational stimuli and seasonal and diurnal conditions should be standardized in studies of measurement in Tourette's disorder.

To address those issues we evaluated the Shapiro Tourette Syndrome Severity (TS-Sev) Scale and a procedure for counting the number and severity of motor and vocal tics using videotape recordings of patients in three standardized stimulus conditions.

Procedures and Methods

The data for this study were derived from a controlled, double-blind crossover study of pimozide versus placebo in 20 patients with a DSM-III diagnosis of Tourette's disorder (Shapiro and Shapiro, 1984). Patients were evaluated at their initial visit, 2 weeks later after withdrawal from previous medication, and for six biweekly revisits while on pimozide or placebo. Dosages were flexibly titrated to maximum effectiveness and minimal adverse effects. All 20 patients completed the study. The dependent improvement variables included: ratings by the physician of the TS-Sev Scale, the Clinical Global Improvement Scale, and Physician Global Evaluation Scale; ratings by the patient of the percent decrease of tic symptoms and Patient Global Evaluation Scale; and ratings of judges of the TS-Sev Scale and frequency counts of tics from videotapes. Other details are reported elsewhere (Shapiro and Shapiro, 1984). A second aim of this study was to evaluate whether the TS-Sev Scale and videotape measures adequately measured Tourette's disorder severity.

Measures

Shapiro Tourette Syndrome Severity Scale

No one measure adequately reflects the severity of Tourette's disorder. Tic severity is influenced by the frequency, intensity, suddenness, type, and location of the tics, interference with the functioning of patients, and the ability to suppress or inhibit tics in various settings. Tourette's disorder severity is also affected by the sensitivity of patients to the tics and by the effect of the tics on other individuals. To encompass these factors we developed a composite rating of severity comprising five factors: the degree to which the tics are noticeable to others, whether they elicit comments or curiosity, whether other individuals consider the patient odd or bizarre, whether the tics interfere with functioning, and whether the patient is incapacitated, home-bound, or hospitalized because of the tics (Table A.2). The ratings for the five items are summed yielding a total sum of ratings that can be converted to a qualitative global severity rating based on the range of scores (in parenthesis) for each severity level (see the last column of Table A.2). The TS-Sev Scale was completed by the treating physician (A.K.S.) and by two judges from videotapes at base line and at each revisit. The TS-Sev Scale has been used in all of our drug studies (Shapiro et al., 1978, 1983a,b,c; Shapiro and Shapiro, 1984).

Videotape Ratings

We videotaped patients at each visit under three different stimulus conditions.

Computation condition

The computation condition was chosen to simulate motor activity for its potential effect on motor tics. Patients were asked to add a series of two numbers as rapidly and correctly as possible for 2.5 min.

Reading condition

The reading condition was selected to simulate vocal activity for its potential effect on vocal tics. Patients were asked to read three standard paragraphs used for the evaluation of reading and language disabilities for 2.5 min.

No-stimulus condition

The no-stimulus condition was designed to remove the inhibiting effect of an observer on symptoms. Patients were told to remain seated after the examiner left the room.

Raters

Raters were a senior Ph.D. psychologist (H. Gurfein, Ph.D.) who had experience with several patients with Tourette's disorder, and a third-year medical student (R. Dworken, M.D.) whose clinical experience was limited to observing 10 hr of videotapes of Tourette's disorder patients and 20 hr of observing the evaluation and treatment of patients at the Mount Sinai School of Medicine Tourette and Tic Laboratory and Clinic, New York City. The two raters discussed recording methods after observing 5 hr of sample tapes of Tourette's disorder patients. The first 12 patients were recorded serially on one tape. However, the raters had difficulty differentiating tics from adventitious movements, and had to observe the recordings many times before they felt confident about their counts and ratings. To simplify and shorten the procedure, the next eight patients were recorded on individual tapes. Once the target symptoms were identified by each judge in the initial session, ratings of subsequent sessions were expedited. Mean tic counts for the two procedures were not significantly different, and intraclass correlation coefficients for the judges were high for both procedures. Ratings were done blindly and independently by the two judges.

Rating of Dependent Measures

Judges' ratings

Tic counts. Tic counts were derived from observing each 2.5-min segment for the three stimulus conditions. Tic counts, expressed as number of tics per minute, were recorded for motor tics, vocal tics and a sum total of both motor and vocal tics under each condition, yielding nine potential scores. Ratings were summed across the three conditions, yielding a total number of motor tics, a total number of vocal tics, and a sum total of both motor and vocal tics.

TS-Sev Scale. The TS-Sev Scale was rated at each visit by the two judges from observation of the videotapes.

Physician ratings

TS-Sev Scale. The TS-Sev Scale was rated at each visit by the physician.

Clinical Global Improvement Scale. The Clinical Global Improvement Scale (CGI) evaluates medication in terms of therapeutic effects on a five-point scale and adverse effects on a four-point scale. The CGI was completed at each revisit after the initial evaluation.

Physician Global Evaluation Scale. The Physician Global Evaluation Scale rates improvement at endpoint after each 6-week treatment segments on a five-point scale.

Patient ratings

Percent decrease of tic symptoms. This measure, derived from the Shapiro Daily Record of Treatment (DROT) (Fig. A.1), is a daily estimate by the patient and family of the percent change for each motor, vocal, and other Tourette's disorder symptom and an overall percent decrease for all symptoms compared to base line. Also recorded each day on the DROT is the dosage of medication, type, and severity of adverse effects, use of other medications, and an overall percent decrease in tic symptoms.

Patient Global Evaluation Scale. The Patient Global Evaluation Scale, completed at home prior to return visits, rates improvement on a four-point scale at endpoint after each 6-week segment of treatment.

Statistical Methods

For each efficacy variable, an ANOVA procedure was used to compare pimozide and placebo according to the approach suggested by Grizzle (1965), and later modified by Grizzle (1974). Other statistical techniques included intraclass correlation coefficients (ricc), generalized Spearman Brown internal consistency reliability (ricr), product moment correlation (r), and t-tests for paired and independent groups. All tests were two-tailed except where specified. All measures and ratings were done at baseline after 2 weeks without medication and at the endpoint of the drug trial.

Results

The results describe the reliability and validity of three measures of initial severity of Tourette's disorder (judges' videotape counts and the TS-Sev Scale rated by judges and physician) at baseline (following a 2-week drug-free period), and for scales used to evaluate the effectiveness of pimozide compared to placebo at endpoint.

Motor and Vocal Tic Counts

Tic counts by the two judges at baseline and endpoint were highly reliable (Table 13.1). Mean counts by the judges of motor and vocal tics for the three conditions were not significantly different. Moreover, the intraclass correlation coefficients averaged 0.85 at baseline and 0.81 at endpoint, ranging from 0.72 to 0.97. Since tic counts were reliable, judges' scores were averaged and are used in subsequent discussion of the results.

Effect of stimulus condition on tic counts

Contrary to expectations, motor and vocal tic counts were not significantly different (repeated ANOVA) in the three stimulus conditions (Table 13.1). However, motor tics were significantly ($p < 0.0001$) more frequent than vocal tics. Moreover, counts of motor and vocal tics were uncorrelated during computation ($r = 0.25$), reading ($r = 0.04$), and no-stimuli ($r = 0.07$) conditions. Therefore, tic counts for the three stimuli conditions were averaged, yielding three variables, total motor tics, total vocal tics, and total motor and vocal tics, which are used in subsequent discussion of the results.

Reliability of the Tourette Syndrome Severity Scale

Rating of videotapes by judges

Judges reliably rated the TS-Sev Scale at baseline and endpoint (Table 13.2). Since the mean scores for the two judges were not significantly different

TABLE 13.1. *Interjudge reliability for ratings by judges at baseline and at endpoint*[a]

Videotape tic counts and ratings[b]	Judge 1 mean (SE)	Judge 2 mean (SE)	Paired t-test[c] t (p)	Intraclass correlation coefficient (ricc)
Base line				
Computation[d]				
Motor tics	9.6(1.9)	9.5(1.8)	0.2(NS)	0.92
Vocal tics	0.8(0.4)	0.8(0.4)	0.5(NS)	0.97
Motor and vocal tics	10.4(1.9)	10.2(1.8)	0.2(NS)	0.92
Reading[d]				
Motor tics	8.6(1.8)	9.1(1.7)	0.6(NS)	0.89
Vocal tics	1.1(0.5)	1.4(0.6)	0.8(NS)	0.72
Motor and vocal tics	9.7(1.9)	10.5(1.8)	0.9(NS)	0.87
No stimuli[d]				
Motor tics	8.7(1.6)	9.6(1.7)	0.8(NS)	0.77
Vocal tics	1.3(0.4)	1.1(0.4)	1.2(NS)	0.84
Motor and vocal tics	9.9(1.7)	10.6(1.7)	0.9(NS)	0.78
Total				
Motor tics	26.9(4.1)	28.2(4.2)	1.0(NS)	0.88
Vocal tics	3.2(1.1)	3.3(1.1)	0.1(NS)	0.86
Motor and vocal tics	30.1(4.2)	31.5(4.4)	0.5(NS)	0.90
Shapiro TS-Severity Scale	4.3(0.7)	4.5(0.8)	0.5(NS)	0.85
Endpoint				
Computation[d]				
Motor tics	5.3(1.5)	5.5(2.1)	1.3(NS)	0.96
Vocal tics	0.5(0.3)	0.4(0.4)	0.1(NS)	0.87
Motor and vocal tics	5.8(1.6)	5.9(1.7)	1.1(NS)	0.96
Reading[d]				
Motor tics	6.0(1.6)	7.2(1.1)	1.3(NS)	0.77
Vocal tics	0.5(0.2)	0.7(0.4)	0.6(NS)	0.76
Motor and vocal tics	6.5(1.7)	7.9(2.2)	2.1(NS)	0.79
No stimuli[d]				
Motor tics	5.6(1.2)	6.8(1.0)	1.1(NS)	0.64
Vocal tics	1.0(0.6)	0.7(0.4)	1.1(NS)	0.83
Motor and Vocal tics	6.6(1.4)	7.5(1.1)	0.3(NS)	0.73
Total				
Motor tics	16.8(3.5)	19.5(4.0)	1.8(NS)	0.86
Vocal tics	2.1(1.1)	1.8(0.8)	0.4(N)	0.88
Motor and vocal tics	18.9(4.1)	21.3(4.3)	2.1(NS)	0.87
Shapiro TS-Severity Scale	2.0(6.5)	2.1(0.6)	2.1(NS)	0.84

[a] $N = 20$.
[b] TS-Sev Scale at base line and pimozide endpoint.
[c] Two-tailed paired *t*-test; NS = not significant.
[d] Average number of tics per minute derived from 2.5 min of observation.

TABLE 13.2 Interjudge reliability for Shapiro TS-Severity Scale at baseline and at endpoint[a]

Variables	Judge 1 mean (SE)	Judge 2 mean (SE)	Judges 1 and 2 mean (SE)	Physician mean (SE)	Judge 1 vs. 2		Judges vs. physician		ricr[d]	
					t(p)[b]	ricc[c]	t(p)[b]	ricc[c]	Judges	Physician
Base line										
Tics noticeable to others	1.9 (0.2)	1.7 (0.2)	1.8 (0.2)	2.2 (0.2)	—	0.81	—	0.42	—	—
Tics elicit comments or curiosity	0.7 (0.1)	0.7 (0.1)	0.7 (0.1)	0.9 (0.1)	—	0.83	—	0.33	—	—
Patient considered odd or bizarre	0.9 (0.2)	1.1 (0.2)	1.0 (0.2)	0.9 (0.2)	—	0.73	—	0.69	—	—
Tics interfere with functioning	0.9 (0.2)	1.1 (0.2)	1.0 (0.2)	0.8 (0.2)	—	0.83	—	0.66	—	—
Total score	4.3 (0.6)	4.5 (0.7)	4.4 (0.7)	4.7 (0.5)	0.5 (NS)	0.85	0.6 (NS)	0.63	0.97	0.82
Endpoint										
Tics noticeable to others	1.0 (0.2)	0.8 (0.2)	0.9 (0.2)	0.9 (0.2)	—	0.83	—	0.43	—	—
Tics elicit comments or curiosity	0.4 (0.1)	0.4 (0.1)	0.4 (0.1)	0.2 (0.1)	—	0.89	—	0.52	—	—
Patient considered odd or bizarre	0.4 (0.1)	0.5 (0.2)	0.4 (0.1)	0.3 (0.1)	—	0.64	—	0.51	—	—
Tics interfere with functioning	0.3 (0.1)	0.4 (0.2)	0.4 (0.1)	0.2 (0.1)	—	0.61	—	0.41	—	—
Total score	2.0 (0.5)	2.1 (0.6)	2.1 (0.6)	1.5 (0.5)	0.5 (NS)	0.84	0.5 (NS)	0.53	0.96	0.92

[a] N = 20.
[b] t(p) = Two-tailed paired t-test.
[c] ricc = Intraclass correlation coefficient.
[d] ricr = Internal consistency reliability.

for the four items and total score, the intraclass correlation for the total score was 0.85 and 0.84, respectively, and the internal consistency reliability was 0.97 and 0.96, respectively; the average of the judges' ratings is used in the discussion of the results.

Clinical rating by physician

The internal consistency reliability of the TS-Sev Scale for the physician was 0.82 at baseline and 0.92 at endpoint, indicating reliability of this measure (Table 13.2).

Interrelationship of Videotape Tic Counts and Ratings of the Tourette Syndrome Severity Scale by Judges and Physicians

Table 13.3 summarizes selected reliability parameters at baseline and endpoint indicating that videotape tic counts and the TS-Sev Scale rated by judges and physician have high intraclass and internal consistency reliability.

Table 13.4 summarizes the interrelationship of tic counts and the TS-Sev Scale ratings by judges, and the TS-Sev Scale by the physician.

TABLE 13.3. *Summary of reliability scores for variables at baseline and at endpoint*[a]

Variables	Paired t-test[b]	Intraclass correlation coefficient	Internal consistency reliability[c]
Baseline			
Video tic counts			
Motor tics[d]	NS	0.88	0.81
Vocal tics[d]	NS	0.86	0.88
Total motor and vocal tics[d]	NS	0.90	0.75
Shapiro TS Severity Scale			
Judges[d]	NS	0.85	0.97
Physician	—	—	0.82
Judges vs. Physician	NS	0.63	—
Endpoint			
Video tic counts			
Motor tics[d]	NS	0.86	0.74
Vocal tics[d]	NS	0.88	0.86
Total motor and vocal tics[d]	NS	0.87	0.79
Shapiro TS-Severity Scale			
Judges[d]	NS	0.84	0.96
Physician	—	—	0.92
Judges vs. physician	NS	0.53	—

[a] $N = 20$.
[b] Paired *t*-test comparing means for judges; NS = not significant.
[c] Averaged ratings of judges.
[d] Judge 1 vs. judge 2.

TABLE 13.4. Summary of reliability data at baseline and endpoint[a]

Variables	Reliability	Reliability of both measures	Correlation between measures	Explained variance	Unexplained variance	Correlation of underlying true scores	Reliability difference scores
Baseline							
Judges' total motor and vocal tic counts[b]	0.75						
Judges' Shapiro TS-Severity Scale[b]	0.97	0.85	0.82	68%	17%	0.96	0.22
Judges' total motor and vocal tic counts[b]	0.75						
Physician Shapiro TS-Severity Scale[c]	0.82	0.78	0.54	29%	49%	0.69	0.53
Endpoint							
Judges' total motor and vocal tic counts[b]	0.87						
Judges' Shapiro TS-Severity Scale[b]	0.84	0.85	0.54	29%	56%	0.64	0.68
Judges' total motor and vocal tic counts[b]	0.87						
Physician Shapiro TS-Severity Scale[c]	0.92	0.89	0.72	52%	37%	0.81	0.63
Judges' Shapiro TS-Severity Scale[b]	0.84						
Physician Shapiro TS-Severity Scale[c]	0.92	0.88	0.67	45%	43%	0.76	0.64

[a]$N = 20$.
[b]Intraclass correlation coefficient.
[c]Internal consistency reliability.

At baseline, tic counts and TS-Sev ratings by judges correlated 0.82, accounting for 68% of the variance. The combined reliability of the two scales is 0.85; thus only 17% of the variability is not accounted for. However, ratings of the TS-Sev by the physician and judges correlated 0.65, accounting for approximately 42% of the variance. Since the combined reliability of the TS-Sev Scale rated by the physician and judges is 0.89, 47% of the variance is unexplained. Similarly, the combined reliability for the physician-rated TS-Sev and counts by judges of the total motor and vocal tics is 0.78, and with a correlation of 0.54 between the two measures, only 29% of the variance is accounted for, and 49% of the variance is not accounted for. Moreover, the lower intraclass correlation of 0.63 for ratings of the TS-Sev Scale by judges and physician (Table 13.3) indicates that judges and physician are rating severity somewhat differently.

Thus, although tic counts by judges are quantitative and have high reliability, only 42% of the variance of the physician-rated TS-Sev Scale is accounted for, leaving 41% unexplained. We concluded, therefore, that tic counts alone are not an adequate measure of severity. The explanation may be that physician-rated severity is based on multiple sources, including previous records, detailed clinical evaluation of the patient, and information obtained from family, whereas judge-rated severity is based on observation of videotapes and tic counts.

At endpoint, however, there is a reversal of the magnitude of explained and unexplained variance for two of the variable pairs (Table 13.4). The correlation between judges' tic counts and the TS-Sev Scale decreases from 0.82 at base line to 0.54 at endpoint, accounting for only 29% of the variance. The decreased correlation is either a chance occurrence, or the TS-Sev Scale and tic counts correlate less strongly when the number of tics and severity decrease with treatment. Correlations between judges' and physician's rating of the TS-Sev Scale at endpoint is 0.67, explaining 45% of the variance, with 43% unexplained. These results are similar to those obtained at base line, again indicating that judges' rating of TS-Sev Scale from videotapes is not useful.

Physician's rating of the TS-Sev Scale and judges' tic counts, however, correlate more strongly at endpoint (0.72) than at base line (0.54), explaining 52% of the variance at endpoint compared to 29% at base line. Again, the correlation may be fortuitous, or the physician's rating of the TS-Sev Scale and judges' tic counts are more highly correlated when the number of tics and severity decrease with treatment.

Test-Retest Reliability

Support for test-retest reliability is derived from the controlled study of pimozide versus placebo (Table 13.5). All patients had base-line ratings at

TABLE 13.5. Results of treatment with placebo and pimozide at endpoint[a]

Variables	Baseline evaluation mean (SE)	Endpoint Placebo[b] mean (SE)	Endpoint Pimozide[b] mean (SE)	Initial vs. placebo[c] p	Initial vs. pimozide[c] p	Placebo vs. pimozide[d] p
Judges' ratings						
Total motor tics	27.6 (4.2)	33.4 (3.8)	18.2 (3.7)	NS	0.001	0.0001
Total vocal tics	3.3 (1.1)	3.4 (1.0)	1.9 (0.9)	NS	0.005	0.0013
Total motor and vocal tics	30.8 (4.3)	36.8 (4.1)	20.1 (4.1)	NS	0.0005	0.0001
Shapiro TS Severity Scale	4.4 (0.7)	4.5 (0.6)	2.1 (0.6)	NS	0.0002	0.0001
Clinician ratings						
Shapiro TS Severity Scale	4.7 (0.5)	4.4 (0.6)	1.5 (0.5)	NS	0.0000	0.0001
Clinical Global Improvement Scale	4.7 (0.5)	3.6 (0.3)	2.2 (0.2)	—	—	0.0001
Physician Global Evaluation Scale	—	3.8 (0.2)	2.0 (0.2)	—	—	0.0001
Patient ratings						
Percent decrease of tic symptoms	—	15.5 (6.2)	59.1 (6.2)	—	—	0.0001
Patient Global Evaluation Scale	—	4.4 (0.3)	2.8 (0.3)	—	—	0.0001

[a] $N = 20$.
[b] Scores at endpoint.
[c] Two-tailed paired t-test.
[d] One-tailed t-test.

visit 2 and ratings after placebo. Mean differences for tic counts and the TS-Sev Scale ratings at baseline and after treatment with placebo were not significantly different. These results provide support for the test-retest reliability of judges' videotape counts of motor and vocal tics and the TS-Sev Scale rated by judges and physician.

Content Validity

The content selected for sampling was based on 20 years of collaborative experience of the two principal authors (E.S., A.K.S.). Previously we observed a marked increase of tics when patients were videotaped without an observer compared to with an observer present. However, in this study, the no-stimulus condition (videotaping alone) did not increase tics either at base line or endpoint. It is possible that we failed to simulate the "alone" or "no-stimulus" condition because patients were aware that they were being videotaped. In addition, the motor task did not increase motor tics, nor did the vocal task increase vocal tics. Patients responded similarly to all three experimental conditions (Table 13.1). Tic counts under these conditions may be a minimal estimate. Moreover, ratings of improvement at endpoint did not vary significantly for the type of tic (motor or vocal tics) or for setting (with close friends, with family, at home and alone, or in school, at work and with strangers) (Table 13.1 and 13.2). The findings may be partially explained by too brief a period of videotaping, the use of low doses of medication, and an acute rather than chronic treatment paradigm.

Construct Validity

Our expectations that severity would significantly decrease after treatment with pimozide and would not significantly change with placebo (Thorndike and Hagen, 1969) were confirmed (Table 13.5). Pimozide was significantly more effective than placebo on all dependent measures: 12 measures of motor and vocal tic counts by judges, the TS-Sev Scale rated by judges and physician, patients' ratings of percent decrease of tic symptoms and Global Evaluation Scale, and physician's rating of the Clinical Global Improvement Scale and Global Evaluation Scale (Table 13.5).

Interrelationships Among Dependent Variables

Several patterns are apparent among the nine dependent variables (Table 13.6). Patient variables tend to correlate more strongly with physician variables than with judges' tic counts. This may be explained as a halo effect because ratings by the physician are based on and influenced by observation of and reports by patients. However, the validity of the TS-Sev Scale rated by the physician is supported by its strong correlation with judges' tic counts (0.63–0.72) and with patient ratings (0.50–0.72) (Table 13.6). Although the evaluation of concurrent validity is limited by the absence of an externally validated criterion variable, concurrent validity for the physician-rated TS-Sev Scale is suggested by its consistently high correlations with all other dependent variables at endpoint (Table 13.6). It should be noted that judges' tic counts, TS-Sev Scale, Clinical Global Improvement, and percent decrease of tic symptoms largely reflect decrease of tics or improvement of symptoms. The influence of adverse effects on improvement is probably better reflected by the Patient and Physician Global Evaluation Scales. Adverse effects may have had a minimal impact, however, because the dosage of pimozide was carefully titrated and kept low to avoid adverse effects.

Discussion

A major difficulty in studies of the validity of Tourette's disorder severity at baseline and during treatment is the absence of an adequate external criterion. Although all of the measures used in this study have high reliability they have different types of validity.

Tic Counts

The frequency, intensity, type, and location of tics markedly vary among patients. Since tic counts measure only frequency and not severity or type of tic they may underestimate or overestimate the severity of Tourette symptoms. For example, if a patient has 30 slight eye tics and 30 low throat-clearing tics in 1 min, the total tic count would be 60 tics/min, whereas for another patient, with a disfiguring facial grimace and one loud barking tic, the total count would be 2 tics/min. Similarly, the type of tic is not accounted for in tic counts. Inconspicuous touching of objects would be rated at less severe compared to touching of genitalia, although both may yield a similar tic count. A just audible "fuh" tic would be a less severe symptom than a loud ejaculatory "fuck." We concluded, therefore, that while tic counts have limited validity as a measure of severity, they are a reliable and valid measure of change of symptoms during therapy.

The carefully controlled conditions, replication of ratings, and results for all seven visits (although only baseline and endpoint measures are described), and the high reliabilities of measurement make it unlikely that a larger sample would substantially increase the reliabilities. Nonetheless, replication on a larger sample, with more adequate statistical power for comparisons and with a range of Tourette's disorder severity from very mild to severe, is necessary.

TABLE 13.6. Intercorrelation matrix for variables at baseline and at endpoint[a]

Variables	Judges' videotape ratings				Clinician's ratings[b]			Patients' ratings	
	Total motor	Total vocal	Total motor and vocal	TS-Sev Scale[c]	TS-Sev Scale[c]	CGI[c]	GES[c]	Percent improved	GES[c]
Base line									
Judges' videotape ratings									
Total motor	(0.81)								
Total vocal tics	−0.06	(0.88)							
Total motor and vocal tics	0.96[d]	0.20	(0.75)						
TS-Sev Scale	0.72[d]	0.41[e]	0.82[d]	(0.97)					
Clinician's ratings	0.42[e]	0.50[f]	0.54[f]	0.65[g]	(0.82)				
Endpoint									
Judges' videotape ratings									
Total motor tics	(0.74)								
Total vocal tics	0.34	(0.86)							
Total motor and vocal tics	0.98[d]	0.53[f]	(0.79)						
TS-Sev Scale	0.50[f]	0.42[e]	0.54[f]	(0.96)					
Clinician's ratings									
TS-Sev Scale	0.64[g]	0.63[g]	0.72[d]	0.67[f]	(0.92)				
Clinical Global Improvement Scale (CGI)	0.34	0.30	0.38	0.29	0.70[d]	—			
Global Evaluation Scale (GES)	0.43[e]	0.40[e]	0.49[f]	0.49[f]	0.68[d]	0.81[d]	—		
Patients' ratings									
Percent decrease of tics	0.52[f]	0.40[e]	0.56[g]	0.36	0.72[d]	0.83[d]	0.71[d]	—	
Global Evaluation Scale (GES)	0.30	0.16	0.31	0.31	0.50[d] 0.61[g]		0.62[g]		—

[a] $N = 20$.
[b] Internal consistency reliability in parentheses in diagonals.
[c] TS-Sev Scale = Shapiro TS-Severity Scale; CGI = Clinical Global Improvement; GES = Global Evaluation Scale.
[d] $p < 0.001$.
[e] $p < 0.10$.
[f] $p < 0.05$.
[g] $p < 0.01$.

The optimum procedure in future studies would be to completely randomize the videotapes when rating them.

Others (Ludlow et al., 1982) have noted that raters routinely record random movements and noises when control samples are compared with Tourette patients. In this study judges had difficulty differentiating tics from random movements and vocal sounds. It may be helpful in future studies, therefore, for the clinician to specify the tics to be counted by the judges at the initial evaluation. Such a procedure was used by Ross and Moldofsky (1978) who reported an intraclass correlation of 0.99. This procedure would be less time-consuming and may increase reliability.

The results of a subsequent preliminary study suggest two other factors that may influence the reliability of videotaped tic counts. As part of a double-blind, cross-over study comparing haloperidol, pimozide, and placebo (study in progress), 17 patients were videotaped at initial evaluation. The tics to be counted by two judges were specified by two clinicians. The first judge, a Ph.D. psychologist with impulsive personality characteristics, who had observed very few Tourette's disorder patients, counted the number of motor and vocal tics occurring in the computation, reading, and alone conditions. The second rater, a psychologist working on a Ph.D. thesis, who has compulsive personality characteristics, had experience testing and counting tics for six to eight visits for 40 patients prior to rating the first 17 patients. T-tests comparing the ratings were not significicantly different for vocal tics, but the second rater counted significantly more motor tics than the first rater. A possible explanation is the different personality characteristics of the raters. The first rater tended to rate a simultaneous head, face, and nose tic as a single tic, whereas the second rater, in some cases when it was not clear that they were simultaneous, rated them as individual tics. These preliminary results suggest that it may be more difficult to reliably count motor tics than vocal tics. This may be due to the difficulty of differentiating between a single tic and a more complex tic and inadvertent movements, but vocal tics are more obvious in patients with Tourette's disorder than inadvertent vocal sounds are in normal subjects. Other possible reasons for the first rater counting less motor tics than the second rater may be due to having less experience counting tics and less contact with patients prior to the tic count.

These results suggest that the optimum conditions for reliable counts of the frequency of tics should include specification of the tics to be counted by clinicians prior to counts by judges, use of experienced judges, a preliminary period in which judges observe patients, conduct practice sessions and discuss the results, random rating of videotapes, no contact of judges with patients, videotaping during the same period of the day and at the same period of time during the patient's visit. Further study is required to determine the most parsimonious procedure for reliably counting tics from videotapes.

Tourette's Disorder Severity Scale

Although the TS-Sev Scale rated by both judges and the clinician have high reliability, judges' ratings have poor validity and are not a good measure of Tourette's disorder severity. Another limitation of this study was the use of internal consistency reliability for evaluating the reliability of the clinician's ratings. A more desirable procedure would be to use intraclass correlation between two independent clinicians. This limitation is offset, however, by the strong relationship of the TS-Sev Scale with dependent measures at endpoint.

Other possible methods of studying the reliability of the TS-Sev Scale have advantages and disadvantages. Ratings could be completed by the patient, members of their family, teachers, friends, etc. However, how patients react to their symptoms varies. Some patients tend to minimize and deny their symptoms and their impact on other individuals; others exaggerate the severity and effect of their symptoms on others. The same variation in response occurs with spouses, teachers, friends, and other informants. To partially control for these distortions, an experienced clinician should interview the patient, observe the symptoms, and use a second informant in addition to the patient, although ratings will be contaminated by and dependent on the patient's behavior and information generated.

Another potential source of variability for the TS-Sev Scale is rater experience. Additional empirical study is necessary to evaluate the reasonable assumption that experienced clinicians might rate Tourette's disorder severity more reliably and validly than inexperienced clinicians and laboratory assistants. This possibility is suggested by the borderline intraclass correlations of 0.63 at base line and 0.53 at endpoint between an experienced clinician (A.K.S.) and less experienced judges.

The TS-Sev Scale should include other important variables such as measures of the patient's subjective discomfort, interference with psychosocial functioning, and impairment of academic, vocational, or professional functioning. The addition of these three variables, using the Spearman Brown Prophecy formula, should increase the reliability from 0.77 to 0.89. In addition, these variables should be measured on a continuous scale with defined ratings varying from mild to severe.

A more comprehensive scale, more consistent with current psychometric principles (Nunnally, 1970), would include many more items identifying different aspects of Tourette's disorder severity, such as effect on school, work, vocational, coordination sports, and social, psychological, marital, and vocational or professional functioning. The scale should be administered to a random sample of at least five, optimum ten, patients per item, so that appropriate and reliable factors can be derived from factor analysis of the scale. A 17-item scale is now included in our Movement Disorder Questionnaire (MDQ) and will be evaluated in the future.

Despite the limitations of the physician-rated TS-Sev Scale, the data indicate that it is a reliable and valid measure of base-line initial severity of Tourette's disorder, and its consistent relationship with other variables at endpoint indicate that it is a reliable and valid measure of symptom change. A major advantage is its simplicity and ease of use.

Dependent Measures at Endpoint

The pattern of the correlations among dependent improvement variables at endpoint (Table 13.6) suggests the following heuristic considerations:

Motor and vocal tic counts, similar to baseline measures, are not significantly correlated. However, judges' counts of motor, vocal, and total motor and vocal tics, and their ratings of the TS-Sev Scale are correlated approximately equally with other dependent measures. It is apparent that the total motor and vocal tic count, which correlates slightly but not significantly with other dependent measures, is the best overall measure used by judges.

Physician- and patient-dependent variables tend to intercorrelate more strongly and consistently with each other than with judges' tic counts. Some of the common variance for the clinical measures may be due to halo effects of physician and patient measures, especially since physician ratings are dependent on patient reports, and physician attitudes may influence patient ratings. The data also indicate, however, that judges and clinical ratings share some but not all of the improvement variance. These measures should not be considered equivalent, therefore, and both should be used because they contribute different facets to measurement.

The pattern of intercorrelations also suggests that the TS-Sev Scale rated by the physician is the best overall measure because of its stronger and more consistent correlation with other dependent variables.

The higher correlations for total motor and vocal tics, the physician TS-Sev Scale and patient percent decrease of tic symptoms compared to the lower correlations of clinical global improvement, Physician Global Evaluation Scale, and Patient Global Evaluation Scale (Table 13.6) may indicate that the first set of variables primarily measures symptomatic improvement or decrease of symptoms, whereas the latter set measures both improvement of symptoms and the effect of adverse effects on total global improvement. This interpretation is supported by the higher intercorrelation within the two sets of variables (Table 13.6), although the difference between correlations was significant only for a comparison between ratings by the physician of the TS-Sev Scale and the Clinical Global Improvement Scale ($t = 2.7$, df = 18, $p < 0.02$) and Patient Global Evaluation Scale ($t = 2.44$, df = 18, $p < 0.03$).

Shapiro Global Improvement Scale

The previous results suggest that a measure incorporating symptomatic improvement and adverse effects should be used for rating improvement in drug studies of Tourette's disorder. Another compelling reason for using such a scale is that the dosages of effective drugs such as haloperidol and pimozide are close to the dosage that induce adverse effects. These drugs, at comparatively low dosages, almost always reduce tics. A major problem is the appearance of many adverse effects (Chapter 12) which are not well tolerated by patients with Tourette's disorder. Therefore, evaluation of therapeutic efficacy requires a measure of improvement that incorporates both therapeutic and adverse effects.

A proposed scale that integrates both therapeutic and adverse effects is the Shapiro Global Improvement Scale (GIS) (Table A.3). The therapeutic effect is rated on a seven-point scale: (5, complete or nearly complete remission of 90 to 100% of symptoms; 4, decided improvement, overall decrease of 70 to 89% of symptoms; 3, considerable improvement, overall decrease of 50 to 69% of symptoms; 2, some improvement, overall decrease of 30 to 49% of symptoms; 1, slight improvement, overall decrease of less than 30% of symptoms; 0, unchanged, no overall change of symptoms; −1, worse, overall increase of symptoms). Adverse effects are rated on a five-point scale: (0, none; 1, do not significantly interfere; 2, slightly interfere; 3, moderately interfere; 4, markedly interfere; 5, nullify therapeutic effect). Subtracting adverse effects from the therapeutic effect ratings yields a numerical rating for the overall therapeutic effect and a qualitative clinical description of the effect of therapy: (5, excellent; 4, marked; 3, moderate; 2, minimum; 1, poor; −1 to −6, worse). The reliability, validity, and clinical usefulness of this proposed integrated scale requires empirical study.

Measures of Psychopathology

As discussed in Chapter 6 the relationship between psychopathology and Tourette's disorder has not been demonstrated. Until the issue is resolved, an established scale measuring behavioral psychopathology which has evidence of reliability and validity, should be used.

Conclusions

The data of this study generated the following conclusions about the use of scales to measure Tourette's disorder severity and tics and suggestions for further research.

Severity of Tourette's Disorder

Counts of motor and vocal tics do not provide an adequate measure of the severity of Tourette's disorder. An adequate measure of severity requires an integrated assessment of the frequency, intensity, type, and location of tics, subjective distress, noticeability of or impact of tics on others, degree of curiosity by others and attitudes toward the patient as being odd or bizarre, and interference with the physical, psychosocial, academic, vocational, or occupational functioning of the patient.

Judges' Videotape Tic Counts

Videotape tic counts have high reliability, adequate validity, and the advantage of being quantitative and independent of other measures. Although our studies (Shapiro et al., 1978, 1983a,b,c; Shapiro and Shapiro, 1984) do not indicate that drugs differentially affect motor and vocal tics (only one methodologically complicated study has reported a differential effect of drugs on motor and vocal tics (Wilson et al., 1982), for heuristic purposes, motor, vocal, and total motor and vocal tic counts should be reported separately.

Contrary to our clinical experience, we found that tic counts did not vary significantly under the three stimulus conditions. We postulated that patients knew they were being videotaped and that the final tic counts were consistent with the number of tics that occur with strangers. The results suggest that the computation condition (adding simple numbers for a 2.5-min period) might provide a simple, adequate, and standardized condition for recording tic counts. It is possible that an even more simple and parsimonious method would be a tic count for random 3-min periods during the second half of the clinical interview. The setting and time of day should be held constant.

Shapiro TS-Severity Scale

The TS-Sev Scale (Table A.2) rated by judges and physician is highly reliable but only the ratings by the physician are valid. The validity of the TS-Sev Scale rated by the physician is demonstrated by the strong and consistent correlations with other dependent variables. The scale should be expanded to include measures of subjective or psychological distress, interference with psychosocial functioning, impairment of academic, vocational, or occupational functioning, and other relevant items. The TS-Sev Scale provides an overall index of severity or improvement, as well as data for assessing severity or improvement of individual parameters. An advantage of the TS-Sev Scale is simplicity of use. The TS-Sev Scale completed by the physician is dependent on and correlates with patient ratings since the ratings are based on clinical inquiry. It would be interesting, nonetheless, to explore the relationship of the TS-Sev Scale completed independently by both the physician and patient.

Global Improvement Scale

There is an heuristic and clinical need for a scale measuring symptom improvement and adverse effects separately and an overall effect integrating both for clinical purposes (Table A.3).

Measures of Psychopathology

Since there are no empirical data supporting the association of psychopathology with Tourette's disorder except in 25% of patients with attention deficit disorder (ADD), hyperactivity, (H) and learning disorders, measures of psychopathology should be rated separately on an established scale which has evidence for its reliability and validity.

Sample

These results are limited by the small sample size of 20 patients. This limitation is possibly offset by the carefully controlled matrix for this study and similar if not identical results for analyses for all visits (1 through 8). Nonetheless, the results should be replicated by other investigators.

EFFECT OF NEUROLEPTICS ON COGNITION

The study was stimulated by an unexpected rejection of a letter to the *Journal of the American Medical Association* (JAMA). The letter described our initial clinical studies in which haloperidol was titrated to high dosages similar to the treatment method used for the psychoses. Although the decrease of tics correlated with dosage, unfortunately so did adverse effects. Moreover, adverse effects occurred at a much lower dosage, unlike the effects reported in other disorders. One adverse effect was cognitive impairment, which was unrecognized at the time because cognitive impairment was not thought to be associated with neuroleptic use. The letter surprisingly was rejected with the usual vague editorial caveat about space limitations and that the findings were clinical. We requested further clarification of the rejection. We were informed that the public health implications were too important for publication as a letter, but that the JAMA would be happy to evaluate the suitability for publication of a carefully controlled study. Although the effectiveness of neuroleptic drugs for the treatment of tics and Tourette's disorder is well established (Shapiro and Shapiro, 1968, 1981, 1984; Bruun et al., 1976; Shapiro et al., 1978, 1981, 1983a,b), 12 years after our rejected letter the adverse effect on cognitive functioning is still largely unrecognized.

We were alerted to the possibility that haloperidol and other neuroleptics interfere with cognitive efficiency during our treatment of hundreds of Tourette patients (Shapiro et al., 1978). Parents reported that their children were not functioning as well as they had before treatment and that school grades had dropped. Adult patients reported that they were not thinking as well as they had before medication. One champion bridge player found that she could no longer play in tournaments. Patients could not identify what aspect of cognitive functioning was affected. Some reported interference with memory, other motivation, attention, or learning. Of particular significance was that the adverse cognitive effects occurred at low dosages of haloperidol, without obvious extrapyramidal signs. These effects persisted through many months of treatment and did not respond to antiparkinsonian agents. With dosage reduction or discontinuation of medication, functioning improved, usually within 2 weeks, or in a range of 4 to 30 days. Similar clinical observations have been reported by other investigators treating both children and adult patients with Tourette's disorder (Cohen et al., 1980; Hagins et al., 1982; O'Quinn and Thompson, 1980).

Review of the Literature

The literature on the cognitive effects of drug treatment revealed considerable variation for drug type, dosage, length of treatment, and test instruments. More important, the samples studied were for the most part patients hospitalized for severe behavior disorders or psychosis.

Seven studies reported an adverse effect on a variety of cognitive tasks (Cunningham et al., 1968; Werry and Aman, 1975; Goldstone and Lhamon, 1976; Helper et al., 1963; Sprague et al., 1970; McAndrew et al., 1972); two reported no adverse effects (Wong and Cock, 1971; Bogomolny et al., 1982); and two reported improved cognitive functioning (Spohn et al., 1977; Campbell et al., 1982). Cognitive impairment was reported more frequently with acute rather than chronic treatment and with high rather than low dosages of neuroleptic drugs.

Methodological problems associated with these studies include the use of samples with different diagnoses, different drugs, dosages, and length of treatment and the use of tests that are insensitive to drug effects, primarily laboratory measures with limited applicability to actual academic performance, and vocational functioning, and for which adequate reliability and validity have not been demonstrated.

Several of these studies provided support for the adverse effect of neuroleptic drugs on cognition in psychotic or schizophrenic hospitalized children or adults and children with learning or behavioral disorders (Cunningham et al., 1968; Werry and Aman, 1975; Helper et al., 1963; Sprague et al., 1970; McAndrew et al., 1972). However, the adverse effects of neuroleptics on cognitive functioning in a nonpsychotic outpatient sample, such as Tourette's disorder, have not been systematically studied. The two studies which evaluated the effect of haloperidol in patients with Tourette's disorder were nonblind, and used variable dosages and different cognitive tasks. Goldstone and Lhamon (1976) reported adverse effects on a time discrimination task in patients taking haloperidol in dosages which varied from 6 to 180 mg/day. Bogolomy et al. (1982), however, reported no adverse effects on higher cognitive processes and motor functioning in 16

Tourette patients treated with a mean dosage of 0.043 mg/kg/day of haloperidol compared to a nondrug condition. Although this study used a comprehensive battery of tests, many of the tests are not generally considered to be sensitive to drug effects. In addition, the mean dosage level was possibly too low to effectively demonstrate a potential negative effect. Patients with Tourette's disorder are nonpsychotic outpatients who are pursuing age-appropriate tasks in school or at work, many of whom require chronic medication. Drug-induced cognitive impairment can be a liability in these patients already burdened with a chronic illness, and may offset potential therapeutic benefit of treatment.

The present study evaluating the effect of pimozide on cognitive functioning was part of a drug study comparing the efficacy of pimozide to placebo in a cross-over, within subjects design, in patients with Tourette's disorder. The results of the drug study indicated that pimozide was significantly superior to placebo in reducing motor and vocal symptoms (Shapiro and Shapiro, 1984). Sixteen patients were rated as having marked to moderate improvement on pimozide compared to placebo, three had no symptomatic benefit, and one was rated as worse. Thus, 80% of patients were significantly improved on pimozide compared to placebo.

Methods

Subjects

Twenty subjects were included in the study: seven females and 13 males. All subjects were evaluated prior to a 2-week drug-free period by two raters, both of whom agreed about the diagnosis of Tourette's disorder and ADD based on DSM-III criteria American Psychiatric Association, 1980. Age of subjects ranged from 11 to 53 (mean 24.65, SD 12.14). Mean age of onset was 7.5 (SD 3.0). ADD or learning difficulties were present in four male subjects. Subjects or guardians signed an informed consent. The study was conducted in the private offices of the authors (E.S. and A.K.S.).

Procedure

The study was a double-blind cross-over (within subject) study comparing pimozide to placebo. The duration of treatment for each patient was 14 weeks with evaluations taking place every 2 weeks. The first 2 weeks consisted of a drug-free period followed by two 6-week periods during which patients randomly received either pimozide or placebo. Twelve patients received pimozide first and eight patients received placebo first. Patients were crossed over to the alternate drug without a drug-free period and treated for a second 6-week period. Cognitive testing was done at visit 2 following a 2-week drug-free period, at the end of the first 6-week drug period (visit 5), and at the end of the second 6-week drug period (visit 8). Testing of visit 2 (base line) was used to familiarize the subjects with the testing procedure, apparatus, and testing room. All testing was done by the same examiner (E.S.), who was not involved in the treatment of patients, and at the same time of day for each subject. These procedures minimized order effects.

All drugs were dispensed in identical capsules and unused medication was returned and counted at each revisit. Standardized drug dosages were not used since the primary purpose of this study was to evaluate the efficacy of pimozide to clinically suppress tic symptoms. The decision to flexibly titrate dosage was also based on our previous work with haloperidol in the treatment of Tourette's disorder (Shapiro et al., 1978). We found, that although dosage was highly correlated with blood level, there was no relationship to therapeutic response, adverse effects, age, sex, weight, chronicity of illness, or length of treatment (Shapiro and Shapiro, 1981a). The initial dosage was 1 mg at bedtime with the dosage increased 1 mg every 2 to 3 days to a potential maximum of 20 mg/day. If adverse side effects occurred, dosage was either reduced, held constant, or benztropine mesylate was added to the drug regimen. The average daily dosage of active medication at endpoint was 6.88 mg/day (SD 1.26). At endpoint, after 6 weeks of treatment, benztropine mesylate was used by 12 patients (60%) on pimozide at an average daily dosage of 1.7 mg/day, and by 7 patients (35%) on placebo.

Test Measures of Cognitive Functioning

Attention

The continuous performance task (CPT) used to measure attention was the Sunrise Systems Yankee I portable microcomputer apparatus (Kornetsky, 1972; Conners, 1972). Alphabetic characters are presented on a screen including a target stimulus X. The subject is instructed to depress a lever immediately when the target stimulus X appears, only if it is preceded by an A, and to refrain from responding if it is not. A dynamic pacing mode was used. This method adjusts the timing parameters every five critical stimuli by increasing or decreasing the interstimulus interval by one-sixteenth of its value depending on the number of late, correct, and omission errors over the last five critical stimuli. Subjects are instructed to maximize stimulus presentation. Test sessions comprised 449 trials. The subject's responses were automatically recorded by a microcomputer and scores were displayed on the face of the instrument. Attention was measured by the number of misses (OE: failure to press the lever at the right time) and the number of incorrects (CE: pressing the lever at the wrong time). Response time was measured by the number of late responses and the interstimulus interval.

Learning

The learning task used a paired associate learning paradigm (PAL) (Conners et al., 1964). The stimuli and instructions were prerecorded on a videotape and presented on a 10-inch video screen. The exposure time for each stimulus was 2 sec. This task required the subject to learn a series of nine pairs of digits from 1 through 9 and an associated symbol. The symbols were taken from the Digit Symbol Subtest of the Wechsler Intelligence Scale for Adults. Each symbol was randomly paired with a single number. The order of the presentation of each digit-symbol pair was randomized during each test session. The subject was initially shown all nine digit-symbol pairs and then each digit individually. The subject was required to recall the symbol paired with the individual digits. Subjects were given 16 trials to correctly recall the entire series of nine digits and symbols at least once. To minimize practice effects, different digit-symbol pairs were used for each test session. Dependent variables on this task are the number of errors and number of trials.

Memory

The Buschke Memory Task (BMT) paradigm was used to test memory (Buschke, 1973). The subjects were presented a list of 16 words in a single category at the rate of one word every 2 sec. Subjects were then given $2\frac{1}{2}$ min to recall the list in any order. On the second presentation subjects were reminded only of the words they failed to recall. This procedure is called selective reminding. Six trials were given to recall the words. To minimize practice effects, a different list was used for each test session. The dependent variable on this task is number of words correctly recalled.

Work Output

The Work Output Task (WOP) was used to measure accuracy and comprehension in copying written material (Wolraich et al., 1978). The paragraphs to be copied were age appropriate. The subjects copied a paragraph and then were asked three questions about the paragraph's content. To minimize practice effects different paragraphs and questions were used for each test session. The dependent variables on this task are the number of errors in copying and number of incorrect responses.

Statistical Methods

The data were first examined to determine whether the sequence of drug administration influenced the estimate of the drug effect. Two-tailed *t*-statistics comparing the responses for the two groups (D/P versus P/D) were used for this purpose, since both an increase or decrease in the drug effect with the sequence was of interest. In the case that a significant interaction is found, the drug effect needs to be analyzed separately for each group. Otherwise, if the effect of the drug does not vary significantly with the sequencing, the drug effect can be estimated pooling the data across the two groups. This was done using the method presented in Hills and Armitage (1979). One-sided tests were done here since the hypothesis of interest is that pimozide decreases cognitive functioning as measured by each of the dependent variables. A significance level of 0.01 was used to provide some compensation for multiple testing.

Results

Subjects performed somewhat worse on all of the tests when they were on pimozide compared to placebo, although significant differences were obtained on selected tests (Table 13.7). There were no significant interactions at the 0.01 level.

Attention

The expectation that the number of misses and incorrect responses would increase significantly with active medication was not supported.

TABLE 13.7. *Effect of drug and placebo on cognitive tests*[a]

Variables	Mean differences		Overall means		SE of Difference	$p =$
	Drug/ placebo	Placebo/ drug	Drug	Placebo		
Continuous Performance Task						
Attention						
Misses	0.583	0.750	4.458	3.79	0.485	0.0952
Incorrect	0.000	4.375	10.87	8.68	2.112	0.1573
Response time						
Late	2.000	1.000	6.229	4.729	0.530	0.0051
Interstimulus interval	3.660[b]	2.75	43.91	40.70	0.682	0.0001
Buschke Memory Task						
Memory						
Recall	0.333	−2.500	13.80	14.79	0.542	0.0302
Paired Associate Learning Task						
Learning						
Errors	−5.500	1.125	5.30	3.95	2.757	0.5477
Trials	−1.166	1.875	4.770	4.415	0.768	0.9201
Work Output Task						
Comprehension and accuracy						
Accuracy	−0.170	−0.125	3.58	3.729	1.290	0.7801
Errors	0.166	−0.625	0.729	0.9583	0.155	0.3284

[a] $N = 20$.
[b] ISI values are milliseconds.

Response Time

As hypothesized, the mean number of late responses significantly increased from 4.729 to 6.229 ($p = 0.005$) when patients were on pimozide compared to placebo. The interstimulus interval was also significantly longer on the drug, 43.91 compared with 40.70 on placebo, ($p = 0.0001$).

Learning

No significant differences were found in the number of errors or the number of trials when pimozide was compared to placebo.

Work Output

No significant differences were found when pimozide was compared to placebo for the number of copying errors and the number of response errors to paragraph meaning.

Memory

Although the t-test combining both drug/placebo and placebo/drug groups resulted in a p value of 0.03 when patients were on pimozide compared to placebo, the significance level did not reach our *a priori* criterion of $p = 0.01$. Because of a possible interaction effect, the effect of pimozide on recall was analyzed separately for each group (Table 13.8). The number of words correctly recalled for patients on active drug was significantly less ($p = 0.003$) than for those receiving placebo first, but not for the group receiving drug first. Although it is possible there may have been a carry-over effect of the drug in the drug/placebo group, the 6-week separation between period one and period two argues against such an explanation. It may be that word lists were not equivalent, although they were derived from categorized word lists. If a more difficult word list was used while patients in the placebo/drug were on drug and a less difficult word list when on placebo, it would result in attenuating the results.

TABLE 13.8. *t-test for effect of pimozide/placebo and placebo/pimozide on memory*

Group	Mean difference (Drug-placebo)	SE of Difference	$p =$
Drug/placebo	0.33	0.864	0.6646
Placebo/drug	−2.50	0.654	0.0032

Discussion

The results of this study indicate that pimozide compared to placebo has a significant depressant effect on some aspects of cognitive functioning and not on others. Pimozide appeared to cause a slowing of performance in the absence of impaired learning. The effect of pimozide on memory, although not significant for the total group, resulted in significant impairment ($p = 0.003$) in the group with only eight subjects.

These results are in agreement with others of the effect of medication on cognitive processes. Cunningham et al. (1968) reported a slowing of reaction time in subjects on 0.1 mg/kg haloperidol, Helper et al. (1963) obtained lower scores on a rote memory task during treatment with chlorpromazine and Sprague et al. (1970) noted increased decision time on a short-term memory task with thioridazine.

Although the results of this study are limited and the precise nature of the cognitive impairment remains elusive, several factors may account for the limited findings of this study in contrast to our clinical experience.

It is possible that a measurable decrease in accuracy (the number of omission errors and commission errors) as a function of taking pimozide would have appeared if the CPT were of longer duration. It is a relatively brief task, lasting about 5 min. In a work or classroom situation, task duration is longer, thus increasing the likelihood of a decline of sustained attention. Some support of this possibility is a study of learning in Tourette children, (Hagins et al., 1982), which demonstrated that children on haloperidol had difficulty sustaining responses over a long period of time.

It is also possible that significant decrements in attention, memory, and learning were not obtained because of the low dosages used in this study. Other studies using higher dosages than used in the present study obtained significant drug effects. Werry and Aman (1975) demonstrated that the higher dosage of haloperidol, 0.05 mg/kg a day compared to 0.025 mg/kg a day impaired attention in 24 hyperactive or unsocialized-aggressive children. Similarly, Goldstone and Lhamon (1976) found a significant impairment of temporal processing in Tourette patients treated with high dosages of haloperidol that ranged from 6 mg/day to 180 mg/day. Dosages of haloperidol that ranged from 0.04 to 0.21 mg/kg produced adverse effects on cognition in a study by Platt et al. (1984) of hospitalized aggressive children. In contrast, Bogomolny et al. (1982), using a lower mean dosage than used in the present study found no adverse effects of haloperidol on cognition.

We did not use fixed high or low dosages in the present study since the primary purpose was to find the appropriate therapeutic dosage that would control tic symptoms without adverse effects. The mean dosage of pimozide at endpoint was 6.88 mg/day, or 0.1 mg/kg/day, within the range we normally use to treat Tourette patients. The dosage equivalence of pimozide and haloperidol is approximately 3:1 (Shapiro et al., 1983a; Shapiro and Shapiro,

1984; Ross and Moldofsky, 1978). Thus, 0.1 mg/kg/day of pimozide is equivalent to 0.03 mg/kg of haloperidol, a lower dosage than was used in the studies demonstrating a depressive effect of medication on cognition.

Another factor that may have negatively affected our results is that the tasks were too simple. In a study of 12 emotionally underachieving boys treated with thioridazine, the number of stimuli presented had a significant effect on decreasing accuracy and increasing reaction time (Sprague et al., 1970).

Could the positive findings be explained by the use of anti-Parkinson drugs to control adverse effects of pimozide in some patients? A *post hoc* analysis was done to determine the effect of benztropine mesylate on CPT and the Buschke Memory Task. Eight subjects who received benztropine mesylate while on both pimozide and placebo were compared to seven subjects who did not receive benztropine mesylate under either treatment condition. Five subjects who received benztropine mesylate during only one segment of the study were not considered in the analysis. Repeated measures (ANOVA) revealed no significant interactions between the treatment effect and benztropine mesylate, nor was the drug a significant main effect for any of the response variables.

We also considered the possibility that the slowed performance was due to sedation or akinesia, a common adverse effect of neuroleptics early in treatment (Shapiro et al., 1978). To evaluate the possible effect of akinesia on the dependent variables for the CPT and the Buschke Memory Task, patients were classified into akinetic and nonakinetic groups. T-tests to determine the mean differences in the responses under pimozide showed no significant differences between the akinetic and nonakinetic groups. We concluded, therefore, that the results in this study were not merely due to sedation or akinesia.

Variables such as age, sex, duration of illness, severity of Tourette's disorder, and diagnosis of ADD, were unrelated to dependent variables since they were controlled for by tic within subject design.

With regard to short-term versus chronic treatment, 6 weeks on active medication may have been too brief. In addition, patients were started on a very low dosage and titrated very slowly to their final dosage at endpoint. Time on the final endpoint dosage may have been too brief for the appearance of more obvious effects. In contrast, clinical patients are maintained on medication for years. For example, in our chronic study of 31 Tourette's disorder patients, treatment averaged 2.8 years, range 0.7 to 5.2 years, the dosage of pimozide at endpoint averaged 13 mg/day with a range of 1 to 64 mg/day (Shapiro et al., 1983a).

Finally, laboratory measures may be insensitive to decreased cognitive functioning which is readily apparent clinically. Perhaps observation of school and work functioning, and reports by teachers or others, may be alternative approaches to obtain insight into the specific nature of the cognitive impairment that has been observed clinically.

Nevertheless, demonstrating a slower response time and a tendency to impaired recall at the low daily dosage of 6.88 mg (0.1 mg/kg) pimozide, equivalent to a daily dosage of 2.3 mg haloperidol, is noteworthy. The limited positive findings confirm our clinical impression that pimozide does adversely affect cognition. There is reason to believe that these results are not limited to pimozide but would apply to haloperidol and other neuroleptic drugs.

Despite the limitation of the findings they have implications for the functioning of chronically treated Tourette's disorder patients. If medication results in slower performance and possible memory impairment, children and adults who must continue to function academically or vocationally will have a potential liability while on medication. This liability may be even greater in Tourette's disorder patients with preexisting neurological impairment and learning disabilities (Shapiro et al., 1978; Hagins et al., 1982).

Treatment with neuroleptics is imperative for some patients with Tourette's disorder because symptoms prevent adequate functioning or cause serious psychosocial problems. Without medication many patients cannot function in school or at work because their symptoms are too disruptive, interfere with funtioning, and often have negative impact on the family and peer group. If medication is required, careful monitoring of academic and vocational performance may alert the treating physician to a decline in functioning before there are negative psychosocial consequences.

Future research on cognitive effects of this class of drugs should establish the dosage above which cognitive effects occur, either generally for patients, or for individual patients. Tests that are relevant to academic and vocational performance, of longer duration, and of greater complexity may enhance the identification of the depressant effects of neuroleptics on cognition. The results of the present study require replication, extension to a larger sample of patients, and the use of measures that will permit precise identification of the adverse cognitive effect. Such a study is currently in progress by our group.

Conclusion

This study demonstrated a slowing response time and a trend toward impaired recall on low dosages of pimozide. While the results are limited, they are consistent with other reports in the literature of neuroleptic induced impairment of selected aspects of cognitive functioning.

14

Conclusions

The status of Tourette's disorder is very different today compared to 10 years ago when we wrote our first edition of *Gilles de la Tourette Syndrome,* and very different compared to 22 years ago when we entered into this field by happenstance when our first patient was referred to us. As a consequence, it has been much more difficult to write this edition than the previous one. The first took 12 months, this one 19 months. The first had 400 references, this one more than 900. In the past only three to four papers were published annually, now six to seven are published monthly. Our sample size and data are much more extensive: 145 patients in the past compared to the present sample of 1,610, yielding 879 variables. Instead of using a hand-held calculator, we needed an IBM AT computer, capable of storing all the data and having the capacity to do sophisticated statistical analyses. Although it required 3 months to learn how to use the computer, the time was well spent because we were able to reduce the variables to 54, to rewrite easily, and to store the whole book on only two high-density floppy disks.

The diagnosis of Tourette's disorder and chronic motor tic has become epidemic in a sense. Clinics treating tic disorders have been established all over the country. The New York-New Jersey-Connecticut area alone has nine such clinics. Paradoxically, it was difficult in the past to collect enough patients to conduct studies because Tourette's disorder was underdiagnosed; today it is still difficult because Tourette's disorder is well known, and patients are widely dispersed and treated by family practitioners, pediatricians and, internists.

INADEQUATE SUPPORT OF RESEARCH

Support for research on tic disorders by the government is miniscule: the all time total is approximately one million dollars to fund six grants. Contrast this amount to that allocated for research in schizophrenia. Congress has earmarked approximately $30,500,000 for research on schizophrenia in 1987 alone, and has allocated relatively the same amount annually since at least 1955 (Barnes, 1987; Holden, 1987). Approximately 1% or 2,400,000 people in the United States are estimated to have schizophrenia, compared to 0.55% or 1,200,000 individuals with Tourette's disorder, 1.0% or 2,400,000 with CMT, and 10% or 24,000,000 with transient tic disorder (TTD). The total expenditure granted for all years is approximately 0.009 cents per person with a tic disorder. The annual research budget for Alzheimer's Disease is even higher, double that for schizophrenia.

A number of factors contribute to the low funding level. Tic and Tourette's disorders are not life-threatening, nor do they result in chronic deterioration or death. Tic disorders have a small consistency with little influence on granting agencies. Tourette's disorder has gained more publicity as a fashionable curiosity, especially because of coprolalia which intrigues the media, more than because it is a serious illness. In addition, drug companies have not supported studies of new drugs because anticipated profits would be less than their investment costs, which would be approximately 30 million dollars. The Orphan Drug Act has not changed the situation; no grants for study of drugs for the treatment of Tourette's disorder have been approved under the Orphan Drug Act.

Another important factor is that research on Tourette's disorder is still in a fact-gathering, exploratory, retrospective, and hypothesis-seeking phase. Granting agencies, with some justification, do not support such studies, but focus on prospective, predictive, or hypothesis-oriented studies with good supporting pilot data suggesting that the hypothesis is tenable. But research to secure pilot data is expensive, funds for this purpose are not available, and meaningful hypotheses and pilot data about Tourette's disorder are not currently available. Research on Tourette's disorder requires development of criteria, definitions, reliable and valid measures and procedures, careful collection of data, and considerable exploratory research. Perhaps because of limited finances and difficulty in securing adequate samples, research will have to be done collaboratively among several centers.

HOMAGE TO RESEARCHERS

Since government and drug company funding is inadequate, and available funds from private individuals and foundations are limited, who pays for the research? Dedicated physicians, neurologists, psychiatrists, psychologists, and basic scientists pay for it by devoting extensive time to these studies, and only after completion of other professional responsibilities or piggybacking funds from other research grants when available. Although we were fortunate to obtain some support at minimal levels for some of our studies and for the publication of over 90 papers, chapters, and books, thousands of hours of unremunerated time were given to these studies. We believe most investigators did the same. And all of this takes unbelievable amounts of time, working late in the evening, on weekends and holidays. The investment in time and money is prodigious and includes reviewing the literature, writing and protocol that will be approved by the Hospital Research Advisory Committee, conducting the research, finding funds to pay for stationery, equipment, etc., to write the paper (typing costs approximately $700), submitting papers to journals, revising them before publication, sometimes taking as long as 1 to 2 years after submission, reprint, and mailing costs (approximately $500). Who would do this? *Funny* people; otherwise why would they do it? Not for money, because any job would be far more profitable. For professional prestige, academic advancement? Yes, but far more important is their curiosity, their need to solve riddles, and to contribute something meaningful to the world.

It is important for us to convey our respect to all the investigators whose papers we reviewed in this book. It is important to state this because at the same time it was necessary to provide a comprehensive critique of the studies and their conclusions. And unfortunately, partly because of absent funding, limited samples and time, and other factors, most of the published studies of Tourette's disorder, including our own, do not fulfill criteria for a scientific study.

CRITIQUE OF RESEARCH IN TOURETTE'S DISORDER

Tourette's disorder studies compared to research on other illnesses such as schizophrenia, depression, and anxiety disorders, have major shortcomings. The limitations include the almost exclusive reporting of retrospective results, infrequently acknowledged, the infrequent use of prospective, predictive, or hypothesis-oriented studies, using small samples without statistical power analysis, absense of controls, or using inadequate or mismatched control groups, not using the double-blind procedure, and using measures and procedures without demonstrated reliability or validity.

Retrospective Versus Prospective Studies

Published studies of Tourette's disorder are, with rare exceptions, retrospective studies which capitalize on chance and lead to type I errors. If hypotheses are not predicted, researchers may be encouraged to repetitively think about, peruse, rearrange, and reanalyze the results of their studies, especially if expectations are not confirmed. The chance of obtaining a significant relationship is increased if the results are examined often enough. If examined 100 times, for example, there is a 500% chance of obtaining a significant relationship or five significant relationships at the 5% probability level. There is then a regrettable tendency to uncritically accept these results as true, whereas, in fact, they are false, and report the positive results and ignore the negative ones. With many such reports, the literature becomes cluttered with results that cannot be replicated and ideas and concepts about which consensus is impossible. It influences the direction of research into fruitless areas, diverts investigators from more meaningful studies and, unfortunately, may result in inadequate, inappropriate, or harmful management and treatment of patients.

The problem is readily apparent from a review of the literature. There are no more than three or four prospective studies in the Tourette's disorder literature. All others are retrospective. Moreover, these studies are often presented as if they were predictive or hypotheses-oriented studies, and without explicit statements that they were postdictive or retrospective.

In our opinion, it is heuristically reasonable to conduct retrospective studies or retrospectively analyze the results of studies, especially for disorders of unknown etiology like Tourette's disorder. However, it is absolutely necessary to describe how many retrospective analyses were done, on how many variables, and to state in the body of the paper that the results are preliminary and if retrospective require replication. Such information about retrospective results are veritably nonexistent in published studies of Tourette's disorder. A few studies appear to be predictive, but the results are often published in such way that it is not possible to distinguish between the hypothesized and restrospective results. The literature on Tourette's disorder is beginning to be flooded by innumerable contradictory findings about which there is little consensual agreement, with different clinicians and researchers clinging to different concepts about Tourette's disorder. There will be much wasted effort unless research becomes predictive rather than postdictive. The importance of predictive studies is indicated in the requirement by National Institutes of Health, National Institutes of Mental Health, and the Food and Drug Administration that proposals be predictive or hypothesis-oriented if they are to be approved.

Sample Size

Because of the limited number of patients available for study, and because the problem is likely to become even more difficult in the future, researchers often had to use small samples and samples with different ages, sexes, demographic, symptoms, and illness variables. Authors frequently acknowledge this limitation, but tend to ignore it in much of the discussion of the results. The results become established and uncritically cited by others in support of their studies.

Small samples may lead to type II errors, that is, rejecting an hypothesis which, in fact, is true. To determine the appropriate size of an experimental and control sample, statistical power analysis is necessary. Only one published study of Tourette's disorder used power analysis. Other sampling problems are the use of samples that include subjects and controls with different demographic, past history and illness variables, and often the use of unmatched patient and control samples.

Control Samples

A cardinal principle of all studies, whether in the physical sciences or clinical medicine, is the requirement that experimental subjects be compared with a control group. Moreover, it is necessary for the control to be as similar as possible to the experimental sample in all respects, except for the variable or issue being studied. Important matching variables include age, sex, and social class, and often a matching type of illness, duration of illness, and motivation for participating in the study.

Control groups are a rarity in published studies of Tourette's disorder. Even more astonishing is the use of inappropriate controls or mismatched samples: Most studies use Tourette's disorder patients who are solicited volunteers. One study used solicited volunteers for both the Tourette's disorder and the control group, but provided no information about the control group. Another study compared ratings of Tourette's disorder subjects by mothers with ratings of normal children by teachers. A third study used a control sample of hospital volunteers without a history of mental illness, which was not stipulated for the Tourette's disorder sample. The control groups used in these studies would tend to yield results in the direction of the investigator's hypothesis. This was especially noteworthy in one study of psychopathology and obsessive-compulsive disorder (OCD) that used a control group of volunteers who were friends and hospital personnel known to the investigators.

Double-Blind Procedure

It has been amply demonstrated that the biases and preconceptions of patients, physicians, and research staff influence the results of studies. Bias in favor of or against a particular drug can influence and determine the outcome of a drug study. Similarly, a study of whether psychopathology or OCD associated with Tourette's disorder can be influenced and determined by the bias or belief of an investigator. This bias may even influence and determine identification and measurement of unknown chemical constituents in qualitative and quantitative chemistry, and is the reason for the requirement that identical controls be used in determinations except for constituents.

The double-blind procedure was developed to minimize the effects of expectations, biases, spontaneous changes, and placebo effects on the results of studies. This is achieved by blinding the patient, physician, or research staff to all experimental conditions. Unfortunately, adequately designed double-blind procedures are used infrequently in studies of Tourette's disorder.

Reliability and Validity

Reliability, consisting of internal consistency, test retest, comparison over time, and rater reliability, is concerned with the precision, repeatibility, or generalizability of measurement. It involves the ability to obtain similar results for a measure, rating, scale, diagnosis, or procedure when repeated over time, administered on different occasions or evaluated by different individuals. Unreliable measures are characterized by error which do not correlate meaningfully with other variables. For example, a diagnostic procedure is unreliable if patients with Tourette's disorder are diagnosed as having OCD by one investigator, and as having a complex tic by another investigator.

Validity, consisting of predictive, concurrent, content, and construct validity, is concerned with the usefulness of measures, what can be inferred from or what is being measured by a test score or other forms of measurement, or how well a measure, rating, or scale reflect a concept that one is trying to measure. For example, a rating of tidiness or the number of complex tics in a Tourette's disorder patient might be reliable, but it would not be a valid measure of OCD. Thus, measures that are not reliable or valid are not useful and result in type II errors, or falsely rejecting a true hypothesis.

This problem has led to the development of procedures for the evaluation of the reliability and validity of measures. Well designed studies require such evidence.

Documentation of the reliability and validity of measures used in published studies of Tourette's disorder are essentially absent. There are only two or three papers that address this problem. Moreover, the procedures used to assess reliability and validity are, for the most part, homespun, unconventional, and inadequate. Methods for evaluating reliability and validity have long been the concern of psychologists who have developed standardized and generally accepted procedures (American Psychological Association, 1974).

The importance of developing reliable and valid measures is often discounted by some researchers and laymen, or is thought to be an academic, wasteful, and easily dismissed exercise when compared with a direct study of potential neurochemical abnormalities. It is not appreciated that the reliability and validity for almost all measures used in study of Tourette's disorder have not been documented. This includes measurement and identification of types of tics, severity of Tourette's disorder, change in severity, and most notably in ratings of behavioral problems, psychopathology, OCD, obsessive-compulsive symptoms (OCS), and mental disorders. Thus, studies of Tourette's disorder are largely or potentially characterized by error and unreplicated results about which there is controversy and little consensus.

As was necessary in the study of other disorders, the highest priority should be given to the development of reliable and valid measures, scales, instruments, and procedures to insure progress in research on Tourette's disorder.

Conclusion

The methodological principles discussed in this section, predictive studies, evaluation of statistical power, adequate controls, double-blind procedure, and acceptable reliability and validity, are only some of the essential requirements for an adequate study. Careful attention and adherence to these methodological principles are essential for future progress in research on Tourette's disorder.

SUMMARY OF RESULTS

The results reported in this volume are based on detailed analysis of the data on 666 consecutive patients with Tourette's disorder who were evaluated from 1965 and 1981, and clinical experience with 944 patients with Tourette's disorder, CMT, TTD, and other movement disorders who were evaluated from 1981 to 1987. The data from these studies are contrasted with the data from studies in the literature. In the following section, we summarize the highlights of the results and our conclusions.

History

The most remarkable historic development is the almost epidemic increase in the number of patients identified as having Tourette's disorder and CMT worldwide. Along with this development has been an extraordinary increase in the publication of clinical reports and studies on Tourette's disorder. In contrast to the past when there were very few physicians who were knowledgeable about tic disorders and their treatment, today most physicians have some knowledge about tic disorders, many are treating these disorders, and clinics specializing in the treatment of Tourette's disorder, tic disorders, and other movement disorders have sprung up all over the country. This development culminated in honoring George Gilles de la Tourette at a Centennial of Tourette Syndrome in 1985 which was held in the clinic in Paris where he trained and worked, and investigators from many countries presented papers to a large audience.

Epidemiology

Published studies underestimate the true prevalence of Tourette's disorder and CMT. Studies done in the past underestimated the prevalence because the diagnostic criteria for Tourette's disorder required coprolalia, echolalia, and intellectual deterioration and dementia. Recent studies underestimate prevalence because samples are limited to clinical patients who tend to have more severe symptoms, and exclude many more nonclinical individuals with mild symptoms in the community. The prevalence of CMT, now thought to be a milder form of Tourette's disorder, is much greater than Tourette's disorder, but has never been directly assessed.

The lifetime prevalence may be as high as 0.55% for Tourette's disorder, 1.0% for CMT, and 1.6% for both Tourette's disorder and CMT. The point prevalence estimate for all tic disorders varies from 4 to 28% for boys and 4 to 20% for girls, and an estimate of the lifetime prevalence of tics in children varies from 16 to 25%. The male-to-female sex ratio is approximately 3:1 in clinical patients with Tourette's disorder, but is approximately equal in nonclinical tic disorder samples in the population. The different sex ratios for the two samples warrant further study. These data only broadly hint at the prevalence of TTD, CMT, and Tourette's disorder in the population, and suggest that the prevalence is much higher than previously estimated. Since there is increasing evidence that the etiology for all tic disorders is similar, the problem may be much more extensive than previously considered.

Patient Characteristics

It is clear that characteristics of patients recently studied are different from earlier samples. Recent patients are younger at the time of initial evaluation (17.4 years), are diagnosed as having Tourette's disorder at a younger age (14.3 years), have a shorter duration between onset and diagnosis (10 years), a shorter duration of illness (10.9 years), less severe forms of Tourette's disorder (mild severity), less coprolalia (32%), have a less frequent diagnosis of attention deficit disorder with hyperactivity (ADD+H) (16%), and have fewer neurological, electroencephalographic, and neuropsychological test abnormalities ($p < 0.05$–0.0001). These changes in sample characteristics suggest that correlates reported for earlier samples are not representative of current clinical samples, and that characteristics for clinical samples may be different from nonclinical samples not identified as patients. The results indicate that studies done in the past of more severely afflicted Tourette's syndrome patients have to be re-evaluated and reinterpreted.

The median age at onset for the typical Tourette patient is 6 years (range 1–17 years, mean 6.7, SD 2.8). Tourette's disorder begins before age 11 in 91%, and before age 15 in 99% of patients. Demographic, family, and patient past history variables are essentially unrelated to Tourette's disorder: racial, ethnic, and religious background, family history of medical and psychiatric illness, parents' age at birth, history of mothers' abortions, pregnancy complications, birth complications, length of labor, birth weight, maturational milestones, birth order, sibling rank, history of head injury, concussion, unconsciousness, convulsion, epilepsy, meningitis, encephalitis, neuromuscular and other neurologic disorders, scarlet fever, rheumatic fever, high fevers over 104°F, Sydenham's chorea, St. Vitus dance, rubella, rubeola, varicella, pertusis, sinusitis, allergy, and total number of childhood illnesses.

Psychosocial, medical, situational, and drug factors preceding the onset of tics were interpreted as random occurrences which were unrelated to the onset of Tourette's disorder. The onset of Tourette's disorder was not associated with head trauma or the use of neuroleptics in any of our patients. The rationale for our conclusion that stimulants do not cause or permanently exacerbate tics or Tourette's disorder is described in Chapter 11.

Initial Tics

Initial tics occurring within 1 week of onset of Tourette's disorder included 82 different tics: simple motor tics 74%, complex motor tics 7%, simple vocal tics 17%, and complex vocal tics 1.3% (coprolalia 1.1%, palilalia 0.2%). The most frequent initial tics in descending order are: eye 37%, horizontal neck 13%, vertical neck 3%, facial grimace 3%, shoulders 3%, arm 2.7%, mouth 2.6%, hands 2.3%, sniff 2.1%, grunt 1.8%, high-pitched sound 1.5%, stuttering or stammering 1.5%, jumping 1.4%,, nose 1.4%, abdomen 1.2%, torso 1.1%, coprolalia 1.1%, and less that 1% for the remaining 65 tics.

Initial Clinical Course

The number, frequency, intensity, or severity of tics varies over time (waxes and wanes) in 97% of patients, and the type or location of tics varies (fluctuates) in 96% of patients. The symptoms fulfill the six criteria for tics listed in Table 10.1. If tics disappear within one year, the diagnosis is TTD. If motor tics persist for more than a year, the diagnosis is CMT disorder. If only vocal tics are present (extremely infrequent) and persist beyond a year, the diagnosis is chronic vocal tic (CVT) disorder. If multiple motor and at least one vocal tic is present for more than 1 year, the diagnosis is Tourette's disorder. Tables 10.8, 10.11, and 10.13 list the diagnostic criteria for tic disorders in DSM-III-R and proposed additions, revisions, and changes suggested by the authors.

Cumulative Lifetime Tics

The cumulatve lifetime number of tics for our sample varied from 2 to 60: 32% with 2 to 10 tics; 61% with 11 to 30 tics; and 6% with 31 to 60 tics. Simple motor tics were present in all patients, simple vocal tics in 99%, complex motor tics in 69%, and complex vocal tics in 33% (coprolalia 32%, echolalia, or palilalia 33%). Eight to 58% of symptoms that were present in the past had disappeared at the time of our initial evaluation. Coprolalia may be an initial symptom (1.1%) or occur 25 years after the onset. The number of cumulative life-time symptoms increase with the duration of the illness (older patients have more chance of developing other symptoms), and are increased in patients with a diagnosis of ADD+H and those with high scores on the Conners Abbreviated Parent Questionnaire (Hyperactivity Index).

Severity of Symptoms

The severity of Tourette's disorder for the total sample, using a rating scale of 1 (very mild severity) to 6 (very severe), averaged 2.67 (SD = 0.87) (mild to moderate severity). Severity has decreased in recent samples compared to earlier samples ($p = 0.0001$). Tourette's disorder is more severe in patients from lower social classes and those with ADHD; high scores on the Conners Hyperactivity Index; fewer intellectual and psychosocial assets, and a history of coprolalia, echolalia, and tics of the legs.

Natural Course and Prognosis

The natural course for Tourette's disorder is not ominous, as once believed, and does not result in intellectual deterioration, psychosis, or chronic hospitalization. Nor is Tourette's disorder associated with any physical or psychological illness, character trait, or type of personality, and the prevalence of other disorders is no different from expectations in individuals without Tourette's disorder. The only possible association, not yet established, and probably related to ascertainment problems, is a greater frequency of ADD among Tourette's disorder patients. The main effect of having Tourette's disorder in our opinion is on psychosocial functioning, which is very much related to the combined effects of severity interacting with the individual's ego resources. The symptoms may secondarily impair psychosocial functioning, cause some patients to withdraw, influence the development of personality traits, but have little or no effect on other patients. Ominous consequences of having Tourette's disorder, although infrequent, include blindness from striking oneself; orthopedic complications from vigorous tics of the joints; temporomandibular complications from neck, head, or jaw tics; excoriation and laceration from biting, scratching, or picking tics; and occasional suicides in predisposed individuals. The symptoms themselves usually do not interfere directly with physical activity and with most academic, vocational, or recreational activities.

Studies of prognosis are infrequent and difficult to conduct, and impressions are limited by methodological problems such as the study of only patient samples, thereby excluding unidentified, nonpatient samples who often have mild symptoms and a better prognosis, patient samples with different age at onset of symptoms, age at initial evaluation and follow-up, duration of illness, length of remission, and treated versus untreated patient samples.

One or more periods of spontaneous remission lasting from 1 month to 19 years occurred in 27.1% of our patients. It should be remembered, however, that Tourette's disorder symptoms may return even after prolonged periods of remission, as demonstrated by several patients whose symptoms disappeared in adolescence and returned in their 60s. In addition, waxing and waning of the severity of symptoms occur spontaneously in 97% of patients, 96% have changes in the type of symptom over time, approximately one-third have spontaneous remission of previous coprolalia, and 8% to 58% of symptoms that were present in the past were not present at the initial evaluation of patients. Moreover, our data indicate that approximately 36% of patients are rated as improved during the first 6 weeks of treatment with placebos. Thus, meaningful improvement would probably have to exceed 36%.

Within these methodological limitations, for children with a tic disorder, complete remissions are estimated to occur in 24 to 61%, improvement in 26 to 68%, and no change or worsening of tics in 3 to 24%.

Another generalization about the natural course of Tourette's disorder is derived from our clinical experience over the past 22 years. Approximately 8% of Tourette's disorder patients are likely to have complete and permanent remissions lasting from 7 to 19 years, usually during puberty and occasionally during adolescence. Remissions in adulthood are unlikely, none having occurred in any of our patients. Of the remainder, the general course during latency, up to approximately age 13, and during adolescence, is the same in approximately 65% of patients. Severity decreases, sometimes markedly, during adolescence in approximately 35% of patients. In adulthood, after 18 or 21 years of age, the severity, waxing, waning, and fluctuation of symptoms decrease. Occasional patients, with a history of very mild symptoms, develop severe symptoms in adulthood, usually in the twenties, occasionally in the early thirties, and frequently for only brief periods of time. Despite these general trends, the natural course is highly variable and it is not possible to predict the clinical course in individual patients. If controlled studies confirm the observation that the natural clinical course for tic disorders cannot be predicted from outwardly observable psychosocial, situational, environmental, or situational events, it would tend to support the concept that it is caused by internal neurochemical changes in the central nervous system.

Behavior Problems and Psychopathology

A broad and extensive range of behavior problems, psychopathology, and mental illness in patients and their families are frequently mentioned in the literature as associated with Tourette's disorder. However, our critical review of the literature indicates that the relationship between psychopathology and Tourette's disorder has not been demonstrated by adequately controlled studies. Moreover, several well controlled studies by our group failed to confirm the hypothesis. We have concluded, as have six other experienced clinicians, that psychopathology among patients with Tourette's disorder is within population estimates, and our guess is that future studies which are necessary to resolve the controversy will confirm our findings.

Obsessive Compulsive Disorder, Symptoms, and Impulsions

Also controversial, is the concept that OCD and OCS occur more frequently than expected in patients with Tourette's disorder and their families. However, documentation is based on several uncontrolled clinical reports and one preliminary, partially controlled study. Moreover, all of the reports and studies erroneously classify symptoms such as touching, smelling, and other complex tics as compulsions. It is obvious that the evidence is circular: If tics are classified as compulsions, many patients with Tourette's disorder will be diagnosed as having cumpulsions, not because they have compulsions but because they have tics. This error has been corrected in DSM-III-R (1987) and these symptoms are now classified as tics and not compulsions. Moreover, many studies use nonrandom, volunteer Tourette's disorder samples who may be more severely afflicted with the disorder and with other psychopathology. In addition, many of these papers use only parts, but not all, of DSM-III and DSM-III-R criteria for the diagnosis of OCD and OCS. Compulsive personality traits were also used as evidence of OCD and and OCS. None of the papers differentiate between OCD and OCS; all use these terms uncritically and interchangeably. None used blind evaluations to control for the bias of investigators. And above all, none used matched control groups to control for the 25 to 60% of OCSs that are reported to be present in nonclinical or normal samples, or they used inappropriate control groups of unmatched volunteer hospital personnel or children of professional colleagues.

It is theoretically and pragmatically important to develop criteria and differential criteria for OCD, OCS, impulsions and tics as suggested in Chapter 6. The main difference between OCD and OCS is that OCD requires marked distress and interference with functioning; in other words it is a clinical disorder, whereas OCS would be reserved for similar symptoms that do *not* cause marked distress or interfere with functioning, that is, symptoms commonly observed in normal individuals. Another group of symptoms resemble OCS, but are different from OCD and OCS because they are an end in themselves, not purposeful, not done to prevent a dreaded consequence, and do not interfere with psychosocial functioning or cause marked distress. They differ from Tourette's disorder symptoms primarily because they are intended rather than involuntary. These symptoms clinically seem to us to be more frequent among Tourette's disorder patients (10–20%) than other individuals. We refer to them as impulsions, as did Tourette, Charcot, and Meige and Feindel. This proposal, developed more fully in Chapters 6 and 10, is proposed for heuristic purposes, because it may be important for studies of both OCD and Tourette's disorder.

Attention-Deficit Disorder with Hyperactivity

Our data suggest that the high percentage of ADD+H reported in studies may be due to ascertainment sampling errors, and that Tourette's disorder and ADHD are unrelated. Ascertainment sampling errors include the greater likelihood of a person with two disorders seeking help than a person with one disorder, and the former having both diagnosed. In addition, the likelihood that Tourette's disorder will be identified in patients evaluated for ADD+H is increased because ADD+H begins at a younger age, disrupts functioning earlier in life, is associated with greater severity of Tourette's disorder, and impairs psychosocial functioning more often than Tourette's disorder. Ascertainment bias may also result from samples in which more severely afflicted Tourette patients predominate, samples using volunteers or questionnaires rather than consecutive patients, samples using clinic populations compared to patients from private practice, and samples from out-of-the-way specialized psychiatric or medical centers.

These problems may explain our early reports, and those of others, that 50 to 60% of Tourette's disorder patients had ADD+H, whereas the percentage is 16% in recent samples. The question is not resolved by family genetic studies since one study concluded that ADD+H is, and another that it is not genetically related to Tourette's disorder. However, since questions have been raised about the independence of Tourette's disorder and ADD+H, it is important for future studies to separate these two groups. It is likely that many previously reported findings (such as neurological, EEG and neuropsychological test abnormalities, learning disorders, psychopathology, and so on) are related more to factors associated with ADD+H than to Tourette's disorder. Combining these groups in studies may result in spurious findings, obscure potentially fruitful hypotheses, and contribute to the problem of heterogeneity in tic disorders.

Central Nervous System Factors

Our conclusion is that current neurological data are inadequate to explain the etiology of Tourette's disorder. Neurological speculations are based on a series of questionable observations, studies, and assumptions. The literature is a potpourri of clinical observations, small samples, inadequate criteria, and reliability for independent and dependent variables, retrospective reports capitalizing on random significance, inadequate controls, and other major methodological problems. The studies are grossly marred by inclusion of high percentages of patients with ADD+H, hyperactivity, learning and other CNS disorders, often with an unknown number of patients on medication, and the absence of appropriate and adequate controls. Despite these limitations, many clinical observations, preliminary findings, and speculations warrant further study.

We have concluded that EEG abnormalities, nonlocalizing neurological signs, ADD+H, hyperactivity and learning disorders, and psychopathology are not intrinsic to Tourette's disorder. Therefore, EEG studies, skull X-rays, computerized axial tomography (CAT), position emission tomography (PET), and magnetic resonance imaging (MRI) studies, chemistries and neuropsychological testing are not necessary for routine evaluation of patients with Tourette's disorder, and should only be done if there are other indications for their use or for research purposes.

Etiology

The use of haloperidol in the 1960s stimulated an interest in an organic etiology for Tourette's disorder, which previously had been attributed to demonic possession in the middle ages, neuropathic antecedents in the nineteenth century and psychodynamic formulations of unconscious conflicts in the twentieth century. Our concept that Tourette's disorder had an organic etiology, first proposed in 1968, although initially resisted, was largely accepted by the middle of the 1970s. Several recent investigators, however, have proposed that the etiology of Tourette's disorder is a disturbance in CNS functioning that requires an environmental or psychological stimulus for its expression, and that attentional and other behavioral problems precede the onset of Tourette's disorder and are invariably associated with the disorder.

Psychological or Organic Etiology

The arguments against a psychological etiology for Tourette's disorder are persuasive. Response to psychological treatment of Tourette's disorder is approximately 35%, which is similar to the range for spontaneous or placebo treatment of Tourette's disorder. Controlled studies of efficacy have not been done and the efficacy of any form of psychological treatment has not been demonstrated. Low dosages of neuroleptics decrease tics in a large proportion of patients without symptom substitution. Situational factors preceding the onset of Tourette's disorder appear to be random events that commonly occur in individuals without the disorder. Etiological concepts of specific psychodynamic conflicts were not confirmed in a well-controlled study, and two studies demonstrated that behavior problems, psychopathology, and mental illness were associated with ADD+H rather than Tourette's disorder, and were not more frequent in Tourette patients without ADD than in a random control sample. Analyses indicate a similar syndromal pattern for the age of onset, symptoms, and clinical course across cultures. Our analyses fail to differentiate patients with Tourette's disorder from individuals without the disorder, except for a higher male to female ratio of 3:1 and a higher than expected family history of tic and Tourette's disorder in probands with the disorder, both of which support a biological etiology. The concordance for tic disorders in monozygotic twins ranges from 77 to 87%.

The hypothesis that the etiology is due to an interaction of organic and psychological factors is unparsimonious and, while possible, has no experimental support.

We have concluded that the available evidence supports the concept that Tourette's disorder is a neurological disorder, and similar to narcolepsy and epilepsy, has no other primary or intrinsic psychological associations, although there may be secondary psychosocial effects.

Tic Disorders as a Continuum or Spectrum

The hypothesis that tic disorders represent an underlying disease with the same etiology (continuum) is supported by the similarity of the initial symptoms, age at onset, sex ratio, signs, symptoms, clinical course (except for the type of symptoms and duration of illness), and the response to treatment with low dosages of haloperidol and other neuroleptics. Factors suggesting that tic disorders are a spectrum disorder are the discordance of 13 to 23% for monozygotic twins for tic disorders and the ineffectiveness of treatment with neuroleptics, even at high dosages, in some patients.

Genetic Factors

Our data and studies in the literature suggest that Tourette's disorder and CMT are similar disorders, and that some forms are inherited. Most studies report that Tourette's disorder and CMT occur more frequently in male patients and family members, but the risks to relatives of affected females are higher than to relatives of affected males. A family history of Tourette's disorder is reported more frequently in selected referrals or volunteer samples than in consecutive clinical patients, and the percentage of affected family members may be higher in samples in which relatives are interviewed, than in samples in which family history is obtained from patients. Our data indicate that a family history of Tourette's disorder or tics is unrelated to the results of treatment with haloperidol, OCD; OCS; impulsions; compulsive personality disorder; psychopathology; ADD+H; a past history of complex, coprolalic, and echophilic tics; or to any other of 54 variables from our data set. Our data suggest that 5% of Tourette patients have one or more primary family members who have Tourette's disorder, 33% have a family history of CMT or TTD, and 35% have a family history of either Tourette's disorder, CMT, or TTD. The corresponding percentages for all family members is 8% for Tourette's disorder, 42% for a tic disorder, and 47% for either Tourette's disorder, CMT, or TTD. The concordance rate for Tourette or CMT in monozygotic twins is approximately 77 to 87%, approximately 25% in same-sex dizygotic twins, and not significantly higher in opposite-sex dyzygotic twins than expectations for non-twin siblings.

Current research indicates that transmission is vertical with one or more intermediate forms of expression. Chromosomal aberrations are infrequent and do not explain the observed familial clustering of Tourette's disorder. The evidence that OCD and ADD + H are related to Tourette's disorder is controversial. A simple Mendelian genetic mechanism and an X-linked and autosomal recessive mechanism have been rejected, polygenic/multifactorial and mixed models have received some support, but a single major locus model best fits the existing data. The mode of inheritance is still unknown, but evidence for an autosomal dominant mode of transmission is increasing.

Dopamine Hypothesis

Circumstantial evidence suggests that the disturbance in Tourette's disorder is the synaptic transmission system in the basal ganglia. Dopaminergic mechanisms are implicated in the pathophysiology of the disorder because tics are suppressed by dopamine-blocking medications and exacerbated by dopamine agonists. The blocking of dopamine at postsynaptic receptors, the effect of L-DOPA on patients with parkinsonism and low levels of CNS homovanillic acid (HVA) reported in some studies, contributes to the hypothesis that Tourette's disorder is caused by supersensitivity of postsynaptic receptors. The effectiveness of neuroleptics known to block dopamine$_2$ receptors provides the most convincing support for the dopamine hypothesis in Tourette's disorder. However, drugs affect many neurotransmitter systems which have significant perturbations and compensatory feedback effects. Hypothesized relationships between clinical response to drugs and underlying neurochemical etiology for tics and Tourette's disorder are indirect, inferential, and problematic. These and other factors lead to the conclusion that the dopamine hypothesis alone, which has also been suggested as the etiology for schizophrenia, manic depressive disorder, tardive dyskinesia, and other hyperkinetic conditions, is probably too simplistic to adequately account for the etiology of Tourette's disorder.

Biochemical Studies

The results of biochemical studies are largely inconsistent or negative. Methodological problems include the use of small samples; different laboratory procedures; variations in methodology; inadequate control for age, sex, diet, diurnal variation, activity level, and many other important variables; inappropriate control samples; and the reporting of retrospective results. Levels of CSF HVA have been reported as high, normal, and low; although low levels have been reported more frequently. Normal levels are reported for CSF 5-hydroxyindoleacetic acid, vanillylmandelic acid (VMA) and 3-methoxy-4-hydroxyphenethyleneglycol (MHPG), urinary VMA and MHPG, cholinesterase activity, plasma dopamine-beta-hydroxylase, norepinephrine and oxidase activity, platelet monoamine oxidase activity, and red blood cell catechol-*O*-methyltransferase (COMT) and choline. Provocative probes using medication with different effects on neurotransmitter systems are largely negative or inconclusive: choline, lecithin, L-tryptophan, 5-hydroxytryptophan, physostigmine, apomorphine, L-DOPA, reserpine, tetrabenzine, disulfiram, dopamine-beta-hydroxylase, benztropine, deanol, methysergide, and clonidine.

The variability of the biochemical, genetic, and treatment results suggests the possiblity of pathophysiologic heterogeneity among Tourette patients.

Neurological Abnormalities

Although higher than expected, nonlocalizing neurological, electroencephalographic, and neuropsychological abnormalities have been reported in the literature, our analyses indicate that these abnormalities are found mainly in patients with Tourette's disorder and ADD+H, and are infrequent in Tourette patients without ADD. Structural lesions in the brains of Tourette patients, using CAT and MRI scans, have not been demonstrated. A preliminary unreplicated study using PET reported decreased glucose utilization in the basal ganglia, suggesting neuronal hypofunction of striatal and cortico-limbic areas.

Postmortem Studies

Only four older postmortem studies have been published, none pointing to a specific etiology for Tourette's disorder. Although approximately a half-dozen brains have become available for study during the past 22 years, preparation was inadequate and the results were inconclusive. Current techniques, not available in the past, include measurement of neurotransmitters in various brain areas. Autopsy studies are obviously very important for study of the anatomy and etiology of Tourette's disorder.

Conclusion

Currently, there is no experimental support for any hypothesis about the etiology of tic and Tourette's disorder.

Nosology and Criteria for Tic Disorders

Although the nosology and criteria for tic disorders have been improved in DSM-III-R, more precise criteria are necessary for research. Based on data from our study and data in the literature, we have proposed specific criteria for motor, vocal, and sensory tics, which have not been described previously. Continued refinement of criteria will be necessary in the future as additional data become available.

Treatment

Our conclusion about the effectiveness of treatment of Tourette's disorder, based on a review of all published studies and clinical reports in the literature, is that neuroleptic drugs with predominant D_2 blocking properties are the most effective drugs. These drugs, cited according to the frequency of their use, include haloperidol, pimozide, fluphenazine, and penfluridol. Less effective and less predictable therapeutic effects are reported in occasional patients for clonazepam. Clonidine is reported as effective by some clinicians and as ineffective by others. All other forms of psychological, behavioral, environmental, physical, and drug treatment are evaluated as ineffective. Surgical treatment has been reported to be effective in a small number of patients but is not used because of the effectiveness of neuroleptic drugs, the seriousness of the surgery, and the potential for serious adverse effects.

We have concluded that the treatment of Tourette's disorder should primarily focus on the alleviation of tics, similar to the control of convulsions in epilepsy, cataplexy in narcolepsy and blood glucose in diabetes. Other medical disorders such as hyperthyroidism, ulcers or fractures, and other psychological problems such as ADD + H, learning disorders, conduct disorders, and other psychopathology should be evaluated separately and treated if indicated. The treatment of Tourette's disorder alone usually requires only the treatment of tics.

The indications for treatment are obvious at the extremes; less indicated if the symptoms are mild and do not interfere with psychosocial functioning, more indicated if the symptoms are severe and interfere with psychosocial functioning, and elective for levels of severity between extremes and determined by the patient based on the degree of distress caused by the symptoms.

The use of neuroleptics for the treatment of Tourette's disorder differs from their use in the psychoses. The dosage is 10 to 50 times higher for the psychoses, and adverse effects interfere with functioning at a much lower dosage in patients with Tourette's disorder. Impaired motivation and cognition are particularly distressing to Tourette patients. These adverse effects are related to dosage but can occur at low dosages. They are difficult to detect and infrequently encountered by most physicians who treat schizophrenic patients with neuroleptics. Management includes dosage reduction and occasional use of stimulant drugs. Slow titration of dosage is recommended for functioning patients because the appropriate dosage, determined by genetic factors, differs among patients, and because the onset of adverse effects can be detected early in treatment and result in minimal interference with functioning. For example, haloperidol, at an initial dosage of 0.25 mg/day, is increased every 4 to 7 days to a final dosage, generally ranging from 1.5 to 10 mg/day, or a dosage that maximally decreases symptoms with minimal adverse effects. The dosage is constantly titrated over time as the clinical course waxes, wanes, and fluctuates. An anti-parkinson drug is always used during the first 3 months of treatment to control dystonic and akinesic adverse effects, and may be necessary for some patients at later stages in treatment. More rapid titration (1–5 mg/hr) is occasionally necessary in emergencies such as retinal detachment from hitting the eye, acute vertebral disc, etc.

These drugs have very few serious adverse effects when slowly titrated to low final dosages, and adverse effects which can be very bothersome to functioning patients can be managed by physicians experienced in the use of neuroleptic drugs for the treatment of patients with Tourette's disorder.

Although, in contrast to the past, we now have several drugs that can effectively control the symptoms in many patients, there is need for even more effective drugs with less adverse effects. More important is identification of the neuropathology for Tourette's disorder which can direct our efforts to the development of even more specific treatment.

MEASUREMENT IN TOURETTE'S DISORDER

The development of reliable and valid measures has high priority for the progress of research in Tourette's disorder. Our preliminary study, which requires replication, indicates that videotape tic counts have high reliability, adequate validity, and the advantage of being more quantitative than and independent of other measures when used as a measure of change with treatment. Although videotape tic counts are reliable, they are not useful as a clinical measure of the severity of Tourette's disorder because the validity is inadequate (correlation with other clinical measures of severity of Tourette's disorder). Although our results did not indicate that drugs differentially affect motor, vocal, or complex tics with treatment, and that the number of tics were not significantly different in three different conditions (computation, reading, and alone conditions), replication and further study of the optimal conditions for recording tics is warranted. Further study is also warranted to determine if there are differences between experienced and inexperienced raters, and the amount of training or experience required for reliable tic counts. Videotape tic counts are not useful as a measure of the severity of Tourette's disorder because the validity is inadequate (low relationship with other clinical measures of the severity of Tourette's disorder).

The Shapiro TS-Severity (TS-Sev) Scale, however, has high reliability and validity as a clinical measure of the severity of the syndrome. The scale rates the degree to which the tics are noticeable to others, elicits comments or curiosity by other people, cause people to think the patient is odd or bizarre, interferes with the functioning of the patient and results in the patient being homebound or requiring hospitalization. Despite the high reliability and validity of the TS-Sev Scale, a more formal psychometric study of a scale reflecting severity of Tourette's disorder should be conducted. This would include rating items reflecting a more comprehensive sampling of the severity domain. In addition, other items should include measures of subjective and objective distress and interference with psychological, social, interpersonal, academic, vocational, occupational, mechanical, athletic, and other relevant areas. The scale should be administered to a large enough sample (ten patients for every item), reliable factors should be derived by factors analysis, the reliability and validity should be evaluated, differences between experienced and inexperienced raters should be assessed, and the study should be conducted at two independent centers.

There is also a heuristic and clinical need for developing a reliable and valid scale for measuring overall improvement which would incorporate symptom improvement and adverse effects. The proposed Shapiro Global Improvement Scale requires empirical study.

Investigators interested in studying the association of behavior problems, OCD, OCS, mental illness, and other psychopathology to Tourette's disorder should use established scales with documented evidence for reliability and validity rather than "homespun" or other scales without such evidence.

Also necessary is the development of more specific definitions of criteria, and reliable and valid measures for simple and complex motor, vocal, sensory, and other types of tics, and more specific data-oriented criteria for atypical tic and other movement disorder categories.

Although the development of sound measures and diagnoses are time consuming and seemingly unimportant compared to direct studies of the etiology of Tourette's disorder, they are essential for further progress in study of the disorder. In the past, it appeared that we could ignore these measurement issues because many feasible hypotheses were available for direct study. We have had over 20 years experience conducting such studies without adequate concern for these psychometric issues, and the reporting of retrospective results, and, in general, conducting a "browsing" type of research. And we are no closer to an understanding of the etiology today than we were 20 years ago. Moreover, ignoring important methodological principles has resulted in many controversial findings and concepts about Tourette's disorder about which there is little consensus. It results in wasted time, fruitless efforts examining irrelevant hypotheses, and diverts research from more meaningful studies.

In schizophrenia, for example, before the development of reliable and valid measures and diagnoses, innumerable studies were concerned with irrelevant etiological issues such as unconscious oral conflicts, family dynamics, interpersonal and societal conflicts, and many other psychological etiologies; and millions of dollars were spent for millions of hours of hundreds of different types of psychotherapy. Like Tourette's disorder, many ineffective drugs were used in treatment for prolonged periods before they faded from use. More careful adherence to methodological principles contributed to focusing research on an organic etiology for schizophrenia, and the development of useful drugs for its treatment.

As in schizophrenia and other disorders of unknown etiology, it is important at this time to focus our efforts on developing reliable and valid measures, procedures for diagnoses, and the use of classical methodological principles in our studies of Tourette's disorder.

Appendix

TABLE A.1. *List of variables*

Variables[a]		Sample size	$\bar{X}$ or %	SD	Range	Factor loadings (R_{xx})[b]
Number	Description					
Demography						
1.	Year evaluated	666	76.4	3.2	1965–1981	—
2.	Age (years)	666	18.8	11.9	4–68	—
3.	Sex: percent males	666	76.3%	42.6	—	—
4.	Social class[c]	666	2.8	1.2	1–5	—
Genetics (family history of:)						
5.	Tourette's disorder[d]	645	7.8%	26.8	—	—
6.	Tic disorder[d]	645	42.0%	49.4	—	—
7.	Other movement disorder[d]	645	9.0%	28.6	—	—
Medical history						
8.	Parents' age at birth FS	666	29.0	5.3	16–49	(0.87)
a.	Fathers' age at birth	666	30.8	6.1	16–54	0.82
b.	Mothers' age at birth	666	27.2	5.1	16–44	0.81
9.	Mothers' abortions	666	0.5	1.0	0–10	—
10.	Pregnancy complications[d]	666	24.7%	42.0	—	—
11.	Birth complications[d]	666	22.7%	41.0	—	—
12.	Length of labor (hours)	666	1.5	7.8	0–72	—
13.	Sit-walk-talk FS	666	3.1	0.8	1.7–9.5	(0.47)
a.	Age walked	666	1.1	0.2	0.6–2	0.27
b.	Age sat	666	0.5	0.1	0.2–1.1	0.26
c.	Age talked	666	1.4	0.6	0.3–8	0.25
14.	Bladder-bowel trained FS	666	4.4	1.4	1.6–22	(0.94)
a.	Age bladder trained	666	2.2	0.8	0.8–12	0.82
b.	Age bowel trained	666	2.2	0.7	0.8–11	0.81
15.	Sibling rank	666	1.9	1.2	1–9	—
16.	History of head trauma FS[d]	666	3.3	0.6	3–6	(0.58)
a.	Concussion[d]	666	3.9%	19.3	—	0.46
b.	Unconscious[d]	666	4.0%	19.7	—	0.44
c.	Head injury[d]	666	20.5%	40.4	—	0.34
17.	History of convulsions[d]	666	4.7%	21.1	—	—
18.	History of epilepsy[a]	666	1.1%	10.2	—	—
19.	History of scarlet fever[a]	666	6.3%	24.3	—	—
20.	History of rheumatic fever[d]	666	1.4%	11.6	—	—
21.	History of chorea[d]	666	0.3%	5.5	—	—
22.	History of allergies[d]	666	30.1%	45.7	—	—

TABLE A.1. *(Continued)*

Variables[a]		Sample size	$\bar{X}$ or %	SD	Range	Factor loadings (R_{xx})[b]
Number	Description					
Behavior						
23.	Hyperactivity FS[e]	318	1.3	0.9	0–3	(0.88)
	a. Constantly fidgeting[e]	318	1.6	1.1	0–3	0.73
	b. Inattentive, easily distracted[e]	318	1.2	1.1	0–3	0.71
	c. Restless or overactive[e]	318	1.5	1.1	0–3	0.70
	d. Short attention span[e]	318	1.2	1.1	0–3	0.69
	e. Excitable, impulsive[e]	318	1.5	1.1	0–3	0.63
	f. Disturbs other children[e]	318	0.8	1.0	0–3	0.49
24.	Learning disorder FS[e]	318	0.6	0.9	0–3	(0.81)
	a. Academic disability[e]	318	0.8	1.0	0–3	0.62
	b. Reading disability[e]	318	0.5	0.9	0–3	0.58
25.	Anger-moodiness FS[e]	318	1.0	0.8	0–3	(0.94)
	a. Temper outbursts, explosive and unpredictable behavior[e]	318	1.0	1.0	0–3	0.84
	b. Explosive anger[e]	318	1.2	1.0	0–3	0.80
	c. Mood changes quickly and drastically[e]	318	1.2	1.0	0–3	0.62
	d. Destructive acts[e]	318	0.5	0.8	0–3	0.53
	e. Demands must be met immediately, easily frustrated[e]	318	1.5	1.2	0–3	0.52
	f. Cries often and easily[e]	318	0.9	1.0	0–3	0.39
26.	Inhibition FS[e]	318	0.7	0.9	0–3	(0.70)
	a. Difficulty expressing anger[e]	318	0.6	1.0	0–3	0.65
	b. Difficulty expressing emotion[e]	318	0.8	1.0	0–3	0.63
27.	Obsessive-compulsive-like symptoms FS[e]	317	0.7	0.7	0–3	(0.73)
	a. Counting things many times, or going through numbers in your head[e]	317	0.5	0.9	0–3	0.65
	b. Checking things that you know you have already done, like doors, switches, etc.[e]	317	0.7	1.0	0–3	0.65
	c. Repetitive thoughts that you cannot turn off, such as worry about germs, fear of accidents to loved ones, violence, etc.[e]	317	0.9	1.1	0–3	0.62

TABLE A.1. *(Continued)*

Variables[a]		Sample size	$\bar{X}$ or %	SD	Range	Factor loadings (R_{xx})[b]
Number	Description					
	d. Even when doing something perfectly, feeling it is not quite right[e]	317	1.1	1.1	0–3	0.51
	e. Touching things over and over again[e]	317	0.3	0.8	0–3	0.41
28.	Compulsive personality FS[e]	317	1.2	0.8	0–3	(0.80)
	a. Cleaning room or home more often than is need to be sure it is clean[e]	317	1.2	1.1	0–3	0.66
	b. Having to keep things in a certain order, or getting dressed in a certain set pattern[e]	317	0.9	1.1	0–3	0.66
29.	Coordination Abilities FS[f]	397	2.3	0.7	1–4	(0.75)
	a. Coordination[f]	397	2.3	0.9	1–4	0.81
	b. Athletic ability[f]	397	2.3	1.0	1–4	0.73
	c. Mechanical ability	397	2.2	0.8	1–4	0.42
30.	Intellectual-psychosocial Assets FS[f]	397	2.4	0.7	1–4	(0.84)
	a. IQ or intelligence[f]	397	2.6	0.8	1–4	0.80
	b. School achievement[f]	397	2.5	1.0	1–4	0.80
	c. Verbal or talking ability[f]	397	2.7	0.9	1–4	0.71
	d. Mathematical ability[f]	397	2.2	0.1	1–4	0.64
	e. Emotional maturity[f]	397	2.0	0.9	1–4	0.52
Illness variables						
31.	Duration of illness FS	666	13.7	11.4	1.3–64	(0.99)
	a. Years from onset to diagnosis	666	11.2	11.4	0–62	0.98
	b. Duration of present illness	666	12.2	11.3	0–62	0.98
	c. Age at diagnosis	666	17.9	12.0	4–68	0.96
32.	Previous diagnosis or consultation FS[d]	666	62.9	33.0	—	(0.44)
	a. Previous diagnosis of TS[d]	666	38.4%	48.7	—	0.56
	b. Previous consultation or treatment[d]	666	87.4	33.2	—	0.40
33.	Age at onset of TS	666	6.7	2.8	1–17	—
Symptoms (history of:)						
34.	Facial tics[d]	666	93.1%	25.4	—	—
35.	Head tics[d]	666	91.1%	28.4	—	—
36.	Upper limb tics[d]	666	68.6%	46.4	—	—

TABLE A.1. *(Continued)*

Variables[a]		Sample size	$\bar{X}$ or %	SD	Range	Factor loadings (R_{xx})[b]
Number	Description					
37.	Lower limb tics[d]	666	40.7%	49.2	—	—
38.	Torso tics[d]	666	46.6%	49.9	—	—
39.	Complex tics[d]	666	68.5%	46.5	—	—
40.	Inarticulate sounds[d]	666	98.5%	12.2	—	—
41.	Coprolalia[d]	666	32.0%	46.7	—	—
42.	Copropraxia[d]	666	12.8%	33.4	—	—
43.	Mental coprolalia[d]	666	3.9%	19.4	—	—
44.	Echophilia[d]	666	32.7%	47.0	—	—
45.	Number of current tics	666	7.0	5.3	0–36	—
46.	Number of cumulative tics	666	15.7	9.2	2–60	—
47.	Rating of TS severity	666	2.7	0.9	1–6	—
Clinical course						
48.	Waxing and waning of tic severity[d]	666	97.1%	16.7	—	—
49.	Fluctuation of tics[d]	666	95.9%	19.7	—	—
50.	Remission of TS FS	666	0.9	1.7	0–8	(0.91)
a.	History of remission[d]	666	27.4%	44.6	—	0.87
b.	Length of remission (years)	666	0.7	1.3	0–7	—
Neurological factors						
51.	Attention deficit disorder[d]	666	25.1%	43.4	—	—
52.	EEG abnormality[g]	325	1.6	0.8	1–3	—
53.	Neurological abnormality[g]	380	1.3	0.6	1–3	—
54.	Right vs. other handedness[d]	666	78.2%	41.2	—	—
Stimuli-induced change of tics						
55.	Interpersonal stimuli FS[h]	394	3.3	0.5	1.3–5.3	(0.62)
a.	Strangers[h]	394	3.2	1.1	1–6	0.70
b.	Family[h]	394	4.6	0.9	1–6	−0.54
c.	School or work[h]	394	3.6	1.1	1–6	0.53
d.	Lectures, church, temple[h]	394	3.7	1.1	1–6	0.46
e.	Sleeping[h]	394	1.0	0.2	1–3	0.38
f.	Automobile[h]	394	4.0	0.9	1–6	0.28
56.	Passive stimuli FS[h]	394	3.9	1.0	1–6	(0.73)
a.	Reading[h]	394	3.7	1.2	1–6	0.70
b.	Movies[h]	394	4.0	1.2	1–6	0.67
c.	Television[h]	394	4.1	1.3	1–6	0.65
57.	Nonanxious absorption stimuli FS[h]	394	3.1	1.0	1–6	(0.80)
a.	Repairing object[h]	394	3.2	1.1	1–6	0.75
b.	Nonanxious absorption[h]	394	2.9	1.1	1–6	0.75

TABLE A.1. *(Continued)*

Variables[a]		Sample size	$\bar{X}$ or %	SD	Range	Factor loadings (R_{xx})[b]
Number	Description					
58.	Anxiety-fatigue FS[h]	394	3.8	0.4	1–6	(0.52)
	a. Evening[h]	394	4.6	1.0	1–6	0.58
	b. Afternoon[h]	394	4.3	0.8	1–6	0.51
	c. Anxiety[h]	394	5.6	0.7	2–6	0.38
	d. Morning[h]	394	3.5	1.1	1–6	−0.32
	e. Pleasurable anticipation[h]	394	4.7	1.2	1–6	0.30
59.	Seasonal stimuli FS[h]	394	3.9	0.4	1–6	(0.49)
	a. Autumn[h]	394	4.1	0.7	1–6	0.64
	b. Winter[h]	394	4.1	0.7	1–6	0.56
	c. Summer[h]	394	3.8	0.9	1–6	−0.32
	d. Spring[h]	394	4.1	0.6	1–6	0.30
Age at onset variables						
60.	Age at onset of muscular tics	666	6.9	2.9	1.2–10	—
61.	Age at onset of vocal tics	666	9.5	4.7	1.2–40	—
62.	Age at onset of coprolalia	209	11.8	5.8	3–36	—
63.	Years from TS onset to coprolalia	209	5.3	5.2	0.25	—
64.	Age at first diagnosis of TS	666	17.9	12.0	4–68	—
65.	Age at first consultation	666	11.9	8.5	2–58	—
Psychological test variables						
66.	Conners Hyperactivity Scale	318	12.0	8.0	0–30	—
67.	Bender-Gestalt Test[g]	170	0.9	0.9	0–2	—
68.	WISC (FSIQ, VIQ, PIQ, V-P Dif.)	131	—	—	—	—
69.	WAIS (FSIQ, VIQ, PIQ, V-P Dif.)	42	—	—	—	—
Other						
70.	Family history of TS or Tics	641	46.7%	49.9	—	—

[a]Variables 1 to 54 are used routinely in data analyses. Variables designated by letter include factor loadings for items in factors and are used for selected analyses referred to in the text. Variables 55 to 70 are used for selected analyses referred to in the text.

[b]R_{xx}: Generalized Spearman Brown internal consistency reliabilities for factor scales specified in parentheses.

[c]Hollingshead and Redlich Social Class Index (1958); 1 = highest social class; 5 = lowest social class.

[d]Yes, 1; No, 0.

[e]Behavioral ratings: none or not at all, 0; just a little, 1; pretty much, 2; very much, 3.

[f]Rating of assets: below average, 1; average, 2; above average, 3; excellent, 4.

[g]Abnormality: normal, 1; borderline, 2; definitely abnormal, 3.

[h]Rating of stimuli-induced change of tic severity: disappear, 1; decrease markedly, 2; decrease slightly, 3; no change, 4; increase slightly, 5; increase markedly, 6.

TABLE A.2 *Shapiro Tourette syndrome severity scale*

Tics noticeable to others[a]	Rating				Sum of ratings[e]	Global severity rating[f,g]	
	Tics elicit comments or curiosity[b]	Patient considered odd or bizarre[c]	Tics interfere with functioning[d]	Incapacitated, homebound, or hospitalized			
No (0)	No (0)	No (0)	No (0)	No (0)	___	___ (0)	= 0 None
Very few (0.5)	No (0)	No (0)	No (0)	No (0)	___	___ (>0–<1)	= 1 Very mild
Some (1)	No (0)	No (0)	No (0)	No (0)	___	___ (1–<2)	= 2 Mild
Most (2)	Possibly (0.5)	No (0)	No (0)	No (0)	___	___ (2–<4)	= 3 Moderate
All (3)	Yes (1)	Possibly (1)	Occasionally (1)	No (0)	___	___ (4–<6)	= 4 Marked
All (3)	Yes (1)	Yes (2)	Yes (2)	No (0)	___	___ (6–8)	= 5 Severe
All (3)	Yes (1)	Yes (2)	Yes (2)	Yes (1)	___	___ (>8–9)	= 6 Very severe
						___ Total	

[a]*Tics noticeable to others:*
0   Tics are not present.
0.5   Tics are infrequent or mild and usually are not noticed by employers, teachers, friends, or strangers, although some family members or very close friends may be aware of the presence of tics. Symptoms can be diminished significantly or controlled completely in public places.

1   Same as above, except tics are noticed by most friends and occasionally by some employers, teachers, or strangers.
  2   Same as above, except tics are noticed by many or most employers, teachers, and strangers.
  3   Same as above, except tics are noticed by all individuals.

bTics elicit comments or curiousity:
  0   Tics are not present or are so infrequent and mild that they are not noticed and do not elicit comments and curiosity from employers, teachers and friends, although they may be apparent to close family members.
  0.5 Tics are more frequent and apparent and possibly elicit comments or curiosity by some individuals.
  1   Tics are frequent and apparent and elicit comments or curiosity by all individuals.

cPatient considered odd or bizarre:
  0   Tics are not present or are infrequent and mild and other individuals would not consider the patient odd or bizarre.
  1   Tics are more frequent, startling, or distort the appearance of the patient, and some observers consider the patient odd or bizarre.
  2   Tics are frequent, startling, or distort the appearance of the patient, and most or all observers consider the patient odd or bizarre.

dTics interfere with functioning:
  0   Tics are absent or are present but do not interfere with academic, vocational, social, or psychological functioning and coordination.
  1   Tics occasionally or somewhat interfere with academic, vocational, social, or psychological functioning or coordination.
  2   Tics frequently, usually, or always interfere with academic, vocational, social, or psychological functioning or coordination.

eTotal sum of ratings: The total sum of ratings is the sum of the ratings of the five factors listed above. The rater has the option of assigning half scores on all factors, e.g., 0.5 for ratings that fall between values.

fGlobal severity ratings: The total sum of ratings is assigned a global severity rating using the ranges (listed in parentheses) in the last column.

gVariables: The Tourette Syndrome Severity Scale yields seven variables that can be used for different clinical and research purposes—tics noticeable to others; tics elicit comments or curiosity; patient considered odd or bizarre; tics interfere with functioning; incapacitated, homebound, or hospitalized; total sum of ratings; and global severity rating.

TABLE A.3 Shapiro global improvement scale

Therapeutic effect[a,c]	Adverse effect[b] (Circle the box under the column that best describes the severity of adverse effects)					
(Circle the phrase in this column that best characterizes the therapeutic effects)	None	Do not significantly interfere	Slightly interfere	Moderately interfere	Markedly interfere	Nullify therapeutic effect
5 Complete or nearly complete remission of 90–100% of tics	5–0	5–1	5–2	5–3	5–4	5–5
4 Decided improvement, overall decrease of 70–89% of tics	4–0	4–1	4–2	4–3	4–4	4–5
3 Considerable improvement, overall decrease of 50–69% of tics	3–0	3–1	3–2	3–3	3–4	3–5
2 Some improvement, overall decrease of 30–49% of tics	2–0	2–1	2–2	2–3	2–4	2–5
1 Slight improvement, overall decrease of less than 30% of tics	1–0	1–1	1–2	1–3	1–4	1–5
0 Unchanged, no overall increase or decrease of tics	0–0	0–1	0–2	0–3	0–4	0–5
−1 Worse, overall increase of tics	(−1)–(0)	(−1)–(1)	(−1)–(2)	(−1)–(3)	(−1)–(−5)	(−1)–(−5)

[a]Rated −1 to 5, corresponding to the phrase in that first column that best characterizes the therapeutic effect.

[b]Rated 0 to 5, corresponding to the phrase in the second column that best describes the severity of adverse effects.

[c]Overall therapeutic effect:
  Therapeutic effect minus adverse effects score = ___ (yields a numerical value for the overall therapeutic effect).
  Qualitative clinical rating = ___ (yields a clinical description of the overall therapeutic effect) derived from therapeutic effect minus adverse effects scores—5 = excellent; 4 = marked; 3 = moderate; 2 = minimum; 1 = poor; 0 = unchanged; −1 to −6 = worse.

SYMPTOM AND TREATMENT RECORD

Patient Identification _____ Age ____ Month ____ Year ____ Page ____

Day of Month →	1	2	3	4	5	6	7	8	9	10	11	12	13	14	15	16	17	18	19	20	21	22	23	24	25	26	27	28	29	30	31
Medication																															
List All Symptoms 1																															
(record the percentage decrease in your symptoms now as compared to before beginning treatment) 2																															
3																															
4																															
5																															
6																															
7																															
8																															
Side Effects of Medication 1																															
(list and record severity of symptoms as follows 3 = marked, 2 = moderate, 1 = slight, 0 = (none) (see key below) 2																															
3																															
4																															
5																															
6																															
7																															
Other Medication 1																															
(name, dosage, purpose, use other side for details) 2																															
3																															
4																															
5																															
Overall percent decrease of tic symptoms now, as compared to before beginning treatment: At home, with family, friends or alone																															
At work, in school, with strangers																															
Average for all symptoms																															

Key for side effects: 1 = slight, do not interfere with my functioning; 2 = moderate, result in some dysfunction and discomfort and require remediation; 3 = marked, result in considerable dysfunction and require immediate remediation

FIG. A.1. Shapiro Daily Record of Treatment: A daily estimate by the patient and family of symptoms, medication, and adverse effects.

Bibliography

Aarons, Z. A. (1958); Notes on a case of *maladie des tics*. *Psychoanal. Q.*, 27:194–204.
Abe K., and Oda, N. (1978): Follow-up study of children of childhood tiqueurs. *Biol. Psychiatry*, 13:629–630.
Abe, K., and Oda, N. (1980): Incidence of tics in the offspring of childhood tiqueurs: A controlled follow-up study. *Dev. Med. Child Neurol.*, 22:649–653.
Aberle, D. F. (1952): 'Arctic hysteria' and latah in Mongolia. *NY Acad. Sci.*, 14:291–297.
Abraham K. (1927): Contributions to a discussion on tic. In: *Selected Papers of Karl Abraham M.D.*, translated by B. D. Strachey. London Hogarth Press, London.
Abuzzahab, F. S. (1981): Clonidine HCL in Gilles de la Tourette syndrome. *First International Gilles de la Tourette Symposium* (abstract, p. 17), New York.
Abuzzahab, F. S., and Anderson, F. O. (1973): Gilles de la Tourette's syndrome: International Registry. *Minn. Med.*, 56:492–496.
Abuzzahab, F. S., and Anderson, F. O. (1974): Gilles de la Tourette's Syndrome: Cross cultural analysis and treatment outcome. *Clin. Neurol. Neurosurg.*, 1:66–74.
Abuzzahab, F. S., and Anderson, F. O. (1976): *Gilles de la Tourette's Syndrome, Vol. 1.* Mason, St. Paul, Minnesota.
Abuzzahab, F. S., and Ehlen, K. J. (1971): The clinical picture and management of Gilles de la Tourette's syndrome. *Child Psychiatry Hum. Dev.*, 2:14–25.
Achenbach, T. M. (1978): The child behavior profile: I. Boys aged 6–11. *J. Consult. Clin. Psychol.*, 46:478–488.
Achenbach, T. M., and Edelbrock, C. S. (1979): The child behavior profile: II. Boys aged 12–16 and girls aged 6–11 and 12–16. *J. Consult Clin. Psychol.*, 47:223–233.
Achenbach, T. M., and Edelbrock, C. S. (1981): Behavioral problems and competencies reported by parents of normal and disturbed children aged 4 through 16. *Monographs of the Society of Research in Child Development*, 46: (Serial No. 188).
Adams, R. D., and Victor, M. (1985): *Principles of Neurology*, 3rd edition. McGraw-Hill, New York.
Aghajanian, G. K. (1981): The modulatory role of seratonin at multiple receptors in brain. In: *Serotonin Neurotransmission and Behavior*, edited by B. L. Jacobs and A. Gelperin. MIT Press, Cambridge.
American Psychiatric Association (1952): *Diagnostic and Statistical Manual of Mental Disorders*, 1st edition. American Psychiatric Association Press, Washington, D.C.
American Psychiatric Association (1965): *Diagnostic and Statistical Manual of Mental Disorders*, 2nd edition. American Psychiatric Association Press, Washington, D.C.
American Psychiatric Association (1980): *Diagnostic and Statistical Manual of Mental Disorders*, 3rd edition. American Psychiatric Association Press, Washington, D.C.
American Psychiatric Association (1987): *Diagnostic and Statistical Manual of Mental Disorders*, 3rd edition, revised. American Psychiatric Association Press, Washington, D.C..
American Psychological Association (1974): *Standards for Educational and Psychological Tests*. American Psychological Association, Washington, D.C.
Anden, N., Butcher, S. G., Corrodl, H., Fuxe, K., and Ungerstedt, U. (1970): Receptor activity and turnover of dopamine and noradrenaline after neuroleptics. *Eur. J. Pharmacol.*, 11:304–314.
Andermann, F., Keene, D. L., Andermann, E., and Quesney, L.F. (1980): Startle disease of hyperekplexia: Further delineation of the syndrome. *Brain*, 103:985–997.
Andreasen, N. C., Endicott, J., Spitzer, R. L., and Winokur, G. (1977): The family history method using diagnostic criteria: Reliability and validity. *Arch. Gen. Psychiatry*, 34:1229–1235.
Ang, L., Borison, R., Dysken, M., and Davis, J. M. (1982): Reduced excretion of MHPG in Tourette syndrome. In: *Advances in Neurology, Vol. 35, Gilles de la Tourette Syndrome*, edited by A. J. Friedhoff and T. N. Chase, pp. 171–175. Raven Press, New York.

Annett, M. (1970): A classification of hand preferences by association analyses. *Br. J. Psychol.*, 61:303–21.
Araneta, E., Magen, J., Musci, M. N., Jr., Singer, P., and Vann, C. R. (1979): Tourette's syndrome symptom onset at age thirty-five. *Int. J. Soc. Psychiatry*, 25:4–9.
Arena, F. P., Chiao, J., Good, R. A., and Shapiro, A. K. (1974): Immunoglobulin levels in the sera of patients with Tourette's syndrome. *Ann. Clin. Res.*, 22:413A.
Asam, U. (1982): A follow-up study of Tourette syndrome. In: *Advances in Neurology, Vol. 35, Gilles de la Tourette Syndrome*, edited by A. J. Friedhoff and T. N. Chase, pp. 285–286. Raven Press, New York.
Asam, U., and Karrass, W. (1981): Gilles de la Tourette syndrome and psychosurgery. *Acta Paedopsychiatr. (Basel)*, 47:39–48.
Ascher, E. (1948): Psychodynamic considerations in Gilles de la Tourette's disease (*maladie des tics*): With a report of five cases and discussion of the literature. *Am. J. Psychiatry*, 105:267–276.
Ascher, E. (1966): Motor syndromes of functional or undetermined origin: tics, cramps, Gilles de la Tourette's disease, and others. In: *American Handbook of Psychiatry*, edited by S. Arieti. Basic Books, New York.
Aston-Jones, G., Foote, S. L., and Bloom, F. E. (1984): Anatomy and physiology of locus coeruleus neurons: Functional implications. In: *Norepinephine*, edited by M. G. Zeigler and C. R. Lake. Williams & Wilkins, Baltimore.
Aston-Jones, G., Ennis, M., Pieribone, V. A., Nickell, W. T., and Shipley, M. T. (1986): The brain nucleus locus coeruleus: Restricted afferent control of a broad efferent network. *Science*, 234:734–737.
Ayd, F. J., Jr. (1961): A survey of drug-induced extrapyramidal reactions. *JAMA*, 175:1054–1060.
Azrin, N. H., Nunn, R. G., and Frantz, S. E. (1980): Habit reversal vs. negative practice treatment of nervous tics. *Behav. Ther.*, 2:169–178.
Bachman, D. S. (1981): Pemoline-induced Tourette's disorder: A case report. *Am. J. Psychiatry*, 138:1116–1117.
Bai, S. (1966): An interesting case report on Gilles de la Tourette's disease. *Indian J. Psychiatry*, 8:228–232.
Baker, E F. W. (1962): Gilles de la Tourette syndrome treated by bimedial frontal leucotomy. *Can. Med. Assoc. J.*, 86:746–747.
Baldessarini, R. J. (1985): Clinical and epidemiologic aspects of tardive dyskinesia. *J. Clin. Psychiatry*, 46:8–13.
Baldessarini, R. J., and Cohen, B. M. (1987): Reply. *Am. J. Psychiatry*, 144:2.
Balthazar, K. (1956): Uber das anatomishe substrat der generalisierten tic-krankeit (maladie des tics, Gilles de la Tourette): Entwicklungshemmung des corpus striatum. *Arch. Psychiatr. Nervenkr.*, 195:531–549.
Barabas, G., and Matthews, W. S. (1983): Coincident infantile autism and Tourette syndrome: A case report. *J. Dev. Behav. Pediatr.*, 4:280–281.
Barabas, G., and Matthews, W. S. (1985): Homogeneous clinical subgroups in children with Tourette syndrome. *Pediatrics*, 75:73–75:
Barabas, G., Matthews, W. S., and Ferrari, M. (1984a): Disorders of arousal in Gilles de la Tourette's syndrome. *Neurology (Cleveland)*, 34:815–817.
Barabas, G., Matthews, W. S., and Ferrari, M. (1984b): Somnambulism in children with Tourette syndrome. *Dev. Med. Child Neurol.*, 26:457–460.
Barabas, G., Matthews, W. S., and Ferrari, M. (1984c): Tourette's syndrome and migraine. *Arch. Neurol*, 41:871–872.
Barabas, G., Matthews, W. S., and Holowinsky, M. (1984d): Electroencephalographic abnormalities in Tourette's syndrome. *Ann. Neurol.*, 16:93.
Barabas, G., Matthews, W. S., and Ferrari, M. (1984e): Letter to the editor: Motion sickness in children with Tourette's syndrome. *Ann. Neurol.*, 15:309.
Barbeau, A. (1979): Lecithin in movement disorders. In: *Nutrition and the Brain, Vol. 5*, edited by A. Barbeau, J. H. Growdon, and R. J. Wurtman. Raven Press. New York.
Barbour, P. F. (1913): "Tic" in children. *Pediatrics*, 25:697–701.
Barlow, C. F. (1974): Soft signs in children with learning disorders. *Am. J. Dis. Child.*, 128:605–606.

Barnes, D. M. (1987): Biological issues in schizophrenia. *Science*, 235:430–433.
Baron, M., Shapiro, E., Shapiro, A. K., and Rainer, J. D. (1981): Genetic analysis of Tourette syndrome suggesting major gene effect. *Am. J. Hum. Genet.*, 33:767–775.
Barr, F F., Lovibond, S. H., and Katsaros, E. (1972): A case of Gilles de la Tourette's syndrome in a brain-damaged child. *Med. J. Aust.*, 2:372–374.
Bateman, D N., Craft, A. W., Nicholson, E., and Pearson, A. D. J. (1983): Dystonic reactions and the pharmacokinetics of metoclopramide in children. *Br. J. Clin. Pharmacol.*, 15:557–559.
Bauer, A. M., and Shea, T. M. (1984): Tourette syndrome: A review and educational implications. *J. Autism Dev. Disord.*, 14:69–80.
Bax, M., and MacKeith, R. (editors) (1963): Minimal cerebral dysfunction. In: *Little Club Clinics in Developmental Medicine*, p. 10. Heineman, London.
Beard, G. M. (1880): *Experiments with the 'Jumpers' of Maine*. Paper read before the American Neurological Association, June, 1880.
Beard, G. M (1886): Experiments with the "jumpers" or "jumping Frenchmen" of Maine. *J. Nerv. Ment. Dis.*, 7:487–490.
Beck, S. J. (1949): *Rorschach Test I: Basic Processes*. Grune & Stratton, New York.
Bender, L. A. (1956): Psychopathology of children with organic brain disorders. Thomas, Springfield, Illinois.
Benedek, L. (1925): Zwangsmässiges schreien in anfällen als postencephalitische hyperkinese. *Z. Ges. Neurol. Psychiatr.*, 98:17–26.
Berecz, J. M., Dysken, M. W., and Davis, J. M. (1979): Nalaxone effect in Tourette syndrome letter. *Neurology (Minneap.)*, 29(1):1316–1317.
Berg, C. J., Rapoport, J. L., and Flament, M. (1986): The Leyton obsessional inventory-child version. *J. Am. Acad. Child Psychiatry*, 25:84–91.
Berg, R. (1985): A case of TS treated with nifedipine. *Acta Psychiatr. Scand.*, 72:400–401.
Bergen, D., Tanner, C. M., and Wilson, R. (1982): The electroencephalogram in Tourette syndrome. *Ann. Neurol.*, 11:382–385.
Bernheim, H. (1889): *Suggestive Therapeutics*. Putnam, New York.
Bernstein, L. (1963): A respiratory tic: "The barking cough of puberty." Report of a case treated successfully. *Laryngoscope*, 73:315–319.
Beumont, P., Bruwer, J., Pimstone, B., Vinik, A., and Utian, W. (1975): Brom-ergocryptine in the treatment of phenothiazine-induced galactorrhea. *Br. J. Psychiatry*, 126:285–288.
Bieren, R. E. (1969): Tourette's disease: Successful treatment. *J. S. Carolina Med. Assn.*, 65:7–8.
Bing, R. (1925): Uber lokale muskelspasmen und tics. *Schweiz. Med. Wochenschr.*, 6:993–997.
Bleeker, H. E. (1978): Gilles de la Tourette's syndrome with direct evidence of organicity. *Psychiatr. Clin.*, 11:147–154.
Bliss, J. (1980): Sensory experiences of Gilles de la Tourette syndrome. *Arch. Gen. Psychiatry*, 37:1343–1347.
Bloomingdale, L. M. (1984): Whither ADD (attention deficit disorder)? *Psychiatr. J. Univ. Ottawa*, 9:175–186.
Bock, R. D., and Goldberger, L. (1985): Tonic, phasic and cortical arousal in Gilles de la Tourette's syndrome. *J. Neurol. Neurosurg. Psychiatry*, 48:535–544.
Bockner, S. (1959): Gilles de la Tourette's disease. *J. Ment. Sci.*, 105:1078–1081.
Bodis-Wollner, I., Yahr, M. D., and Mylin, L. H. (1980): Visual evoked potential latency changes due to neurotransmitter deficiency in humans. *Trans. Am. Neurol. Assoc.*, 105:215–218.
Bogomolny, A., Erenberg, G., and Rothner, A. D. (1982): Behavioral effects of haloperidol in young Tourette syndrome patients. In: *Advances in Neurology, Vol. 35, Gilles de la Tourette Syndrome*, edited by A.J. Friedhoff and T. N. Chase, pp. 427–432. Raven Press, New York.
Boncour, G. P. (1910): Les tic chez l'ecolier et leur interpretation. *Prog. Med.*, 26:495–596.
Bonheim, C. (1930): Uber den tic im kindesalter. *Klin. Wochenschr.*, 9:2005–2011.
Borak, W. (1969): Przypadek encefalopatii Z tikami Tourette's zespolem anankastycznym i impulsywymi tendencjami do Samovszkodzen. *Psychiatr. Pol.*, 3:111–114.
Borenstein, P., Dabba, M., and Bles, G. (1962): Etude electroencephalographique de la thioproperazine. *Rev. Neurol. (Paris)*, 106:238–243.
Boris, M. (1968): Gilles de la Tourette's syndrome: Remission with haloperidol. *JAMA*, 205:102–103.

Borison, R. L., and Davis, J. M. (1983): Amantadine in Tourette syndrome. *Curr. Psychiatr. Ther.*, 22:127–130.
Borison, R. L., Ang, L., Chang, S., Dysken, M., Comaty, J. E., and Davis, J. M. (1982): New pharmacological approaches in the treatment of Tourette syndrome. In: *Advances in Neurology, Vol. 35, Gilles de la Tourette Syndrome*, edited by A. J. Friedhoff and T. N. Chase, pp. 377–382. Raven Press, New York.
Borison, R. L., Ang, L., Hamilton, W. J., Diamond, B. I., and Davis, J. M. (1983): Treatment approaches in Gilles de la Tourette syndrome. *Brain Res. Bull.*, 11:205–208.
Bornstein, R. A., Carroll, A., and King, G. (1985): Relationship of age to neuropsychological deficit in Tourette syndrome. *Dev. Behav. Pediatr.*, 6:284–286.
Bosco, J. J., and Robin, S. S. (1980): Hyperkinesis: Prevalence and treatment. In: *Hyperactive Children: The Social Ecology of Identification and Treatment*, edited by C. K. Whalen and B. Henker, pp. 173–187. Academic Press, New York.
Bouteille, E. M. (1810): *Traite de Chorée*. Vincard, Paris.
Boyer, W. F., Honeycutt-Bakalar, N., and Lake, C. R. (1987): Anticholinergic prophylaxis of acute haloperidol-induced acute dystonic reactions. *J. Clin. Psychopharmacol.*, 7:164–166.
Bradnan, W. A. (1972): Familial communicating patterns of a patient with Gilles de la Tourette's syndrome. *J. Nerv. Ment. Dis.*, 154:60–68.
Brain, W. R. (1928): The treatment of tic. *Lancet*, 1:1295–1296.
Bremnes, A. B., and Sverd, J. (1979): Methylphenidate induced Tourette syndrome. *Am. J. Psychiatry*, 136:1334–1335.
Bresler, V. O. (1896): Beitrag zur lehre von der maladie des tics convulsifs. *Neurol. Centralbl.*, 15:965–972.
Bresnahan, J. L., and Shapiro, M. M. (1966): A general equation and technique for the exact partitioning of Chi-square contingency tables. *Psychol. Bull.*, 66:252–262.
Brissaud, E. (1899): Chorée variable. *Presse Medicale*, 13:73–74.
Brodde, O. E., Anlauf, M., Graben, N., and Bock, K. D. (1982): *In vitro* and *in vivo* downregulation of human platelet alpha$_2$-adrenoreceptors by clonidine. *Eur. J. Clin. Pharmacol.*, 23:403–409.
Bromberg. W. (1954): *Man Above Humanity-A History of Psychotherapy*. J. B. Lippincott Co., Philadelphia.
Brown, E. E. (1957): Tic (habit spasms) secondary to sinusitis. *Arch. Pediatr.*, 74:39–46.
Brown, W. A., and Laughren, T. P. (1981): Tolerance to the prolactin-elevating effect of neuroleptics. *Psychiatry Res.*, 5:317–322.
Bruch, H,. and Thum, L. C. (1968): *Maladie des tics* and maternal psychosis. *J. Nerv. Ment. Dis.*, 146:446–456.
Bruun, R. D. (1982): Clonidine treatment of Tourette syndrome. In: *Advances in Neurology, Vol. 35, Gilles de la Tourette Syndrome*, edited by A.J. Friedhoff and T. N. Chase, pp. 403–405. Raven Press, New York.
Bruun, R. D., Shapiro, A. K., Shapiro, E., Sweet, R. D., Wayne, H., and Solomon, G. E. (1976): A follow-up of 78 patients with Gilles de la Tourette's syndrome. *Am. J. Psychiatry*, 133: 944–947.
Buck, S. H., and Yamamura, H. I. (1982): Neuropeptides in normal and pathological basal ganglia. In: *Advances in Neurology, Vol. 35, Gilles de la Tourette Syndrome*, edited by A. J. Friedhoff and T. N. Chase. Raven Press, New York.
Buckwald, N. A. Hull, D. C., and Levine, M. S. (1979): Basal ganglia neuronal activity and behavioral set. *Appl. Neurophysiol.*, 42:109–12.
Bullen, J. G., and Hemsley, D. R. (1983): Sensory experience as a trigger in Gilles de la Tourette's syndrome. *J. Behav. Ther. Exp. Psychiatry*, 14:197–201.
Bunney, B. S. (1984): Antipsychotic drug effects on the electrical activity of dopaminergic neurons. *Trends Neurosci.*, 7:212–215.
Bunney, B. S., and Aghajanian, G. K. (1978): d-Alphetamine-induced depression of central dopamine neurons: evidence for mediation by both autoreceptors and a striato-nigral feedback pathway. *Naunyn Schmiedebergs Arch. Pharmacol.*, 304:255–261.
Bunney, B. S., and DeRiemer, S. (1982): Effect of clonidine on dopaminergic neuron activity in the substantia nigra: Possible indirect mediation by noradrenergic regulation of the serotonergic raphe system. In: *Advances in Neurology, Vol. 35, Gilles de la Tourette Syndrome*, edited by A. J. Friedhoff and T. N. Chase. Raven Press, New York.

Burd, L., and Kerbeshian, J. (1985): Tourette syndrome, atypical pervasive developmental disorder and Ganser syndrome in a 15-year-old, visually impaired, mentally retarded boy. *Can. J. Psychiatry*, 30:74–76.
Burd L., Kerbeshian, J., Fisher, W., and Gascon, G. (1986a): Anticonvulsant medications: An iatrogenic cause of tic disorders. *Can. J. Psychiatry*, 31:419–423.
Burd, L., Kerbeshian, J., Wikenheiser, M., and Fisher, W. (1986b): Prevalence of Gilles de la Tourette's syndrome in North Dakota adults. *Am. J. Psychiatry*, 143:787–788.
Burd, L., Kerbeshian, L., Wikenheiser, M., and Fisher, W. (1986c): A prevalence study of Gilles de la Tourette syndrome in North Dakota school-age children. *J. Am. Acad. Child Psychiatry*, 25:552–553.
Buschke, H. (1973): Selective reminding for analysis of memory and learning. *Verbal Learning Verbal Behavior* 12:543–550.
Butler, I. J., Koslow, S. H. Seifert, W. E., Jr., Caprioli, R. M., and Singer, H.S. (1979): Biogenic amine metabolism in Tourette syndrome. *Ann. Neurol.*, 6:37–39.
Butler, M. (1985): Review of developmental-behavioral pediatrics. *Am. J. Psychiatry*, 142:876–877.
Bytheway, B. (1974): A statistical trap associated with family size. *J. Biosoc. Sci.*, 6:67–72.
Caine, E. D. (1985): Gilles de la Tourette's syndrome. A review of clinical and research studies and considerations of future directions for investigation. *Arch. Neurol.*, 42:393–397.
Caine, E. D., and Polinsky, R. J. (1979): Haloperidol induced dysphoria in patients with Tourette syndrome. *Am. J. Psychiatry*, 136:1216–1217.
Caine, E. D., and Polinsky, R. J. (1981): Letter to the editor: Tardive dyskinesia in persons with Gilles de la Tourette's disease. *Arch. Neurol.*, 38:471–472.
Caine, E. D., Margolin, D. I., Brown, G. L., and Ebert, M. H. (1978): Gilles de la Tourette's syndrome, tardive dyskenesia, and psychosis in an adolescent. *Am. J. Psychiatry*, 135:241.
Caine, E. D., Polinsky, R. J., Ebert, M. H., Rapoport, J. L., and Mikkelsen, E. J. (1979a): Trial of chlorimipramine and desipramine for Gilles de la Tourette syndrome. *Ann. Neurol.*, 5:305–306.
Caine, E. D., Polinsky, R. J., Kartzinel, R., and Ebert, M. H. (1979b): The trial use of clozapine for abnormal involuntary movement disorders. *Am. J. Psychiatry*, 136:317–320.
Caine, E. D., Polinsky, R. J., Ludlow, C. L., Ebert, M. H., and Nee, L. E. (1982): Heterogeneity and variability in Tourette's syndrome. In: *Advances in Neurology, Vol. 35, Gilles de la Tourette Syndrome*, edited by A. J. Friedhoff and T. N. Chase, pp. 437–442. Raven Press New York.
Caine, E. D., Ludlow, C. L., Polinsky, R. J., and Ebert, M. H. (1984): Provocative drug testing in Tourette's syndrome: d- and l-amphetamine and haloperidol. *J. Am. Acad. Child Psychiatry*, 23:147–152.
Caine, E. D., McBride, M. C., Chiverton, P., Bamford, K. A., Rediess, S., and Shiao, J. (1985): *Tourette Syndrome in Monroe County School Children.* Talk presented at Tourette Clinical Symposium, October 1985, Mt. Sinai Medical Center, New York.
Caine, E. D., Weltkamp, L. R., Chiverton, P., Guttormsen, S., Yagnow, R., Hempfling, S., and Kennelly, D. (1985): Tourette syndrome and HLA. *J. Neurol. Sci.*, 59:201–206.
Campbell, A., and Baldessarini, R. J. (1985): Letter to the editor: Prolonged pharmacologic activity of neuroleptics. *Arch. Gen. Psychiatry*, 46:637.
Campbell, M. (1985): On the use of neuroleptics in children and adolescents. *Psychiatric Ann.*, 15:101–107.
Campbell, M., Anderson, L. T., Small, A. M., Perry, R., Green, W. H., and Caplan, R. (1982): The effects of haloperidol on learning and behavior in autistic children. *J. Autism Dev. Disord.*, 12:167–175.
Campbell, M., Perry, R., Palij, M., Nobler, M., and Shore, H. (1985): Naltrexone in infantile autism: An acute dose trial. In: *Proceedings of the Annual Meeting of the American Academy of Child Psychiatry*, edited by L. Greenhill, p. 29.
Canavan, A. G. M., and Powell, G. E. (1981): The efficacy of several treatments of Gilles de la Tourette's syndrome as assessed in a single case. *Behav. Res. Ther.*, 19:549–556.
Cantwell, D. (1984): Discussions. In: *Attention Deficit Disorder: Diagnostic, Cognitive, and Therapeutic Understanding*, edited by L. M. Bloomingdale, pp. 127–130. Spectrum, New York.
Caparulo, B. K., Cohen, D. J., Rothman, S. L., Young, D. G., Katz, J. D., Shaywitz, S. E., and Shaywitz, B. A. (1981): Computed tomographic brain scanning in children with developmental neuropsychiatric disorders. *J. Am. Acad. Child Psychiatry*, 20:338–357.

Caprini, G., and Melotti, V. (1961): Un grave sindrome ticcosa guarita con haloperidol. *Riv. Sper. Freniat.*, 85:191–196.
Carroll, W. J. (1974): Gilles de la Tourette's syndrome. *Virginia Med. Monthly*, 101:672–674.
Casamenti, F., Bianci, C., Beani, L., et al. (1980): Effect of haloperidol and pimozide on acetylcholine output from the cerebral cortex in rats and guinea pigs. *Eur. J. Pharmacol.*, 65:279–284.
Castellan, N. J., Jr. (1965): On the partitioning of contingency tables. *Psychol. Bull.*, 64:330–338.
Catrou, J. (1890): Etude sur la maladie des tics convulsifs (jumping, latah, myriachit). *Doctoral thesis, Faculte de Médecine de Paris*. Henri Jouve, Paris.
Chabbert, L. (1893): De la maladie des tics (tics, chorée, hysterie: diagnostique). *Arch. Neurol.*, 25:10–41.
Challas, G., and Brauer, W. (1963): Tourette's disease: Relief of symptoms with R1625. *Am. J. Psychiatry*, 120:283–284.
Challas, G., Chapel, J. L., and Jenkins, R. L. (1967): Tourette's disease: Control of symptoms and its clinical course. *Int. J. Neuropsychiatry*, 3(Suppl. 1):96–109.
Chang, R. J., Laufer, L., and DeFazio, J. (1982): Bromocriptine therapy of hyperprolactinemia. *Drug Ther.*, May: 67–75.
Chapel, J. L. (1970): Latah, myriachit, and jumpers revisited. *NY State J. Med.*, 70:2201–2204.
Chapel, J. L., Brown, N., and Jenkins, R. L. (1964): Tourette's disease: Symptomatic relief with haloperidol. *Am. J. Psychiatry*, 121:608–610.
Charcot, J. M. (1885): Intorno ad alcuni casi di tic convulsivo con coprolalia ed echolalia. Reported by G. Melotti. *La Riforma Medica*, pp. 184–186.
Charcott, J. M. (1888–1889): *Leçons du Mardi à la Salpêtrière-Polyclinique*, 2:13–17.
Chase, T. N., Foster, N. L., Fedio, P., Brooks, R., Mansi, L., Kessler, R., and DiChiro, G. (1984): Gilles de la Tourette syndrome: Studies with the fluorine-18-labeled fluorodeoxyglucose positron emission tomographic method. *Ann. Neurol. (Suppl.)*, 15:175.
Chouinard, G., and Annable, L. (1977): Phenothiazine-induced ECG abnormalities. *Arch. Gen. Psychiatry*, 34:951–954.
Clauss, J. L., and Balthasar, K. (1954): Zur kenntnis der generalisierten tic-krankheit (maladie des tics, Gilles de la Tourette' sche krankheit). *Arch. Psychiatr. Nervenkr.*, 191:398–418.
Clement, P. W. (1974): Parents, peers, and child patients make the best therapists. In: *Clinical Child Psychology*, edited by G. J. Williams and S. Gordon. Behavioral Publications, New York.
Clements, R. O. (1972): Gilles de la Tourette's syndrome—an overview of development and treatment of a case using hypnotherapy, haloperidol, and psychotherapy. *Am. J. Clin. Hypn.*, 14:167–172.
Clements, S. (1966): Minimal brain dysfunction in children. In: *NINBD Monograph No. 3*. United States Public Health Service, Washington, D.C.
Clements, S. O., and Peters, J. E.: (1962): Minimal brain dysfunctions in the school-age child. *Arch. Gen. Psychiatry*, 6:185–197.
Cloninger, C. R., Reich, T., and Yokoyama, S. (1983): Genetic diversity, genome organization, and investigation of the etiology of psychiatric diseases. *Psychiatr. Dev.*, 3:225–246.
Cohen, D. J., Shaywitz, B. A., Johnson, W. T., and Bowers, M. B., Jr. (1974): Biogenic amines in autistic and atypical children. *Arch. Gen. Psychiatry*, 31:845–853.
Cohen, D. J., Dibble, E., Grawe, J. M., and Pollin, W. (1973): Separating identical from fraternal twins. *Arch. Gen. Psychiatry*, 29:465–469.
Cohen, D. J., Dibble, E., Grawe, J. M., and Pollin, W. (1975): Reliably separating identical from fraternal twins. *Arch. Gen. Psychiatry*, 32:1371–1375.
Cohen, D. J., Shaywitz, B. A., Caparulo, B., Young, J. G., and Bowers, M. B., Jr. (1978): Chronic, multiple tics of Gilles de la Tourette's disease: CSF acid monoamine metabolites after probenecid administration. *Arch. Gen. Psychiatry*, 35:245–250.
Cohen, D. J., Shaywitz, B. A., Young, J. G., Carbonari, C. M., Nathanson, J. A., Lieberman, D., Bowers, M. B., Jr., and Maas, J. W. (1979a): Central biogenic amine metabolism in children with the syndrome of chronic multiple tics of Gilles de la Tourette: Norepinephrine, serotonin, and dopamine. *J. Am. Acad. Child Psychiatry*, 18:320–341.
Cohen, D. J., Young, J. G., Nathanson, J. A., and Shaywitz, B. A. (1979b): Clonidine in Tourette's syndrome. *Lancet*, 2:551–533.

Cohen, D. J., Detlor, J., Young, J. G., and Shaywitz, B. A. (1980): Clonidine ameliorates Gilles de la Tourette syndrome. *Arch. Gen. Psychiatry*, 37:1350–1357.
Cohen, D. J., Detlor, J., Shaywitz, B. A., and Leckman, J. F. (1982): Interaction of biological and psychological factors in the natural history of Tourette syndrome: A paradigm for childhood neuropsychiatric disorders. In: *Advances in Neurology, Vol. 35, Gilles de la Tourette Syndrome*, edited by A. J. Friedhoff and T. N. Chase, pp. 31–40. Raven Press, New York.
Cohen, D. J., Leckman, J. F., and Shaywitz, B. A. (1983): Tourette syndrome: Assessment and treatment. In: *Diagnosis and Treatment in Pediatric Psychiatry*, edited by D. Shaffer, A. A. Ehrhardt, and L. Greenhill. MacMillan Free Press, New York.
Cohen, D. J., Ort, S., Caruso, K. Anderson, G. M., Hunt, R. D., Shaywitz, B. A., Kremenitzer, M., and Leckman, J. F. (1987): Parotid gland salivary secretion in Tourette's syndrome and attention deficit disorder: A model system for the study of neurochemical regulation. *J. Am. Acad. Child Adolescent Psychiatry*, 26:65–68.
Cohen, J., and Cohen P. (1983): *Applied Multiple Regressional Correlation Analysis for the Behavioral Sciences*, 2nd edition. Lawrence Erlbaum Associates, Hillsdale, New Jersey.
Cohen, P., and Cohen, J. (1984): The clinician's illusion. *Arch. Gen. Psychiatry*, 41:1178–1182.
Cohn, R. (1947): *Clinical Electroencephalography*. McGraw-Hill, New York.
Comings, D. E., and Comings, B. G. (1984): Tourette syndrome and attention deficit disorder with hyperactivity—are they due to the same gene? *J. Am. Acad. Child Psychiatry*, 23:138–146.
Comings, D. E., and Comings, B. G. (1985): Tourette Syndrome: Clinical and psychological aspects of 250 cases. *Am. J. Hum. Genet.*, 37:435–450.
Comings, D. E., and Comings, B. G. (1986): Evidence for an X-linked modifier gene affecting the expression of Tourette syndrome and its relevance to the increased frequency of speech, cognitive, and behavioral disorders in males. *Proc. Natl. Acad. Sci. USA*, 83:2551–2555.
Comings, D. E., Goetz, I. E., Holden, J., and Holtz, J. (1981): Huntington disease and Tourette syndrome. II. Uptake of glutamic acid and other amino acids by fibroblasts. *Am. J. Hum. Genet.*, 33:175–186.
Comings, E. E., Gursey, B. T., Hecht, T., and Blume, K. (1982a): HLA typing in Tourette Syndrome. In: *Advances in Neurology, Vol. 35, Gilles de la Tourette Syndrome*, edited by A. J. Friedhoff and T. N. Chase, pp. 251–253. Raven Press, New York.
Comings, D. E., Gursey, B. T., Avelino, E., Kopp, U., and Hanin, I. (1982b): Red blood cell choline in Tourette syndrome. In: *Advances in Neurology, Vol. 35, Gilles de la Tourette Syndrome*, edited by A. J. Friedhoff and T. N. Chase, pp. 255–258. Raven Press, New York.
Comings, D. E., Comings, B. G., Devor, E. J., and Cloninger, C. R. (1984): Detection of a major gene for Gilles de la Tourette syndrome. *Am. J. Hum. Genet.*, 36:586–600.
Connell, P. H., Corbett, J. A., Horne, D. I., and Mathews, A. M. (1967): Drug treatment of adolescent ticqueurs: A double-blind trial of diazepam and haloperidol. *Br. J. Psychiatry*, 113:375–381.
Connors, C. K. (1969): A teacher rating scale for use in drug studies with children. *Am. J. Psychiatry*, 126:152:156.
Connors, C. K. (1970): Symptom patterns in hyperkinetic, neurotic and normal children. *Child Dev.*, 41:667–682.
Connors, C. K. (1972): Pharmacotherapy of psychopathology in children. In: *Psychopathology Disorders of Children*, edited by H. C. Quay and J. S. Werry, pp. 316–347. Wiley, New York.
Connors, C. K. (1985a): Issues in the study of adolescent ADD-H/hyperactivity. *Psychopharmacol. Bull.*, 21:243–250.
Connors, C. K. (1985b): Methodological and assessment issues in pediatric psychopharmacology. In: *Diagnosis and Psychopharmacology of Childhood and Adolescent Disorders*, edited by J. M. Wiener, pp. 69–110. Wiley, New York.
Connors, C. K., Eisenberg, L., and Sharpe, L. (1964): Effect of methylphenidate (ritalin) on paired-associate learning and Porteus maze performance in emotionally disturbed children. *J. Consult. Psychiatry*, 28:14–22.
Cooper, I. S. (1969): *Involuntary Movement Disorders*. Hoeber Medical Division, Harper & Row, New York.
Cooper, J. R., Bloom, F. E., and Roth, R. H. (1986): *The Biochemical Basis of Neuropharmacology*, 5th edition. Oxford University Press, New York.

Corbett, J. A. (1976): Tics and Tourette syndrome. In: *Child Psychiatry Modern Approaches*, edited by M. Rutter and L. Hersov, pp. 674–687. Lippincott, Philadelphia.
Corbett, J. A., Mathews, A. M., Connell, P. H., and Shapiro, D. A. (1969): Tics and Gilles de la Tourette's syndrome: A follow-up study and critical review. *Br. J. Psychiatry*, 115:1229–1241.
Corbin, K. B. (1970): Common neuro-physiologic factors reported in the literature. *NY State J. Med.*, 70:2193–2197.
Cote, L., and Crutcher, M. D. (1985): Motor functions of the basal ganglia and diseases of transmitter metabolism. In: *Principles of Neural Science*, 2nd edition, edited by E. R. Kandel and J. H. Schwartz. Elsevier, New York.
Craven, E. M. (1969): Letter to the editor: Gilles de la Tourette's syndrome treated with haloperidol. *JAMA*, 210:134.
Creak, M., and Guttman, E. (1935): Chorea, tics, and compulsive utterances. *J. Ment. Sci.*, 81:834–839.
Creese, I., Sibley, D. R., Hamblin, M. W., and Leff, S. E. (1983): The classification of dopamine receptors: Relationship to radioligand binding. *Annu. Rev. Neurosci.*, 6:43–71.
Crosley, C. J. (1979): Decreased seratonergic activity in Tourette syndrome. *Ann. Neurol.*, 5:596–597.
Cruchet, R. (1901): Etude critique sur le tic convulsif et son traitment gymnastic. *Doctoral Thesis, University of Bordeaux*.
Culver, C. M., and Gert, B. (1982): *Philosophy in Medicine*, Chapter 6. Oxford University Press, London.
Cummings, J. L., and Frankel, M. (1985): Gilles de la Tourette syndrome and the neurological basis of obsessions and compulsions. *Biol. Psychiatry*, 20:1117–1126.
Cunningham, M. A., Pillai, V., and Rogers, W. T. (1968): Haloperidol in treatment of children with severe behavioral disorders. *Br. J. Psychiatry*, 114:845–854.
Dana, C. L., and Wilkin, W. P. (1886): On convulsive tic with explosive disturbance of speech (so called Gilles de la Tourette's disease). *J. Nerv. Ment. Dis.*, 13:407–409.
Daube, J. R., and Peters, H. A. (1966): Hereditary essential myoclonus. *Arch. Neurol.*, 15:587–594.
Davidenkow, S. (1926): Auf hereditar-abiographischer Grundlage Akut auftretende, regressierende und episodische Erkrankungen des Nervensystems und Bemerkungen über die famillare subakute, myoklonische. *Dystonie Z. Neurol. Psychiatr.*, 104:596–622.
Debray-Ritzen, P., and Dubois, H. (1980): Maladie des tics de l'enfant. A propose de 93 cas. *Rev. Neurol. (Paris)*, 136:15–18.
Debray, P., Messerschmitt, P., Lonchap, D., and Herbault, M. (1972): L'utilization du pimozide en pedopsychiatrie. *Nouv. Presse Med.*, 1:2917–2918.
Denckla, M. B., Bemporad, J. R., and McKay, M. C. (1976): Tics following methylphenidate administration. A report of 20 cases. *JAMA*, 235:1379–1381.
Desai, A. B., Doongaji, D. R., and Satoskar, R. S. (1983): Metoclopramide in Gilles de la Tourette's syndrome (a case report). *J. Postgrad. Med.*, 29:181–183.
DeVeaugh-Geiss, J. (1980): Letter to the editor: Tardive Tourette syndrome. *Neurology*, 30:562–563.
Devinsky, O. (1983): Neuroanatomy of Gilles de la Tourette's syndrome: Possible midbrain involvement. *Arch. Neurol.*, 40:508–514.
Devor, E. J. (1984): Complex segregation analysis of Gilles de la Tourette syndrome: further evidence for a major locus mode of transmission. *Am. J. Hum. Genet.*, 36:704–709.
Dewulf, A., and van Bogaert, L. (1940): Etudes anatomo-cliniques de syndromes hypercinétiques complexes. *Mschr. Psychiatr. Neurol.*, 104:53–61.
Diamond, B. I., Reyes, M. G., and Borison, R. (1982): A new animal model for Tourette syndrome. In: *Advances in Neurology, Vol. 35, Gilles de la Tourette Syndrome*, edited by A. J. Friedhoff and T. N. Chase, pp. 221–225. Raven Press, New York.
DiGiacomo, J. N., Fahn, S., Glass, J. B., and Westlake, R. J. (1971); A case with Gilles de la Tourette's syndrome: recurrent refractoriness to haloperidol and unsuccessful treatment with L-dopa. *J. Nerv. Ment. Dis.*, 152:115–117.
Dillon, D. C., Salzman, I. J., and Schulsinger, D. A. (1985): The use of imipramine in Tourette's syndrome and attention deficit disorder: Case report. *J. Clin. Psychiatry*, 46:348–349.
Director, K. L., and Muniz, C. E. (1982): Diazepam in the treatment of extra-pyramidal symptoms: A case report. *J. Clin. Psychiatry*, 43:160.

Dolmierski, R., and Kloss, M. (1962): De la maladie de Gilles de la Tourette. *Ann. Med. Psychol.,* 1:225–232.
Domino, E. F., Piggott, L., Demetriou, S., and Culbert, J. (1982): Visually evoked responses in Tourette syndrome. In: *Advances in Neurology, Vol. 35, Gilles de la Tourette Syndrome,* edited by A. J. Friedhoff and T. N. Chase, pp. 115–120. Raven Press, New York.
Donnelly, M., and Rapoport, J. L. (1985): Attention deficit disorders. In: *Diagnoses and Psychophamacology of Childhood and Adolescent Disorders,* edited by J. M. Wiener, pp. 179–197. Wiley, New York.
Dorsey, R. (1981): Letter to the editor: Clonidine and Gilles de la Tourette syndrome. *Arch. Gen. Psychiatry,* 38:1185.
Downing, R. W., Comer, N. I., and Ebert, J. N. (1984): Family dynamics in a case of Gilles de la Tourette's syndrome. *J. Nerv. Ment. Dis.,* 138:548–557.
Drage, W. (1963): Mary Hall of Gadsden in Hertford. In: *300 Years of Psychiatry,* edited by R. Hunter and I. McAlpine, pp. 174–177. OUP, London.
Drury, L., Mellinger, J. F., and Michels, V. V. (1986): Letter to the editor: Episodic Tourette's syndrome in a patient with citrullinemia. *Ann. Neurol.,* 19:612.
DSM-III-R Task Force (1986): Consensus meeting on diagnostic criteria for tic disorders.
Dunlap, J. R. (1960): A case of Gilles de la Tourette's disease (*maladie des tics*): A study of the intrafamily dynamics. *J. Nerv. Ment. Dis.,* 130:340–344.
Dyer, R. S., Howell, W. E., and McPhail, R. C. (1981): Dopamine depletion slows retinal transmission. *Exp. Neurol.,* 7:326–340.
Dysken, M. W., Berecz, J. M., Samarza, A., and Davis, J. M. (1980): Letter to the editor: Clonidine in Tourette syndrome. *Lancet,* 2:926–927.
Edlund, M. J., and Craig, T. J. (1984): Antipsychotic drug use and birth defects: An epidemiologic reassessment. *Compr. Psychiatry,* 25:32–36.
Eeg-Olofsson, O. (1971): The development of the electroencephalogram in normal adolescents from the age of 16 through 21 years. *Neuropaediatrie,* 3:11–45.
Eeg-Olofsson, O., Petersen, I., and Sellden, U. (1971): The development of the electroencephalogram in normal children from the age of 1 through 15 years. Paroxysmal activity. *Neuropaediatrie,* 2:375–404.
Eggers, C., Olbricht, T., and Rotherberger, A. (1983): Neurobiological findings in children with tics and Gilles de la Tourette syndrome. In: *Special Aspects of Psychopharmacology,* edited by M. Ackenheil and N. Matussek, pp. 191–202. Expansion Scientifique Francaise, Paris.
Eisenberg, L. Ascher, E., and Kanner, L. (1959): A clinical study of Gilles de la Tourette's disease (*maladie des tics*) in children. *Am. J. Psychiatry,* 115:715–723.
El-Defrawi, M. H., and Greenhill, L. L. (1984): Substituting stimulants in treating behavior disorders. *Am. J. Psychiatry,* 141:610–611.
Eldridge, R. (1976): Discussion. In: *Advances in Neurology, Vol. 14, Dystonia,* edited by R. Eldridge and S. Fahn, p. 281. Raven Press, New York.
Eldridge, R., Sweet, R. D., Shapiro, A. K., and Arena, F. (1975): Clinical and genetic observations of 21 families and Gilles de la Tourette syndrome (abstract). *Neurology,* 25:379.
Eldridge, R., Sweet, R. D., Lake, C. R., Ziegler, M., and Shapiro, A. K. (1977): Gilles de la Tourette syndrome: Clinical, genetic, psychological and biochemical aspects of 21 selected families. *Neurology,* 27:115–124.
Elkins, R., Rapoport, J. L., and Lipsky, A. (1980): Obsessive-compulsive disorder of childhood and adolescence: A neurobiologic viewpoint. *J. Am. Acad., Child Psychiatry* 19:511–524.
Elkisch, P. (1968): Nonverbal, extraverbal and austistic verbal communication in the treatment of a child tiqueur. *Psychoanal. Study Child,* 23:423–437.
Ellison, R. M. (1964): Gilles de la Tourette's syndrome. *Med. J. Aust.,* 153:155.
Erenberg, G. (1982): Letter to the editor. *JAMA,* 248:1062.
Erenberg, G. (1985): Letter to the editor: Sleep disorders in Gilles de la Tourette's syndrome. *Neurology,* 35:1397.
Erenberg, G., and Rothner, A. D. (1978): Tourette syndrome: A childhood disorder. *Cleve. Clin. Q.,* 45:207–212.
Erenberg, G., Cruse, R. P., and Rothner, D. (1985): Gilles de la Tourette syndrome: Effects of stimulant drugs. *Neurology,* 35:1346–1348.
Erenberg, G., Cruse, R. P., and Rothner, A. D. (1986): Tourette syndrome: An analysis of 200 pediatric and adolescent cases. *Cleve. Clin. Q.,* 53:127–31.

Erickson, H. M. (1964): Experimental hypnotherapy in Tourette's disease. *Am. J. Clin. Hypn.*, 7:325–331.
Erickson, H. M., Goggins, J. E., and Messiha, F. S. (1976): Comparison of lithium and haloperidol therapy in Gilles de la Tourette syndrome. In: *Advances in Experimental Medicine and Biology, Vol. 90*, edited by F. S. Messiha and A. D. Kenny, pp. 197–205. Plenum Press, New York.
Eriksson, B., and Persson, T. (1969): Gilles de la Tourette's syndrome, two cases with an organic brain inquiry. *Br. J. Psychiatry*, 115:351–353.
Escalar, G., Majeron, M. A., Finavcra, L. and Zamberletti, P. (1972): Contributo alla conoscenza della sindrome de Gilles de la Tourette: Studio su due gemelli, *Minerva Med.*, 63:3517–3522.
Esecover, H., Malitz, S., and Wilkens, D. (1961): Clinical profiles of paid normal subjects volunteering for hallucinogenic drug studies. *Am. J. Psychiatry*, 117:910.
Evarts, E. V., Kimura, M., Wurtz, R. H., and Hikosaka, O. (1984): Behavioral correlates of activity in basal ganglia neurons. *Trends Neurosci.*, 7:447–453.
Fahn, S. (1982a): A case of post-traumatic tic syndrome. In: *Advances in Neurology, Vol. 35, Gilles de la Tourette Syndrome*, edited by A. J. Friedhoff and T. N. Chase, pp. 349–350. Raven Press, New York.
Fahn, S. (1982b): The clinical spectrum of motor tics. In: *Advances in Neurology, Vol. 35, Gilles de la Tourette Syndrome*, edited by A. J. Friedhoff and T. N. Chase, pp. 341–344. Raven Press, New York.
Fahn, S., and Eldridge, R. (1976): Definition of dystonia and classification of the dystonic states. *Adv. Neurol.*, 14:1–5.
Fahn, S., Marsden, C. D., and Van Woert, M. H. (1986): Definition and classification of myoclonus. In: *Advances in Neurology, Vol. 43, Myoclonus*, edited by S., Fahn, D. Marsden, and M. H. Van Woert, pp. 1–5. Raven Press, New York.
Faux, E. J. (1966): Gilles de la Tourette Syndrome, social psychiatric management. *Arch. Gen. Psychiatry*, 14:139–142.
Fayer, S. A. (1986): Letter to the editors: Torsades de pointes ventricular tachyarrhythmia associated with haloperidol. *J. Clin. Psychopharmacol.*, 6:375–376.
Feild, J. R., Corbin, K. B., Goldstein, N. P., and Klass, D. W. (1966): Gilles de la Tourette's syndrome. *Neurology*, 16:453–462.
Feinberg, M., and Carroll, B. J. (1979): Effects of dopamine agonists and antagonists in Tourette's disease. *Arch. Gen. Psychiatry*, 36:979–985.
Feinberg, T. E., Shapiro, A. K., and Shapiro, E. (1986): Paroxysmal myoclonic dystonia with vocalizations: New entity or variant of preexisting syndromes? *J. Neurol. Neurosurg, Psychiatry*, 49:52–57.
Fenichel, O. (1945): *The Psychoanalytic Theory of Neurosis*. Norton Press, New York.
Ferenczi, S. (1921): Psycho-analytical observations on tic. *Int. J. Psychoanal.*, 2:1–30.
Fernando, S. J. M. (1967): Gilles de la Tourette's syndrome. *Br. J. Psychiatry*, 113:607–617.
Fernando, S. J. M (1976): Six cases of Gilles de la Tourette's syndrome. *Br. J. Psychiatry*, 128:436–441.
Ferrari, M., Mathews, W. S., and Barabas, G. (1984): Children with Tourette syndrome: Results of psychological tests given prior to drug treatment. *Dev. Behav. Pediatr.*, 5:116–119.
Field, J. G. (1960): Two types of tables for use with Wechsler's intelligence scales. *J. Clin. Psychol.*, 16:3–7.
Finegold, L. (1985): Allergy and Tourette's syndrome. *Ann. Allergy*, 55:119–121.
Finney, J. W., Christophersen, E. R., and Ziegler, D. K. (1981): Letter to the editor: Deanol and Tourette syndrome. *Lancet*, 2:989.
Fisarova, M. (1968): Lecba choroby Gilles de la Touretteovy frenolenem. *Bratisl. Lek. Listy*, 49:670–672.
Fisarova, M. (1972): Choraba Gilles de la Touretteova. *Cesk. Neurol. Neurochir.*, 35:202–208.
Fisarova, M. (1976): Gilles de la Tourette's disease. In: *Gilles de la Tourette's Syndrome, Vol. I*, edited by F. Abuzzahab Sr. and F. Anderson, pp. 89–98. Mason, St. Paul, Minnesota.
Flaherty, J. A., and Lahmeyer, H. W. (1978): Letter to the editor: Laryngeal-pharyngeal dystonia as a possible cause of asphyxia with haloperidol treatment. *Am. J. Psychiatry*, 135:1414–1415.
Fleischner, E. C. (1911): The treatment of tic in childhood. *J. Calif. State Med.*, 9:379–382.

Foa, E. B., Grayson, J. B., Skeketee, G. S., Doppelt, H. G., Turner, R. M., and Latimer, P. R. (1983): Success and failure in the behavioral treatment of obsessive-compulsives. *J. Consult. Clin. Psychol.*, 51:287–297.

Fog, R., and Pakkenberg, H. (1980): Theoretical and clinical aspects of the Tourette syndrome (chronic multiple tics). *J. Neural Transm. (Supp.)*, 16:211–215.

Fog, R., Pakkenberg, H., Regeur, L., and Pakkenberg, B. (1982): "Tardive" Tourette syndrome in relation to long-term neuroleptic treatment of multiple tics. In: *Advances in Neurology, Vol. 35, Gilles de la Tourette Syndrome*, edited by A. J. Friedhoff and T. N. Chase, pp. 419–421. Raven Press, New York.

Ford, C. V., and Gottlieb, F. (1969): An objective evaluation of haloperidol in Gilles de la Tourette's syndrome. *Dis. Nerv. Syst.*, 30:328–332.

Frank, S. M. (1978): Psycholinguistic findings in Gilles de la Tourette syndrome. *J. Commun. Disord.*, 11:349–363.

Frankel, M., Cummings, J. L., Robertson, M. M., Trimble, M. R., Hill, M. A., and Benson, D. F. (1986): Obsessions and compulsions in Gilles de al Tourette syndrome. *Neurology*, 36:378–382.

Fras, I. (1978): Gilles de la Tourette's syndrome. Effects of tricyclic antidepressants. *NY State J. Med.*, 78:1230–1232.

Fras, I., Karlavage, J. (1977): The use of methylphenidate and imipramine in Gilles de la Tourette disease in children. *Am. J. Psychiatry*, 134:195–199.

Freud, S. (1966): Pre-psycho-analytic publications and unpublished drafts (1886–1899). In: *Complete Psychological Works, Standard Edition, Vol. 1*, edited by J. Strachey. London Hogarth Press, London.

Friedhoff, A. J. (1982): Receptor maturation in pathogenesis and treatment of Tourette syndrome. In: *Advances in Neurology, Vol. 35, Gilles de la Tourette Syndrome*, edited by A. J. Friedhoff and T. N. Chase, pp. 133–140. Raven Press, New York.

Friedman, S. (1980): Self-control in the treatment of Gilles de la Tourette's syndrome: Case study with 18-month follow up. *J. Consult. Clin. Psychol.*, 48:400–402.

Friedrich, N. (1881): Uber koordinierte erinnerungskrampfe. *Virchows Arch. Pathol. Anat. Physio. Klin. Med.*, 86:430–434.

Friel, P. B. (1973): Familial incidence of Gilles de la Tourette's disease, with observations on aetiology and treatment. *Br. J. Psychiatry*, 122:655–658.

Friend, J. (1701): De spasmi rerioris historia. In: *Philosophical Transactions*, pp. 799–804.

Frost, N., Feighner, J., and Schuckit, M. A. (1976): A family study of Gilles de la Tourette syndrome. *Dis. Nerv. Syst.*, 37:537–538.

Fuster, J. M. (1984): Behavioral electrophysiology of the prefrontal cortex. *Trends Neurosci.*, 7:408–414.

Gadoth, N. (1974): Gilles de la Tourette's syndrome. *Harefuach*, 86:371–373.

Gamstorp, I. (1970): *Pediatric Neurology*. Appleton-Century-Crofts, New York.

Gardos, G., Cole, J. O., and Tarsy, D. (1978): Withdrawal syndromes associated with antipsychotic drugs. *Am. J. Psychiatry*, 135:1321–1324.

Gardos, G., Cole, J. O., Rapkin, R. M., LaBrie, R. A., Baquelod, E., Moor, P., Sovner, R., and Doyle, J. (1984): Anticholinergic challenge and neurologic withdrawal. *Arch. Gen. Psychiatry*, 41:1030–1035.

Gestaut, H., and Villeneuve, A. (1967): The startle disease or hyperekplexia: Pathological surprise reaction. *J. Neurol. Sci.*, 5:523–542.

Gastfriend, D. R., Biederman, J., and Jellinek, M. S. (1984): Desipramine in the treatment of adolescents with attention deficit disorder. *Am. J. Psychiatry*, 141:906–908.

Gerard, M. W. (1946): The psychogenic tic in ego development. *Psychoanal. Study Child*, 2:133–162.

Ghadirian, A. M. Chouinard, G., and Annable, L. (1982): Sexual dysfunction and plasma prolactin levels in neuroleptic-treated schizophrenic outpatients. *J. Nerv. Mentl. Dis.*, 170:463.

Ghez, C. (1985): Introduction to the motor system. In: *Principles of Neural Sciences*, 2nd edition, edited by E. R. Kandel and J. H. Schwartz. Elsevier, New York.

Ghez, C., and Fahn, S. (1985): The cerebellum. In: *Principles of Neural Sciences*, 2nd edition, edited by E. R. Kandel and J. H. Schwartz. Elsevier, New York.

Giller, E. L., Jr., Young, J. G., Breakefield, X. O., Carbonari, C., Braverman, M., and Cohen, D. J. (1980): Monoamine oxidase and catechol-*o*-methyltransferase activities in cultured fibro-

blasts and blood cells from children with autism and the Gilles de la Tourette syndrome. *Psychiatry Res.*, 2:187–197.
Gilles de la Tourette, G. (1884): Jumping, latah, myriachit. *Arch. Neurol.*, 8:68–84.
Gilles de la Tourette, G. (1885): Étude sur une affection nerveuse caractérisée par de l'incoordination motrice accompagnée d'echolalie et de copralalie. *Arch. Neurol.*, 9:19–42, 158–200.
Gilles de la Tourette, G. (1899): La maladie des tics convulsifs. *La Semaine Medicale*, 19:153–156.
Gillies, D. R., and Forsythe, W. I. (1984): Treatment of multiple tics and the Tourette syndrome. *Dev. Med. Child Neurol.*, 26:830–833.
Gillman, M. A., and Sandyk, R. (1984): Tourette syndrome: Effect of analgesic concentrations of nitrous oxide and naloxone. *Br. Med. J.*, 288:114.
Gillman, M. A., and Sandyk, R. (1985): Letter to the editor: Tourette syndrome and the opioid system. *Psychiatry Res.*, 15:161–162.
Gillman, M. A., and Sandyk, R. (1986): The endogenous opioid system in Gilles de la Tourette syndrome. *Med. Hypotheses*, 19:371–378.
Gittleman, R., and Mannuzza S. (1985): Diagnosing ADD-H in adolescents. *Psychopharmacol. Bull.*, 21:237–242.
Glaze, D. G., Frost, J. D., Jr., and Jankovic, J. (1983): Sleep in Gilles de la Tourette's syndrome: Disorder of arousal. *Neurology*, 33:586–592.
Goetz, C. G., Tanner, C. M., and Klawans, H. L. (1982): Compressive neuropathies in Tourette syndrome. In: *Advances in Neurology, Vol. 35, Gilles de la Tourette Syndrome*, edited by A. J. Friedhoff and T. N. Chase, pp. 345–347. Raven Press, New York.
Goetz, C. G., Tanner, C. M., and Klawans, H. L. (1984): Fluphenazine and multifocal tic disorders. *Arch. Neurol.*, 41:271–272.
Goetz, I. E., Roberts, E., and Warren, J. (1981): Skin fibroblasts in Huntington disease. *Am. J. Hum. Genet.*, 33:187–196.
Goff, D. (1986): The stimulant challenge test in depression. *J. Clin. Psychiatry*, 47:538–543.
Goforth, E. G. (1974): Gilles de la Tourette's syndrome: a 25 year follow-up study. *J. Nerv. Ment. Dis.*, 158:306–309.
Goggins, J. E., and Erickson, H. M. (1979): Dilemmas in diagnosis and treatment of Gilles de la Tourette syndrome. *J. Pers. Assess.*, 43:339–346.
Goldberg, L. I. (1985): Dopamine: receptors and clinical applications. *Clin. Physiol. Biochem.*, 5:120–126.
Golden, G. S. (1974): Gilles de la Tourette's syndrome following methylphenidate administration. *Dev. Med. Child Neurol.*, 16:76–78.
Golden, G. S. (1977a): The pediatric perspective. *Am. J. Dis. Child.*, 131:531–534.
Golden, G. S. (1977b): The effect of central nervous system stimulants on Tourette syndrome. *Ann. Neurol.*, 2:69–70.
Golden, G. S. (1978a): Tics, twitches and habit spasms. *Curr. Probl. Pediatr.*, 8:29–41.
Golden, G. S. (1978b): Tics and Tourette's: A continuum of symptoms. *Ann. Neurol.*, 4:145–148.
Golden, G. S. (1979): Tics and Tourette syndrome. *Hosp. Pract.*, 14:91–93, 96–97.
Golden, G. S. (1982): Tourette syndrome in children: Ethnic and genetic factors and response to stimulant drugs. In: *Advances in Neurology, Vol. 35, Gilles de la Tourette Syndrome*, edited by A. J. Friedhoff and T. N. Chase, pp. 287–289. Raven Press, New York.
Golden, G. S. (1983): Tics in childhood. *Pediatr. Ann.*, 12:821–824.
Golden, G. S. (1984): Book review: Tourette's syndrome and attention deficit disorder. *J. Dev. Behav. Prob.*, 5:226–227.
Golden, G. S. (1985): Tardive dyskinesia in Tourette syndrome. *Pediatri. Neurol.*, 1:192–194.
Golden, G. S., and Greenhill, L. (1981): Tourette syndrome in mentally retarded children (review). *Ment. Retard.*, 19:17–19.
Golden, G. S., and Hood, O. J. (1982): Tics and tremors. *Pediatr. Clin. North Am.*, 29:95–103.
Goldfried, M. R., Stricker, G., and Weiner, I. B. (1971): *Rorschach Handbook of Clinical and Research Applications*. Prentice-Hall, New Jersey.
Goldman-Rakic, P. S. (1984): The frontal lobes: Uncharted provinces of the brain. *Trends Neurosci.*, 7:425–429.

Goldstein, J. A. (1984): Letter to the editor: Nifedipine treatment of Tourette's syndrome. *J. Clin. Psychiatry*, 45:360.
Goldstone, S., and Lhamon, W. T. (1976): The effects of haloperidol upon temporal information processing by patients with Tourette's syndrome. *Psychopharmacologia*, 50:7-10.
Gonce, M., and Barbeau, A. (1977): Seven cases of Gilles de la Tourette's syndrome: Partial relief with clozapan: A pilot study. *Can. J. Neurol. Sci.*, 4:279.
Gonce, M., and Dugas, M. (1981): Tourette syndrome versus minor tics; Clinical and therapeutical differences. *First International Gilles de la Tourette Symposium* (abstract), New York.
Goyot, C., Debray, Q., Dugas, M., Guay, C., Giraud, J., and Grenier, J. (1985): Haloperidol. Surveillance plasmatique et incidence hormonale du traitement. *Pathol. Biol. (Paris)*, 33:999-1004.
Grad, G., Pelcovitz, D., Mathews, M., Olson, M., and Grad, L. (1984): Psychopathology of children with Tourette's syndrome. *Annual Meeting of the American Psychiatric Association* (presentation), Los Angeles.
Grasset, J. (1890): Leçons sur un cas de maladie des tics et un cas de tremblement singulier de la tête et des membres gauches. *Arch. Neurol.*, 20:27-45,187-211.
Grimes, J. D., Hassan, M. N., and Preston, D. N. (1982): Adverse neurologic effects of metoclopramide. *Can. Med. Assoc. J.*, 126-23-25.
Grizzle, J. E. (1965): The two-period change-over design and its use in clinical trails. *Biometrics*, 21:467-480.
Grizzle, J. E. (1974): Corrections. *Biometrics*, 30:727.
Gross, M. D., and Wilson, W. C. (1974): *Minimal Brain Dysfunction*. Brunner/Mazel, New York.
Grossman, H. Y., Mostofsky, D. I., and Harrison, R. H. (1986): Psychological aspects of Gilles de la Tourette syndrome. *J. Clin. Psychol.*, 42:228-235.
Groves, P. M., and Young, S. J. (1985): Neurons, networks, and behavior: An introduction. In: *Psychiatry, Vol. 3*, edited by R. Michels and J. O. Cavenar, Chapter 42. Lippincot, Philadelphia.
Gualtieri, C. T., and Patterson, D. R. (1986): Neuroleptic-induced tics in two hyperactive children, *Am. J. Psychiatry*, 143:1176-1177.
Guggenheim, M. A. (1979): Familial Tourette syndrome. *Ann. Neurol.*, 5:104.
Guggenheim, M. A., and Dodge, P. R. (1970); Unusual arm movements with onset in childhood—a nosologic entity. *Trans. Am. Neurol. Assoc.*, 95:182-186.
Guggenheim, P., and Haynal A. (1964): Über electroencephalographishe untersuchungen bein der maladie Gilles de la Tourette. *Schweiz. Arch. Neurol. Neurochir. Psychiatr.*, 94:265-278.
Guinon, G. (1886): Sur la maladie des tics convulsifs. *Rev. Med.*, 6:50-80.
Guinon, G. (1887): Tics convulsifs et hysterie. *Rev. Med.*, 7:509-519.
Haber, S. N., Kowall, N. W., Vonsattel, J. P., Bird, E. D., and Richardson, E. P. (1986): Gilles de la Tourette's syndrome: A postmortem neuropathological and immunohistochemical study. *J. Neurol. Sci.*, 75:225-241.
Hagins, R. A., Beecher, R., Pagano, G., and Kreeger, H. (1982): Effect of Tourette syndrome on learning. In: *Advances in Neurology, Vol. 35, Gilles de la Tourette Syndrome*, edited by A. J. Friedhoff and T. N. Chase, pp. 323-328. Raven Press, New York.
Hajal, F., and Leach, A. M. (1981): Familial aspects of Gilles de la Tourette syndrome. *Am. J. Psychiatry*, 138:90-92.
Hallett, M. (1987): The pathophysiology of myoclonus. *Trends Neurosci.*, 10:69-73.
Hammond, G. M. (1892): Convulsive tic: Its nature and treatment. *Medical Record*, 41:236-239.
Hammond, W. A. (1884): Myriachit, a newly described disease of the nervous system and its analogues. *Br. Med. J.*, 2:758-759.
Hamra, B. J., Dunner, F. H., and Larson, C. (1983): Remission of tics with lithium therapy: Case report. *J. Clin. Psychiatry*, 44:73-74.
Han-bai, C., and Han-quin, L. F. (1983): Tourette syndrome: Report of 19 cases. *Chinese Med. J.*, 96:45-50.
Hanin, I., Merikangas, J. R., Merikangas, K. R., and Kopp, U. (1979): Letter to the editor: Redcell choline and Gilles de la Tourette syndrome. *N. Engl. J. Med.*, 301:661-662.
Harcherik, D. F., Carbonari, C. M., Shaywitz, S. E., Shaywitz, B. A., and Cohen, D. J. (1982):

Attentional and perceptual disturbances in children with Tourette's syndrome, attention deficit disorder, and epilepsy. *Schizophr. Bull.*, 8:356–359.
Harcherik, D. F., Leckman, J. F., Detlor, J., and Cohen, D. J. (1984): A new instrument for clinical studies of Tourette's syndrome. *J. Am. Acad. Child Psychiatry*, 23:153–160.
Harcherik, D. F., Cohen, D. J., Ort, S., Paul, R. Shaywitz, B. A., Volkmer, F. R., Rothman, S. L. J., and Leckman, J. F. (1985): Computed tomographic brain scanning in 4 neuropsychiatric disorders of childhood. *Am. J. Psychiatry*, 142:731–734.
Hare, E. H., and Moran, A. P. (1979): Parental age and birth order in homosexual patients: A replication of Slater's study. *Br. J. Psychiatry*, 134:178–182.
Hart, Z., Rennick, P. M., Klinge, V., and Schwartz, M. (1974): A pediatric neurologist's contribution to evaluation of school underachievers. *Am. J. Dis. Child.*, 128:319–323.
Hartshorn, E. A. (1975): Interactions of < NS drugs: Psychotherapeutic agents—the antipsychotic drugs. *Drug Intel. Clin. Pharmacol.*, 9:536–552.
Hashimoto, T., Endo, S., Fukuda, K. Hiura, K., Kawano, N., Suzue, J., Kokawa, T., and Miyao, M. (1981): Increased body movements during sleep in Gilles de la Tourette syndrome. *Brain Dev.*, 3:31–35.
Hassler, R., and Dieckmann, G. (1970): Traitement stéréotaxique des tics et cris inarticulés ou coprolalique considérés comme phénomène d'obsession notrice au cours de la maladie Gilles de la Tourette. *Rev. Neurol. (Paris)*, 123:89–100.
Healy, C. E. (1970): Gilles de la Tourette's syndrome (*maladie des tics*). *Am. J. Dis. Child.*, 120:62–63.
Healy, N. M., and Fisher, I. (1965): Gilles de la Tourette's syndrome in an autistic child. *J. Irish Med.*, 57:93–94.
Hecaen, H., and Ajuriaguerra, J. (1964): *Left-Handedness: Manual Superiority and Cerebral Dominance*. Grune & Stratton, New York.
Helper, M. M., Wilcott, R. C., and Garfield, S. L. (1963): Effects of chlorpromazine on learning and related processes in emotionally disturbed children. *J. Consult. Psychol.*, 27:1–9.
Heuscher, J. E. (1953): Intermediate states of consciousness in patients with generalized tics. *J. Nerv. Ment. Dis.*, 117:29–38.
Hills, M., and Armitage, P. (1979): The two-period cross-over clinical trial. *Br. J. Clin. Pharmacol.*, 8:7–20.
Hillyard, S. A., Picton, T. W., and Regan, D. (1978): Sensation, perception and attention: Analysis using ERPs. In: *Event-Related Brain Potentials in Man*, edited by E. Callaway, P. Tueting, and S. H. Koslow, pp. 223–321. Academic Press, New York.
Hinsie, L. E., and Campbell, R. J. (1960): *Psychiatric Dictionary*, 3rd edition. Oxford University Press, New York.
Hinsie, L. E., and Campbell, R. J. (1970): *Psychiatric Dictionary*, 4th edition. Oxford University Press, New York.
Hoge, S. K., and Biederman, J. (1986): A case of Tourette's syndrome with symptoms of attention deficit disorder treated with desipramine. *J. Clin. Psychiatry*, 47:478–479.
Holden, C. (1987): A top priority at NIMH. *Science*, 235:431.
Hollandsworth, J. G., and Bausinger, L. (1978): Unsuccessful use of massed practice in the treatment of Gilles de la Tourette's syndrome. *Psychol. Rep.*, 43:671–677.
Hollingshead, A. B., and Redlich, F. C. (1958): *Social Class and Mental Illness*. Wiley, New York.
Hollister, L. E., Bennett, J. L., Kalm, S. C., and Kimball, I. (1963): Drug-induced EEG abnormalities as predictors of clinical responses to thiopropazate and haloperidol. *Am. J. Psychiatry*, 119:887–888.
Holmes, O. W. (1891): *Medical Essays, 1842–1882*. The Riverside Press, Cambridge.
Holomboe, R. (1977): *Sixth World Congress of Psychiatry* (presentation), Honolulu, Hawaii.
Hoogduin, K. (1986): On the diagnosis of obsessive-compulsive disorder. *Am. J. Psychother.*, 40:36–51.
Hubbard, J. W., Ganes, D., and Midha, K. K. (1987): Letter to the editor: Prolonged pharmacologic activity of neuroleptic drugs. *Arch. Gen. Psychiatry*, 44:99–100.
Hunt, R. D., Cohen, D. J., Anderson, G. M., and Clark, L. (1984): Possible change in noradrenergic receptor sensitivity following methylphenidate treatment: Growth hormone and MHPG response to clonidine challenge in children with attention deficit disorder and hyperactivity. *Life Sci.*, 35:885–897.

Hunt, R. D., Minderaa, R. D., and Cohen, D. J. (1985): Clonidine benefits children with attention deficit disorder and hyperactivity: Report of a double-blind placebo cross-over therapeutic trial. *J. Am. Acad. Child Psychiatry*, 24:617–629.
Incagnoli, T., and Kane, R. (1982): Neuropsychological functioning in Tourette syndrome. In: *Advances in Neurology, Vol. 35, Gilles de la Tourette Syndrome*, edited by A. J. Friedhoff and T. N. Chase, pp. 305–309. Raven Press, New York.
Incagnoli, T., and Kane, R. (1983): Developmental perspective of the Gilles de la Tourette syndrome. *Percept. Mot. Skills*, 57:1271–1281.
Ingram, T. T. S. (1973): Soft signs. *Dev. Med. Child Neurol.*, 15:527–529.
Insel, T. R. (1982): Obsessive compulsive disorder—five clinical questions and a suggested approach. *Comp. Psychiatry*, 23:241–251.
Insel, T. R. (editor) (1984): *New Findings in Obsessive-Compulsive Disorder*. American Psychiatric Press, Washington, D.C.
Insel, T. R., Zahn, T., and Murphy, D. L. (1985): Obsessive-compulsive disorder: An anxiety disorder? In: *Anxiety and the Anxiety Disorders*, edited by A. H. Tuma and J. Maser, pp. 2–22. Lawrence Erlbaum Press, Hillside, New Jersey.
Itard, J. M. G. (1825): Memoire sur quelques fonctions involuntaires des appareils de la locomotion de la prehension et de la voix. *Arch. Gen. Med.*, 8:385–407.
Itard, J. M. G. (1962): *The Wild Boy of Aveyron*. Appleton, New York.
Ito, M. (1986): Neural systems controlling movement. *Trends Neurosci.*, 9:515–518.
Izmeth, A. (1979): Gilles de la Tourette syndrome. *J. Ment. Defic. Res.*, 23:25–27.
Jacobs, B. L., Trulson, M. E., Heym, J., and Steinfels, G. F. (1982): On the role of CNS serontonin in the motor abnormalities of Tourette syndrome: Behavioral and single-unit studies. In: *Advances in Neurology, Vol. 35, Gilles de la Tourette Syndrome*, edited by A. J. Friedhoff and T. N. Chase, pp. 93–98. Raven Press, New York.
Jagger, J., Prusoff, B. A., Cohen, D. J., Kidd, K. K., Carbonari, C. M., and John, K. (1982): The epidemiology of Tourette's syndrome: A pilot study. *Schizophr. Bull.*, 8:267–278.
Janet, P. (1924): *Principles of Psychotherapy*. MacMillan, New York.
Janet, P. (1925): *Psychological Healing: A Historical and Clinical Study, Vol. 1*. George Allen and Unwin, London.
Jankovic, J., and Glass, J. P. (1985): Metoclopramide-induced phantom dyskinesia. *Neurology*, 35:432–435.
Jankovic, J., Glaze, D. G., and Frost, J. D. (1984): Effect of tetrabenazine on tics and sleep of Gilles de la Tourette's syndrome. *Neurology*, 34:688–692.
Jenkins, R. L., and Ashby, H. B. (1983): Gilles de la Tourette's syndrome in identicial twins, *Arch. Neurol.*, 40:249–251.
Jenkins, R. L., and Fine, B. N. (1976): Experience in 20 cases of Tourette syndrome. In: *Gilles de la Tourette's Syndrome, Vol. 1: International Registry*, edited by F. Abuzzahab, R., and F. Anderson. Mason, St. Paul, Minnesota.
Jenner, P., and Marsden, C. D. (1983): Neuroleptics. In: *Psychopharmacology I: Part 1: Preclinical Psychopharmacology*, edited by D. G. Grahame-Smith and P. J. Cowen, pp. 180–247. Excerpta Medica, Amsterdam.
Jeste, D. V., Sule, S. M., Apte, J. S., and Vahia, N. S. (1973): Gilles de la Tourette's disease. *Indian J. Pediatr.*, 40:435.
Jeste, D. V., Wisniewski, A. A., and Wyatt, R. J. (1986): Neuroleptic-associated tardive syndromes (review). *Psychiatr. Clin. North Am.*, 9:183–192.
Johnson, G. C., Pepple, J. M., Singer, H. S., and Littlefield, J. W. (1977): HGPRT in the Gilles de la Tourette syndrome. *N. Engl. J. Med.*, 297:339.
Johnson, J. (1905): A case of maladie des tics convulsion. *Br. Med. J.*, 2:810.
Joschko, M., and Rourke, B. P. (1982): Neuropsychological dimensions of Tourette syndrome: Test-retest stability and implications for intervention. In: *Advances in Neurology, Vol. 35, Gilles de la Tourette Syndrome*, edited by A. J. Friedhoff and T. N. Chase, pp. 297–304. Raven Press, New York.
Kaim, B. (1983): Gilles de la Tourette's syndrome treated with clonazepam. *Brain. Res. Bull.*, 11:213–214.
Kanner, L. (1957): *Child Psychiatry*. Thomas, Springfield, Illinois.
Karson, C. N., Kaufmann, C. A., Shapiro, A. K., and Shapiro, E. (1985): Eye-blink rate in Tourette's syndrome. *J. Nerv. Ment. Dis.*, 173:566–569.

Keepers, G. A., Clappison, V. J., and Casey, D. E. (1983): Initial anticholinergic prophylaxis for neuroleptic-induced extrapyramidal syndromes. *Arch. Gen. Psychiatry,* 40:1113–1117.
Kehne, J. H., Gallagher, D. W., and Davis, M. (1985): Spinalization unmasks clonidine's d_1-adrenergic mediated excitation of the flexor reflex in rats. *J. Neurosci.,* 5:1583–1590
Kelman, D. H. (1965): Gilles de la Tourette's disease in children. A review of the literature. *J. Child Psychol. Psychiatry,* 6:219–226.
Kennard, M. (1960): Value of equivocal signs in neurological diagnosis. *Neurology,* 10:753–764.
Kerbeshian, J., and Burd, L. (1985): Auditory hallucinosis and atypical tic disorder: Case reports. *J. Clin. Psychiatry,* 46:398–399.
Kerbeshian, J., and Burd, L. (1986–87): A second visually impaired, mentally retarded male with pervasive developmental disorder, Tourette disorder and Ganser's syndrome: diagnostic classification and treatment. *Int. J. Psychiatry Med.,* 16:67–75.
Kerbeshian, J., Burd, L., and Martsolf, J. T. (1984): Fragile X syndrome associated with Tourette symptomatology in a male with moderate mental retardation and autism. *Dev. Behav. Pediatr.,* 5:201–203.
Kerlinger, F. N., and Pedhazar, E. J. (1973): *Multiple Regression in Behavioral Research.* Holt, Reinhart and Winston, New York.
Kidd, K. K., Prusoff, B. A., and Cohen, D. J. (1980): The familial pattern of Tourette syndrome. *Arch. Gen. Psychiatry,* 37:1336–1339.
Kidd, K. K., and Pauls, D. L. (1982): Genetic hypotheses for Tourette syndrome. In: *Advances in Neurology, Vol. 35, Gilles de la Tourette Syndrome,* edited by A. J. Friedhoff and T. N. Chase, pp. 243–249. Raven Press, New York.
Kinsbourne, M. (1973): School problems. *Pediatrics,* 52:679–710.
Klawans, H. L., and Barr, A. (1985): Recurrence of childhood multiple tic in late adult life. *Arch. Neurol.,* 42:1079–1080.
Klawans, H. L., Falk, D. A., Nausieda, P. A., and Weiner, W. J. (1978): Tourette syndrome after long-term chlorpromazine therapy. *Neurology (Minneap.),* 28:1064–1065.
Klawans, H. L., Goetz, C. G., and Perlik, S. (1980): Tardive dyskinesia: Review and update. *Am. J. Psychiatry,* 137:900–907.
Klawans, H. L., Nausieda, P. A., Goetz, C. C., Tanner, C. M. and Weiner, W. J. (1982): Tourette-like symptoms following chronic neuroleptic therapy. In: *Advances in Neurology, Vol. 35, Gilles de la Tourette Syndrome,* edited by A. J. Friedhoff and T. N. Chase, pp. 415–418. Raven Press, New York.
Klein, M. (1925): Zur genese des tics. *Int. Psychoanal.,* 11:332.
Klempel, K. (1974): Gilles de la Tourette's symptoms induced by L-dopa. *S. Afr. Med. J.,* 48:1379–1380.
Klopfer, B., and Kelley, D. M. (1946): *The Rorschach Technique.* World Book, New York.
Knott, P. J., and Hutson, P. H. (1982): Stress-induced stereotype in the rat: Neuropharmacological similarities to Tourette syndrome. In: *Advances in Neurology, Vol. 35, Gilles de la Tourette Syndrome,* edited by A. J. Friedhoff and T. N. Chase, pp. 233–238. Raven Press, New York.
Koester, G. (1899): Uber die maladie des tics impulsifs (mimische krampfneurose). *Dtsch. Z. Nervenkr.,* 15:147–159.
Kondo, K., and Kabasawa, T. (1978): Letter to the editor: Improvement in Gilles de la Tourette syndrome after corticosteroid therapy. *Ann. Neurol.,* 4:387.
Kondo, K., and Nomura, Y. (1982): Tourette syndrome in Japan: Etiologic considerations based on associated factors and familial clustering. In: *Advances in Neurology, Vol. 35, Gilles de la Tourette Syndrome,* edited by A. J. Friedhoff and T. N. Chase, pp. 271–276. Raven Press, New York.
Koranyi, E. K. (1977): Remarkable etiology in Gilles de la Tourette's disease. *Psychiatr. J. Univ. Ottawa,* 1:507.
Kornetsky, C. (1972): The use of a simple test of attention as a measure of drug effects in schizophrenic patients. *Psychopharmacologia,* 24:99–106.
Kornhuber, H. H., and Deecke, L. (1965): Hirnpotentialanderungen bei Wilkurbewegungen und passiven Bewegungen des Menschen: Bereitschaftspotential und reafferente Potentiale. *Pfluegers Arch.,* 284:1–17.
Korten, J. J., Notermans, S. L. H., Frenken, C. W. G. M., Gabreels, F. J. M., and Joosten, E. M. G. (1974): Familial essential myoclonus. *Brain,* 97:131–138.

Koslow, S. H., and Cross, C. K. (1982): Cerebrospinal fluid monoamine metabolites in Tourette syndrome and their neuroendocrine implications. In: *Advances in Neurology, Vol. 35, Gilles de la Tourette Syndrome*, edited by A. J. Friedhoff and T. N. Chase, pp. 185–197. Raven Press, New York.

Krumholz, A., Singer, H. S., Niedermeyer, E., Burnite, R., and Harris, K. (1983): Electrophysiological studies in Tourette's syndrome. *Ann. Neurol.*, 14:638–641.

Krumholz, A., Singer, H. S., and Niedermeyer, E. (1984): Reply. *Ann. Neurol.*, 16:94.

Kunkle, E. C. (1967): The 'jumpers' of Maine: A reappraisal. *Arch. Intern. Med.*, 119:355–358.

Kurczynski, T. W. (1983): Hyperekplexia. *Arch. Neurol.*, 40:246–248.

Kurlan, R., Behr, J., Medved, L., Shoulson, L., Pauls, D., Kidd, J. R., and Kidd, K K. (1986): Familial Tourette's syndrome: Report of a large pedigree and potential for linkage analysis. *Neurology*, 36:772–776.

Kurlan, R., Behr, J., Medved, L., Shoulson, I., Pauls, D., and Kidd, K. K. (1987): Severity of Tourette's syndrome in one large kindred: Implication for determination of disease prevalence rate. *Arch Neurol.*, 44:268–269.

Kurland, M. L. (1965): Gilles de la Tourette's syndrome: the psychotherapy of two cases. *Compr. Psychiatry*, 6:298–309.

Kurtz, D. (1976): The EEG in acute and chronic drug intoxications. In: *Clinical EEG: Handbook of Electroencephalography and Clinical Neurophysiology, Vol. 15*, edited by D. D. Daly, G. H. Glaser, and A. Remond, pp. 88–104. Elsevier, Amsterdam.

Kutcher, S. P., Mackenzie, S., Galarraga, W., and Szalal, J. (1987): Letter to the editor: Clonazepam treatment of adolescents with neuroleptic-induced akathisia. *Am. J. Psychiatry*, 144:823–824.

Lacoursiere, R. B., Spohn, H. E., and Thompson, K. (1976): Medical effects of abrupt neuroleptic withdrawal. *Compr. Psychiatry*, 17: 285–294.

Lahey, B. B., Schaughency, E. A., Strauss, C. C., and Frame, C. L. (1984): Are attention deficit disorders with and without hyperactivity similar or dissimilar disorders? *J. Am. Acad. Child Psychiatry*, 23:302–309.

Lake, C. R., Ziegler, M. G., Eldridge, R., and Murphy, D. L. (1977): Catecholamine metabolism in Gilles de la Tourette's syndrome. *Am. J. Psychiatry*, 134:257–260.

Lal, S., and Al Ansari, E. (1986): Tourette-like syndrome following low dose short-term neuroleptic treatment. *Can. J. Neurol. Sci.*, 13:125–128.

Lang, A. E., Moldofsky, H., and Awad, A. G. (1983): Letter to the editor: Long latency between the onset of motor and vocal tics in Tourette's syndrome. *Ann. Neurol.*, 14:693–694.

Lanier, Bob (1985): Alternative approaches to Tourette syndrome. *Symposium on Tourette Syndrome* (presentation), Mt. Sinai School of Medicine, New York.

Lapouse, R., and Monk, M. (1958): An epidemiologic study of behavior characteristics in children. *Am. J. Public Health*, 48:1134–1144.

Lapouse, R., and Monk, M. (1964): Behavior deviations in a representative sample of children; Variation by sex, age, race, social class, and family size. *Am. J. Orthopsychiatry*, 34:436–446.

Laron, Z., Gil-Ad, I., Topper, E., Kaufman, H., and Josefsberg, Z. (1982): Low oral dose of clonidine: An effective screening test for growth hormone deficiency. *Acta Paediatr. Scand.*, 71:847–848.

Lasagna, L., Mosteller, F., Von Felsinger, J., and Beecher, H. A. (1954): A study of the placebo response. *Am. J. Med.*, 16:770–779.

Latimer, R. H., (1945): The parent child relationship in children afflicted with tics. *Nerv. Child*, 4:353–358.

Laursen, A. M. (1963): The corpus striatum. *Acta. Physiol. Scand.*, 59: Suppl. 211:1–106.

Lawden, M. (1986): Gilles de la Tourette syndrome: a review. *J. R. Soc. Med.*, 79:282–288.

Lechin, F., van der Dijs, B., Gomez, F., Acosta, E., and Arocha, L. (1982): On the use of clonidine and thioproperazine in a woman with Gilles de la Tourette's disease. *Biol. Psychiatry*, 17:103–108.

Leckman, J. F., and Cohen, D. J. (1983): Recent advances in Gilles de la Tourette syndrome: Implications for clinical practice and future research. *Psychiatr. Dev.*, 3:301–316.

Leckman, J. F., Scholomskas, D., Thompson, W. D., Belanger, A., and Weissman, M. M. (1982a): Best estimate of lifetime psychiatric diagnoses: A methodological study. *Arch. Gen. Psychiatry*, 39:879–883.

Leckman, J. F., Cohen, D. J., Detlor, J., Young, J. G., Harcherik, D., and Shaywitz, B. A.

(1982b): Clonidine in the treatment of Tourette syndrome: A review of data. In: *Advances in Neurology, Vol. 35, Gilles de la Tourette Syndrome,* edited by A. J. Friedhoff and T. N. Chase, pp. 391–401. Raven Press, New York.
Leckman, J. F., Detlor, J., Harcherik, D. F., Young, J. G., Anderson, G. M., Shaywitz, B. A., and Cohen, D. J. (1983): Acute and chronic clonidine treatment in Tourette's syndrome: A preliminary report on clinical response and effect on plasma and urinary catecholamine metabolites, growth hormone, and blood pressure. *J. Am. Acad. Child Psychiatry,* 22:433–440.
Leckman, J. F., Cohen, D. J., Gertner, J. M., Ort, S., and Harcherik, M. S. (1984a): Growth hormone response to clonidine in children ages 4–17: Tourette's syndrome vs children with short stature. *J. Am. Acad. Child Psychiatry,* 23:174–181.
Leckman, J. F., Cohen, D. J., Price, R. A., Minderaa, R. B., Anderson, G. M., and Pauls, D. L. (1984b): The pathogenesis of Gilles de la Tourette's syndrome. A review of data and hypotheses. In: *Movement Disorders,* edited by A. B. Shah, N. S. Shah, and A. G. Donald. Plenum Press, New York.
Leckman, J. F., Anderson, G. M., Cohen, D. J., Ort, S., Harcherik, D. F. Hoder, E. L., and Shaywitz, B. A. (1984c): Whole blood serotonin and tryptophan levels in Tourette's disorder: Effects of acute and chronic clonidine treatment. *Life Sci.,* 35:2497–2503.
Leckman, J. F., Detlor, J., Harcherik, D. F., Ort, S., Shaywitz, B. A., and Cohen D. J. (1985): Short and long-term treatment of Tourette's syndrome with clonidine: A clinical perspective. *Neurology,* 35:343–351.
Leckman, J. F., Ort, S., Caruso, K. A., Anderson, G. M., Riddle, M. A., and Cohen, D. J. (1986): Rebound phenomena in Tourette's syndrome after abrupt withdrawal of clonidine: Behavioral cardiovascular, and neurochemical effects. *Arch. Gen. Psychiatry,* 43:1168–1176.
Leckman, J. F., Price, R. A., Walkup, J. T., Ort, S., Pauls, D. L., and Cohen, D. J. (1987): Letter to the editor: Nongenetic factors in Gilles de la Tourette's syndrome. *Arch. Gen. Psychiatry,* 44:100.
Lee, S. H., and Sul, C. K. (1968): A case of Gilles de la Tourette syndrome. *Neuropsychiatry,* 7:33–36.
Lees, A. J. (1985): *Tics and related disorders. Clinical Neurology and Neurosurgery Monographs, Vol. 7.* Churchill Livingstone, New York.
Lees, A. J., Robertson, M., Trimble, M. R., and Murray, N. M. F. (1984): A clinical study of Gilles de la Tourette syndrome in the United Kingdom. *J. Neurol. Neurosurg. Psychiatry,* 47:1–8.
Lefkowitz, R. J., Caron, M. G., and Stiles, G. L. (1984): Mechanisms of membrane-receptor regulation: Biochemical physiological, and clinical insights derived from studies of the adrenergic receptors. *N. Engl. J. Med.,* 310:1570–1579.
Leopold, N. A. (1984): Prolonged metoclopramide-induced dyskinetic reaction. *Neurology,* 34:238–239.
Lerman, P., and Nussbaum, E. (1974): Treatment with haloperidol in "*Maladie des tics*" in children. *Harefuah,* 86:241–242.
Levine, J. (editor) (1979): *Coordinating Clinical Trials and Psychopharmacology: Planning, Documentation, and Analysis.* DHEW Publication No. (ADM) 79–803, Washington, D.C.
Levine, J., Schiele, B. C., and Bouthelet, L. (editors) (1971): *Principles and Problems in Establishing the Efficacy of Psychotropic Agents.* Public Health Service Publication No. 2138, Washington, D.C.
Levy, B. S., and Ascher, E. (1968): Phenothiazines in the treatment of Gilles de la Tourette's disease. *J. Nerv. Ment. Dis.,* 146:36–40.
Lewis, A. (1935/1936): A problem of obsessional illness. *Proc. R. Soc. Med., 29:235–245.*
Lewis, J. A., and Bertorini, T. E. (1982): Letter to the editor: Duchenne muscular dystrophy and Tourette syndrome. *Neurology (NY),* 32:329.
Licamele, W. L., and O'Leary, J. H. (1986): Letter to the editor: Tourette's syndrome and attention deficit disorder. *J. Clin. Psychiatry,* 47:330.
Liebenfeld, A. M. (1976): *Foundations of Epidemiology.* Oxford University Press, New York.
Lieberman, J. (1984): Evidence for a biological hypothesis of obsessive-compulsive disorder. *Neuropsychobiology,* 11:14–21.
Lieh-Mak, F., Luk, S. L., and Leung, L. (1979): Gilles de la Tourette syndrome: Report of five cases in the Chinese. *Br. J. Psychiatry,* 134:630–634.
Lieh-Mak, F., Chung, S. Y., Lee, P., and Chen, S. (1982): Tourette syndrome in the Chinese: A

follow-up of 15 cases. In: *Advances in Neurology, Vol. 35, Gilles de la Tourette Syndrome,* edited by A. J. Friedhoff and T. N. Chase, pp. 281–283. Raven Press, New York.

Lindenmulder, F. G. (1933): Familial myoclonus occurring in three successive generations. *J. Nerv. Ment. Dis.,* 77:489–491.

Lindner, H., and Stevens, H. (1967): Hypnotherapy and psychodynamics in the syndrome of Gilles de la Tourette. *Int. J. Clin. Exp. Hypn.,* 15:151–155.

Linet, L. S. (1985): Tourette syndrome, pimozide and school phobia: The neuroleptic separation anxiety syndrome. *Am. J. Psychiatry,* 142:613–615.

Lipcsey, A. (1983): A propos de la maladie de Gilles de la Tourette. *Sem. Hop. Paris,* 59:695–696.

Lipinski, J. F., Zubenko, G. S., Cohen, B. M., and Barreira, P. J. (1984): Propranolol in the treatment of neuroleptic-induced akathisia. *Am. J. Psychiatry,* 141:412–415.

Lishman, W. A., and McMeekan, E. R. L. (1976): Hand preference patterns in psychiatric patients. *Br. J. Psychiatry,* 129:158–166.

Logue, P. E., Platzek, D., Hutzell, R., and Robinson, B. (1973): Neurological, neuropsychological and behavioral aspects of Gilles de la Tourette's syndrome: A case. *Percept. Mot. Skills,* 37:855–861.

Louis, J. A. and Bertorini, T. E. (1982): Duchenne muscular dystrophy and Tourette syndrome. *Neurology,* 32:329.

Lowe, T. L., Cohen, D. J., Detlor, J., Kremenitzer, M. W., and Shaywitz, B. A. (1982): Stimulant medications precipitate Tourette's syndrome. *JAMA,* 247:1168–1169.

Lucas, A. R. (1964): Gilles de la Tourette's disease in children: treatment with phenothiazine drugs. *Am. J. Psychiatry,* 121:606–608.

Lucas A. R. (1967): Gilles de la Tourette's disease in children: treatment with haloperidol. *Am. J. Psychiatry,* 124:146–149.

Lucas, A. R. (1973): A report of Gilles de la Tourette's disease in two succeeding generations. *Child Psychiatry Hum. Dev.,* 3:231–233.

Lucas, A. R., and Rodin, E. A. (1973): EEG in Gilles de la Tourette's disease. *Dis. Nerv. Syst.,* 34:85–89.

Lucas, A. R., Kauffman, P. E., and Morris, E. M. (1967): Gilles de la Tourette's disease, a clinical study of 15 cases. *J. Am. Acad. Child Psychiatry,* 6:700–722.

Lucas, A. R., Beard, C. M., Rajput, A. H., and Kurland, L. T. (1982): Tourette syndrome in Rochester, Minnesota, 1968–1979. In: *Advances in Neurology, Vol. 35, Gilles de la Tourette Syndrome,* edited by A. J. Friedhoff and T. N. Chase, pp. 267–269. Raven Press, New York.

Ludlow, C. L., Polinsky, R. J., Caine, E. D., Bassich, C. J., and Ebert, M. H. (1982): Language and speech abnormalities in Tourette syndrome. In: *Advances in Neurology, Vol. 35, Gilles de la Tourette Syndrome,* edited by A. J. Friedhoff and T. N. Chase, pp. 351–361. Raven Press, New York.

Lynch, G., and Baudry, M. (1984): The biochemistry of memory: A new and specific hypothesis. *Science,* 224:1057–1063.

MacDonald, I. J. (1963): A case of Gilles de la Tourette's syndrome, with some aetiological observations. *Br. J. Psychiatry,* 109:206–210.

MacFarlane, J. W., Allen, L., and Honzik, M. P. (1954): *A Developmental Study of Behavior Problems of Normal Children Between Twenty-One Months and Fourteen Years.* University of California, Berkeley.

McAndrew, J. B., Quentin, C., and Treffert, D. A. (1972): Effects of prolonged phenothiazine intake on psychotic and other hospitalized children. *J. Autism Child Schizophr.,* 2:75–91.

McDanal, C. E., Jr. (1981): Haloperidol and laryngeal-pharyngeal dystonia. *Am. J. Psychiatry,* 138:1262–1263.

McGee, R., Williams, S., and Silva, P. A. (1985): Factor structure and correlates of ratings of inattention, hyperactivity, and antisocial behavior in a large sample of 9 year old children from the general population. *J. Consult. Clin. Psychol.,* 53:480–490.

McHenry, L. C., Jr. (1967): Samuel Johnson's tics and gesticulations. *J. Hist. Med.,* 22:152–168.

McKeith, I. G., Williams, A., and Nicol, A. R. (1981): Clonidine in Tourette syndrome letter. *Lancet.,* 8214:270–271.

McNeil Pharmaceutical (1985): ORAP Prescribing Information. Spring House, Pennsylvania.

Mahler, M. S. (1944): Tics and impulsions in children: a study of motility. *Psychoanal. Q.,* 13:430–444.

Mahler, M. S. (1949): Psychoanalytic evaluation of tics: A sign and symptom in psychopathology. *Psychoanal. Study Child.*, 3–4:279.
Mahler, M. S., and Gross, I. H. (1945): Psychotherapeutic study of a typical case with tics syndrome. *Nerv. Child.*, 4:359–373.
Mahler, M. S., and Luke, J. A. (1946): Outcome of the tic syndrome. *J. Nerv. Ment. Dis.*, 103:433–445.
Mahler, M. S., and Rangell, L. (1943): A psychosomatic study of maladie des tics (Gilles de la Tourette's disease). *Psychiatr. Q.*, 17:579–603.
Mahler, M. S., Luke, J. A., and Daltroff, W. (1945): Clinical and follow-up study of the tic syndrome in children. *Am. J. Orthopsychiatry*, 15:631–647.
Mahloudji, M., and Pikielny, R. T. (1967): Hereditary essential myoclonus. *Brain*, 90:669–674.
Mansdorf, I. J. (1986): Assertiveness training in the treatment of a child's tics. *J. Behav. Ther. Exp. Psychiatry*, 17:29–32.
Maragos, W. F., Greenamyre, J. T., Penney Jr., J. B., and Young, A. B. (1987): Glutamate dysfunction in Alzheimer's disease: An hypothesis. *Trends Neurosci.*, 10:65–68.
Marks, I. M. (1981): Review of behavioral psychotherapy, I: Obsessive-compulsive disorders. *Am. J. Psychiatry*, 138:5.
Marneros, A. (1984): Gilles de la Tourette's syndrome. *Fortschr. Neurol. Psychiatr.*, 52:250–257.
Marra, T. R., Reynolds, N. C., Jr., and Dahl, D. S. (1980): Tourette syndrome, an acquired encephalopathy? A report of two cases with epileptiform dysrhythmia. *Clin. Electroencephalogr.*, 11:118–123.
Marsden, C. D. (1976): The problem of adult-onset idiopathic torsion dystonia and other isolated dyskinesias in adult life. In: *Advances in Neurology, Vol. 14, Dystonia,* edited R. Eldridge and S. Fahn. Raven Press, New York.
Marsden, C. D., Hallett, M., and Fahn, S. (1982): The nosology and pathophysiology of myoclonus. In: *Movements Disorders,* edited by C. D. Marsden and S. Fahn, pp. 196–248. Butterworth, London.
Marsden, C. D., Obeso, J. A., and Rothwell, J. C. (1983): Clinical neurophysiology of muscle jerks: myoclonus, chorea, and tics. *Adv. Neurol.*, 39:865–881.
Marti-Masso, J. F., and Obeso, J. A. (1985): Coprolalia associated with hemiballismus: Response to tetrabenazine. *Clin. Neuropharmacol.*, 8:189–190.
Martin, R. R., Ebert, M. H., Gordon, E. K., Linnoila, M., and Kopin, I. J. (1984): Effects of clonidine on central and peripheral catecholamine metabolism. *Clin. Pharmacol. Ther.*, 35:322–327.
Martindale, C. (1976): The grammes of the tic in Gilles de la Tourette's syndrome. *Lang. Speech*, 19:266–275.
Matthews, K. L. (1981): Familial Gilles de la Tourette's syndrome associated with tuberous sclerosis. *Tex. Med.*, 77:46–49.
Matthysee, S. (1973): Antipsychotic drug actions: A clue to the neuropathology of schizophrenia? *Fed. Proc.*, 32:200–205.
Mazur, W. P. (1953a): Gilles de la Tourette's disease. *Can. Med. Assoc. J.*, 69:520–522.
Mazur, W. P. (1953b): Gilles de la Tourette's disease. *Edinburgh Med. J.*, 60:427–433.
Meige, H., and Feindel, E. (1907): *Tics and Their Treatment.* Translated and edited by S. A. K. Wilson. William Wood, New York.
Menaker, E. (1945): Hypermotility and transitory tic in a child of seven. *Nerv. Child*, 4:335–341.
Mendelson, W. B., Caine, E. D., Goyer, P., Ebert, M., and Gillin, J. C. (1980): Sleep in Gilles de la Tourette syndrome. *Biol. Psychiatry*, 15:339–343.
Menuck, M. (1981): Letter to the editor: Laryngeal-pharyngeal dystonia and haloperidol. *Am. J. Psychiatry*, 138:394–395.
Merikangas, J. R., Merikangas, K. R., Kopp, U., and Hanin, I. (1985): Blood choline and response to clonazepam and haloperidol in Tourette's syndrome. *Acta Psychiatr. Scand.*, 72:395–399.
Merrill, C. R., Leavitt, J., Van Keuren, M. L., Ebert, M. H., and Caine, E. D. (1979): Hypoxanthine guanine phosphoribosyltransperase (HGPRT) in Gilles de la Tourette syndrome. *Neurology (Minneap.)*, 29:131–134.
Merskey, H. (1974): A case of multiple tics with vocalization (partial syndrome of Gilles de la Tourette) and XYY karyotype. *Br. J. Psychiatry*, 125:593–594.

Mesnikoff, A. M. (1959): Three cases of Gilles de la Tourette's syndrome treated with psychotherapy and chlorpromazine. *Arch. Neurol. Psychiatry*, 81(6):710.

Messerschmitt, P. L. (1972): L'utiilization du pimozide en pédopsychiatrie (apropos de 186 malades). *Thesis, Faculté de Médécine de Paris.*

Messiha, F. S., and Knopp, W. (1976): A study of endogenous dopamine metabolism in Gilles de la Tourette's disease. *Dis. Nerv. Syst.*, 37:470–473.

Messiha, F. S., Knopp, W., Vanecko, S., O'Brien, V., and Corson, S. A. (1971): Haloperidol treatment in Tourette's syndrome: Neurophysiological, biochemical, and behavioral correlations. *Life Sci.*, 10:449–457.

Meyerhoff, J. L., and Snyder, S. H. (1973): Gilles de la Tourette's disease and minimal brain dysfunction: Amphetamine isomers reveal catecholamine correlates in an affected patient. *Psychopharmacologia*, 29:211–220.

Michael, R. P. (1957): Treatment of a case of compulsive swearing. *Br. Med. J.*, 1:1506–1508.

Mikkelsen, E. J., Detlor, J., and Cohen, D. J. (1981): School avoidance and social phobia triggered by haloperidol in patients with Tourette's disorder. *Am. J. Psychiatry*, 138:1572–1576.

Milman, D. H. (1960): Multiple tics. *Am. J. Psychiatry*, 116:935–936.

Milman, D. (1975): Gilles de la Tourette syndrome. *NY State J. Med.*, 75:892–895.

Milner, B., and Petrides, M. (1984): Behavioral effects of frontal-lobe lesions in man. *Trends Neurosci.*, 7:403–407.

Miltenberger, R. C., Fuqua, R. W., and McKinley, T. (1985): Habit reversal with muscle tics: Replication and component analysis. *Behav. Ther.*, 16:39–50.

Min, S. K. (1983): Gilles de la Tourette's syndrome: Report on 24 Korean cases. *Yonsei Med. J.*, 24:76–82.

Minnigerode, B., and Polyzoidis, T. (1981): The barking cough of puberty. *J. Fr. Otorhinolaryngol.*, 30:391–393.

Mitchell, E., and Matthews, K. L. (1980): Gilles de la Tourette's disorder associated with Pemoline. *Am. J. Psychiatry*, 137:1618–1619.

Mizrahi, E. M., Holtzman, D., and Tharp, B. (1980): Haloperidol-induced tardive dyskinesia in a child with Gilles de la Tourette's disease. *Arch. Neurol.*, 37:780.

Modestin, J., Krapf, R., and Boker, W. (1981): A fatality during haloperidol treatment: Mechanism of sudden death. *Am. J. Psychiatry*, 138:1616–1617.

Moldofsky, H. (1971): A psychophysiological study of multiple tics. *Arch. Gen. Psychiatry*, 25:79–87.

Moldofsky, H., and Brown, G. M. (1982): Tics and serum prolactin response to pimozide in Tourette syndrome. In: *Advances in Neurology, Vol. 35, Gilles de la Tourette Syndrome*, edited by A. J. Friedhoff and T. N. Chase, pp. 387–390. Raven Press, New York.

Moldofsky, H., and Sandor, P. (1983): Lecithin in the treatment of Gilles de la Tourette's syndrome. *Am. J. Psychiatry*, 140:1627–1629.

Moldofsky, H., Tullis, C., and Lamon, R. (1974): Multiple tic syndrome (Gilles de la Tourette's syndrome). *J. Nerv. Ment. Dis.*, 159:282–291.

Montgomery, M. A., Clayton, P. J., and Friedhoff, A. J. (1982): Psychiatric illness in Tourette syndrome patients and first-degree relatives. In: *Advances in Neurology, Vol. 35, Gilles de la Tourette Syndrome*, edited by A. J. Friedhoff and T. N. Chase, pp. 335–339. Raven Press, New York.

Morphew, J. A., and Sim, M. (1969): Gilles de la Tourette's syndrome: A clinical and psychopathological study. *Br. J. Med. Psychol.*, 42:293–301.

Morrison, J. R. (1983): Early birth order in Briquet's syndrome. *Am. J. Psychiatry*, 140:1596–1598.

Morselli, P. L., Bianchetti, G., Durand, G., Le Heuzey, M. F., ZariFian, E., and Dugas, M. (1979): Haloperidol plasma level monitoring in pediatric patients. *Therapeutic Drug Monitoring*, 1:35–46.

Mueller, J., and Aminoff, M. J. (1982): Tourette-like syndrome after long-term neuroleptic drug treatment. *Br. J. Psychiatry*, 141:191–193.

Munetz, M. R., Slawsky, R. C., and Neil, J. F. (1985): Tardive Tourette's syndrome treated with clonidine and mesoridazine. *Psychosomatics*, 26:254–257.

Murray, T. J. (1978): Tourette's syndrome: A treatable tic. *Can. Med. Assoc. J.*, 118:1407–1410.

Murray, T. J. (1979): Dr. Samuel Johnson's movement disorders. *Br. Med. J.*, 1:1610–1614.

Murray, T. J. (1982): Doctor Samuel Johnson's abnormal movements. In: *Advances in Neurology, Vol. 35, Gilles de la Tourette Syndrome,* edited by A. J. Friedhoff and T. N. Chase, pp. 25–30. Raven Press, New York.
Myers, R. D., and Knott, P. J., editors (1986): *Neurochemical Analysis of the Conscious Brain: Voltammetry and Push-Pull Perfusion.* Annals of the New York Academy of Science, Vol. 473. New York Academy of Science, New York.
Nadvornik, P., Sramka, M., Lisy, L., and Svicka, I. (1972): Experiences with dentatotomy. *Confin. Neurol.,* 34:320–324.
Navia, B. A., Cho, E-S, Petito, C. K., Price, R. W. (1986): AIDs dementia complex: II. Neuropathology. *Ann. Neurol.,* 19:525–535.
Nee, L. E., Caine, E. D., Polinsky, R. J., Eldridge, R., and Ebert, M. H. (1980): Gilles de la Tourette syndrome: Clinical and family study of 50 cases. *Ann. Neurol.,* 7:41–49.
Nee, L. E., Polinsky, R. J., and Ebert, M. H. (1982): Tourette syndrome: Clinical and family studies. In: *Advances in Neurology, Vol. 35, Gilles de la Tourette Syndrome,* edited by A. J. Friedhoff and T. N. Chase, pp. 291–295. Raven Press, New York.
Negishi, Y. (1983): Psychotherapeutic study of tics in childhood—on relationship between family dynamics and onset. *Folia. Psychiatr. Neurol. Jpn.,* 37:1–23.
Neglia, J. P., Glaze, D. G., and Zion, T. E. (1984): Tics and vocalizations in children treated with carbamazepine. *Pediatrics,* 73:841–844.
Nomura, Y., and Segawa, M. (1979): Gilles de la Tourette syndrome in oriental children. *Brain Dev.,* 1:103–111.
Nomura, Y., and Segawa, M. (1982): Tourette syndrome in oriental children: Clinical and pathophysiological considerations. In: *Advances in Neurology, Vol. 35, Gilles de la Tourette Syndrome,* edited by A. J. Friedhoff and T. N. Chase, pp. 227–280. Raven Press, New York.
Norton, A. (1952): Incidence of neurosis related to maternal age and birth order. *Br. J. Soc. Med.,* 6:253–258.
Nose, T., and Takemoto, H. (1975): The effect of penfluridol and some psychotropic drugs on monoamine metabolism in central nervous system. *Eur. J. Pharmacol.,* 31:351–359.
Nuwer, M. R. (1982): Coprolalia as an organic symptom. In: *Advances in Neurology, Vol. 35, Gilles de la Tourette Syndrome,* edited by A. J. Friedhoff and T. N. Chase, pp. 363–368. Raven Press, New York.
Nyback, H., Schubert, J., and Sedvall, G. (1970): Effect of apomorphine and pimozide on synthesis and turnover of labelled catecholamines in mouse brain. *J. Pharm. Pharmacol.,* 22;622–624.
Oberndorf, C. P. (1916): Simple tic mechanism. *JAMA,* 16:99–100.
Obeso, J. A., Rothwell, J. C., and Marsden, C. D. (1981): Simple tics in Gilles de la Tourette's syndrome are not prefaced by a normal premovement EEG potential. *J. Neurol. Neurosurg. Psychiatry,* 44:735–738.
Obeso, J A., Rothwell, J. C., and Marsden, C. D. (1982): The neurophysiology of Tourette syndrome. In: *Advances in Neurology, Vol., 35, Gilles de la Tourette Syndrome,* edited by A. J. Friedhoff and T. N. Chase, pp. 105–114. Raven Press, New York.
Obeso, J. A., Rothwell, J. C., Lang, A. E., and Marsden, C. D. (1983): Myoclonic dystonia. *Neurology (NY),* 33:825–830.
O'Brien, J. A. (1883): Latah. *J. Br. Asiat. Soc.,* 1:381.
Onofrj, M., and Bodis-Wollner, I. (1982): Dopaminergic deficiency causes delayed visual evoked potentials in rat. *Ann. Neurol.,* 11:484–490.
O'Quinn, A. N., and Thompson, R. J., Jr. (1980): Tourette's syndrome: An expanded view. *Pediatrics,* 66:420–424.
Orne, M. T. (1962): On the social psychology of the psychological experiment: With particular reference to demand characteristics and their implications. *Am. Psychol.,* 17:776–783.
Orvaschel, H., Thompson, W. D., Belanger, A., Prusoff, B. A., and Kidd, K. K. (1982): Comparison of the family history method to direct interview: factors affecting the diagnosis of depression. *J. Affective Disord.,* 4:49–59.
Osler, W. (1891): *On Chorea and Choreiform Affections.* H. K. Lewis, London.
Osler, W. (1905): Medicine in the nineteenth century. In: *Aequanimatas.* P. Blakeston, Philadelphia.
Oxford English Dictionary (compact edition) (1971): Oxford University Press, Glasgow, Scotland.

Parikh, M. D., Abhyanka, R. R., Bajaj, N., and Doongaji, D. R. (1979): Penfluridol in the treatment of Gilles de la Tourette's syndrome. *Neurology (India)*, 27:174–177.
Parker, K. (1985): Helping school-age children cope with Tourette syndrome. *J. Sch. Health*, 55:30–32.
Parker, W. B. (1908, 1909): *Psychotherapy, A Course of Reading in Sound Psychology, Sound Medicine and Sound Religion, Vol. 3*. Centre, New York.
Pasamanick, B., and Kawi, A. (1956): A study of the association of prenatal and paranatal factors in the development of tics in children. *J. Pediatr.*, 48:596–601.
Pasquier, C., and Pouplard, F. (1977): Some thoughts on tics in children resulting from a therapeutic test. *Rev. Neuropsychiatr. Infant.*, 25:645–651.
Patel, M. (1986): Letter to the editor: Long-term neurologic complications of metaclopramide. *NYS J. Med.*, 3:210.
Patrick, H. T. (1905): Convulsive tic. *JAMA*, 44:437–442.
Pauls, D. L., Towbin, K. E., Leckman, J. F., Zahner, G. E. P., and Cohen, D. J. (1986b): Gilles de la Tourette's syndrome and obsessive-compulsive disorder. *Arch. Gen. Psychiatry*, 43:1180–1182.
Pauls, D. L., Cohen, D. J., Heimbuch, R., Detlor, J., and Kidd, K. K. (1981): Familial pattern and transmission of Gilles de la Tourette syndrome and multiple tics. *Arch. Gen. Psychiatry*, 38:1091–1093.
Pauls, D. L., Kruger, S. D., Leckman, J. F., Cohen, D. J., and Kidd, K. K. (1984): The risk of Tourette's syndrome and chronic multiple tics among relatives of Tourette's syndrome patients obtained by direct interview. *J. Am. Acad. Child Psychiatry*, 23:134–137.
Pauls, D. L., Hurst, C. R., Kruger, S. D., Leckman, J. F., Kidd, K. K., and Cohen, D. J. (1986a): Evidence against a genetic relationship between Tourette syndrome and attention deficit disorder. *Arch. Gen. Psychiatry*, 43:1177–1179.
Pauls, D. L., and Kurlan, R. (1986): A genetic linkage study of Gilles de la Tourette's syndrome (Abstract). In: *Scientific Proceedings of the Annual Meeting of the American Academy of Child and Adolescent Psychiatry*, edited by L. L. Greenhill, pp. 24.
Pauls, D. L., Leckman, J. F., Towbin, K. E., Zahner, G. E. P., and Cohen, D. J. (1986c): A possible genetic relationship exists between Tourette's syndrome and obsessive–compulsive disorder. *Psychopharmacol. Bull.*, 22:730–733.
Pauls, D. L., and Leckman, J. F. (1986): The inheritance of Gilles de la Tourette's syndrome and associated behaviors: Evidence for autosomal dominant transmission. *New Engl. J. Medicine*, 315:993–997.
Penney, J. B., Jr., and Young, A. B. (1983): Speculations on the functional anatomy of basal ganglia disorders. *Annu. Rev. Neurosci.*, 6:73–94.
Perlin, S., Pollin, W., and Butler, R. N. (1958): The experimental subject. *Arch. Neurol. Psychiatry*, 80:65.
Peters, J. E., Romine, J. S., and Dykman, R. A. (1975): A special neurological examination of children with learning disabilities. *Dev. Med. Child Neurol.*, 17:63–78.
Petersen, I., and Eeg-Olofsson, O. (1971): The development of the electroencephalogram in normal children from the age of 1 through 15 years. Non-paroxysmal activity. *Neuropaediatrie*, 2:247–304.
Philpott, R. (1975): Recent advances in the behavioral measurement of obsessional illness: difficulties common to these and other measures. *Scot. Med. J. (Suppl.)*, 20:33–40.
Physicians' Desk Reference, 39th edition (1985): Medical Economics, Oradell, New Jersey.
Picat, J., Lae, D., and Goulffes, A. (1983): Maladie d'ethique, le syndrome de Gilles de la Tourette et l'obsession de la perfection. *LARC Med.* 3:426–429.
Pinta, E. R. (1977): Deanol in Gilles de la Tourette syndrome: A preliminary investigation, *Dis. Nerv. Syst.*, 38:214–215.
Piotrowski, Z. A. (1937): The Rorschach ink blot method for organic disturbances of the central nervous system. *J. Nerv. Ment. Dis.*, 86:525–537.
Piotrowski, Z. A. (1945): Rorschach records of children with a tic syndrome. *Nerv. Child.*, 4:342–352.
Pitman, R. K. (1987): Pierre Janet on obsessive-compulsive disorder (1903). *Arch. Gen. Psychiatry*, 44:226–232.
Plaisted, J. R. (1984): Intellectual, achievement, and neuropsychological correlates in Tourette Syndrome. *Int. J. Clin. Neuropsychol.*, 6:75.

Platt, J. E., Campbell, M., Green, W. H., and Grega, D. M. (1984): Cognitive effects of lithium carbonate and haloperidol in treatment-resistant aggressive children. *Arch. Gen. Psychiatry*, 41:657–662.
Polinsky, R. J., Ebert, M. H., Caine, E. D., Ludlow, C., and Bassich, C. J. (1980): Letter to the editor: Cholinergic treatment in the Tourette syndrome. *N. Engl. J. Med.*, 302:1310.
Polites, D. J., Kruger, D., and Stevenson, I. (1965): Sequential treatments in a case of Gilles de la Tourette's Syndrome. *Br. J. Med. Psychiatry*, 38:43–52.
Pollack, M. A., Cohen, N. L., and Friedhoff, A. J. (1977): Gilles de la Tourette syndrome: Familial occurrence and precipitation by methylphenedate therapy. *Arch. Neurol.*, 34:630–632.
Pollera, C. F., Cognetti, F., Nardi, M., and Mazza, D. (1984): Letter to the editor: Sudden death after acute dystonic reaction to high-dose metoclopramide. *Lancet*, 2:460–461.
Pollin, W., and Perlin, S. (1958): Psychiatric evaluation of "normal control" volunteers. *Am. J. Psychiatry*, 115:129–133.
Prabhakaran, N. (1970): A case of Gilles de la Tourette's syndrome with some observations on etiology and treatment. *Br. J. Psychiatry*, 116:539–541.
Price, A. R., Kidd, K. K., Cohen, D. J., Pauls, D. L., and Leckman, J. F. (1985): A twin study of Tourette syndrome. *Arch. Gen. Psychiatry*, 42:815–820.
Price, A. R., Leckman, J. F., Pauls, D. L., Cohen, D. J., and Kidd, K. K. (1986): Tics and central nervous system stimulants in twins and non-twins with Tourette syndrome. *Neurology*, 36:232–237.
Price, J. S., and Hare, E. H. (1969): Birth order studies: Some sources of bias. *Br. J. Psychiatry*, 115:633–646.
Prince, M. (1906): Case of multiform tic including automatic speech and purposive moments. *J. Nerv. Ment. Dis.*, 33:29–34.
Pringle, M. L., Butler, N. R., and Davie, R. (1967): *11,000 Seven Year Olds*. National Bureau of Cooperation in Child Care, London.
Przuntek, H., and Muhr, H. (1983): Essential familial myoclonus. *J. Neurol.*, 230:153–162.
Psychopharmacology Bulletin (1985): National Institute of Mental Health, Vol. 21, No. 2, pp. 159–257. U.S. Department of Health and Human Services, Washington, D.C.
Pulst, S. M., Walshe, T. M., and Romero, J. A. (1983): Carbon monoxide poisoning with features of Gilles de la Tourette's syndrome. *Arch. Neurol.*, 40:443–444.
Quay, H. C., and Werry, J. S. (1972): *Psychopathological Disorders of Childhood*. Wiley, New York.
Quitkin, F., Rifkin, A., and Klein, D. F. (1976): Neurologic soft signs in schizophrenia and character disorders: Organicity in schizophrenia with premorbid asociality and emotionally unstable character disorders. *Arch. Gen. Psychiatry*, 33:845–853.
Rachman, S. J., and deSilva, P. (1978): Abnormal and normal obsessions. *Behav. Res. Ther.*, 16:233–248.
Rachman, S. J., and Hodgson, R. J. (1980): *Obsessions and Compulsions*. Prentice-Hall, Englewood Cliffs, New Jersey.
Railton, T. C. (1886): Notes on a case of involuntary muscular movements accompanied by coprolalia. *Med. Chron. Manchester*, 4:24–29.
Rapaport, D. (1946): *Diagnostic Psychological Testing, Vol. II*. Year Book, Chicago.
Rapoport, J. L. (1959): Maladie des tics in children. *Am. J. Psychiatry*, 116:177–178.
Rapoport, J. L., Quinn, O., and Lamprecht, F. (1974): Minor physical anomalies and plasma dopamine-beta-hydroxylase activity in hyperactive boys. *Am. J. Psychiatry*, 131:4.
Rapoport, J. L., Nee, L., Mitchell, S., Polinsky, R., and Ebert, M. (1982): Hyperkinetic syndrome and Tourette syndrome. In: *Advances in Neurology, Vol. 35, Gilles de la Tourette Syndrome*, edited by A. J. Friedhoff and T. N. Chase, pp. 423–426. Raven Press, New York.
Rapoport, J. L., Langer, D. H., Sceery, W., Buchsbaum, M. S., Murphy, D. L., Zahn, T. P., Lake, R., Ludlow, C., and Mendelson, W. (1987): Childhood obsessive compulsive disorder. *Am. J. Psychiatry*, 138:1545–1554.
Rasmussen, S. A., and Tsuang, M. T. (1984): The epidemiology of obsessive compulsive disorder. *J. Clin. Psychiatry*, 45:450–457.
Rasmussen, S. A., and Tsuang, M. T. (1986): Epidemiological and clinical findings of significance to the design of neuropharmacologic studies of obsessive–compulsive disorder. *Psychopharmacol. Bull.*, 22:723–729.

Realmuto, G. M., and Main, B. (1982): Coincidence of Tourette's disorder and infantile autism. *J. Autism Dev. Disord.*, 12:367–72.

Reguer, L., Pakkenberg, B., Fog, R., and Pakkenberg, H. (1986): Clinical features and long-term treatment with pimozide in 65 patients with Gilles de la Tourette's syndrome. *J. Neurol. Neurosurg. Psychiatry*, 49:791–795.

Reiger, D. A., Myers, J. K., Kramer, M., Robins, L. N., Blazer, D. G., Hough, R. L., Eaton, W. W., and Locke, B. Z. (1984): The NIMH epidemiologic catchment area (ECA) program: Historical context, major objectives, and study population characteristics. *Arch. Gen. Psychiatry*, 41:934–941.

Reitan, R. M. (1975): Assessment of brain-behavior relationships. In: *Advances in Psychological Assessment.* Vol. 3, pp. 186–242, edited by P. McReynolds. Josey-Bass, Inc., San Francisco.

Richards, T. W. (1960): Personality of subjects who volunteer for research on a drug (mescaline). *J. Project Techn.*, 24:424–428.

Richardson, E. P., Jr. (1982): Neuropathological studies of Tourette syndrome. In: *Advances in Neurology, Vol. 35, Gilles de la Tourette Syndrome*, edited by A. J. Friedhoff and T. N. Chase, pp. 83–87. Raven Press, New York.

Riddle, M., Hardin, M. T., Towbin, K. E., Leckman, J. F., and Cohen, D. J. (1987): Letter to the editor: Tardive dyskinesia following haloperidol treatment in Tourette's syndrome. *Arch. Gen. Psychiatry*, 44:98–99.

Risch, S. C., Groom, G. P., and Janowsky, D. S. (1981): Interfaces of psychopharmacology and cardiology. Part two. *J. Clin. Psychiatry*, 42:47–59.

Robins, L. N., Helzer, J. E., Weissman, M. M., Orvaschel, H., Gruenberg, E., Burke, J. D., Jr., and Regler, M. D. (1984): Lifetime prevalence of specific psychiatric disorders in three sites. *Arch. Gen. Psychiatry*, 41:949–958.

Robinson, R. J. (1966): Gilles de la Tourette's disease. *Dev. Med. Child. Neurol.*, 8:599–612.

Robbins, T. W. (1984): Cortical noradrenaline, attention, and arousal. *Psychol. Med. (London)*, 14:13–21.

Rodin, E., Lucas, A., and Simson, C. A. (1963): A study of behavior disorders in children by means of general purpose computers. In: *Proceedings of the Conference on Data Acquisition and Processing in Biology and Medicine*, pp. 115–124. Pergamon, New York.

Rosenheim, F. (1948): Animal identification in a ticquer. *Am. J. Orthopsychiatry*, 18:529–535.

Rosenthal, R. T., and Rosnow, R. L. (1975): *The Volunteer Subject.* Wiley, New York.

Ross, D. M., and Ross, S. A. (1982): *Hyperactivity: Theory, Research, and Action*, 2nd edition. Wiley, New York.

Ross, M. S., and Moldofsky, H. (1977): Comparison of pimozide with haloperidol in Gilles de la Tourette's syndrome. *Lancet*, 1:103.

Ross, M. S., and Moldofsky, H. (1978): A comparison of pimozide and haloperidol in the treatment of Gilles de la Tourette's syndrome. *Am. J. Psychiatry*, 135:585–587.

Ross, T. W. E. (1909): A case of convulsive tic. *Br. Med. J.*, 2:135–136.

Roth, D. C. (1850): *Histoire de la Masculation Irrésistible ou de la Chorée Anormale.* Germer-Baillière, Paris.

Roth, R. H. (1984): CNS dopamine autoreceptors: Distribution, pharmacology, and function. *Ann. NY Acad. Sci.*, 430:27–53.

Rothenberger, A., and Kemmerling, S. (1982): Bereitschaftspotential in children with multiple tics and Gilles de la Tourette syndrome. In: *Event-Related Potentials in Children*, edited by A. Rothenberger. Elsevier, Amsterdam.

Rubin, R. T., Forsman, A., Heykants, J., Ohman, R., Tower, B., and Michiels, M. (1980): Serum haloperidol determinations in psychiatric patients. *Arch. Gen. Psychiatry*, 37:1069–1074.

Rutter, M., Graham, P., and Yule, W. (1970): *A Neuropsychiatric Study in Childhood.* Spastics International Medical Publications, London.

Rutter, M. (1982): Syndromes attributed to "minimal brain dysfunction" in childhood. *Am. J. Psychiatry*, 139:21–33.

Rutter, M. (1983): Behavioral studies: Questions and findings on the concept of a distinctive syndrome. In: *Developmental Neuropsychiatry*, edited by M. Rutter. Guilford Press, New York.

Sacks, O. W. (1982): Acquired Tourettism in adult life. In: *Advances in Neurology, Vol. 35, Gilles*

de la Tourette Syndrome, edited by A. J. Friedhoff and T. N. Chase, pp. 89–92. Raven Press, New York.
Sacks, O. W. (1987): Tics. *NY Rev. Books,* Jan. 29:37–41.
Sadger, J. (1914): Ein beitrag zum verständnis des tics. *Int. Z. Psychoanal.,* 2:354–366.
Saint-Hilaire, M. H., Saint-Hilaire, J. M., and Granger, L. (1986): Jumping Frenchmen of Maine. *Neurology,* 36:1269–1271.
Saletu, B. (1977): The evoked potential in pharmacopsychiatry. *Neuropsychobiology,* 3:75–104.
Saletu, B., Saletu, M., Itil, T., and Marasa, J. (1971): Somatosensory-evoked potential changes during haloperidol treatment of chronic schizophrenics. *Biol. Psychiatry,* 3:299–307.
Salmi, K. (1961): Gilles de la Tourette's syndrome: The report of a case and its treatment. *Acta Psychiatr. Scand.,* 36:156–162.
Salzman, L., and Thaler, F. H. (1981): Obsessive compulsive disorders: A review of the literature. *Am. J. Psychiatry,* 138:286–296.
Sand, P. (1972): Neuropsychological test performance before and after symptom removal in a child with Gilles de la Tourette syndrome. *J. Clin. Psychol.,* 28:596–600.
Sand, P. L., and Carlson C. (1973): Failure to establish control over tics in the Gilles de la Tourette sydrome with behavior therapy techniques. *Br. J. Psychiatry,* 122:665–670.
Sanders, D. G. (1973): Familial occurrence of Gilles de la Tourette's syndrome: Report of the syndrome occurring in a father and son. *Arch. Gen. Psychiatry,* 28:326–328.
Sandoval, J., Lambert, N. M., and Sassone, D. (1980): The identification and labeling of hyperactivity in children: An interactive model. In: *Hyperactive Children,* edited by C. K. Whalen and B. Henker. Academic Press, Inc., New York.
Sandras, C. M. S. (1851): *Traite Pratique des Maladies Nerveuses.* Germer-Bailliere, Paris.
Sandyk, R. (1985a): The endogenous opioid system in neurological disorders of the basal ganglia. *Life Sci.,* 37:1655–1663.
Sandyk, R. (1985b): Letter to the editor: The opioid system in Gilles de la Tourette's syndrome. *Neurology,* 35:449–450.
Sandyk, R. (1985c): Letter to the editor: The effects of naloxone in Tourette's syndrome. *Ann. Neurol.,* 18:367–368.
Sandyk, R. (1986): Letter to the editor: Naloxone withdrawal exacerbates Tourette syndrome. *J. Clin. Psychopharmacol.,* 6:58–59.
Sandyk, R., Iacono, R. P., and Allender, J. (1986): Naloxone ameliorates compulsive touching behavior and tics in Tourette's syndrome. *Ann. Neurol.,* 20:437.
Sarna, S., Kaprio, J., Sistonen, P., and Koskenvuo, M. (1978): Diagnosis of twin zygosity by mailed questionnaire. *Hum. Hered.,* 28:241–254.
SAS/STAT Guide for Personal Computers (1985): Version 6 edition. SAS Institute, Cary, North Carolina.
Savin, L. H. (1961): Remarks on spasm and tics in ophthalmic practice with notes on four cases of the syndrome on Gilles de la Tourette. *Trans. Ophthalmol. Soc. UK,* 31:39–52.
Schafer, R. (1953): Content analysis in the Rorschach test. *J. Project Tech.,* 17:335–339.
Schaltenbrand, Georges (1975a): The effects on speech and language of stereotactical stimulation in thalamus and corpus callosum. *Brain Lang.,* 2:70–77.
Schaltenbrand, Georges (1975b): The effects of stereotactic electrical stimulation in the depth of the brain. *Brain,* 88:835–840.
Schmitt, B. D. (1975): The minimal brain dysfunction myth. *Am. J. Dis. Child.,* 129:1313–1318.
Schneck, J. M. (1960): Gilles de la Tourette's disease. *Am. J. Psychiatry,* 117:78.
Schneider, R. H., Smith, C. B., and Zweifler, A. J. (1984): Clonidine treatment decreases platelet alpha$_2$-adrenoreceptors in hypertensive patients. *Fed. Proc.,* 43:839.
Schoenberg, B. S. (1982): Neuroepidemiologic approach to Tourette syndrome. In: *Advances in Neurology, Vol. 35, Gilles de la Tourette Syndrome,* edited by A. J. Friedhoff and T. N. Chase, pp. 259–265. Raven Press, New York.
Seeman, M. V., Patel, V., and Pyke, J. (1981): Tardive dyskinesia with Tourette-like syndrome. *J. Clin. Psychiatry,* 42:357–358.
Seeman, P., and Lee, T. (1975): Antipsychotic drugs: Direct correlations between clinical potency and presynaptic action on dopamine neurons. *Science,* 188:1217–1219.
Seignot, M. J. N. (1961): Un cas de maladie des tics de Gilles de la Tourette gueri par le R-1625. *Ann. Med. Psychol.,* 119:578–579.
Selinger, D., Cohen, D. J., Ort, S., Anderson, G. M., Caruso, K. A., and Leckman, J. F. (1984):

Parotid salivary response to clonidine in Tourette's syndrome: Indications of adrenergic responsivity. *J. Am. Acad. Child Adolescent Psychiatry*, 23:392–398.

Selling, L. (1929): The role of infection in the aetiology of tics. *Arch. Neurol. Psychiatry*, 22:1163–1171.

Shaenboen, M. I., Nigro, M. A., and Martocci, R. J. (1984): Letter to the editor: Colpocephaly and Gilles de la Tourette's syndrome., *Arch. Neurol.*, 41:1023.

Shaffer, D., and Schonfeld, I. (1984): A critical note on the value of attention deficit as a basis for a clinical syndrome. In: *Attention Deficit Disorder: Diagnostic, Cognitive, and Therapeutic Understanding*, edited by L. M. Bloomingdale, pp. 119–131. Spectrum, New York.

Shaffer, D., O'Connor, P. A., Shafer, S. Q., and Prupis, S. (1983): Neurological "soft signs": Their origins and significance for behavior. In: *Developmental Neuropsychiatry*, edited by M. Rutter. The Guilford Press, New York.

Shaffer, D., Schonfeld, I., O'Connor, P. A., Stokman, C., Fraulman, P., and Shafer, S. (1985): Neurological soft signs: Their relation to psychiatric disorders and intelligence in childhood and adolescence. *Arch. Gen. Psychiatry*, 42:342–358.

Shapiro, A. K. (1959): The placebo effect in the history of medical treatment: Implications for psychiatry. *Am. J. Psychiatry*, 116:298–304.

Shapiro, A. K. (1960): A contribution to a history of the placebo in treatment. *J. Nerv. Ment. Dis.*, 130:200–211.

Shapiro, A. K. (1964): A historic and heuristic definition of the placebo. *Psychiatry*, 27:52–58.

Shapiro, A. K. (1970a): Dangers of premature psychological diagnosis. *NY State J. Med.*, 70:2193–2213.

Shapiro, A. K. (1970b): Gilles de la Tourette's syndrome. *NY State J. Med.*, 70:2193–2214.

Shapiro, A. K. (1970c): Symposium on Gilles de la Tourette's syndrome. *NY State J. Med.*, 70:2193–2214.

Shapiro, A. K. (1971): Placebo effects in medicine, psychotherapy, and psychoanalysis. In: *Handbook of Psychotherapy and Behavior Change: Empirical Analysis*, edited by A. E. Bergin and S. L. Garfield, pp. 439–473. Wiley, New York.

Shapiro, A. K. (1972): Letter to the editor: Gilles de la Tourette's disease. *Am. J. Psychiatry*, 129:99.

Shapiro, A. K. (1974): Contribution to a history of the placebo effect. In: *Biofeedback and Self Control—1973*, edited by N. E. Miller, Aldine, Chicago.

Shapiro, A. K. (1976a): The behavior therapies: Therapeutic breakthrough or latest fad? *Am. J. Psychiatry*, 133:154–159.

Shapiro, A. K. (1976b): Psychochemotherapy. In: *Biological Foundations of Psychiatry*, edited by R. G. Grenell and S. Gabay, pp. 793–836. Raven Press, New York.

Shapiro, A. K. (1978): The placebo effect. In: *Principles of Psychopharmacology*, edited by W. G. Clark and J. Del Guidice. Academic Press, New York.

Shapiro, A. K. (1981): Letter to the editor: Pimozide induced enuresis. *Am. J. Psychiatry*, 138:123–124.

Shapiro, A. K., and Morris, L. (1977a): The placebo response. In: *Practice of Medicine*, edited by M. D. Hagerstown. Harper & Row, New York.

Shapiro, A. K., and Morris, L. (1977b): Placebos in psychiatric therapy. In: *Current Psychiatric Therapies, Vol. 17*, pp. 157–163, edited by J. H. Masserman. Grune and Stratton, New York.

Shapiro, A. K., and Morris, L. (1978): The placebo effect in healing. In: *Handbook of Psychotherapy and Behavior Change*, edited by S. L. Garfield and A. E. Bergin, pp. 477–536. Aldine, New York.

Shapiro, A. K., and Shapiro, E. (1968): Treatment of Gilles de la Tourette's syndrome with haloperidol. *Br. J. Psychiatry*, 114:345–350.

Shapiro, A. K., and Shapiro, E. (1971): Clinical dangers of psychological theorizing. *Psychiatr. Q.*, 45:159–171.

Shapiro, A. K., and Shapiro, E. (1974): Questions and answers about Tourette's syndrome. *Fam. Physician*, 9:94–96.

Shapiro, A. K., and Shapiro, E. (1980): *Tics, Tourette Syndrome and Other Movement Disorders: A Pediatrician's Guide*. Tourette Syndrome Association, New York.

Shapiro, A. K., and Shapiro, E. (1981a): The treatment and etiology of tics and Tourette syndrome. *Compr. Psychiatry*, 22:193–205.

Shapiro, A. K., and Shapiro, E. (1981b): Do stimulants provoke, cause or exacerbate tics and Tourette's syndrome? *Compr. Psychiatry*, 22:265–273.
Shapiro, A. K., and Shapiro, E. (1981c): "Embarrassed." In: *DSM-III Case Book*, edited by R. L. Spitzer, A. E. Skodol, M. Gibbon, and J. B. W. Williams. American Psychiatric Association, Washington, D.C.
Shapiro, A. K., and Shapiro, E. (1981d): *Tics, Tourette Syndrome and Other Movement Disorders: A Physician's Guide*. Tourette Syndrome Association, Cleveland, Ohio.
Shapiro, A. K., and Shapiro, E. (1982a): Clinical efficacy of haloperidol, pimozide, penfluridol, and clonidine in the treatment of Tourette syndrome. In: *Advances in Neurology, Vol. 35, Gilles de la Tourette Syndrome*, edited by A. J. Friedhoff and T. N. Chase, pp. 383–386. Raven Press, New York.
Shapiro, A. K., and Shapiro, E. (1982b): Tourette syndrome: History and present status. In: *Advances in Neurology, Vol. 35, Gilles de la Tourette Syndrome*, edited by A. J. Friedhoff and T. N. Chase, pp. 17–23. Raven Press, New York.
Shapiro, A. K., and Shapiro, E. (1982c): An update on Tourette syndrome. *Am. J. Psychother.*, 36:379–390.
Shapiro, A. K., and Shapiro, E. (1982d): Tourette syndrome: Clinical aspects, treatment and etiology. *Semin. Neurol. Movement Disorders*, 2:373–385.
Shapiro, A. K., and Shapiro, E. (1983): "Teased." In: *Psychopathology: A Case Book*, edited by R. L. Spitzer, A. E. Skodol, M. Gibbon, and J. B. W. Williams. McGraw-Hill, New York.
Shapiro, A. K., and Shapiro, E. (1984): Controlled study of pimozide vs. placebo in Tourette syndrome. *J. Am. Acad. Child Psychiatry*, 23:161–173.
Shapiro, A. K., and Shapiro, E. (1985a): Patient-provider relationships and the placebo effect. In: *Behavioral Health: Handbook of Health Enhancement and Disease*, edited by J. D. Matarazzo, N. E. Miller, S. M. Weiss, and J. A. Herd, pp. 371–383, Wiley, New York.
Shapiro, A. K., and Shapiro, E. (1985b): Guidelines for treatment. *Pediatrics for Parents*.
Shapiro, A. K., and Shapiro, E. (1985c): Debate: Use of stimulant medications as adjuncts to standard drugs. *Tourette Clinical Symposium*, October 14, 1985, Mount Sinai Medical Center, New York.
Shapiro, A. K., and Shapiro, E. (1987): Treatment of tic disorders. In: *Antimanics, Anticonvulsants and Other Drugs in Psychiatry*, edited by G. D. Burrows, T. R. Normand, and B. Davies, pp. 267–289. Elsevier/North-Holland and Biomedical Press, Amsterdam.
Shapiro, A. K., and Shapiro, E. (1987): Tic disorders. In: *Comprehensive Textbook of Psychiatry*, 5th Edition, edited by H. I. Kaplan and B. J. Sadock. Williams & Wilkins, New York (*in press*).
Shapiro, A. K., Shapiro, E., Wayne, H. L., and Clarkin, J. (1972a): The psychopathology of Gilles de la Tourette's syndrome. *Am. J. Psychiatry*, 129:427–434.
Shapiro, A. K., Shapiro, E., and Wayne, H. L. (1972b): Birth, developmental and family histories and demographic information in Tourette's syndrome. *J. Nerv. Ment. Dis.*, 155:335–344.
Shapiro, A. K., Shapiro, E., and Wayne, H. L. (1973a): Treatment of Gilles de la Tourette's syndrome with haloperidol: Review of 34 cases. *Arch. Gen. Psychiatry*, 28:92–96.
Shapiro, A. K., Shapiro, E., and Wayne, H. L. (1973b): The symptomatology and diagnosis of Gilles de la Tourette's syndrome. *J. Am. Acad. Child Psychiatry*, 12:702–723.
Shapiro, A. K., Shapiro, E., Wayne, H. L., and Clarkin, J. (1973c): Organic factors in Gilles de la Tourette's syndrome. *Br. J. Psychiatry*, 122:659–664.
Shapiro, A. K., Shapiro, E., Wayne, H. L., Clarkin, J., and Bruun, R. D. (1973d): Tourette's syndrome: Summary of data on 34 patients. *Psychosom. Med.*, 35:419–435.
Shapiro, A. K., Mike, V., Barten, H., and Shapiro, E. (1973e): Study of the placebo effect with a test of placebo reactivity. *Compr. Psychiatry*, 15:535–548.
Shapiro, A. K., Shapiro, E., Bruun, R. D., Sweet, R., Wayne, H., and Solomon, G. (1976): Gilles de la Tourette's syndrome: Summary of clinical experience with 250 patients and suggested nomenclature for tic syndromes. In: *Advances in Neurology, Vol. 14, Dystonia*, edited by R. Eldridge and S. Fahn, pp. 277–283. Raven Press, New York.
Shapiro, A. K., Shapiro, E., Bruun, R. D., and Sweet, R. D. (1978): *Gilles de la Tourette Syndrome*. Raven Press, New York.
Shapiro, A. K., Shapiro, E., and Sweet, R. D. (1981): Treatment of tics and Tourette syndrome. In: *Disorders of Movement*, edited by A. Barbeau, pp. 105–132. MTP Press, Lancaster, England.

Shapiro, A. K., and Shapiro, E., and Eisenkraft, G. J. (1983a): Treatment of Gilles de la Tourette syndrome with pimozide. *Am. J. Psychiatry*, 140:1183–1186.
Shapiro, A. K., and Shapiro, E., and Eisenkraft, G. J. (1983b): Treatment of Tourette disorder with penfluridol. *Compr. Psychiatry*, 24:327–331.
Shapiro, A. K., and Shapiro, E., and Eisenkraft, G. J. (1983c): Treatment of Gilles de la Tourette's syndrome with clonidine and neuroleptics. *Arch. Gen. Psychiatry*, 40:1235–1240.
Shapiro, A. K., Baron, M., Shapiro, E., and Levitt, M. (1984): Enzyme activity in Tourette's syndrome. *Arch. Neurol.*, 41:282–285.
Shapiro, E., and Shapiro, A. K. (1975): Sexuality in Tourette's syndrome. *Human Sexuality*, 9:100–120.
Shapiro, E., and Shapiro, A. K. (1979): Tic disorders. In: *Clinician's Handbook of Childhood Psychopathology*, edited by M. M. Josephson and R. T. Porter, pp. 323–336. Jason Aronson, New York.
Shapiro, E., and Shapiro, A. K. (1980a): Tic, Tourette or movement disorder? A guide to early diagnosis. *Diagnosis*, 2:76–84.
Shapiro, E., and Shapiro, A. K. (1980b): Patient with a tic: Neurologic or psychiatric problem? *Consultant*, 20:159–169.
Shapiro, E., and Shapiro, A. K. (1981a): Tic disorders. *JAMA*, 245:1583–1585.
Shapiro, E., and Shapiro, A. K. (1981b): Application of data oriented psychiatry to Tourette syndrome. *Interaction*, 4:33–38.
Shapiro, E., and Shapiro, A. K. (1982a): Tardive dyskinesia and chronic neuroleptic treatment of Tourette patients. In: *Advances in Neurology, Vol. 35, Gilles de la Tourette Syndrome*, edited by A. J. Friedhoff and T. N. Chase, p. 413. Raven Press, New York.
Shapiro, E., and Shapiro, A. K. (1982b): The role of the school nurse in tic and Tourette syndromes. *School Nurse*, Fall:6–7.
Shapiro, E., and Shapiro, A. K. (1984a): Tourette syndrome. In: *The World Book Encyclopedia*. World Book—Childcraft International, Chicago.
Shapiro, E., and Shapiro, A. K. (1984b): Tourette syndrome and female sexual behavior. *Med. Aspects of Hum. Sexuality*, 18:71–72.
Shapiro, E., and Shapiro, A. K. (1984c): Tourette syndrome. In: *Collier's Encyclopedia*, edited by T. Zinn and E. E. Rosenblum. MacMillan, New York.
Shapiro, E., and Shapiro, A. K. (1984d): A biography of Georges Gilles de la Tourette. In: *International Encyclopedia of Psychiatry, Psychology, Psychoanalysis, and Neurology*, edited by B. Wolman. Aesculapius, New York.
Shapiro, E., and Shapiro, A. K. (1985a): Tourette syndrome. In: *International Encyclopedia of Psychiatry, Psychology, Psychoanalysis, and Neurology*. Aesculapius, New York.
Shapiro, E., and Shapiro, A. K. (1985b): Tourette syndrome. In: *Movement Disorder*, edited by A. Donald and N. Shah, Plenum, New York.
Shapiro, E., and Shapiro, A. K. (1986): Semiology, nosology and criteria for tic disorders. *Rev. Neurol. (Paris)*, 142:824–832.
Shapiro, E., Shapiro, A. K., and Clarkin, J. (1974): Clinical psychological testing in Tourette's syndrome. *J. Pers. Assess.*, 38:464–478.
Shapiro, E., Shapiro, A. K., Sweet, R. D., and Bruun, R. D. (1975): The diagnosis, etiology, and treatment of Gilles de la Tourette's syndrome. In: *Mental Health in Children, Vol. 1*, edited by S. Sanker, PJD, Westbury, New York.
Shapiro, T., and Perry, R. (1976): Latency revisited. *Psychoanal. Study Child*, 31:79–105.
Shapiro, T., Burkes, L., Petti, T. A., and Ranz, J. (1978): Consistency of "nonfocal" neurological signs. *J. Am. Acad. Child Psychiatry*, 17:70–79.
Shaywitz, S. E., Cohen, D. J., and Shaywitz, B. A. (1984): Pharmacotherapy of attention deficit disorder. *Pediatrics Update*, 43–60.
Shepherd, M., Oppenheim, B., and Mitchell, S. (1971): *Childhood Behavior and Mental Health*. Grune and Stratton, New York.
Shostak, M., and Perel, J. (1976): Radioimmune assay for haloperidol. *Fed. Proc.*, 35:531.
Silverstein, F., Smith, C. B., and Johnston, M. V. (1985): Effect of clonidine on platelet alpha$_2$-adrenoreceptors and plasma norephinephrine of children with Tourette syndrome. *Dev. Med. Child Neurol.*, 27:793–799.
Simons, R. C. (1980): The resolution of the latah paradox. *J. Neurol. Ment. Dis.*, 168:195–206.

Singer, H. S., Oshida, L., and Coyle, J. T. (1984): CFS cholinesterase activity in Gilles de la Tourette's syndrome. *Arch. Neurol.*, 41:756–757.
Singer, H. S., Pepple, J. M., Ramage, A. L., and Butler, I. J. (1978): Gilles de la Tourette syndrome: Further studies and thoughts. *Ann. Neurol.*, 4:21–25.
Singer, H. S., Rabins, P., Tune, L. E., and Coyle, J. T. (1981): Serum haloperidol levels in Gilles de la Tourette syndrome. *Biol. Psychiatry*, 16:79–84.
Singer, H. S., Butler, I. J., Tune, L. E., Seifert, W. E., Jr., and Coyle, J. T. (1982a): Dopaminergic dysfunction in Tourette syndrome. *Ann. Neurol.*, 12:361–366.
Singer, H. S., Tune, L. E., Butler, I. J., Zaczek, R., and Coyle, J. T. (1982b): Clinical symptomatology, CSF neurotransmitter metabolities, and serum haloperidol levels in Tourette syndrome. In: *Advances in Neurology, Vol. 35, Gilles de la Tourette Syndrome*, edited by A. J. Friedhoff and T. N. Chase, pp. 177–183. Raven Press, New York.
Singer, K. (1963): Gilles de la Tourette's Disease. *Am. J. Psychiatry*, 120:80–81.
Singer, W. D. (1981): Transient Gilles de la Tourette syndrome after chronic neuroleptic withdrawal. *Dev. Med. Child Neurol.*, 23:518–521.
Singh, D. N., Howe, H. L., Jordan, H. W., and Hara, S. (1982): Tourette's syndrome in a black woman with associated triple x and 9p mosaicism. *J. Natl. Med. Assoc.*, 74:675–682.
Skirboll, L. R., Grace, A. A., and Bunney, B. S. (1979): Dopamine auto- and post-synaptic receptors: Electrophysiological evidence for differential sensitivity to dopamine agonists. *Science*, 206:80–82.
Slater, E. (1962): Birth order and maternal age of homosexuals. *Lancet*, 1:69–71.
Sleator, E. K. (1980): Deleterious effects of drugs used for hyperactivity on patients with Gilles de la Tourette syndrome. *Clin. Pediatr. (Phila.)*, 19:453–454.
Snyder, S. H., Taylor, K. H., Coyle, J. T., and Meyerhoff, J. L. (1970): The role of brain dopamine in behavioral regulation and the actions of psychotropic drugs. *Am. J. Psychiatry*. 127:199–207.
Spitz, M. C., Jankovic, J., and Killian, J. M. (1985): Familial tic disorder, parkinsonism, motor neuron disease, and acanthocytosis: A new syndrome. *Neurology*, 35:366–370.
Spohn, H. E., Lacoursiere, R. B., Thompson, K., and Lolafaye, C. (1977): Phenothiazine effects on psychological and physiological dysfunction in chronic schizophrenics. *Arch. Gen. Psychiatry*, 34:633–644.
Sprague, R., Barnes, K., and Werry, J. (1970): Methylphenidate and thioridazine: Learning, activity, and behavior in emotionally disturbed boys. *Am. J. Orthopsychiatry*, 40:615–628.
Sprenger, J. (1489): *Malleus Maleficarum*. Translated by Montague Summers (1948). Pushkin Press, London.
Sramek, J. J., Simpson, G. M., Morrison, R. L., and Heiser, J. F. (1986): Anticholinergic agents for prophylaxis of neuroleptic-induced dystonic reactions: A prospective study. *J. Clin. Psychiatry*, 47:6.
Stahl, S. M. (1980): Tardive Tourette syndrome in an autistic patient after long-term neuroleptic administration. *Am. J. Psychiatry*, 137:1267–1269.
Stahl, S. M., and Berger, P. A. (1980): Cholinergic treatment in the Tourette syndrome. *N. Engl. J. Med.*, 302:1311.
Stahl, S. M., and Berger, P. A. (1981): Physostigmine in Tourette syndrome: Evidence for cholinergic underactivity. *Am. J. Psychiatry*, 138:240–242.
Stahl, S. M., and Berger, P. A. (1982a): Cholinergic and dopaminergic mechanisms in Tourette syndrome. In: *Advances in Neurology, Vol. 35, Gilles de la Tourette Syndrome*, edited by A. J. Friedhoff and T. N. Chase, pp. 141–150. Raven Press, New York.
Stahl, S. M., and Berger, P. A. (1982b): Neuroleptic effects in Tourette syndrome predict dopamine excess and acetylcholine deficiency. *Biol. Psychiatry*, 17:1047–1053.
Stam, F. C. (1971): Gilles de la Tourette's disease. *Ned. Tijdschr. Geneeskd.*, 115:541–543.
Stedman's Medical Dictionary (1966): 21st edition. Williams & Wilkins, Baltimore.
Stefl, M. E. (1983): *The Ohio Tourette Study: An Investigation of the Special Service Needs of Tourette Syndrome Patients*. University of Cincinnati, Cincinnati, Ohio.
Stefl, M. E. (1984): Mental health needs associated with Tourette syndrome. *Am. J. Public Health*, 74:1310–1313.
Stefl, M. E., and Rubin, M. (1985): Tourette syndrome in the classroom: Special problems, special needs. *J. Sch. Health*, 55:72–75.

Stevens, H. (1964): The syndrome of Gilles de la Tourette and its treatment: Report of a case. *Medical Annals of the District of Columbia,* 33:277–279.
Stevens, J. R., and Blachly, P. H. (1966): Successful treatment of the *maladie des tics. Am. J. Dis. Child.,* 112:541–545.
Stevens, J. R., Sachder, K., and Milstein, V. (1968): Behavior disorders of childhood and the electroencephalogram. *Arch. Neurol.,* 18:160–177.
Stevens, H. (1971): Gilles de la Tourette and his syndrome by serendipity. *Am. J. Psychiatry,* 128:489–492.
Stewart, M. A., Pitts, I. N., Jr., Craig, A. G., and Dieruf, W. (1966): The hyperactive child syndrome. *Am. J. Orthopsychiatry,* 36:861–867.
Still, G. F. (1902): Some abnormal psychical conditions in children. *Lancet,* 1:1077–1082.
Storms, L. (1985): Massed negative practice as a behavioral treatment for Gilles de la Tourette's syndrome. *Am. J. Psychother.,* 39:277–281.
Strauss, A. A., and Lehtinen, L. E. (1947): *Psychopathology and Education of the Brain-Injured Child.* Grune and Stratton, New York.
Subrahmanya, B., Channabasavanna, S. M., and Pradhan, N. (1983): Gilles de la Tourette syndrome. *J. Indian. Med. Assoc.,* 80:17–18.
Suhren, O., Bruyn, G. W., and Tuynman, J. A. (1966): Hyperekplexia: A hereditary startle syndrome. *J. Neurol. Sci.,* 3:577–605.
Surwillo, W. W. (1981): Cortical evoked potentials in Gilles de la Tourette's syndrome: A single case study. *Psychiatry Res.,* 4:31–38.
Surwillo, W. W., Shafii, M., and Barrett, C. L. (1978): Gilles de la Tourette syndrome: A 20-month study of the effects of stressful life events and haloperidol on symptom frequency. *J. Nerv. Ment. Dis.,* 166:812–816.
Sutherland, R. J., Kolb, B., Schoel, W. M., Whishaw, I. Q., and Davies, D. (1982): Neuropsychological assessment of children and adults with Tourette syndrome: A comparison with learning disabilities and schizophrenia. In: *Advances in Neurology, Vol. 35, Gilles de la Tourette Syndrome,* edited by A. J. Friedhoff and T. N. Chase, pp. 311–322. Raven Press, New York.
Sverd, J., and Kupietz, S. (1984): Letter to the editor: Effects of high dose propranolol in Tourette syndrome. *J. Clin. Psychopharmacol.,* 4:359–361.
Sverd, J., Cohen, S., and Camp, J. A. (1983): Brief Report: Effects of propranolol in Tourette syndrome. *J. Autism Dev. Disord.,* 13:207–13.
Swanson, P. D., Lutterell, C. N., and Magladery, J. W. (1962): Myoclonus—A report of 67 cases and review of the literature. *Medicine,* 44:339–356.
Sweeney, D., Pickar, D., Redmond, D. E., Jr., and Maas, J. (1978): Letter to the editor: Noradrenergic and dopaminergic mechanisms in Gilles de la Tourette syndrome. *Lancet,* 8069:872.
Sweet, R. D., Solomon, G. E., Wayne, H. L., Shapiro, E., and Shapiro, A. K. (1973): Neurological features of Gilles de la Tourette's syndrome. *J. Neurol. Neurosurg. Psychiatry,* 36:1–9.
Sweet, R. D., Bruun, R. D., Shapiro, A. K., and Shapiro, E. (1976): The pharmacology of Gilles de la Tourette's syndrome (chronic multiple tic). In: *Clinical Neuropharmacology, Vol. 1,* edited by H. L. Klawans. Raven Press, New York.
Tallman, J. F., and Gallager, D. W. (1985): The GABA-ergic system: A locus of benzodiazepine action. *Annu. Rev. Neurosci.,* 8:21–44.
Tanner, C. M., Goetz, C. G., and Klawans, H. L. (1982): Cholinergic mechanisms in Tourette syndrome. *Neurology (NY),* 32:1315–1317.
Tasman, A., Hale, M. S., and Simon, R. H. (1981): Neuroleptic drug effects on average evoked response augmentation-reduction in rats. *Neuropsychobiology,* 7:292–296.
Teoh, J. L. (1974): Gilles de la Tourette's syndrome: A study of the treatment of six cases by mass negative practice and with haloperidol. *Singapore Med. J.,* 15:139–146.
Thompson, M. W. (1986): *Genetics in Medicine,* 4th edition, W. B. Saunders Company, Philadelphia.
Thompson, R. J., O'Quinn, A. N., and Logue, P. E. (1979): A review and neuropsychological aspects of four cases. *J. Pediatr. Psychol.,* 4:371.
Thorndike, R. L., and Hagen, E. (1969): *Measurement and Evaluation in Psychology and Education,* 3rd edition. Wiley, New York.

Tibbets, R. W. (1981): Neuropsychiatric aspects of tics and spasms. *Br. J. Hosp. Med.*, 25:454, 456–457, 459.
Tiller, J. W. (1978): Brief family therapy for childhood tic syndrome. *Fam. Process*, 17:217–223.
Tobin, W. G., and Reinhardt, J. B. (1961): Tic de Gilles de la Tourette. *Am. J. Dis. Child.*, 101:778–783.
Torgersen, S., (1980): The oral obsessive, and hysterical personality syndromes: A study of hereditary and environmental factors by means of the twin method. *Arch. Gen. Psychiatry*, 37:1272–1277.
Torup, E. (1962): A follow-up study of children with tics. *Acta Paediatr. Scand.*, 51:261–268.
Trousseau, A. (1873): *Clinique médical de l'hôtel Dieu de Paris*, 2:267.
Turner, S. M., Beidel, D. C., and Nathan, R. S. (1985): Biological factors in obsessive compulsive disorders. *Psychol. Bull.*, 97:430–450.
Turpin, G., and Powell, G. E. (1984): Effects of massed practice and cue-controlled relaxation on tic frequency in Gilles de la Tourette's syndrome. *Behav. Res. Ther.*, 22:165–178.
Uhr, S. B., Berger, P. A., Pruitt, B., and Stahl, S. M. (1984): R022-1319, a D-2 receptor antagonist for treatment of Tourette's syndrome. *N. Engl. J. Med.*, 311:989.
Uhr, S. B., Pruitt, B., Berger, P. A., and Stahl, S. M. (1986): Case report of four patients with TS treated with piquindone, a D_2 receptor antagonist. *J. Clin. Psychopharmacol.*, 6:128–130.
Ullman, D. G., Egan, D., Fiedler, N., Jurenec. G., Pliske, R., Thompson, P., and Doherty, M. E. (1981): The many faces of hyperactivity: Similarities and differences in diagnostic policies. *J. Consult. Clin. Psychol.*, 49:694–704.
Van Bogaert, L., and Nyssen (1925): Mouvements bradysyncinétiques de la langue, crampes toniques, labiopalato phyrangées cervicales et troubles respiratoires dans le parkinsonisme postencephalitique. *J. Neurol. (Brussels)*, 25:386–400.
Van de Wetering, B. J. M., Martens, C. M. C., Fortgens, C., Slaets, J. P. J., and Van Woerkom, T. C. A. M. (1985): Late components of the auditory evoked potentials in Gilles de la Tourette syndrome. *Clin. Neurol. Neurosurg.*, 87:3.
Van Lancker, D. (1975): Heterogeneity in language and speech: Neurolinguistic studies. Working Papers in Phonetics 29, University of California, Los Angeles.
Van Woert, M. H., Jutkowitz, R., Rosenbaum, D., and Bowers, M. B., Jr. (1976): Gilles de la Tourette's syndrome: Biochemical approaches. In: *The Basal Ganglia*, edited by M. D. Yahr. Raven Press, New York.
Van Woert, M. H., Rosenbaum, Howieson, J., and Bowers, M. B., Jr. (1977a): Long-term therapy of myoclonus and other neurologic disorders with L-5-hydroxytryptophan and carbidopa. *N. Engl. J. Med.*, 296:70–75.
Van Woert, M. H., Yip, L. C., and Balis, M. E. (1977b): Purine phosphoribosyltransferase in Gilles de la Tourette syndrome. *N. Engl. J. Med.*, 296:210.
Van Woert, M. H., Rosenbaum, D., and Enna, S. J. (1982): Overview of pharmacological approaches in therapy for Tourette syndrome. In: *Advances in Neurology, Vol. 35, Gilles de la Tourette Syndrome*, edited by A. J. Friedhoff and T. N. Chase, pp. 369–375. Raven Press, New York.
Varma, S. K., and Messiha, F. S. (1983): Endocrine aspects of lithium therapy in Tourette's syndrome. *Brain Res. Bull.*, 11:209–211.
Verma, N. P., Syrigoupapavasiliou, P., and LeWitt, P. A. (1986): Electroencephalographic findings in unmedicated, neurologically and intellectually intact Tourette syndrome patients. *Electroencephalogr. Clin. Neurophysiol.*, 64:12–20.
Vogel, F., and Motulsky, A. G. (1982): *Human Genetics: Problems and Approaches.* Springer-Verlag, Berlin.
Volkmar, F. R., Leckman, J. F., Detlor, J., Harcherik, D. F., Prichard, J. W., Shaywitz, B. A., and Cohen, D. J. (1984): EEG abnormalities in Tourette's syndrome. *J. Am. Acad. Child Psychiatry*, 23:352–353.
Volkmar, F. F., Hoder, E. L., and Cohen, D. J. (1985): Inappropriate uses of stimulant medications. *Clin. Pediatr. (Phila.)* 24:127–130.
Von Economo, C. (1917): Encephalitis lethargica. *Wein Klin. Wochenschr.*, 30:581–585.
Von Economo, C. (1931): *Encephalitis Lethargica.* Oxford, New York.
Voulters, L., Bressman, S. B., and Fahn, S. (1985): Treatment of tic disorders with clonazepam. *J. Can. Sci. Neurol.*, 12:172–173.

Wagner, E. E. (1970): Results of psychological testing on a child with Gilles de la Tourette's disease. *J. Clin. Psychol.*, 26:52–57.
Walsh, P. J. F. (1962): Compulsive shouting and Gilles de la Tourette disease. *Br. J. Clin. Pract.*, 16:651–655.
Walsh, T. L., Lavenstein, B., Licamele, W. L., Bronheim, S., and O'Leary, J. O. (1986): Calcium antagonists in the treatment of Tourette's disorder. *Am. J. Psychiatry*, 143:1467–1468.
Waserman, J., Lal, S., and Gauthier, S. (1983): Gilles de la Tourette's syndrome in monozygotic twins. *J. Neurol. Neurosurg. Psychiatry*, 46:75–77.
Wassman, E. R., Eldridge, R., Abuzzahab, I. S., Sr., and Nee, L. (1978): Gilles de la Tourette syndrome: Clinical and genetic studies in a midwestern city. *Neurology (Minneap.)*, 28:304–307.
Wayne, H. L., Shapiro, A. K., and Shapiro, E. (1972): Gilles de la Tourette's syndrome: Electroencephalographic investigation and clinical correlation. *Clin. Electroencephalogr.*, 3:160–168.
Webster's Third New International Dictionary (1961): Merriman, Springfield, Massachusetts.
Wechsler, D. (1944): *The Measurement of Adult Intelligence*, 3rd edition. Williams and Wilkins, Baltimore, Maryland.
Wechsler, I. S. (1952): *Clinical Neurology*, 7th edition. Saunders, Philadelphia.
Weiner, A., Reich, T., Robins, E., Fishman, R., and Van Doren, T. (1976): Obsessive-compulsive neurosis: Record, follow-up, and family studies. *Compr. Psychiatry*, 17:527–539.
Weingarten, K. (1968): Tics. In: *Handbook of Clinical Neurology*, Vol. 6, edited by P. J. Vinken and G. W. Bruyn, pp. 782–808. North-Holland, Amsterdam and Wiley, New York.
Weiss, G., and Hechtman, L. (1979): The hyperactive child syndrome. *Science*, 205:1348–1353.
Weissman, M. M., Myers, J. K., and Harding, P. S. (1978): Psychiatric disorders in a U.S. urban community: 1975–1976. *Am. J. Psychiatry*, 135:489–492.
Weissman, M. M., Merikangas, K. R., John, K., Wickramaratane, P., Prusoff, B. A., and Kidd, K. K. (1986): Family genetic studies of psychiatric disorders. *Arch. Gen. Psychiatry*, 43:1104–1116.
Wenar, C. (1963): The reliability of developmental histories. *Psychosom. Med.*, 23:505–509.
Wender, P. H. (1971): *Minimal Brain Dysfunction in Children*. Wiley, New York.
Wender, P. H., Reimherr, F. W., and Wood, D. R. (1981): Attention deficit disorder ('minimal brain dysfunction') in adults. *Arch. Gen. Psychiatry*, 38:449–456.
Wender, P. H., Reimherr, F. W., Wood, D., and Ward, M. (1985): A controlled study of methylphenidate in the treatment of attention deficit disorder, residual type, in adults. *Am. J. Psychiatry*, 142:547–552.
Werry, J. S. (1968): Studies of the hyperactive child. *Arch. Gen. Psychiatry*, 19:9–16.
Werry, J. S., and Aman, M. G. (1975): Methylphenidate and haloperidol in children. *Arch. Gen. Psychiatry*, 32:790–795.
Werry, J. S., Minde, K., Guzman, A., Weiss, G., Dogan, K., and Hoy, E. (1972): Studies on the hyperactive child: VII. *Am. J. Orthopsychiatry*, 42:441–450.
Williams, T. A. (1912): Interpretation of "professional cramp-neurosis" as a tic. *J. Abnorm. Psychol.*, 7:161–166.
Wilson, R. S., Garron, D. C., and Klawans, H. L. (1978): Significance of genetic factors in Gilles de la Tourette syndrome: A review. *Behav. Genet.*, 8:503–510.
Wilson, R. S., Garron, D. C., Tanner, C. M., and Klawans, H. L. (1982): Behavior disturbance in children with Tourette syndrome. In: *Advances in Neurology, Vol. 35, Gilles de la Tourette Syndrome*, edited by A. J. Friedhoff and T. N. Chase, pp. 329–333. Raven Press, New York.
Wilson, S. A. K. (1927): Tics and allied conditions. *J. Neurol. Psychopathol.*, 8:93–109.
Wilson, S. A. K. (1940): *Neurology*. Williams & Wilkins, Baltimore.
Winsberg, B. G., and Yepes, L. E. (1978): Antipsychotics (major tranquilizers, neuroleptics). In: *Pediatric Psychopharmacology: The Use of Behavior Modifying Drugs in Children*, edited by J. S. Werry, pp. 234–273. Brunner/Mazel, New York.
Winslow, R. S., Stillner, V., Coons, D. J., and Robinson, M. W. (1986): Prevention of acute dystonic reactions in patients beginning high-potency neuroleptics. *Am. J. Psychiatry*, 143:706–710.
Wise, S. P. (1985): The primate premotor cortex: Past, present, and preparatory. *Annu. Rev. Neurosci.*, 8:1–19.
Wise, S. P., and Strick, P. L. (1984): Anatomical and physiological organization of the non-primary motor cortex. *Trends Neurosci.*, 7:442–446.

Wohlfart, G., Ingvar, D. H., and Hellberg, A. M. (1961): Compulsory shouting (Benedek's 'Klazomania') associated with oculogyric spasm in chronic epidemic encephalitis. *Acta Psychiatr. Scand.*, 36:369–377.
Wolraich, M., Drummond, T., Salomon, M. K., O'Brien, M. L., and Sivage, C. (1978): Effects of methylphenidate alone and in combination with behavior modification procedures on the behavior and academic performance of hyperactive children. *J. Abnorm. Child Psychol.*, 6:149–161.
Wong, G. H., and Cock, R. J. (1971): Long-term effects of haloperidol on seventy emotionally disturbed children. *Aust. J. Psychiatry*, 5:296–300.
Woodrow, K. M. (1974): Gilles de la Tourette's disease—a review. *Am. J. Psychiatry*, 131:1000–1004.
World Health Organization (1978): *Mental Disorders: Glossary and Guide to Their Classification in Accordance with the Ninth Revision of the International Classification of Diseases.* World Health Organization, Geneva.
World Health Organization (1977): *Manual of the International Statistical Classification of Diseases, Injuries and Causes of Death, Ninth Revision, Vol. 1.* World Health Organization, Geneva.
Yap, P. M. (1952): The latah reaction, its pathodynamics and nosological position. *J. Ment. Sci.*, 413:515–564.
Yaryura-Tobias, J. A. (1975): Chlorimipramine in Gilles de la Tourette's disease. *Am. J. Psychiatry*. 132:1221.
Yaryura-Tobias, J. A. (1979): Gilles de la Tourette syndrome. Interactions with other neuropsychiatric disorders. *Acta Psychiatr. Scand.*, 599–16.
Yaryura-Tobias, J. A., and Neziroglu, F. (1974): The action of chlorimipramine in obsessive compulsive neurosis: a pilot study. *Curr. Ther. Res., 17:111–116.*
Yaryura-Tobias, J. A., and Neziroglu, F. A. (1977): Gilles de la Tourette syndrome: A new clinicotherapeutic approach. *Prog. Neuropsychopharmacol.*, 1:335–338.
Yaryura-Tobias, J. A., Neziroglu, F., Howard, S., and Fuller, B. (1981): Clinical aspects of Gilles de la Tourette syndrome. *Orthomolec. Psychiatry*, 10:263–268.
Yeragani, V. K., Blackman, M., and Baker, G. E. (1983): Biological and psychological aspects of a case of Gilles de la Tourette's syndrome. *J. Clin. Psychiatry*, 44:27–29.
Young, J. G., Cohen, D. J., Kavanagh, M. E., Landis, H. D., Shaywitz, B. A., and Maas, J. W. (1981a): Cerebrospinal fluid, plasma, and urinary MHPG in children. *Life Sci.*, 28:2837–2845.
Young, J. G., Cohen, D. J., Hattox, S. E., Kavanagh, B. S., Anderson, G. H., Shaywitz, B. A., and Maas, J. W. (1981b): Plasma free MHPG and neuroendocrine responses to challenge doses of clonidine in Tourette's syndrome: Preliminary report. *Life Sci.*, 29:1467–1475.
Young, J. G., Leven, L. I., Knott, P. J., Leckman, J. F., and Cohen, D. J. (1985): Tourette's syndrome and tic disorders. In: *Diagnosis of Psychopharmacology of Childhood and Adolescence Disorders*, edited by J. M. Weiner, pp. 215–247, John Wiley and Sons, New York.
Zausmer, D. M. (1954): The treatment of tics in childhood: A review and follow-up study. *Arch. Dis. Child.*, 29:537–542.
Zawadski, A. (1972): Treatment of *maladie des tics* with carbamazepine. *Pediatr. Pol.*, 47:1105–1110.

Subject Index

A

Abilities, assets and, 39,119,122
Abnormalities
  chromosomal, 293
  electroencephalographic, 123,125,270–280
  neurological, 117,123,125,280–282,497
  perinatal, 98–99
  psychological test, 123,125,241–250
Abortions, history of, 95
Achievements, over past 25 years, 26–27
Acute dystonia, haloperidol and, 430
ADD, *see* Attention deficit disorder
Addiction, to haloperidol, 436
Adopted probands, family history of tic disorders in, and in nonadopted probands, 90–91
Adverse effects, management of, 430–441
  amantadine, use of, 439–440
  anticholinergics, use of, 439–440
  benzodiazepines, use of, 431
  benztropine, use of, 439–440
  bromocriptine, use of, 436
  by dosage reduction, 440
  propranolol, use of, 431
Adverse effects, recognition of, 430–441
  acute dystonia, 430
  akathisia, 431
  akinesia, 430–431
  anticholinergic
    constipation, 435
    impaired near vision, 435
    mydriasis, 435
    xerostomia, 435
  blood dyscrasia, 439
  cardiovascular, 442–443
  cognitive impairment, 432
  depression, 436
  dysphoria, 436
  extrapyramidal, 431–432
    hand–finger mannerism, 432
  fog states, 436–437
  hyperthermia, 438
  jaundice, 439
  metabolic and endocrine, 435–436
    appetite, 435
    galactorrhea, 435
    gynecomastia, 435
    hypoglycemia, 435
    libido, loss of, 435–436
    menstruation, 435
    weight gain, 435
  miscellaneous, 438–439
  paranoid states, 437–438
  phobias, 436
  tardive akinesia, 431
  tardive dyskinesia, 432–435
  tardive dystonia, 431
  tardive Tourette's disorder, 431
  teratogenicity, 435
  unexpected death, 438
Age, 64–65
  and ADD, interaction of, with sex ratio, 71–72
  and diagnosis of ADD, 112
  effect of, on EEG, 274–275
  at onset, 127–131
    for coprophilia, 156,158
    genetics and, 292–293
  of parent, at birth, 95
Agreement, and controversies, consensual areas of, 27
Akathisia, haloperidol and, 431
Akinesia, haloperidol and, 430–431
Allergic desensitization, 401
Amantadine, 439–440
Amino acid neurotransmitters, 326–327
Amitriptyline, 395
Antecedents, hereditary, history of, 1–10
Antianxiety-sedative-hypnotics, 397–398
Anticholinergic adverse effects, of haloperidol, 435
Anticholinergic medication, use of, for adverse effects of haloperidol, 439–440
Anticonvulsants, 396–397
Antidepressants, 393,394–396
Apomorphine, 391
Arousal, disturbance of, 286–287
Assets and abilities, 39,119,122
Attention, testing of, 474,476
Attention deficit disorder (ADD)
  confidence scale, 213
  diagnosis of, 110–111
    age and, 112
    private versus clinic patients and, 113
  effect of, on EEG, 275
  with hyperactivity
    diagnostic criteria for, 34–35
    effect of
      on reports, 169

SUBJECT INDEX

ADD, with hyperactivity, effect of *(contd.)*
  on stimuli-induced change in tics, 184–187
  increased severity of Tourette's disorder with, 113–115,116–120
  stimulants and, 404–406,407
  summary of, 493
  without hyperactivity, diagnostic criteria for, 35
  interaction of age and, with sex ratio, 71–72
  with organic stigmata, 106–115
  prevalence of, 111
  and psychopathology, 211–212
  rating scale, 213
  residual type, diagnostic criteria for, 25–26
  sample changes over time associated with, 112–113
  and sex ratio, 70–71,111–112
  and Tourette's disorder, possible genetic relationship between, 305–308
Atypical disorder, diagnostic criteria for, 34
Auditory evoked potential, 282–283

B

Background, ethnic and religious, 74,76–78
Baclofen, 400
Basal ganglia
  and coordination, 314–320
  and coprolalia, 160
Behavior therapy, 415–417
Behavioral problems
  psychotherapy or counseling for associated, 445–449
  summary of, 491–492
  and symptoms, 38–39
    associated disorders, 336
    psychopathology, as criteria, 363–364
    study of, 115–124,195–241
Bender-Gestalt Test, 245
Benzodiazepines, 398
Benztropine mesylate
  adverse effects of, 435
  as cholinergic antagonist, 394
  for control of adverse effects, 425,428–432, 439
Bereitschafts potential, 284–286
Biological probands, family history of tic disorders in nonbiological and in, 90–91
Birth complications, 97–98
Birth control pills, effect of, on tics, 187
Birth history, 95–100
Birth order, 99–100,101
Birth, place of, 74,76
Birth weight, 95
Brain–mind dualism, 347
Brief tics, 348
Butyrophenones, 384–387

C

Calcium channel blockers, 400
Carbamazepine, 396–397
Catabolic enzymes, 334
Central nervous system, 253–341
  and coprolalia, 160
  summary, 493–494
Cerebellum, and coordination, 314
Change(s)
  of diagnostic classification, from stereotyped movement disorders to tic disorders, 345
  sample, over time, 61–64
  associated with ADD, 112–113
  in severity of symptoms, stimuli-induced, 179–187
  stimuli-induced, in tics, 349
Child behavior checklist (CBCL), 38,212–220
Childhood illnesses, 100–102
Children
  of patients with Tourette's disorder, 83
  siblings and, who have sibling and parent with tic disorders, increased risk of tic disorders to, 86–88
Chlorimipramine, 395
Choline, 393–394
Cholinergic agonists, 393–394
Cholinergic antagonists, 394
Cholinergic function, clinical research in, 331
Cholinergic neuronal systems, 326
Chorea, 262
Choreic syndromes, 263
Chromosonal abnormalities, 293
Chronic cough of adolescence, 371,372
Chronic motor tic disorder
  criteria for, 365,367–370
  diagnostic, 33–34
  epidemiology of, 58–59
  Tourette's disorder and, combination of, epidemiology of, 59
Chronic vocal tic disorder, criteria for, 370–371
Clinic patients, private versus, and diagnosis of ADD, 113
Clinical course, 169–176
  of coprophilia, 158
  initial, summary of, 489
Clinical samples
  and nonclinical, relationship of, to sex ratio, 69–72
  questionnaire survey and, differences between, 190–193
Clinical studies, of tic disorders, epidemiologic compared with, sex ratio in, 65–68
Clinical use, of EEGs in Tourette's disorder, 280
Clonazepam, 397–398,444
Clonidine, 398–399,443–444
Clonidine challenge, response to, 331–333

SUBJECT INDEX

Clozapine, 390
Cognitive functioning, test measures of, 474–475
Cognitive impairment, haloperidol and, 432
  study of, 471–480
Complex motor tics
  copropraxic, 356
  criteria for, 351–352
  cumulative, 139,141–144
  echophilic, criteria for, 355
Complex vocal tics
  coprophilic, criteria for, 355
  criteria for, 354
  echophilic, criteria for, 354–355
Complications
  birth, 97–98
  perinatal, 256,257
  possible, in clinical course, 175–176
  pregnancy, 95,97
Compulsions, 220–240; *see also* Obsessive-compulsive *entries*
Computation condition, in videotaping, 454
Computerized axial tomography (CAT), 285
Conners Abbreviated Parent–Teacher Questionnaire, 35,213
Consensual areas of agreement and controversies, 27
Construct validity, 463
Content validity, 463
Continuum, or spectrum, tic disorders as, 378–380,495
Contrast samples, 41
Controlled study, of psychopathology, 212–220
Control, regulatory, and coordination, of motor system, 314–321
Control samples, 485
Controversies
  agreement and, consensual areas of, 27
  about attention deficit disorder, 106–124, 362–363
  about atypical tic or movement disorder, 375–377
  about chronic motor and vocal tic disorder, 365–371
  about clonidine, 398–399
  about coprolalia, 159–164
  about etiology, 494–497
  about family psychopathology, 197–198
  about impulsions, 362
  about obsessive–compulsive disorder or symptoms, 220–241,361–362
  about patient psychopathology, 198–220, 363–364
  about sensory tics, 356–361
  about stimulants and tic disorders, 402–413, 440–441
  about tardive dyskinesia, 432–435
  about tic disorders as continuum or spectrum, 378–380
Coordination, regulatory control and, of motor system, 314–321
Coprolalia, 151–156
  effects of, 153
  frequency and persistence of, 155–156
  mental, 156
  pitfalls in identifying, 153–155
  types of, 151,153
Coprophilia, 151–164
  aberrant stimulation of neurons as explanation for, 164
  age at onset for, 156,158
  clinical course for, 158
  criteria for, 355–356
  cumulative, 151
  etiology for, psychophysiological, 162–164
  as organic symptom, 159–161
  psychological etiology for, 161–162
  puzzle of, 159
  relationship of, to other variables, 158–159
Copropraxia, 156,157
Copropraxic complex motor tics, criteria for, 356
Corticosteroids, 400
Cough, chronic, of adolescence, 371,372
Counseling, psychotherapy or, for associated behavioral problems, 445–449
Course
  clinical, *see* Clinical course
  natural, of tic and Tourette disorders, 187–190
  prognosis and, summary of, 490–491
Criteria
  diagnostic
    for attention deficit disorder, 34–36
    for chronic motor or vocal tic disorder, 33–34,365,367–372
    for complex motor tics, 351–352
    for complex vocal tics, 354–356
    for impulsions, 240–241
    for movement disorder not otherwise specified, 34,375–376
    for obsessive–compulsive disorder or symptoms, 232–240
    for sensory tics, 34,356–360
    for simple motor tics, 350–351
    for simple vocal tics, 352–354
    for tic disorder not otherwise specified, 34,375
    for tics, 345–349
    for Tourette's disorder, 33,364–367
    for transient tic disorder, 33,371–375
  summary of, 498
  history of, 343–345
Critique of research in Tourette's disorder, 483–487

Cumulative lifetime prevalence of symptoms (tics), 138–151,164–165,166–167
summary of, 489–490

D

Data management, 36–40
Data, missing, 40
Data-oriented approach to study of tic disorders, 43–44
Deanol, 393
Depressive adverse effects, of haloperidol, 436
Desensitization, allergic, 401
Desimipramine, 395–396
for treatment of ADD, 396
Developmental disorders, 256,257
Diagnostic classification, change of, from stereotype movement disorders to tic disorders, 345
Diet, 401
Diphenylbutylpiperidines, 384–387
Direct family interview method, 300–303
Disorder(s)
attention deficit, see Attention deficit disorder
behavioral symptoms and, associated, 336
chronic motor tic, see Chronic motor tic disorder
developmental, 256,257
genetic, types of, 290
movement, 34,345,375–378,379
neurological, 256,259–268
obsessive–compulsive, see Obsessive–compulsive disorder
psychiatric, associated, 304–310
tic, see Tic disorder(s)
tic-like symptoms associated with other, 255–268
Tourette's, see Tourette's disorder
Disulfiram, 391
Diurnal variation, effect of, on symptoms, 183
Dopamine agonists, 391–392
Dopamine antagonists, 384–391
Dopamine-blocking drugs, effect of, on evoked potentials, 284
Dopamine hypothesis, 496
Dopaminergic function, clinical research in, 327–329
Dopaminergic neuronal systems, 322–324
Dosages of drugs used in tic disorders, 444
Double-blind procedure, 485–486
Drug challenge procedures, dynamic, neuroendocrine indices and, 335–336
Drugs
dopamine-blocking, effect of, on evoked potentials, 284
potentiation of other, by haloperidol, 436
Duration of illness, 61,131–132
change of, 61–64

effect of, on reports, 168
Dyskinesia, tardive, haloperidol and, 432–435
Dysphoric adverse effects, of haloperidol, 436
Dystonia, 262
acute, haloperidol and, 430
paroxysmal myoclonic, with vocalization, 376–377
tardive, haloperidol and, 431

E

Early history, of treatment, 381–383
Echoing, mental, 149–150
Echokinesis, cumulative, 150
Echolalia, 145,148
Echophilia
correlates of, 151
criteria for, 354–355
cumulative, 145,148–150
Ejaculatory tics, 348
Electroencephalography, 38,270–280
abnormalities reported in, 123,125,270–273
compared with controls, 279–280
effect of ADD on, 275–276
effect of age on, 274–275
effect of medication on, 276–280
Endocrinological adverse effects, of haloperidol, 435–436
Environment, genes and, 293,311
Enzyme activities, 333–334
Epidemiology, 45–59
history of, 17–18
studies, compared with clinical studies of tic disorders, sex ratio in, 65–68
summary of, 487–488
Ethnic background, 74,77,78
Etiology
family dynamics, 197–198
genetic and hereditary, 1–2,4,7,78–91,92–94,289–312,495–496
impaired inhibition, 162–163
learned habits, 415–417
medical illness, 100–103
neuropsychological, 241–251
obsessive–compulsive, 220–241
organic, physiological, neurological or central nervous system, 11,105–124,159–161,253–288,313–341,346,350,362–363,378–380,421,493–495
paranatal, 95–99
precipitating events, 124–126
psychoanalytic theories, 11,13–17,347
psychological, 10,99–100,115–123,161–163,195–251,363–364,413–415,445–447,491–495
for coprophilia, 161–162
history of, 10–13
psychophysiological, for coprophilia, 162–163

SUBJECT INDEX

summary of, 494–497
Evoked potentials, 282–284
Examination, neurological, 37,280–282,283
Extrapyramidal parkinsonian adverse effects, of haloperidol, 431–432
Extrapyramidal parkinsonian hand–finger mannerism, haloperidol and, 432

F

Familial syndromes, 256,258
Families of female patients, higher frequency of tic disorders in, 86
Family aggregation, in Tourette's disorder, clinical research on, 293–300
Family history, of tic disorders
  in adopted probands and in nonadopted probands, 90–91
  in children, 83
  in one or more family members, 80,82,83–84,85
  in siblings, 80–83
  and Tourette's, correlates of, 92–94
Family interview, direct, method of, 300–303
Family members, history of tic disorders in one or more, 82,83–84,85
Family psychopathology, 197–198,199
Female patients
  higher frequency of tic disorders in families of, 86
  male and, differences between, 74,75
Females versus males, *see* Male to female ratio
Fluctuation of symptoms (tics), 349
  spontaneous, 169–170,174–175
Fluphenazine, 387–388,443
Fog states, with haloperidol, 436–437
Freudian unconscious motivation, 347

G

Genes, and environment, 293,311
Genetic disorders, types of, 290
Genetic factors, 495–496
Genetic heterogeneity, 291
Genetic markers, 91–92
Genetic relationship, possible
  between ADD and Tourette's disorder, 305–308
  between obsessive–compulsive disorder and Tourette's disorder, 308–310
Genetic syndromes, 256,258
Genetics, 78–94,289–312
Genotype, clinical expression of, variation in, pedigree patterns and, 290–291

H

Hallervorden-Spatz disease, 256,259
Haloperidol
  action of, 327–331,384–385
  adverse effects of, 430–439
    cognitive impairment, 432
    antiparkinsonian drug use with, 439–440
    benztropine mesylate and, 439–440
    blood levels of, 426–427
    clinical response to, 384–385
    complications and side-effects of, 430–439
    effects on EEG activity, 276–280
    effects on evoked potentials, 282–284
    general principles of treatment, 423–425
    increases in, indications and guidelines for, 423–426
    rapid, advantages and methods for, 427–429
    slow, advantages of, 426
  indications for treatment, 422
  potentiated effects of, 436
  side-effects of, 430–441
    akathesia, 431
  treatment regime, 425–426
    gradual, 425–426
    rapid, 427–429
  withdrawal effects, 433–434
Handedness, 105–106
Hand–finger mannerism, extrapyramidal parkinsonian, haloperidol and, 432
Hereditary antecedents, 1–10
History
  of abortions, 95
  birth, 95–100
  of criteria, 343–345
  early, of treatment, 381–383
  family, *see* Family history
  medical, 39,100–103
  of psychopathology, 195–197,198,200–203
  summary of, 487
  of Tourette and tic disorders, 1–27
  treatment, of patients in current study, 417, 418–419
Homage to researchers, 482–483
Hospital records, review of, 18–24
Huntington's chorea, 262–263
L-5-hydroxytryptophan (5-HTP), 392
Hyperactivity
  ADD with, *see* Attention deficit disorder, with hyperactivity
  ADD without, diagnostic criteria for, 35
  diagnostic criteria for, 35
Hyperekplexias, 259–262
Hypnosis, 415

I

Illness(es)
  adult, 102–103
  childhood, 100–102
  duration of, effect of, on reports, 168
  present, characteristics of, 131–132
Illness variables, 40

Imipramine, 395
Impulses, impaired inhibition of, 162
Impulsions, 240–241
 criteria for, 362
 summary of, 492–493
Impulsivity, diagnostic criteria for, 35
Inadequate support of research, 481–482
Inarticulate vocal tics, cumulative, 144–145, 146–147
Inattention, diagnostic criteria for, 34
Indications for treatment, 423
Inhibition of impulses, impaired, 162
Inhibitory neuronal circuits, excitatory and, 315–318
Initial clinical course, summary of, 489
Initial symptoms, 133–138
Initial tics, summary of, 489
Interaction
 of age and ADD with sex ratio, 71–72
 gene, and environment, 293,311
Intercourse, effect of, on tics, 187
Interview, family, direct, method of, 300–303
Involuntary movement, vocalization or sensory tics, criteria for, 346–348

J

Judges' ratings, in videotaping, 455,456,458, 459–461,470

L

Laboratory testing, with haloperidol, 439
Language, speech and, 250–251
Learning, testing of, 475,477
Lecithin, 394
Levodopa, 392
Lifetime prevalence of symptoms (tics)
 cumulative, 138–141,164–165,166–167
 summary of, 489–490
 variables affecting reports of, 168–169
List of variables, 503–507
Lithium, 396
Local axon collaterals, 318
Localization, neuronal, of neurotransmitters, 322–327

M

Magnetic resonance imaging (MRI), 286
Male patients, and female, differences between, 74,75
Male to female ratio, 65–69; see also Sex ratio
 other variables and, 73
 for Tourette's-alone group, 72
Management, data, 36
Marital status, 104–105
Markers, genetic, 91–92
Maturational milestones, 105,106

Measurement
 effect of, on reports, 169
 in tic disorders, 451–480
 in Tourette's disorder
  reliability and validity of, 451–471,486–487
  summary of, 499–501
Measures, 453–455
 of psychopathology, 469,471
 test, of cognitive functioning, 474–475
 videotaping, 455,459–461,468
Medical history, 39,100–103
Medication, see Drugs
Megavitamins, 401
Memory, testing of, 475,477
Mental coprolalia, 156
Mental echoing, 149–150
α-Methylparatyrosine, 390–391
Methysergide, 393
Metoclopramide, 389
Mineral therapy, orthomolecular, 401
Missing data, 40
Monoamine enzymes, 333
Monoamine oxidase inhibitors, 396
Motor cortex, nonprimary, 320–321
Motor system
 general organization of, 313–314
 regulatory control and coordination of, 314–321
Motor tic counts, 456
Motor tic disorder, chronic, see Chronic motor tic disorder
Motor tics
 complex, cumulative, 139,141–144
 criteria for, 349–352
 simple, cumulative, 139,140
Movement disorder questionnaire, 32,213,503
Myoclonic dystonia, paroxysmal, with vocalization, 376–377
Myoclonus, 263–264

N

Naloxone, 399–400
Natural course, of tic and Tourette disorders, 187–190
 summary of, 490–491
Neural mechanisms, 313–341
Neuroacanthocytosis, 263
Neuroanatomical perspectives, hypothesis of, 340–341
Neurochemical research, clinical, 327–336
Neuroendocrine indices, and dynamic drug challenge procedures, 335–336
Neurological abnormalities, 123,125,280–283,497
Neurological disorders, 256,259–268
Neurological examination, 37,280–282,283
Neurology, 253–288

SUBJECT INDEX

Neuronal circuits, excitatory and inhibitory, 315–318
Neuronal localization, of neurotransmitters, 322–327
Neuronal systems
  cholinergic, 326
  dopaminergic, 322–324
  noradrenergic, 324–325
  serotonergic, 326
Neurons
  aberrant stimulation of, coprophilia and, 164
  spiny, and differential refinement of motor regulation, 319–320
Neuropathology, of stimuli-induced tics or Tourette's disorder, 411–412
Neuropharmacological methods, in clinical research, 327–331
Neuropharmacology, neurotransmitters and, 322–327
Neuropsychological tests, 247–250
Neurosurgery, 268,269
Neurotransmitter function, hypothesis of, 337–340
Neurotransmitters
  amino acid, 326–327
  neuronal localization of, 322–327
Nonprimary motor cortex, 320–321
Nonspecific effects, 417,419–420
Noradrenergic function, clinical research in, 329–331
Noradrenergic neuronal systems, 324–325
Nosology; see also Criteria
  proposed, 343–380
  for tic disorders, summary of, 498
Nutrition, 401

O

Obsessions, 220–240
Obsessive–compulsive disorder
  criteria for, 361
    diagnostic, 232–233,234–238
  in population, 228
  summary of, 492–493
  and Tourette's disorder, possible genetic relationship between, 308–310
  in Tourette's disorder, review of clinical reports and studies of, 225–228
  Tourette's versus, 233–240
  versus obsessive–compulsive symptoms, 233,234–238
Obsessive–compulsive-like symptoms, 39
Obsessive–compulsive symptoms
  criteria for, 362
  obsessive–compulsive disorder versus, 233, 234–238
  in population, 228–232
  summary of, 492–493

  in Tourette's disorder, studies of
    problems in, 224–225
    review of clinical reports and, 225–228
  Tourette's disorder versus, 233–240
Obsessive–compulsive syndrome, history of, 220–224
Onset
  age at, see Age at onset
  of Tourette's disorder, situational events preceding, 124–126
Opioid peptidergic function, clinical research in, 331
Organic etiology, 494–495
Organic factors, as criteria, 362–363
Organic stigmata, 105–124,125
Organic symptom, coprophilia as, 159–161
Organization, general, of motor system, 313–314
Orthomolecular mineral therapy, 401
Ovarian cycle, effect of, on tics, 187
Overlapping syndromes, 264

P

Palilalia, 145,149
Paranoid state(s), with haloperidol, 437–438
Parent(s)
  age of, at birth, 95
  recommendations to, 447–449
  sibling and, with tic disorders, increased risk of disorders to siblings and children who have, 86–88
Paroxysmal myoclonic dystonia, with vocalization, 376–377
Pathophysiology, neurotransmitters and, 322–327
Patient characteristics, 61–126,127–132; see also Sample(s)
  summary of, 488–489
Patient Global Evaluation Scale, 455
Patient psychopathology, 198
Patient ratings, in videotaping, 455
Patients
  in current study, treatment history of, 417, 418–419
  female
    higher frequency of tic disorders in families of, 86
    male and, differences between, 74,75
    private versus clinic, and diagnosis of ADD, 113
  with Tourette's disorder alone and Tourette's disorder with ADD, comparison of, 115,121–123
Pedigree patterns, difficulties in interpretation of, 290–293
Penetrance, concept of, 292
Penfluridol, 386–387,443
Percent decrease of tic symptoms, 455

Perinatal abnormalities, 98–99
Perinatal complications, 256,257
Pharmacotherapy, 26,268,270,384–402
  see also specific drug names
Phenothiazines, 387–389
Phobic adverse effects, of haloperidol, 436
Physician Global Evaluation Scale, 455
Physician ratings, in videotaping, 455,459–461
Physostigmine, 393
Pimozide, 385–386,441–443
  cardiovascular effects, 442–443
  FDA recommendation for use of, 441–442
Piquindone, 391
Piribedil, 391
Placebo effects, 417,419–420
Place of birth, 74,76
Pleiotropy, 291–292
Population, obsessive–compulsive symptoms and disorder in, 228–232
Population surveys, 17–18
Positron emission tomography (PET), 285
Postinfectious syndromes, 264,266
Postmortem studies, neurological, 253–255
  summary of, 497
Potentiation of other drugs, by haloperidol, 436
Prefrontal cortex, 321
Pregnancy, effect of, on tics, 187
Pregnancy complications, 95,97
Premotor cortex, 320–321
Premovement potential, 284–286
Present illness, characteristics of, 131–132
Prevalence
  of ADD, 111
  difficulty of establishing, 51,54
  of symptoms (tics)
    cumulative lifetime, 138–151,164–165, 166–167
    summary of, 489–490
Private versus clinic patients, and diagnosis of ADD, 113
Probands, adopted, family history of tic disorders in, and in nonadopted probands, 90–91
Procedure, clinical, 32
Prognosis, for Tourette's disorder, 190
  summary of, 490–491
Propranolol, 399
Prospective studies, retrospective versus, 483–484
Psychiatric disorders, associated, 304–310
Psychoanalysis, history of, 13–17
Psychochemotherapy, history of, 26
Psychological etiology, 494–495
  for coprophilia, 161–162
  history of, 10–13
Psychological test abnormalities, 123,125, 241–250

Psychometric tests, 242–247
Psychopathology, 38–39,195–220
  ADD and, 211–212
  behavioral symptoms and, as criteria, 363–364
  controlled study of, 212–220
  family, 197–198,199
  general, 198,200–211
  history of, 195–197,198,200–203
  measures of, 469,471
  obsessions and compulsions, 220–241
  patient, 198
  summary of, 491–492
Psychophysiological etiology, for coprophilia, 162–163
Psychotherapy, 413–417
  or counseling, for associated behavioral problems, 445–449

Q

Questionnaire survey and clinical samples, differences between, 190–193

R

Race, 74,76
Raters, in videotaping, 454–455
Rating of dependent measures, in videotaping, 455,459–461,468
Reading condition, in videotaping, 454
Receptor binding research, 334–335
Recommendations to parents, 447–449
Records, hospital reviews of, 18–24
Regulatory control and coordination, of motor system, 314–321
Relatives, with tic disorders
  sex ratio of, 86
  or Tourette's disorder, 80,81
Reliability
  of diagnoses, 36
  test–retest, 461–463
  and validity, of measurement in Tourette's disorder, 451–471
  summary of, 486–487
Religious background, 74,77,78
Remission, spontaneous, of symptoms, 171–175
Reports
  clinical, and studies, of obsessive–compulsive symptoms and disorder in Tourette's disorder, review of, 225–228
  of lifetime symptoms, variables affecting, 168–169
  and studies, citing psychopathology, 203–211
Research
  critique of, 483–487
  inadequate support of, 481–482
Researchers, homage to, 482–483

SUBJECT INDEX

Residual type ADD, diagnostic criteria for, 25–26
Response time, 477
Retrospective studies, versus prospective, 483–484
Reviews
 of clinical reports and studies of obsessive–compulsive symptoms and disorder in Tourette's disorder, 225–228
 of hospital records, 18–24
 of literature, 24–25
 on effect of neuroleptics on cognition, 472–473
 on epidemiology of tics, 48–51,52–53
Risk of tic disorder, increased, to siblings and children who have sibling and parent with tic disorders, 86–88

S

Sample(s), 29–32
 changes in, over time, 61–64
 associated with ADD, 112–113
 clinical
  and nonclinical, relationship of, to sex ratio, 69–72
  questionnaire survey and, differences between, 190–193
 comparison of sensory tic with Tourette, 359–360
 contrast, 41
 control, 485
Sample size, 484–485
Sampling problems, in studies of Tourette's disorder, 165,168–169
Seasonal effect, on tics, 183
Segregation analysis, familial aggregation, classic pedigree method and, 290–303
Semantic factors, 347–348
Sensation, involuntary, tics of, criteria for, 346–348
Sensory tics, criteria for, 34,356–360
Serotonergic function, clinical research in, 329
Serotonergic neuronal systems, 326
Serotonin agonists, 392–393
Severity of symptoms, 176–179
 relationship of, to sex ratio, 70
 spontaneous waxing and waning of, 170–171,174–175
 stimuli-induced changes in, 179–187
 summary of, 490
Severity of Tourette's disorder, 469–470
 increased, with ADD and hyperactivity, 113–115,116–120
Sex-limited and sex-influenced traits, 292
Sex ratio, 65–74
 in ADD and tic disorders, 111–112
 relationship of clinical and nonclinical samples to, 69–72

of relatives with tic disorders, 86
Shapiro Daily Record of Treatment, 511
Shapiro Global Improvement Scale, 455,468, 470,510
Shapiro Tourette's Syndrome Severity Scale, 40,214,453–454,455,456,458,459–461, 467–468,470,508–509
Siblings, 80–83
 and children, who have sibling and parent with tic disorders, increased risk of tic disorders to, 86–88
Side-effects, see Adverse effects
Signs, 127–193; see also Clinical course; Symptoms
Simple motor tics
 criteria for, 350–351
 cumulative, 139,140
Simple vocal tics, criteria for, 353–354
 cumulative, 144–145
Situational events, preceding onset of Tourette's disorder, 124–126
Sleep
 disturbance of, 286
 effect of, on symptoms, 181
 tics during, 287–288
Social class, 103,213
Somatosensory evoked potential, 284
Somatotopic organization, 318–320
Source of information, relationship of, to sex ratio, 69
Spectrum, continuum or, tic disorders as, 378–380,495
Speech, and language, 250–251
Spiny neurons, and differential refinement of motor regulation, 319–320
Spontaneous effects, 417,419–420
Spontaneous fluctuation of symptoms, 169–170,174–175
Spontaneous remission of symptoms, 171–175
Spontaneous waxing and waning of severity of symptoms, 170–171,174–175
Statistical analysis, 41–42
Stereotyped movement disorders, change of diagnostic classification from, to tic disorders, 345
Stereotypic tics, 348
Stigmata, organic, 105–124,125
Stimulants, 394
 to control adverse effects of haloperidol, 440–441
 and tic disorders, controversy about, 402–413
Stimulation of neurons, aberrant, coprophilia and, 164
Stimuli-induced changes
 in severity of symptoms, 179–187
 in tics, 349
Stimulus condition, effect of, on tic counts, 456,457

SUBJECT INDEX

Supplementary motor cortex, 320–321
Support of research, inadequate, 481–482
Surgical procedures, 268–269,401–402
Surveys, population, 17–18
Sydenham's chorea, 262
Symptom(s)
  behavioral, 38–39
  initial, 133–138
  lifetime, see Lifetime prevalence of symptoms
  obsessive–compulsive, see Obsessive–compulsive symptoms
  obsessive–compulsive-like, 39
  organic, coprophilia as, 159–161
  severity of, see Severity of symptoms
  spontaneous fluctuation of, 169–170,174–175
  spontaneous remission of, 171–175
  tic-like, associated with other disorders, 255–268
  variables of, 40
Symptomatology, 132–165
Syndrome
  definition of, 78
  Tourette's, see Tourette's disorder

T

Tardive akinesia, 431
Tardive dyskinesia, 432–435
Tardive dystonia, 431
Teratogenicity, haloperidol and, 438
Test(s)
  neuropsychological, 247–250
  psychological, abnormalities in, 123,125
  psychometric, 242–247
Test measures, of cognitive functioning, 474–475
Tetrabenazine, 389
Thalamus, and coprolalia, 160–161
Tiapride, 389–390
Tic(s)
  characteristics of, 349
  criteria for, 345–349
  effect of ovarian cycle, pregnancy, birth control pills, and intercourse on, 187
  effect of specific stimuli on, 179,181–187
  as end in itself, 349
  epidemiology of, 45–55
  inarticulate vocal, cumulative, 144–145, 146–147
  initial, summary of, 489
  motor, see Motor tic entries
  prevalence of
    difficulty of establishing, 51,54
    lifetime, see Lifetime prevalence of symptoms (tics)
  sensory
    criteria for, 356–360
  subtype of, of Tourette's disorder, diagnostic criteria for, 34
  stimulants and, 407–413
  stimuli-induced, neuropathology of, 411–412
  vocal, see Vocal tic entries
Tic counts, 455,456,457,459–461,464,466, 470
Tic disorder(s), see also Tourette's disorder
  atypical, diagnostic criteria for, 34
  change of diagnostic classification from stereotyped movement disorders to, 345
  chronic motor, see Chronic motor tic disorder
  as continuum or spectrum, 378–380,495
  criteria for, see Criteria
  epidemiologic compared with clinical studies of, sex ratio in, 65–68
  in families of female patients, higher frequency of, 86
  family history of, in adopted probands and in nonadopted probands, 90–91
  history of, 1–27
  increased risk of, to siblings and children who have sibling and parent with tic disorders, 86–88
  measurement in, 451–480
  motor tic, see Chronic motor tic disorder
  natural course of, 187–190
  nosology for, summary of, 498
  not otherwise specified, criteria for, 375
  in one or more family members, history of, 82,83–84,85
  relatives with, 80,81
  sex ratio of, 86
  sex ratio in, 111–112
  spontaneous remission of, 171–172,173
  stimulants and, controversy about, 402–413
  and Tourette's disorder
    family history of, correlates of, 92–94
    genetics and relationship between, 84, 86
  transient, criteria for, 371–375
    diagnostic, 33
  vocal, chronic, criteria for, 370–371
Tic-like symptoms, associated with other disorders, 255–268
Tourette samples, comparison of sensory tic with, 359–360
Tourette's disorder; see also Tic disorders
  ADD and possible genetic relationship between, 305–308
  alone
    group with, male to female ratio for, 72
    and Tourette's disorder with ADD, comparison of patients with, 115,121–123

and chronic motor disorder
  combination of, epidemiology of, 59
  preliminary study of, 368–370
clinical use of EEGs in, 280
criteria for, 364–365,366
  diagnostic, 33
epidemiology of, 45–59
genetics and, *see* Genetic *entries*
with haloperidol, 431
history of, 1–27
measurement in, *see* Measurement, in Tourette's disorder
natural course of, 187–190
  summary of, 490–491
neural mechanisms in, 313–341
  hypotheses for research in, 337–340
neurology and, 253–288
nosology, criteria and differential diagnosis in, 343–380
obsessive–compulsive disorder and, possible genetic relationship between, 308–310
obsessive–compulsive symptoms in, *see* Obsessive–compulsive symptoms
onset of, *see* Onset
patient characteristics in, 61–126
  summary of, 488–489
prognosis for, 190
psychology, psychopathology, and neuropsychology in, 195–251
relatives with, 80,81
research in, *see* Research
samples, procedures and variables in, 29–44
sensory tic subtype of, diagnostic criteria for, 34
severity of, 469–470
  increased, with ADD and hypersensitivity, 113–115,116–120
signs, symptoms, and clinical course of, 127–193
spontaneous remission in, 172–174
stimulants and, 403–413
stimuli-induced, neuropathology of, 411–412
studies of, 165,168–169
and tic disorders
  family history of, correlates of, 92–94
  genetics and relationship between, 84, 86
treatment in, *see* Treatment *entries*
versus obsessive–compulsive disorder and obsessive–compulsive symptoms, 233–240
Tourette's Syndrome Severity Scale, *see* Shapiro Tourette's Syndrome Severity Scale
Toxic syndromes, 264

Transient tic disorder, criteria for, 371–375
  diagnostic, 33
Treatment; *see also* specific drug names
  allergic desensitization, 401
  antianxiety-sedative-hypnotic drugs, 397
  anticonvulsants, 396–397
  antidepressants, 394–396
  behavior therapy, 415–417
  calcium channel blockers, 400
  clonazepam, 444
  clonidine, 443–444
  corticosteroids, 400
  diet and nutrition, 401
  early history of, 381–383
  fluphenazine, 443
  general principles of, 423–425
  haloperidol, 425–430
  hypnosis, 415
  indications for, 423
  megavitamins, 401
  miscellaneous, 401
  orthomolecular, 401
  penfluridol, 443
  pimozide, 441–443
  psychotherapy, 413–415
  studies of, 381–421
  summary of, 498–499
  surgical procedures, 268–269,401–402
  of tic disorders, 423–449
Treatment history, of patients in current study, 417,418–419
Treatment interventions, 268–270
Tricyclic antidepressants, 393
L-Tryptophan, 392–393
TS, *see* Tourette's disorder *entries*
Twinship, 88–90
  research on, 303–304
  stimulants and, 406

U

Unconscious motivation, Freudian, 347

V

Validity
  construct, 463
  content, 463
  reliability and, 451–471
  summary of, 486–487
Verbal-Performance Difference Scores (V-P), 246
Videotape tic counts
  effect of stimuli on, 451–461,464–466, 470
  reliability and validity of, 456–466,470
  ratings of, 454,456,458–461,470
Visual evoked potential, 284

Vocalization
    involuntary, tics of, criteria for, 346–348
    paroxysmal myoclonic dystonia with, 376–377
Vocal tic disorder, chronic, criteria for, 370–371
Vocal tics
    criteria for, 352–354
    inarticulate, simple, complex, cumulative, 144–159

W

Waxing and waning
    of severity of symptoms, spontaneous, 170–171, 174–175
    of tics, 349
Weschler Intelligence Scale for Children (WISC), 246
Weight, birth, 95
Wilson's disease, 259
Withdrawal, from haloperidol, 436
Work output, testing of, 475, 477